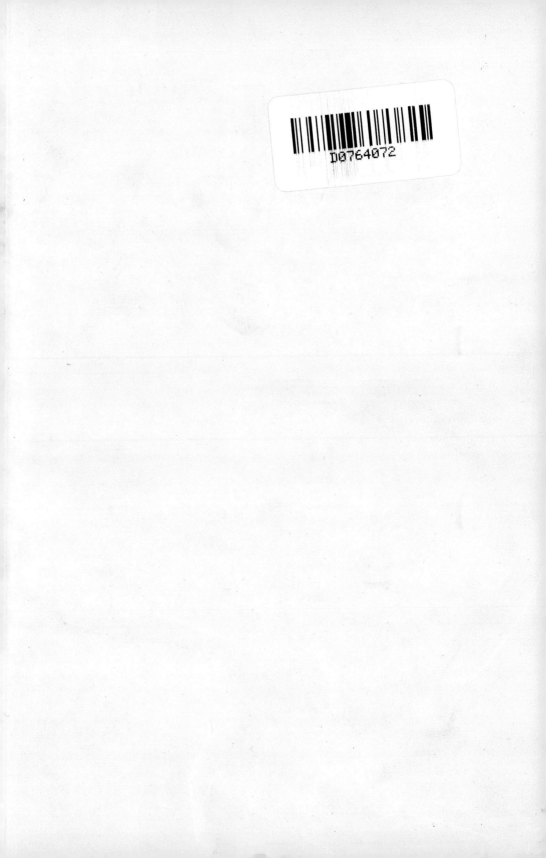

THE INFLAMMATORY PROCESS

Second Edition

VOLUME I

CONTRIBUTORS

Gunnar D. Bloom

Zanvil A. Cohn

Robert H. Ebert

Peter Elsbach

Lester Grant

James G. Hirsch

Rochelle Hirschhorn

Edward D. Korn

W. J. Mergner

W. Scott Ramsey

Ralph M. Steinman

B. F. Trump

Marjorie B. Zucker

THE INFLAMMATORY PROCESS

SECOND EDITION

EDITED BY

Benjamin W. Zweifach, Ph. D.

*Department of Applied and
Mechanical Engineering Sciences
University of California, San Diego
La Jolla, California*

Lester Grant, M. D.

*Department of Medicine
School of Medicine
New York University
New York, New York*

Robert T. McCluskey, M. D.

*Department of Pathology
Harvard Medical School and
The Children's Hospital Medical Center
Boston, Massachusetts*

VOLUME I

1974

ACADEMIC PRESS   New York   San Francisco   London
A Subsidiary of Harcourt Brace Jovanovich, Publishers

ACADEMIC PRESS, INC.
111 Fifth Avenue, New York, New York 10003

United Kingdom Edition published by
ACADEMIC PRESS, INC. (LONDON) LTD.
24/28 Oval Road, London NW1

Library of Congress Cataloging in Publication Data

Zweifach, Benjamin William, Date   ed.
    The inflammatory process.

    Includes bibliographies.
    1.   Inflammation.   I.   Grant, Lester, joint ed.
II.   McCluskey, Robert T., joint ed.   III.   Title.
[DNLM: 1.   Inflammation.   QZ150 Z9671]
RB131.Z753   616.07'2   73-21716
ISBN 0–12–783401–X (v. 1)

CONTENTS

PART I. INFLAMMATORY PROCESS AT THE MOLECULAR LEVEL

Chapter 1. The Experimental Approach to the Study of Inflammation

Robert H. Ebert and Lester Grant

Chapter 6.   Phagocytosis

Peter Elsbach

PART II.   INFLAMMATORY PROCESS AT THE CELL LEVEL

Chapter 7.   Neutrophil Leukocytes

James G. Hirsch

Chapter 8.   The Metabolism and Physiology of the Mononuclear Phagocytes

Ralph M. Steinman and Zanvil A. Cohn

Chapter 9.   Platelets

Marjorie B. Zucker

Chapter 10.   Structural and Biochemical Characteristics of Mast Cells

Gunnar D. Bloom

LIST OF CONTRIBUTORS

Numbers in parentheses indicate the pages on which the authors' contributions begin.

GUNNAR D. BLOOM (545), Department of Histology, University of Umeå, Umeå, Sweden

ZANVIL, A. COHN (449), Laboratory of Cellular Physiology and Immunology, The Rockefeller University, New York, New York

ROBERT H. EBERT (1), Harvard Medical School, Boston, Massachusetts

PETER ELSBACH (363), Department of Medicine, School of Medicine, New York University, New York, New York

LESTER GRANT (1,287), Department of Medicine, School of Medicine, New York University, New York, New York

JAMES G. HIRSCH (411), Laboratory of Cellular Physiology and Immunology, The Rockefeller University, New York, New York

ROCHELLE HIRSCHHORN (259), Department of Medicine, School of Medicine, New York University, New York, New York

EDWARD D. KORN (51), Section of Cellular Biochemistry and Ultrastructure, Laboratory of Biochemistry, National Heart and Lung Institute, National Institutes of Health, Bethesda, Maryland

W. J. MERGNER (115), Department of Pathology, University of Maryland School of Medicine, Baltimore, Maryland

W. SCOTT RAMSEY (287),* Department of Biology, Yale University, New Haven, Connecticut

*Present address: Research and Development Laboratories, Corning Glass Works, Corning, New York 14830.

Ralph M. Steinman (449), Laboratory of Cellular Physiology and Immunology, The Rockefeller University, New York, New York

B. F. Trump (115), Department of Pathology, University of Maryland School of Medicine, Baltimore, Maryland

Marjorie B. Zucker (511), Department of Pathology, New York University Medical Center, New York, New York

PREFACE

Since publication of the first edition of "The Inflammatory Process," investigators have unearthed an enormous amount of basic information about inflammation, much of it relevant to clinical states. In addition, the biologic probe has moved closer and closer to the cell, its wall and contents, which has brought some insight into molecular mechanisms and their derangements in inflammatory states. In a sense, in the last decade the direction of research in the inflammatory reaction seems to have changed, with a shift toward molecular biology, but this is more apparent than real. Research has been moving in this direction not only in this field but in others as well for many years.

These would be reasons enough for a second edition of this treatise which deals with the commonest pathologic reaction in the animal kingdom. The first edition received favorable critical comment, characterizing it as a scholarly work that made a reasonably successful attempt to synthesize a sprawling literature and to invest the subject with some directional guidelines.

Fortified by this encouraging response we had no difficulty in reaching a decision that a second edition of this work was necessary. In planning this edition it became clear that new material on a subject as broad as inflammation could not possibly be compressed into a single volume without running the risk of superficiality. Space had to be reserved for an analysis of cell surface phenomena; for a fuller treatment of connective tissue; for an extensive discussion on the role of the formed elements of the blood in inflammatory states, particularly in the light of the rapidly burgeoning literature on platelet physiology; for an extended discussion of the life history and functional capacities of the leukocytes; for a synthesis of the vast inchoate bits and pieces of literature dealing with chemotaxis; for a summation of phagocytosis, which biochemists have been exploring vigorously for a decade and which is now yielding new insights at a molecular level, many of them carrying strong clinical implications; and for an analysis of the mechanisms responsible for tissue damage in inflammation, especially in immunologically induced reactions. These are among the aspects of the subject that demanded special treatment over and above briefer references to them in the first edition. Thus, the second edition is comprised of three volumes.

It is fitting to conclude such an edition with a chapter by Dr. Lewis Thomas, who offers the laconic suggestion that there is some question about whether there does exist in Nature an inflammatory process as commonly understood. There are inflammatory reactions to be sure, and this could mean only that there are inflammatory processes. In our zeal to put trees together in well-tended and nicely pruned forests, we may have succumbed to the occupational hazard, a pitfall for scientists and theologians alike, of rearranging Nature as we imagine was intended in the first place but conceivably setting on a construction quite wide of the mark.

Benjamin W. Zweifach
Lester Grant
Robert T. McCluskey

PREFACE TO FIRST EDITION

At a time when journals and textbooks are proliferating so rapidly that the scientific community is hard pressed to keep up with them, it is fair to ask why another book is needed now in an area where the literature is voluminous. Since the early nineteenth century, the inflammatory process has been one of the most intensively investigated fields of experimental medicine. At the turn of the century textbooks of pathology devoted fully one third of their contents to the subject of inflammation, and today it still bulks large in most texts. Yet it is a curious commentary that, aside from relatively short review articles, few attempts have been made to sort out the extensive literature in this important field to bring it up to date in a critical and coherent way. The last such effort, indeed, was that of Adami, of McGill, who in 1909 brought out a monograph, "Inflammation—An Introduction to the Study of Pathology" in an effort to deal with, and unify, the many interrelated and often contradictory aspects of this subject. It is of some interest that the monograph was 249 pages long, carried 226 references and, most remarkable of all, was written without collaboration. In the intervening half-century a substantial number of symposia and treatises emerged but these were directed largely to special viewpoints and circumscribed aspects of the problem. Perhaps the closest approach to a current, objective review can be found in Florey's "General Pathology," in which the subject is covered in many of its significant aspects.

The editors and publishers of "The Inflammatory Process" believe that with the enormous multiplication of research in this field the need exists for a more comprehensive volume which would include analyses of the major immunologic mechanisms which give rise to inflammatory reactions. Investigations of the immune process tend, in a sense, to move toward a common meeting ground with studies of inflammatory mechanisms, one supporting the other. One of the major objectives of the present volume is to explore areas where these two approaches converge.

Aside from the convenience of an encyclopedic background for research in this field, the value of this volume depends in part on its success in correlating new and old facts. The contributors were asked, therefore, to organize the material in such a way that pressing questions could be raised against a background of the apparent acceptable, hard core of experimental facts. Such an assignment is a difficult one. The very nature of the research process requires a constant challenging and modifying of hypotheses; new facts are accepted as significant or are discarded, depending on whether they provide a further insight into biologic mechanisms. Inevitably, in dealing with a sprawling literature, a selection of data has to be made. The editors know that the choices of each essayist were thoughtful ones and appropriate in the design of this volume.

The realization that much current material may not stand the test of time seemed no deterrent for a work that runs to more than 800 pages. It is intended that the treatment be comprehensive enough to serve as a reference work, with the main lines of research in the field placed in an historical perspective. This militated against a treatise of monograph size. It its present form, the volume can serve equally well as an authoritative reference for graduate students and medical students, for experimental biologists, and for others who wish to examine the experimental background of current theories of inflammation. Inevitably there is an overlap in some of the chapters, but where this serves to maintain continuity in the development of the author's theses, it has been considered important to preserve it. The book covers comprehensively both the morphologic and the dynamic aspects of the problem. It starts with a discussion of the experimental approach to the study of inflammation in which the emphasis is on the importance of a changing technology in providing new viewpoints on old problems. An attempt is made then to establish the morphologic basis of the problem as a prelude to a discussion of dynamic events and an analysis of the participation of white blood cells in the inflammatory process. The roles of mast cells, chemical mediators, lysosomes, and hemostatic mechanisms lead to two general chapters on fever and wound healing, as expressions of inflammation, followed by a discussion of anti-inflammatory agents and their contributions to an understanding of inflammatory reactions. The later chapters deal with the complexities of complement and the mechanisms of inflammation resulting from immunologic processes. It is hoped that the emphasis on pathophysiology and mechanisms of the inflammatory process will cast the discussion in a meaningful context for serious students and at the same time provide others who are interested in this area of experimental pathology with an authoritative introduction to the subject.

The editors would like to thank the publishers and the contributors for an extraordinary sense of responsibility in meeting a tight deadline for this volume, the revisions and editing of which, including new bibliography, continued almost to the point of publication.

Benjamin W. Zweifach
Lester Grant
Robert T. McCluskey

CONTENTS OF OTHER VOLUMES

THE INFLAMMATORY PROCESS

Second Edition

VOLUME I

Part I

INFLAMMATORY PROCESS AT THE MOLECULAR LEVEL

Chapter 1

THE EXPERIMENTAL APPROACH TO THE STUDY OF INFLAMMATION

ROBERT H. EBERT AND LESTER GRANT

I. Introduction

A. Definition of Inflammation

Grawitz (1890) defined inflammation as the reaction of irritated and damaged tissues which still retain vitality, and Adami (1909) in quoting this definition emphasized that inflammation is a *process* and not a *state*. Certainly the dynamic nature of the process is important to emphasize, but the definition given above is perhaps too limited, for it neglects several aspects of inflammation. First, it fails to include healing as a part of the process, and second, it insists that damaged tissues must still retain their vitality. Surely it must be recognized that tissue destruction may be the end result of inflammation and one can hardly separate the caseation necrosis of a tubercle from the inflammatory reaction which surrounds it. Even the caseous tubercle may be in a state of dynamic change with healing occurring in one portion of the tubercle and extension of caseation necrosis in another (Ebert, 1952). Permanent destruction of tissue is evident in the stable walled-off caseous tubercle or cavity in the human lung, and it is important to emphasize that the end result of the inflammatory process, even in response to an infectious agent, may be deleterious. Thus it is difficult to construct a definition of inflammation which is neither so all-inclusive as to be meaningless nor so specific that it ignores the protean nature of this intriguing biological phenomenon. Perhaps the following definition will suffice: Inflammation is a process which begins following sublethal injury to tissue and ends with permanent destruction of tissue or with complete healing.

The definition above offers something more important than a mere quibble over terminology. By including the definition all the events from sublethal injury to wound healing, one includes many pieces of a biological puzzle, enabling one to get some phylogenetic perspective on a process that probably represents a primordial character of living cells. For example, chemotaxis and phagocytosis are as integral a sequences in the inflammatory response as other widely investigated phenomena, such as alterations in capillary permeability. If this is so, then aspects of the inflammatory process have roots so deep in the evolutionary scheme that the process itself can be linked with the most elementary functions of living cells, antedating, possibly by evolutionary eons, the immunological response. Metchnikoff (1885, 1892), for example, described as "phagocytes" certain cells which have the capacity to ingest and sometimes absorb food particles. He gave many examples of this in both invertebrate and vertebrate species, pointing out, among other things, that in sponges a great part of the nutritional mechanism is performed by amoeboid cells of the mesoderm and stated that in such forms as Bipinnaria and Phyllirhoe such cells function indirectly as absorben organs (1885). Although nineteenth-century literature is saturated with examples of the phagocytic and extrusive powers of one-celled organisms, Metchnikoff apparently saw this, better than anyone, in an evolutionary context. He took the entire world —the plant and animal kingdoms—as his laboratory, ranging across phyla and species to demonstrate in a brilliant series of studies the chemotactic, phagocytic, and excretory properties of primitive cell form (1892). He probably overrated the locomotive properties of endothelial cells and he certainly underrated the role of the endothelial cell in mediating intravascular inflammatory reactions, but he saw with a clarity that almost blinded his critics the dynamic interrelationships among cells, and he did not shudder, as many of his contemporaries did, at the charge that his vitalist theory assumed psychical activity on the part of leukocytes. Metchnikoff quotes Frankel (1892, p. 192) as stating that "the phagocyte theory presupposes extraordinary powers on the part of the protoplasm of leucocytes, to which are attributed sensations, thoughts and actions, in fact a kind of psychical activity." Metchnikoff answered that the sensibility of the phagocytes is not an hypothesis which can be admitted or rejected at will, but an established fact which cannot be ignored. Metchnikoff wrote:

> Whether they possess powers of thought and volition, as this author (Frankel) accuses me of assuming, is quite beside the question, though we are justified in considering that they possess a germ of these qualities and that their sensibility, like that of various vegetable and animal unicellular organisms represents the lowest stage in the long series of phenomena which culminate in the psychical activities of man.

Given, then, the assumption that phagocytic and chemotactic properties of primitive cells represent early examples of the inflammatory response, it would appear that this response antedates, by a considerable time span on the evolutionary scale, the immune response. Day and his colleagues (1970a,b) demonstrated that activities such as those associated with complement are present in lower vertebrates, e.g., the frog, and similar activities are present in representative of several lines of invertebrates specifically chosen to be widely divergent phylogenetically. These investigators point out that many studies have been done to determine whether invertebrates have classic adaptive immune responses (see Good and Papermaster, 1964; Tripp, 1969). As yet, even though suggestive evidence has been obtained for the existence of cellular immunity in the earthworm (Cooper, 1969), no clear evidence of immunoglobulin or true adaptive antibody responses has been presented for invertebrates. Day et al. (1970a,b) note that such a conclusion involves the hazards of negative evidence, but from studies thus far the burden remains on those who contend that invertebrates possess adaptive immunity comparable to that of mammals. Studies from Good's laboratory (Gewurz et al., 1967; Page et al., 1968) and by others (Cochrane, 1969; Willoughby et al., 1969; Ward, 1967; Ward and Hill, 1970) indicate that the complement system may play a role in inflammatory reactions under circumstances where initiation by the classic immune pathway is not involved. One can think, therefore, of the complement system as being more primitive than the immune system itself, suggesting that another fragment of the inflammatory response may be associated with quite elementary forms of life.

However, one defines inflammation, the temptation is irresistible to consider it fundamental to the survival of the organism. It seems to be nothing more than common sense to appreciate that without the protection of an inflammatory reaction there would be no defense against noxious external stimuli nor would there be a mechanism to repair damaged tissue. Take, for example, the difference between the effects of inoculating a small number of pneumococci under the skin of a normal rabbit and under the skin of a rabbit in which the inflammatory response has been altered by acute alcohol intoxication (Pickrell, 1938). In the normal animal a small local lesion is produced and the animal survives. In the alcoholic rabbit there is spread of the infection often with septicemia and sometimes death. This example may have its counterpart in human disease, as in the case of the increased severity of pneumonia in the alcoholic. Another example in which the host response has been altered by some unknown mechanism is that of the fatal septicemia seen in the patient in whom the inflammatory process has been modified by unusually large doeses of corticosteroids; or the case where an abscess of the hand is not localized in skin but spreads through the vasculature, or tissue planes, disseminating infection to distant organs.

It is not surprising, however, that inflammation, similar to other vital processes, may become aberrant and considerably more harmful to the body than the noxious stimulus which originated the reaction. Thus horse serum is an innocuous agent when injected into the skin of a rabbit for the first time, but after repeated injections it is capable of producing a violent and destructive inflammatory response. Similarly, diseases which are thought to be immunological in origin, such as rheumatic fever, rheumatoid arthritis, and disseminated lupus erythematosus, are associated with diffuse inflammatory reactions which appear to provide nor protection to the host. Another way to formulate the problem is as follows: Within certain limits the inflammatory reaction is sterotyped and it cannot distinguish between those instances in which the process protects the host and those in which the host is harmed.

Thus, biologists believe, almost universally, that the many inflammatory sequences, mediators, and mechanisms available to injured tissue are present to subserve one objective—the maintenance of the integrity of the organism. Metchnikoff believed this, too, but because his critics read into his phagocytic concept elements of vitalism and animism, he couched his reading of the inflammatory process in precise terms (1892) and he chose his words carefully:

It is equally erroneous to attribute a teleological character to the theory that inflammation is a reaction to the organism against injurious agencies. This theory is based on
the law of evolution according to which the properties that are useful to the organism
survive while those which are harmful are eliminated by natural selection. Those of the
lower animals which were possessed of mobile cells to englobe and destroy the enemy
survived, whereas others whose phagocytes did not exercise their function were necessarily destined to perish. In consequence of this natural selection, the useful characteristics, including those required for inflammatory reaction, have been established and transmitted, and we need not invoke the assistance of a designed adaptation to a predestined
end, as we should from the teleological point of view.

Metchnikoff then cited criticism (Baumgarten, 1884; Sanderson, 1891)
that if the phagocytic reaction has been developed in order to protect the
organism from danger, how is it that the phagocytes refuse to act just when
the organism is most threatened? "This objection again arises from an
insufficient knowledge of the principles of the theory," Metchnikoff answered.

It is just because the defense by the phagocytes is developed according to the law of
natural selection and is not a designed adaptation to a particular end, that cases naturally
occur where the phagocytes do not fulfill their functions, a neglect followed by the most
serious danger or death of the organism. In nature the organism is possessed of many
characteristics, which may be either useful or injurious to their owner. The former causes
the survival, the latter the death of the possessor. Let us take two organisms: one in which
the phagocytes are readily repulsed by the microbe, the other whose phagocytes show a
positive sensibility causing considerable phagocytosis. The former will soon fall prey to
the parasite and be eliminated by natural selection, whereas the latter will resist the infection, survive and put forth progeny possessed of the same phagocytic properties. Under
these conditions, the activity of the phagocytes will increase with every successive generation. But the curative force of nature, the most important element of which is the inflammatory reaction, is not yet perfectly adapted to its object. The frequence of the disease and
the instances of premature death are a sufficient proof of this. The phagocytic mechanism
has not yet reached its highest stage of development and is still undergoing inprovement.
In too many cases, the phagocytes flee before the enemy or destroy the cells of the body to
which they belong (as in the scleroses). It is this imperfection in the curative forces of
nature which has necessitated the active intervention of man.

The rationality of Metchnikoff's argument has dominated thinking in this
area in this century. Assuming merit for the view and granting what seems
to be obvious—that the inflammatory process, although often morbid, is
nonetheless a bastion of defense against the spread of disease—it does not
follow that all the concoctions of the scientific enterprise explain biological
events. Often such constructions may explain only something about artifi-
cially arranged systems which have the symmetry of technical reproducibility
but quite conceivably lack biological relevance. Scientists often may be in the
position of the inebriated gentleman who was noticed to be searching for
something under a lighted pole on a street corner. On being asked if he had
lost something under the pole, he explained that he had not lost something

there but had in fact lost something down the street a distance. Asked why he did not search for the lost object down the street, he answered that there was no light down the street. Technology often is the handmaiden of science, and technology can, at times, simply study itself rather than biological systems. It is conceivable, therefore, that the imposition of grand designs on natural phenomena may really be nothing more than an overreading of Nature's message; or, as Dr. Thomas points out in Volume III, Chapter 12, the independent component mechanisms involved in what is considered to be the classic inflammatory process may each represent an intelligent defense mechanism, but when they occur simultaneously, the host, subjected to the net effect, may suffer inappropriate degrees of tissue injury. One possible result, then, of all the things that happen in inflammation occurring at once may not be that of an orderly sequential cascade of events, each designed to limit the injury, but can be that of several mechanisms working at once and, in a sense, coming into play out of phase with each other. This view leaves intact the Metchnikoff hypothesis that the inflammatory process is a mechanism of defense against environmental assault on the host, but it questions the rationality of the expression, "the inflammatory process," and implies that it might be more logical to think of "inflammatory processes." The formulation leaves open the view that inflammation is a process, not a static state, but it accommodates the possibility that the sum of the individual parts may, on occasion, be greater than the whole.

B. The Current State of Knowledge of Inflammation

It is the purpose of this treatise to evaluate our current knowledge of the inflammatory process. Obviously, if inflammatory mechanisms were completely understood, such a review would be written in quite a different way. It would start at the beginning with a statement of the molecular events which characterize cellular changes when tissue is damaged and then it would proceed to a relationship between thise changes and the gross changes that ensue in the organism. Because of gaps in our knowledge, many such areas are explored in succeeding chapters but not necessarily in a rigidly scientific order.

For this reason, this chapter will concern itself with those methods and approaches which have had a major impact on the study of inflammation. It is not intended to make this a comprehensive review but rather to point out how some of our knowledge about inflammation has been acquired and how method, to a degree, has influenced our preoccupation with one or another aspect of the inflammatory process. It should be noted, however, that this second edition of *The Inflammatory Process* carries much more strongly an emphasis on molecular events than the first edition did. This is reflected in several chapters but none more emphatically than in Dr. Korn's treatment of cell membranes which follows as Chapter 2 in a volume that in general is confined to molecular and cellular considerations. As Dr. Korn points out, the animal cell is a maze of membranes and membranous organelles and these membranes are not just static barriers demarcating cellular space as sheet rock demarcates the walls of a house. Membranes are dynamic structures, and major biochemical events of the cell occur in, on, or through them. An increasingly sophisticated technology has permitted such exploration of the inflammatory process at a level not possible a generation ago. There is no doubt that in the next decade this will be one of the most vigorously pursued experimental lines of attack on the problem, and the mining of it should yield some rich ore.

The subdivisions of this chapter are somewhat arbitrary, but they reflect the influence of classic methodology, beginning with the gross pathology of inflammation and proceeding through *in vivo* studies with light microscopy. An attempt is made to weave into these changes in technology the impact of various disciplines, and shifting emphases, including significant contributions of the microbiologists and immunologists, and of biochemical technology of recent decades. There are instances of overlap but, to a degree, they will serve to demonstrate how method influences the status of scientific knowledge.

II. The Gross Pathology of Inflammation

A. Prehistoric

There is no direct way of knowing whether prehistoric man was familiar with inflammation since there are no written records, but it is probable that he recognized inflammation of the skin in the form of ulcers or abscesses and certainly he had familiarity with wounds and possibly with the healing of wounds. What he knew is lost to us, but, if one can infer something about primitive man from the study of the North American Indian, it is probable that he had a rudimentary kind of medical knowledge which preceded the dawn of civilization.

B. Ancient

In the recorded history of all ancient peoples there is evidence that certain types of inflammation were clearly recognized, and as one might expect, inflammatory reactions involving the skin or external organs were described in each culture. The Babylonians were evidently familiar with certain disease states, for in the Code of Hammurabi, thought to have been composed about 1950 B.C., specific rules were imposed for opening an abscess of the eye with a bronze lancet (Major, 1954). The concern seems to have been for the patient, since the physician was warned that if he destroyed the man's eye in the process of opening the abscess the physician would have his fingers cut off.

Two important records of ancient Egypt have permitted historians to reconstruct something of medical knowledge of the times. The Edwin Smith Surgical Papyrus was written in the seventeenth century B.C., but was thought by James Breasted (1930), who was the translator, to have been copied from a more ancient manuscript written in 3000–2500 B.C. In it are mentioned a number of diseases including various types of abscesses and ulcers. In addition, adhesive plaster was suggested to draw together the edges of a wound, intimating that the ancient Egyptians had knowledge of the healing of wounds by first intention. The Papyrus Ebers, written in the sixteenth century B.C., was also believed to be a compilation of more ancient knowledge, and it also deals with a number of kinds of inflammation including erysipelas, carbuncles, and suppurating lymph glands. In the Ebers papyrus it is advised to allow wounds to heal by granulation.

Medicine made giant steps forward during the flowering of Greek civilization and Hippocrates' name stands out as one of the great physicians of all time. His description of disease was particularly accurate, and he identified pneumonia, pleurisy, pulmonary tuberculosis, malaria, and typhoid fever, among other diseases. He noted the association of kyphosis with hard and soft tubercles of the lung as well as purulent abscesses about the lumbar region and groin which were chronic and hard to cure. It is apparent that he was describing tuberculosis of the spine associated with pulmonary tuberculosis and cold abscesses draining into the lumbar and femoral regions. He wrote about the healing of wounds after drawing the edges together either with sutures or bandages and was familiar with wound healing by first intention.

Greek medicine had a profound influence on Roman medicine and in fact many of the physicians of ancient Rome were Greek. The outstanding treatise of the Roman era, however, was written in Latin by a Roman and was a compilation of much of the medical knowledge of the time. The author was Cornelius Celsus whose life spanned the turn of the Christian era (see translation of 1831). He probably was not a physician but was an encyclopedist who wrote on many subjects. In book three of the treatise *De Medicina* the famous descriptive sentence is found: "Now there are four diagnostic marks of inflammations, redness and swelling, with heat and pain." These have become known as the cardinal signs of inflammation and represent a classic description of the inflammatory process. It is of interest that Celsus also wrote at length about wound healing and recommended suturing of wounds, but only after the internal surface of the wound was cleansed. He noted that if this were not done and clotted blood remained it would be coverted to pus and excite inflammation.

Galen (130–200 A.D.), a Greek physician and a man who perhaps had more influence on medicine during the Middle Ages than Hippocrates, added loss of function as the fifth cardinal sign of inflammation. Galen propounded the concept that disease was the result of a cause acting locally and this produced disturbance of function. In other words, corruption produced an abscess which caused interference with function.

C. Renaissance to Modern Times

One way to examine the historical development of our knowledge about inflammation is to use tuberculosis as an example, since it was prevalent in urban areas from the dawn of history and is identifiable from the description of its gross pathology. The ancient Greeks knew a good deal about tuberculosis or "phthisis" although descriptions were largely clinical. It will be recalled that Hippocrates described the association of cold abscesses with tuberculosis of the spine, and he as well as others carefully described the fever, night sweats, blood spitting, and other symptoms of pulmonary tuberculosis. Galen was convinced that the exhalations from patients with phthisis were dangerous, which is the first suggestion that tuberculosis was a contagious disease.

Little was added to our knowledge of medicine in general and tuberculosis in particular during the Middle Ages. What medical knowledge was available was based on the writings of the great Greco-Roman physicians. Beginning with Clovis in the Fifth Century, the kings of France were believed to have a divine power to heal scrofula (tuberculosis of the lymph gland) by touch, and perhaps some might consider the "King's touch" an early contribution to psychotherapy; but aside from this dubious therapeutic advance, the Middle Ages were remarkably barren as far as contributions from Western Europe were concerned.

With the development of interest in anatomical dissection in Italy during the Renaissance, there was a concomitant increase in knowledge of tuberculosis. In part this was hindered by fear of contagion, so Morgagni and other anatomists avoided doing autopsies on known cases of tuberculosis for fear of contracting the disease (Dubos and Dubos, 1952). In 1679, however, Franciscus Sylvius described characteristic nodules in the lung and elsewhere which he called tubercles. He noted that these might suppurate and cause ulcers. In 1700, Manget described tubercles which looked similar to millet seeds, and this was the first description of miliary tuberculosis. If one recalls the variegated pathology of tuberculosis, it is not surprising that there was considerable disagreement about the unity of the disease process. Certianly there was much discussion about the differences between those lesions which were rocklike or chalky and those which were cheesy and full of pus. In 1689, Morton proposed that tubercles in other organs were the same as those found in the lung, and in 1760, Stark suggested that the solid tubercles could give rise to cavities and that the variety of types of inflammatory reaction did not preclude a common etiology (see Dubos and Dubos, 1952, for all the above).

At the end of the Eighteenth Century and the beginning of the Nineteenth Century, Paris became a great center for study of pathological anatomy. At the same time, tuberculosis was more rampant than ever before and it is not surprising that much attention was paid to the pathology of this disease. Gaspard Bayle published in 1810 his *Recherches sur la phthisie pulmonaire* and in it he described with great precision a variety of manifestations of tuberculosis, including miliary tuberculosis, tuberculous laryngitis, and enteritis. He concluded that he had described six different diseases. Laënnec, a close friend, was profoundly influenced by Bayle's work and traced the course of tuberculosis in 200 autopsies from the smallest tubercle to the largest caseous area. He believed that a tubercle began as a gray semitransparent lesion which later liquefied, and if a bronchus were nearby, the softened material would be expelled, leaving a tuberculous excavation. One of the ironies of history is that both Bayle and Laënnec, who made such careful descriptions of the gross pathology of the disease, were victims of tuberculosis. Sharing as they did the popular view of the day that tuberculosis was not contagious, they took no precautions at the autopsy table. Finally, in 1839, Schonlein of Zurich suggested the word tuberculosis as the generic term for all manifestations of phthisis (see Dubos and Dubos, 1952, for all the above).

As will be noted a little later, these studies did not finally establish the unity of the disease, for this was not accomplished conclusively until Koch's great discovery, but certainly a great deal was learned about the basic pathology of tuberculosis by careful observation at the autopsy table.

III. The Light Microscope and the Study of Inflammation

A. The Discovery of the Light Microscope

The magnifying power of a lens was known to the Romans and was described in the writing of both Pliny and Seneca. But the discovery that two convex lenses placed at an appropriate distance apart would produce much greater magnification was not made until the end of the Sixteenth Century (Major, 1954). The Jansens, father and son, of Middleburg, Holland, are credited with this great advance, and in 1624, Galileo, hearing of the discovery, introduced the microscope to Italy. It remained something of a curiosity, and not until shortly after the middle of the Seventeenth Century did Malpighi begin his work with the microscope. He made a number of notable discoveries, among them being the identification of capillary communications between small arteries and veins in the lung. Malpighi saw erythrocytes but incorrectly called them fat globules.

Shortly after the publication of these discoveries by Malpighi, a Dutch dry-goods proprietor, Antony van Leeuwenhoek, began his remarkable observations with microscopes which he constructed. These were set forth in a series of letters to the Royal Society, and among his numerous observations he described the capillary circulation in the tail of the eel, described red blood cells, and was the first man to visualize bacteria (see Major, 1954, for all the above).

B. The Use of the Microscope in the Field of Pathology

It is curious that there was such a long hiatus between the discovery of the microscope and its extensive use in the field of pathology, but it was not until the Nineteenth Century that it came into general use, and the great pathologists of the period such as Rokitansky and Virchow used the instrument for the routine study of the disease. Rokitansky in 1855 first discovered the giant cell, the microscopic anatomy of which was further elaborated by Langhans, but it was Virchow who propounded the cellular concept of disease. It was he who emphasized that pathological cells are derived from normal cells and propounded the modern idea that disease is an aberration of normal physiology. Among his other accomplishments, he carefully described the histology of the tubercle, although he believed that the small semitransparent tubercle and large caseous lesions had different etiologies (see Major, 1954).

C. In Vivo Studies of Inflammation

The use of the microscope during the Nineteenth Century to describe the *in vivo* changes associated with inflammation gave an enormous impetus to our understanding of the process. Dutrochet, in 1824, and William Addison, in 1843, were the first to describe the adherence of white cells to vascular endothelium. Waller in 1846 and Thoma in 1878 made similar observations (Florey, 1962).

However, it was Julius Friedrich Cohnheim who provided us with a simple yet classic description of the events of inflammation as he saw them in the mesentery and tongue of the frog. One can do no better than to quote from his *Lectures on General Pathology* (1882), for in his words events take place "which are well calculated to fully engross your attention." He proceeds:

> The first thing you notice in the exposed vessels is a dilatation which occurs chiefly in the arteries, then in the veins, and least of all in the capillaries. With the dilatation which is gradually developed, but which during the space of fifteen to twenty minutes has usually attained considerable proportions (often exceeding twice the original diameter) there immediately sets in in the mesentery an acceleration of the blood stream, most striking again in the arteries, but very apparent in the veins and capillaries also. Yet this acceleration never lasts long; after half an hour or an hour, or sometimes after a shorter or longer interval, it invariably gives place to a decided retardation, the velocity of the stream falling more or less below the normal standard, and so continuing as long as the vessels occupy their exposed situation.

Cohnheim goes on to describe the fact that many more capillaries become visible than are seen in normal tissue, following which he states: "But it is the veins rather than the capillaries that attract the notice of the observer; for slowly and gradually there is developed in them an extremely characteristic condition; the originally plasmatic zone becomes filled with innumerable colourless corpuscles." He notes that the white corpuscles do not remain entirely motionless but advance a little, and then states:

> Yet this does not lessen the striking contrast presented by the central column of red blood corpuscles, flowing on in an uninterrupted stream of uniform velocity, and the peripheral layer of resting colourless cells; the internal surface of the vein appears paved with a single but unbroken layer of colourless corpuscles without the interposition at any time of a single red one.

Further on comes a description of the emigration of white blood cells:

> A pointed projection is seen on the external contour of the vessel wall; it pushes itself further outwards, increases in thickness, and the pointed projection is transformed into a colourless rounded hump; this grows longer and thicker, throws out fresh points, and gradually withdraws itself from the vessel wall, with which at last it is connected only by a long thin pedicle. Finally this also detaches itself, and now there lies outside the vessel a colourless, faintly glittering contractile corpuscle with a few short processes and one long one, of the size of a white blood cell and having one or more nuclei, in a word, a colourless blood corpuscle.

Cohnheim goes on to describe an increased transudation of fluid causing infiltration and swelling of the tissue of the tongue or mesentery. He also notes that white cells migrate away from vessels and become distributed throughout the tissue.

It was Cohnheim's view that the most important event of inflammation was a change in the vessel wall and he states:

> According to this view we have here to deal with a molecular change of the vessel walls, whose highest degree involves death of the latter, but whose slighter degrees, on the other hand, call forth a certain typical series of abnormal events in connection with the motion of the blood and the transudation.

chnikoff). If this is true, and it seems to be, then Cohnheim was incorrect in his assertion that white cell emigration is passive (and Metchnikoff was right) and endothelial mobility in these reactions (Metchnikoff's assertion), whether correct or not, and it is probably incorrect, is unnecessary. It is interesting that what remains to be demonstrated 75 years after this argument was waged is absolute proof that the products of cell lysis and dematured proteins of inflammatory reactions *in vivo* are, in fact, chemotactic for white blood cells. There is some evidence that this is so (see discussion in Chapter 5 on Chemotaxis by Ramsey and Grant), but scientifically the point remains open to dispute.

IV. Bacteriology and Immunology

A. Specificity of Infection

Although it is true that a number of infectious diseases including smallpox, cow pox, and syphilis had been clearly recognized prior to the discovery of the specific agents causing these diseases, there was still considerable confusion about many infections, and even Virchow did not consider tuberculosis to be one disease. For this reason, Pasteur's study of infected wounds in 1870 and his enunciation of the principle of the specificity of infection had an enormous impact on our understanding of a large group of diseases (Murray, 1948). Robert Koch clarified further the thinking about the specificity of infection and the relationship of specific infection to different types of inflammation. He discovered the organism which caused anthrax and in so doing developed the technique of isolating pure bacterial cultures. Subsequently he developed methods of isolating pure cultures from mixed infections and, by introducing aniline dyes as stains, he was able to identify the morphology of various bacteria with greater accuracy (see Murray, 1948, for all above).

Koch's greatest triumph was his discovery, announced in 1882, of the cause of tuberculosis. By injecting guinea pigs and rabbits with infected material from humans, Villemin, a French Army surgeon, had demonstrated that tuberculosis was a transmissible disease (Dubos and Dubos, 1952). About the time that Koch made his discovery, several other investigators had observed tubercle bacilli in tuberculous lesions, but the demonstration by Koch of the cause and effect relationship between the tubercle bacillus and tuberculosis was so elegant in its method that it overshadowed the work of all others. He demonstrated the constant presence of tubercle bacilli in tuberculous lesions, he cultivated these organisms in pure culture from infected material, he produced the disease in animals with pure cultures of tubercle bacilli, and finally he was able to recover the organisms in pure culture from infected animals. This process of deriving absolute proof of cause-and-effect relationships in infectious disease became embodied in a biological formula known as Koch's Postulates, a lodestar for investigators for the past 90 years.

B. Exotoxins and Endotoxins

With the development of the concept of specific infection, it was natural that there should be interest in the cause of the signs and symptoms of clinical infectious diseases, and attempts were made to relate these to the specific bacteria involved (van Heyningen, 1962). In 1883, Klebs discovered the diphtheria bacillus and a year later Loeffler (1884) demonstrated that it was responsible for the disease diphtheria. In 1888, Roux and Yersin discovered that the diphtheria bacillus produced a soluble exotoxin which caused the manifestations of diphtheria, and shortly thereafter von Behring and Kitasato (1890) found that a specific antitoxin could be produced which would neutralize the effects of this toxin. Subsequently, other exotoxins were found and a number of these had considerable significance in relation to inflammation. It was discovered that *Staphylococcus aureus* produced a number of different exotoxins, including several which damaged leukocytes, and streptolysin, released by *Streptococcus pyogenes*, was also found to be leukocidal.

Exotoxins to which specific antitoxins could be produced were formed by gram-positive bacteria, but another group of toxins were described by Pfeiffer and Bessau (1910) that were called endotoxins. These toxins were released after autolysis or drying of bacterial cells and were associated with gram-negative bacteria. They did not have the specificity of the exotoxin and were not neutralized by immune sera. Boivin (see van Heyningen, 1962) demonstrated that the toxicity of smooth strains of a gram-negative enteric group of bacilli was due to a complex containing phospholipids and polysaccharides. Endotoxins are capable of producing inflammatory reactions and have been of interest in studies of fever, thier association with certain types of experimental shock, and their relationship to the Shwartzman reaction, a process of disseminated intravascular coagulation (Thomas, 1959).

C. Altered Cell and Tissue Reactivity

An inflammatory reaction can be induced by a great number of offending agents and laboratory maneuvers ranging from direct trauma through ionizing radiation and infections. The reaction is essentially an expression of tissue damage through a final common pathway irrespective of the cause and is characterized more by similarity among lesions caused by different agents than by differences among these lesions. Of the lesions to be mentioned here for purposes of illustration, three types will be discussed in a general way, but later chapters in this treatise deal in some detail with mechanisms of these reactions.

In all three types of these reactions the host must be "prepared" for the inflammatory reaction by previous exposure to the specific agent. It is the "sensitizing" or original exposure that predetermines the response of the host. These responses show certain differences depending on whether the hypersensitivity reaction is of the "immediate" or "delayed" type, but in either case an inflammatory reaction of the immune type presumes prior exposure to the agent. In the case of endotoxin there are some differences, as well as certain events in common with classic immune reactions. These lesions are discussed in detail later in this edition (see Volume III, Chapters 3 on the Arthus reaction by Cochrane and Janoff, 5 on anaphylaxis by Stechschulte and Austen, 7 on delayed hypersensitivity by Dvorak, and other discussions of related material. The reader is also referred to Chapter 5 on chemotaxis by Ramsey and Grant and Chapter 6 on phagocytosis by Elsbach).

1. BACTERIAL HYPERSENSITIVITY OF THE TUBERCULIN TYPE (DELAYED HYPERSENSITIVITY)

Edward Jenner first described the phenomena of delayed hypersensitivity (1800). He related, as follows, the case history of Mary Barge of Woodford who was inoculated with variolous material in the year 1791:

An efflorescence of a palish red colour soon appeared about the parts where the matter was inserted, and spread itself rather extensively, but died away in a few days without producing any variolous symptoms. She has since been repeatedly employed as a nurse to Small-Pox patients, without experiencing any ill consequences. This woman had the Cow Pox when she lived in the service of a Farmer in this parish thirty-one years before.

In a footnote Jenner then states:

It is remarkable that variolous matter, when the system is disposed to reject it, should excite inflammation on the part to which it is applied more speedily than when it produces the Small Pox. Indeed it becomes almost a criterion by which we can determine whether the infection will be received or not. It seems as if a change, which endures through life, had been produced in the action, or disposition to action, in the vessels of the skin; and it is remarkable too, that whether this change has been effected by the Small Pox, or the Cow Pox, that the disposition to sudden cuticular inflammation is the same on the application of variolous matter.

The scientific world had little interest in the phenomenon described by Jenner until Robert Koch emphasized the fact that the skin of a tuberculous animal reacts quite differently to inoculation with tubercle bacilli than does the skin of a normal animal (Rich, 1946). He noted that there was little reaction for 10–14 days after subcutaneous injection of tubercle bacilli in the normal guinea pig, after which time a nodule formed and ultimately ulcerated. In contrast, the injection of a pure culture of tubercle bacilli into a previously infected animal caused the appearance of an inflamed area in 1–2 days and shortly thereafter necrosis and ulceration.

In 1890, Koch announced the discovery of a brownish liquid which would protect against the disease and even cure it. This was the introduction of tuberculin to the scientific community, and while it was doomed to heart-breaking failure as a therapeutic tool, it did ultimately assume a vital role as a diagnostic method. It remained for von Pirquet (1907) to develop the tuberculin test which bears his name and to describe the delayed inflammatory response in the skin of tuberculous patients. Koch had fully appreciated the altered response of tuberculous patients to tuberculin but was more interested in the systemic response and the flare up of old tuberculous lesions after systemic tuberculin therapy.

The expression delayed hypersensitivity was an invention of Hans Zinsser (1921), but the critical fact about these reactions—that they depend on sensitized lymphocytes—was a discovery of Landsteiner and Chase (1942), a landmark finding that altered the course of immunology.

2. ANAPHYLACTIC HYPERSENSITIVITY: THE ARTHUS REACTION

Arthus (1903) demonstrated that repeated injections of horse serum into the skin of a rabbit could ultimately produce a hemorrhagic and necrotic reaction. He noted, as had others, that at first there was the rapid development of a wheal with erythema, but this reaction subsided quickly. He found that after each succeeding injection the reaction became more intense until finally the necrotic lesion noted above was produced. The intensity of this reaction, which has come to be known as the "Arthus phenomenon," is related to the level of circulating antibody.

There is evidence that the Arthus reaction is complement dependent, but there is evidence that it may not necessarily be so (see discussion by Cochrane and Janoff in Volume III, Chapter 3, by Ramsey and Grant, Chapter 5, and by Grant, Volume II, Chapter 7). As noted above, the classic view of the Arthus reaction as an intravascular phenomenon may depend less on the nature of the reaction than it does on the way the experiment to achieve it is performed (Grant *et al.*, 1967). It is possible that the spraying of reactive immunological materials into a tightly compressed intradermal compartment sets up foci of injury, in and outside of blood vessels, that unloose chemotactic materials which draw white blood cells into the damaged arena. This view of the reaction, however, as in the case of other formulations of the Arthus reaction, creates the implication that the reaction can move in one direction only— toward the piling up of degranulating white blood cells which are engaged in a mounting process of self-destruction with no provision for a mechanism that shuts off the reaction. Recent evidence, however, points to inflammatory agents themselves as potential mediators of a system that causes extravascular lesions to wind down, but the molecular signals that herald this event have not yet been defined clearly.

Here then are two types of inflammatory reactions which can produce necrosis: the one caused by hypersensitivity seemingly unrelated to circulating antibody and the other dependent on it. Another type of reaction associated with local hemorrhage and necrosis is the so-called "Shwartzman reaction," which requires that the tissue be prepared for the reaction with bacterial filtrates.

3. The Phenomenon of Local Tissue Reactivity or the So-Called "Shwartzman Reaction"

In 1927, Gregory Shwartzman first described the phenomenon which bears his name, and in 1937, he published a monograph entitled *Phenomenon of Local Tissue Reactivity* which exhaustively reviewed the subject. Shwartzman (1937) discovered that if a filtrate of *Bacillus typhosus* was injected into the skin of a rabbit, it produced relatively little reaction. If this was followed 24 hours later by an intravenous challenge with the same bacterial filtrate, a hemorrhagic and often necrotic lesion was produced at the original site of intradermal injection. He subsequently described the same phenomenon with filtrates from a variety of gram-negative bacteria and later with more purified preparations of endotoxin.

V. Chemotaxis

The name of Elie Metchnikoff is associated with another phenomenon called chemotaxis. Pfeffer, a botanist, coined the name "chemotaxis" to describe the attraction of fern spermatozoids by malic acid (Florey, 1962). As described above, Metchnikoff used *Bipinnaria asterigera* and *Daphnia* and noted how amoeboid cells were actively attracted by microorganisms. He was of the opinion that chemotaxis was responsible for the mobilization of phagocytic cells whatever the stimulus. Leber (1888) first applied the term chemotaxis to phenomena involving leukocytes [for a further discussion of chemotaxis, see Chapters 5 by Ramsey and Grant, 7 by Hirsch, 8 by Steinman and Cohn, 7 (Volume II) by Grant, 2 (Volume III) by Nelson, and 3 (Volume III) by Cochrane and Janoff].

It is generally accepted that bacteria and starch granules can be shown to be chemotactic for neutrophils *in vitro* (Harris, 1954), and more recently Boyden (1962) and many others have demonstrated that antigen–antibody complexes act similarly, in many cases mediated by complement [see extensive discussions of this matter by Ramsey and Grant (Chapter 5), and by Cochrane and Janoff (Volume III, Chapter 3)]. There is a recurrent theme in the literature that tissue breakdown products are also chemotactic, a point affirmed by Menkin (1956), who claimed to have isolated a polypeptide, leukotaxine, a chemotactic agent. However, Harris (1953) found no evidence *in vitro* that dead or dying tissue has any such property. It is interesting, however, that this issue will not die because its rationality has great appeal for biologists, although unambiguous evidence to support the idea is meager (see discussion in Grant *et al.*, 1967). Another vexing problem in the study of chemotaxis is that volumes of evidence have accumulated, most of it *in vitro*, to demonstrate the launching of the chemotactic mechanism, but only recently have investigators turned up suggested modifiers of the reaction come into prominence. It is a fair guess that if the 1960's was a decade of the study of factors that turn chemotaxis on, the 1970's will be a decade of the study of factors that turn it off. Perhaps within the decade there will be a reconciliation of the dynamism of the reaction and some understanding of the events that shift inflammatory reactions toward necrosis and the events that shift them toward healing. (For a discussion of this point, see Chapter 5).

VI. Phagocytosis

To Metchnikoff (1905) must go the credit for emphasizing the importance of phagocytosis in the inflammatory process. It surprised him to learn that the great bacteriologists and pathologists of the period, including Klebs, Koch, Waldeyer, and even Virchow, were entirely familiar with the presence of microorganisms within white corpuscles and yet misinterpreted the significance of this phenomenon. The teaching of the period was that microorganisms found the interior of leukocytes a particularly favorable environment in which to survive, and it was believed that leukocytes favored the dissemination of microorganisms to lymphatic tissue and throughout the body.

Metchnikoff thought the reverse must be true, and he was quite excited to learn about Cohnheim's observations of the emigration of white cells during inflammation, for to Metchnikoff this suggested that leukocytes could be mobilized in this way in order to protect the host. He describes how he set about proving this hypothesis as follows (Metchnikoff, 1905):

> This reflection led me to make the following experiment: to wound and introduce spines beneath the skin of very transparent marine animals; if my hypothesis should be well founded this should bring about an accumulation of amoeboid cells at the injured spot. I selected for this purpose the large Bipinnaria larvae of star-fish, so abundant at Messina, and inserted prickles of the rose into their bodies. Very shortly these prickles were found to be surrounded by a mass of amoeboid cells such as seen in human exudation as the result of the introduction of a spine or other foreign body. The whole process took

place under my eyes in a transparent animal possessing neither blood nor other vessels, nor a nervous system. The first point was settled. The inflammatory exudation must be considered as a reaction against all kinds of lesions, the exudation being a more primitive and more ancient phenomenon in inflammation than are the functions of the nervous system or of the vessels.

At the time Metchnikoff did these experiments in 1882 he was aware that pathologists thought that most, if not all, inflammation was caused by microorganisms and so he felt that he must do further experiments of a similar nature using microorganisms. Accordingly, he introduced various kinds of bacteria into lower animals and demonstrated that the bacteria were ingested and destroyed by amoeboid cells.

Metchnikoff distinguished between microphages (polymorphonuclear leukocytes), which he suggested were the first cells to emigrate during the inflammatory process, and macrophages, which followed later. He believed that the microphages were most active in combating microorganisms, whereas macrophages engulfed larger objects such as blood corpuscles. He noted, however, that macrophages did engulf microorganisms responsible for more chronic diseases such as leprosy, tuberculosis, and actinomycosis. He looked on the inflammatory reaction as protective and noted that it could occur in response to a variety of stimuli including sterile foreign bodies (for a further discussion of phagocytosis, see Chapter 6 by Elsbach).

The ideas proposed by Metchnikoff were not warmly received, and he spent many years in dispute with other scientists. It is difficult to understand why he was opposed so violently. Possibly it was because he was an enthusiast who was not medically qualified and because there was so much interest in humoral immunity during the same period. Perhaps the great advances being made in the study of toxins and antitoxins made Metchnikoff's idea seem unimportant; yet with the perspective of time, Metchnikoff contributed greatly to our understanding of the evolution of the inflammatory process and the importance of phagocytosis.

The battle between those favoring Metnikoff's theory of cellular defense and those favoring the humoral theory of defense was not without its useful by-products, however, for it stimulated more work in the field of phagocytosis. In 1885, Denys and Leclef showed that immunization enhanced phagocytosis, and in 1903, Wright gave the name opsonin to the activity of immune sera which enhanced specific phagocytic activity (see Murray, 1948).

VII. The Physiological Approach to Problems of Inflammation

The term "physiological" is used here in its broadest sense and is meant to convey a mode of thinking and experimental approach to biological problems which fostered much of the scientific progress of the latter part of the

Nineteenth Century and the first half of the Twentieth Century. Obviously the same kind of thinking was involved in the developments made in the field of bacteriology and immunology and this arbitrary separation is made only for emphasis.

A. The Microcirculation

1. ANATOMICAL AND FUNCTIONAL CONSIDERATIONS

Early in the chapter it was noted that the popular method of the moment, and to a degree the current scientific fashion, dictated what aspect of the inflammatory process was considered important, and this is quite evident if one traces the interest of biologists in the microcirculation. It will be recalled that Cohnheim (1882) gave a vivid description of the events which occur in the microcirculation of the frog's tongue and mesentery, and certainly he was concerned with what happened to the altered capillary wall, even postulating that there were molecular changes which altered and permeability of endothelium. It is of interest, therefore, to note Adami's comments about the role of blood vessels in inflammation in his monograph published in 1909.

It is apparent that Adami was profoundly influenced by the work of Metchnikoff, and he devoted considerable attention to the phenomenon of phagocytosis. In describing the role of blood vessels in the inflammatory process, Adami (1909) asserted:

> The study of the action and function of the leucocytes in inflammation has profoundly modified our conception of the inflammatory process. When the leucocytes were regarded as purely passive agents, and their diapedesis as purely secondary to modified conditions of the blood current and of the vascular walls, Cohnheim's hypothesis was that most generally accepted; this hypothesis regarded the changes in the vessels as of the first importance. Thus it was that for several years our attention was mainly concentrated upon the determination of the various changes of the vessel walls, and of the mechanism whereby these changes were brought about. Nowadays less attention is directed to this side of the inflammatory process . . .

But new fashion becomes outmoded and old fashion returns to favor, and the work of Ebbecke (1917), Krogh (1924), and Lewis (1927) revived interest in the changes in the small blood vessels. Gradually the concept arose that the microcirculation could be considered as a functioning unit which provided for the exchange of gases, salts, water, and metabolites according to tissue needs. It was recognized that the microcirculation was to a degree specialized to meet the particular needs of different tissues, but that there were certain basic units involved.

Krogh (1924), more than anyone else, emphasized the importance of the anatomy and physiology of the capillary bed, and he began his studies on capillaries because he was concerned with how oxygen was supplied to striated muscle. One of Krogh's earliest papers dealt with actual counts of the number of capillaries per square millimeter of muscle. Using the gastrocnemius of the horse, he discovered that there were 1350 ± 31 capillaries/mm^2 in the transverse section of muscle. He found that in cold-blooded animals, such as the frog, the number of capillaries per square millimeter of muscle was 400 and in small mammals, such as the guinea pig, the number was closer to 4000. He calculated that if the muscle of a man weighs 50 kg and there are 2000 capillaries/mm^2, the total available capillary surface would be in the neighborhood of 6300 m^2. These calculations emphasized the enormous surface available for exchange of metabolites in muscle, and also made it perfectly clear that at any one time only a fraction of the capillary bed was open.

Krogh then turned his attention to the control of capillary circulation, noting that the idea of independent contractility of capillaries, which had been accepted toward the end of the Nineteenth Century, had given way to the idea that capillary circulation was entirely passive and was controlled by arterial and arteriolar tone. Krogh mobilized considerable evidence from his own work and that of others to prove that the capillary circulation was not in fact an entirely passive process, and concluded from his studies that capillaries could contract independently. He rejected the idea that this was because of inherent contractility of capillary endothelium and proposed instead that perivascular cells tightly adherent to capillary endothelium, the so-called Rouget cells, were contractile units. He thought that these cells could respond to both sympathetic nerve stimulation and to humoral factors.

Krogh was struck by the fact that something circulating in the blood controlled the contractility of the Rouget cells. It was a common observation that reactive hyperemia ensued when the blood supply to the ear of a rabbit was obstructed and then released, and it was assumed that capillary dilation was because of lack of oxygen. Krogh studied the same phenomena in the tongue of the frog following obstruction to the lingual arteries. He observed that the erythrocytes in the stagnant vessels retained their oxygen throughout the period of obstruction, and yet reactive hyperemia ensued when the obstruction was released. Even if the frog was kept in an atmosphere of pure oxygen the results were the same. In both experiments normal tone was restored 20–30 minutes after circulation was reinstated. On the basis of these studies, Krogh assumed that something circulating in the blood was necessary for normal tone of capillaries, and he drew the conclusion that no capillary could remain closed for an indefinite period since the tonus of a capillary receiving no blood will diminish and, finally, becoming relaxed, will admit a current of blood again.

In summary, Krogh looked on the capillary bed as an important organ of response to tissue needs. He felt that capillary blood flow could vary independently of arteriolar tone. The capillary bed could respond to oxygen lack, to tissue metabolities, and to ill-defined factors in the blood responsible for normal tone. He thought that changes in capillary circulation as the result of inflammation could be primary because of direct injury to the capillary wall or secondary to tissue damage.

For a time there was general acceptance of the concept that Rouget cells were contractile units, but doubts arose and it remained for Zweifach and Chambers (Zweifach, 1961) to clarify the functional control of the microcirculation (see Volume II, Chapter 1). In a series of carefully controlled experiments on the living circulation, Zweifach concluded that the microcirculation was somewhat more complex anatomically than the classic view of an undifferentiated capillary bed connected to the arterial circulation on one side and the venous circulation on the other. He pointed out that in the normal resting circulation there are preferential pathways of flow—the so-called preferential channels—and branching off these channels at sharp angles are capillaries which open or close as tissue needs require. He was unable to confirm Krogh's observations that the pericapillary Rouget cell was a contractile element and pointed out that muscular sphincters exist at the point of bifurcation of the capillaries from the thoroughfare channel. He found that there is not an abrupt change from a muscular arteriole to a non-muscular capillary but that scattered muscle cells are found along the terminal arterioles or metarterioles and changes in capillary blood flow are mediated by muscle cells, especially the muscle of the precapillary sphincters. He described a rhythmic opening and closing of precapillary sphincters which he called vasomotion and emphasized the importance of the physiological control of the microcirculation in meeting tissue needs. He also found that normal vasomotion disappears when tissue becomes inflamed. Thus the studies of Zweifach have extended the concept of the microcirculation as a functioning unit and have modified Krogh's approach to the capillary bed.

2. Vascular Permeability

In 1896, Starling proposed a theory to explain the exchange of fluid in the capillary bed (Starling, 1896). He calculated the total osmotic pressure of blood plasma to be in the range of 7 atm and noted that most of this was owing to substances of small molecular size which could easily pass the capillary membrane. He calculated the colloidal osmotic pressure of plasma proteins to be about 30 mm of mercury, a value which although small was probably significant in terms of filtration. He postulated that this pressure balanced the pressure in the capillary circulation and proposed that if capillary pressure exceeded the colloid osmotic pressure of the blood that there would be outward filtration, and if the reverse were true, inward filtration would occur. The truth of this premise was based on the assumption that the capillary wall acted as an inert filter relatively impermeable to proteins.

In order to verify Starling's theory of capillary filtration, it was necessary to measure capillary pressure, and beginning in 1875, a variety of attempts were made to accomplish such measurements either indirectly by skin blanching or by observing capillaries directly and noting cessation of flow on applying pressure with a rigid surface or with an elastic capsule (Landis, 1934). None of the methods used was exact, and values from 3 to 71 mm of mercury were obtained for the capillary pressure in man. In 1922, Carrier and Rehberg attempted direct cannulation of capillaries in order to accomplish more precise measurement, but they were handicapped by the size of the pipettes used, lack of rigid support for pipettes, and the brief periods that intubation of capillaries could be accomplished. The result was that they obtained falsely low readings of 3.3–5.5 mm of mercury.

In 1926, Landis began a series of much more accurate measurements using micropipettes and a Chambers microinjection apparatus (Landis, 1934). He found that the intubation of capillaries could be accomplished for long enough periods to arrive at a true equilibrium so that no fluid moved in or out of the tip of the pipette. He was able to measure the pressure in both arteriolar and venous capillaries and found a consistent pressure gradient higher on the arteriolar side and lower on the venous side. He found a consistent relationship between the colloid osmotic pressure of plasma and the capillary pressure in various species. For example, in the frog the average arteriolar capillary pressure was 14 cm of water, whereas the colloid osmotic pressure was reported to range between 5.5 and 13.4 cm of water. In man the arteriolar capillary pressure was 45 cm of water, the venous capillary pressure 22 cm of water, and the colloid osmotic pressure about 36 cm of water. Thus Landis made the point that on the arterial side the capillary pressure tends to be higher than the colloid osmotic pressure, and, therefore, outward filtration is favored, whereas capillary pressure is lower than osmotic pressure on the venous side, and, therefore, inward filtration is more likely to occur.

Landis noted that capillary pressure could be quite variable and that it reflected changes in local temperature, arterial pressure, and venous outflow. He particularly emphasized that capillary pressure was likely to be higher if there was arteriolar dilation and that capillary pressure did not reflect the height of the systemic blood pressure.

The considerations of Starling and Landis do not come to grips with the structural basis of blood tissue exchange. Since capillary endothelium is permeable not only to water and electrolytes but to larger molecules such as sucrose and inulin, it behaves quite differently from the cell membrane proper. For this reason Pappenheimer (1953) and his colleagues found it convenient to think of the capillary endothelium as having pores. They have calculated on the basis of experimental work that these theoretical pores should be in the range of 30 to 45 Å. They found that the capillary permeability of a graded series of lipid-insoluble molecules decreased with increasing molecular size and postulated that the progressive decrease in free diffusibility with increasing size was a measure of the mechanical restriction to free diffusion of each molecule (Renkin, 1959).

It has also been found that the transport of molecules soluble in lipids is very much more rapid than for lipid-insoluble molecules, and he proposed that the whole capillary wall is permeable to lipid-soluble molecules, whereas lipid-insoluble molecules pass through pores presumably between cells. Pappenheimer has calculated that only a small fraction of the capillary surface is in fact available for filtration or diffusion of lipid-insoluble molecules. Despite the attractiveness of the physiological model of capillary pores, such holes in the endothelium or between endothelial cells have not been demonstrated by electron microscopy.

(For an attempted reconciliation of the various viewpoints on vascular permeability, see Volume II, Chapter 2, by Luft).

3. INCREASED CAPILLARY PERMEABILITY

One of the most characteristic aspects of inflammation is increased capillary permeability. The swelling of an inflamed part is evidence of this, and Cohnheim (1882) described in detail the increase in extravascular fluid as the result of altered permeability of small blood vessels in an inflamed area. He also noted that the fluid more nearly corresponds to serum and has a solid residue of 6–7%. He attributed this to albumen and noted the difference between the transudation owing to mechanical hyperemia in which there was very little albumen and that caused by inflammation which was rich in albumen. This observation has been repeatedly confirmed, and the protein-rich nature of the fluid of the inflammatory transudate can only be explained on the basis of a change in the vessel wall allowing larger molecules to pass freely. The nature of this defect has been a matter of experimentation and speculation for many years.

Landis (1934) found by direct measurement that the capillary pressure was increased in inflamed areas and attributed in part the accumulation of extravascular fluid to this and to increased blood flow. At the same time he noted that there had to be some additional injury to explain the protein-rich nature of the fluid.

Hoyer (1877) stained endothelium with silver nitrate and demonstrated a network of blackened lines outlining endothelial cells. Arnold (1876) repeated these experiments, and by staining mesentery with indigo blue postulated that there was a cement substance which was present between endothelial cells that was responsible for the normal adherence of endothelium. Until relatively recently this concept of an intracellular cement substance was generally accepted, and alterations in cement substance were thought to be responsible for changes in vascular permeability. Additional evidence for a cement substance was presented by Chambers and Zweifach (1940), who found that if an isolated mesentery preparation was perfused with calcium-deficient medium, endothelial cells became less firmly attached to one another and could be separated easily with microneedles. This phenomenon could be reversed by perfusing once again with medium containing the normal amount of calcium. Florey and his colleagues (1959) were unable to find an anatomical structure corresponding to "cement" in the sense used by previous workers, although they thought that the space between adjacent cells no doubt contains some substance. (See further discussion of this matter by Luft, Volume II, Chapter 2.)

4. EMIGRATION OF CELLS

Closely related to the changes in permeability of endothelium resulting from inflammation is the emigration of cells, and there has been much specu-lation about how this occurs. Arnold (1873) made drawings of small blood vessels and showed leukocytes migrating through areas of the capillary wall, associated with what he described as "intercellular cement" and "stigmata" between the cells. Other investigators also suggested that migration occurred between cells but as the result of an alteration in the intercellular cement.

One of the most striking changes to occur in inflammation is the apparent "stickiness" of leukocytes which adhere to endothelium (see Volume II, Chapter 7 by Grant). Adami in discussing the sticky nature of leukocytes pointed out that the same phenomenon can be seen in the organism *Daphnia* which is without a vascular system. Leukocytes move freely in health, but if injury is incurred the leukocytes tend to adhere to the walls of the body cavity beneath the region of injury and elsewhere. Clearly, Adami associated this change with stickiness of the leukocytes, but it has also been suggested that the endothelial wall itself becomes "sticky."

It is of interest to observe this phenomenon in the rabbit ear chamber after the local injection of any number of noxious agents, of which bradykinin can serve as an example.

Within a few minutes after the injection there is striking margination of white cells, chiefly in venules, and leukocytes roll slowly along the endothel-ium. Within 4 minutes appreciable numbers of white cells adhere tightly to the endothelial surface and cannot be dislodged by the rapid flow of blood through the venule. The persistence of sticking is a function of dose, and with a concentration of 2 μg/ml the fixed sticking gives way to rolling in about one-half an hour and no cells emigrate. With higher concentrations the fixed sticking is more persistent and emigration occurs. It would appear that this adherence of leukocytes is a necessary prelude to diapedesis, but migration need not necessarily occur. Careful study of the phenomenon with the electron microscope has not explained this apparent stickiness of leukocytes or of endothelium, but it seem clear that endothelial injury alone, all other factors remaining unchanged, can cause thrombotic phenomena in blood vessels. Grant and Epstein (1974) have demonstrated this point by perfusing the rabbit ear chamber with neutral solutions and then inflicting laser lesions on blood vessels at a time when the plasma, red cells, white cells, and platelets were not in the field. When blood flow was permitted to return, white cells and/or platelets adhered to the vessel wall, apparently depending on the severity of the stimulus, the white cells but not the platelets adhering with minimal stimuli, and the platelets dominating the reaction shearing injuries.

B. Lymphatics and the Inflammatory Process

Some idea of the richness of the capillary plexus of lymphatics can be obtained by injecting a dye such as Patent blue V intradermally. Hudack and McMaster (1933) took movies of this procedure, and the rapid filling of fine network of lymphatics is striking. Lymphatic capillaries are similar to blood capillaries, their most striking difference being the absence of a basement membrane. Leukocytes apparently migrate into lymphatics with ease.

Since lymphatics are concerned with normal movement of fluid from tissues to lymph node and finally via afferent lymphatics to the thoracic duct and back to the bloodstream, it is not surprising that the lymphatics should play a role in the inflammatory process. It will be recalled that Cohnheim in his analysis of the inflammatory process performed experiments to discover whether swelling was due to transudation of fluid or to blocking of lymphatic flow. He discovered that in an inflamed limb of a dog not only was there no obstruction to lymphatic flow but that it was much increased. This has been confirmed by others, and the careful studies by Drinker and Yoffey (1941) have proved how important lymphatics are to the process of inflammation.

Since lymphatics are little more than endothelial tubes, it might be supposed that they would collapse as the result of the edema and increased tissue pressure which occur as a part of the inflammatory process. That this is not the case was demonstrated in an elegant experiment by Pullinger and Florey (1935). These investigators injected the lymphatic of the mouse ear with a fine suspension of carbon so that the lymphatic vessels might be recognized easily and then produced swelling of the ear. Sections of the ear revealed dilated lymphatics, and attached to the walls were connective tissue fibers continuous with the surrounding connective tissue. The greater the swelling, the more pull was exerted by the connective tissue bands connected with the vessel walls and the greater was the lymphatic dilatation. (For a full review of factors important in lymphatic physiology and pathology, see Volume II, Chapter 6 by Casley-Smith. See also Volume III, Chapter 10 by Dumont on repair and Volume III, Chapter 1 on lymphocytes by McGregor and Mackaness.)

C. The Origin and Function of the Cells found in Inflammatory Exudates

There is perhaps no more a confused chapter in the history of medicine than that which concerns the origin of cells of the inflammatory exudate, and it would be fruitless to review all the various theories which have been proposed and the experimental work done to support or refute these theories. Perhaps the most popular theory for many years was the unitarian concept proposed by Maximow (1906). He believed that all mesenchymal cells derived from an undifferentiated blast cell which in the bone marrow was a free mesenchymal cell or hemocytoblast and in other tissues was the fixed undifferentiated mesenchymal cell. He proposed that the large lymphocyte was such a multipotential cell and that it could transform normally into macrophages or fibroblasts and under certain conditions such as extramedullary hematopoiesis into myeloid cells and erythrocytes. There are numerous objections to this concept and they are treated in some detail in other chapters of this treatise (see Chapter 7, on neutrophils, by Hirsch, Chapter 8 on mononuclear cells by Cohn, Chapter 9 on platelets by Zucker, Chapter 10 on mast cells by Bloom, and Volume III, Chapter 1 on lymphocytes by McGregor and Mackaness, as well as Volume III, Chapter 6 on chronic inflammation by Spector).

1. THE POLYMORPHONUCLEAR LEUKOCYTE

Metchnikoff termed this cell the "microphage" and noted its activity in the first line of defense against infection. It has been uniformly observed that the polymorphonuclear leukocyte is the first cell to appear in the acute inflammatory exudate. The polymorph is an actively motile cell, but seems to survive for a relatively short time in exudate. Just how long it persists in a living active state is unclear, but it is probably a matter of 24 hours or less.

Since the polymorphonuclear leukocyte is a scavenger cell, it is not surprising that it should contain a number of biologically active agents, many of them enzymatic in nature. A growing list of such agents already includes enzymatic, nonenzymatic, and bactericidal agents of various types (see

Chapter 7 by Hirsch), as well as other constituents that influence permeability, chemotaxis, the induction of fever, and the alteration of coagulation factors (see Volume III, Chapter 3 by Cochrane and Janoff).

During the past decade there has been an enormous increase in knowledge of the phagocytic events which begin with chemotaxis (see Chapter 5, Ramsey and Grant) and end with contact of the particle with the cell membrane, ingestion, and digestion or killing of the particle (see Chapter 6 by Elsbach and Chapter 7 by Hirsch). On contact with the cell surface a vesicle (or phagosome) derived from plasma membrane is formed which encapsulates the particle and carries it internally. The granules of the leukocyte fuse with the phagosome, and the contents of the granule are discharged into the enlarged vacuole which harbors the particle. This "degranulation" is a central event in the mobilization of bactericidal substance contained in the granules. Much work has been done with living bacteria to define the role of various bactericidal agents found within the granules of the leukocyte, including acid hydrolases, myeoloperoxidase, lysosyme, and phagocytin. There has been particular interest in the H_2O_2-myeloperoxidase-halogen system in bacterial killing because this system is implicated in the clinical syndrome of chronic granulomatous disease.

It is interesting that the considerable literature of the last decade on the contents of white cell organelles was stimulated by an observation by de Duve and his associates (Berthet and de Duve, 1951; Berthet *et al.*, 1951) that the activity of the enzymatic acid phosphatase appeared to be relatively low in freshly prepared homogenates of liver but was increased when these homogenates were "aged" or left in storage. (See discussion by Hirshhorn, Chapter 4.) They had at their disposal several possible explanations for these changes but they chose to imagine that the enzyme was membrane bound in the cell and that during aging the membrane was disrupted, allowing the enzyme free access to substrate and altering the sediment able characteristics of the material. This bit of prescience enabled them to postulate the existence of an intracellular organelle which was membrane bound, between 0.2 and 0.8 μm in size and which contained at least five hydrolytic enzymes. Because these enzymes are lytic, they proposed the name lysosome. From that point on, the search for and identification of lysosomes became one of the biological preoccupations of the decade, and it has yielded an enormous dividend in the understanding of the pathogenesis of the inflammatory response.

2. THE MACROPHAGE

The most persistent scavenger cell which appears in inflammatory exudate is a large mononuclear cell which Metchnikoff called the macrophage. It was first described by von Recklinghausen in 1863 in the course of study of experimentally induced inflammation of the cornea. It is this cell which has been given such a wide variety of origins by investigators. A list of these will suffice to make the point (Ebert, 1939).

    a. Origin from fixed tissue histiocytes: von Recklinghausen, 1863; Ziegler, 1890; Grawitz, 1890.

    b. Origin from adventitial cells: Marchand, 1890; Kiyono, 1914; Foot, 1925; von Möllendorf and von Möllendorf, 1926; Bauer, 1929.

    c. Mesothelium: Weidenreich, 1909; Schott, 1909; Szecsi, 1912; Downey, 1915.

    d. Fibroblast: von Möllendorf and von Möllendorf, 1926; Koll, 1927; Knake, 1927; Stockinger, 1928; Parker, 1932.

    e. Lymphocytes: Ranvier, 1890; Maximow, 1902; Dominici, 1902; Renaut, 1906; Dubreil, 1913; Downey, 1917.

    f. Monocytes and histiocytes as variations of the same cell type: Kiyono, 1914; Carrel and Ebeling, 1922; Lewis and Lewis, 1924; Clark and Clark, 1930; Seeman, 1930.

    g. Monocytes and histiocytes as different cell types and giving rise to exudate cells of different types: Sabin *et al.*, 1925.

    h. Endothelial origin: Mallory, 1898; Herzog, 1916; Permar, 1920; McJunkin, 19191; Foot, 1919.

The confusion about this cell is attested to by the many names which have been used to describe it. These include macrophage, polyblast, histiocyte, clasmatocyte, resting wandering cell, rhagiocrine cell, pyrrhol cell, carmine cell, adventitial cell, endothelial leukocyte, blood histiocyte, blood clasmatocyte, and monocyte.

One of the reasons for the confusion is the fact that so-called transitional forms seen in exudates were interpreted as metamorphosis from one cell type to another. Ebert and Florey (1939) described the change of monocytes which migrated from the bloodstream first into macrophages and then into cells indistinguishable from fixed tissue histiocytes. These observations were made *in vivo* and individual cells marked with ingested carbon particles were followed for weeks and months. They also found that in the rabbit ear chamber the monocyte appeared to be the cell which became the actively motile macrophage in new areas of inflammation, although the fixed histiocyte retained its phagocytic activity.

Just as in the case of the neutrophil, renewed interest in the macrophage was stimulated by de Duve's demonstration of the existence of membrane-bound organelles in liver cells. The macrophage has an abundance of lysosomes (see Chapter 8 by Steinman and Cohn) and, in addition, a highly sophisticated complement of defense mechanisms for isolating and killing foreign invaders. While the role of the macrophage in the induction of an immune response is not clear, the evidence is good that macrophages can destroy antigen and they may play an important role, as noted by Steinman and Cohn, Chapter 8, in the development of immunity and tolerance.

3. THE LYMPHOCYTE

The life history and function of the lymphocyte was obscured for many years by difficulties in separating these cells by morphological criteria from other cells (i.e., monocytes which often appear to look similar to lymphocytes. The discovery by Gowans (1957, 1959a,b, 1962; see also Gowans and Knight, 1964) of the extraordinary fact that small lymphocytes circulate through the body by a route that is different from all other cell types stimulated an interest in the reexamination of this cell. Further evidence that the small lymphocyte is a mediator of the immune response and more recent studies identifying lymphocytes as memory cells (Gowans and Uhr, 1966; McGregor et al., 1971; Miller and Sprent, 1971; Collins and Mackaness, 1971) has generated, among immunologists, an enormous interest in this cell, stimulated in no small measure by the implication of the lymphocyte in the rejection of skin grafts (Billingham et al., 1960; Gowans, 1961, 1962; Porter and Cooper, 1962a,b). Thus the lymphocyte has emerged as a mediator or the source of mediators (lymphokines) of one important aspect of the inflammatory response. (For fuller discussion of these facts, see Volume III, Chapter 1 by McGregor and Mackaness; Volume III, Chapter 7 by Dvorak; and, for an earlier historical treatment of the subject, Chapter 7, first edition of *The Inflammatory Process*, 1965.)

4. THE PLATELET

The platelet plays a prominent role in intravascular inflammatory reactions (see review by Mustard and Packham, 1971, and Chapter 9 by Dr. Zucker). A series of studies by Born and his colleagues that adenosine derivatives influence a fundamental step in platelet aggregation (Gaarder et al., 1961; Born and Cross, 1963; Clayton et al., 1963) opened a new approach to platelet physiology. This was followed by the observation that collagen particles can aggregate platelets, and this is induced by ADP released by the platelets (Hovig, 1963; Spaet and Zucker, 1964). More recent evidence suggests that platelets can also adhere to basement membrane (Stemmerman et al., 1971). However, a critical observation by Moe and Jorgensen (1967, 1968) showed that deposits on the syncytium of villi and chorion plate in the normal human placenta are thrombi derived from material blood, beginning as platelet thrombi. In this case the thrombosis is not initiated by an interaction between platelets and exposed basement membrane, or collagen fibers, since the platelets adhere to an uninterrupted syncytium with no possibility of contact with the underlying connective tissue components. Grant and Epstein have demonstrated (1974) that in microburns of blood vessels mild stimuli seem to evoke white cell sticking, whereas more severe stimuli, notably those that create shearing reactions of the vessels, elicit massive platelet sticking. They also showed, by electon microscopy, platelet approximation of endothelial surfaces without evidence that the platelets had breached the vessel wall or were in contact with basement membrane. It is not clear, then, that the platelet needs exposure either to collagen or basement membrane for adherence to vessel walls, but there seems to be ample confirmation in modern studies for the classic view of the platelet as filling a role of a thumb in a dike to prevent the escape of intravascular contents when shearing reactions are imposed on the vessel wall. [For a further discussion of these points and related matters, see Majno *et al.* (1969, 1971) and Volume II, Chapter 7 on white cell sticking by Grant.]

5. THE ENDOTHELIAL CELL

The origin of the endothelial cell is obscure, its chemical properties virtually unknown, and the nature of its remarkable luminal membrane still a cause of speculation. In vertebrates, endothelial tissue first appears in relation to the yolk sac wall as isolated cellular cords which later develop a lumen. Confluence of the lumina of separate cords results in the formation of an endothelial network of vitelline vessels. By extension and growth, this network progressively approaches, and is eventually found within, the embryonic body. Primitive blood cells are found within the endothelial lining of the network, but the histogenetic relation between the endothelial and the blood cells has not yet been established. It is widely accepted that the endothelial cells lining the vitellin vessels are of splanchnopleuric mesodermal origin; the endothelium may, however, arise from "yolk cells" lying between the endoderm and mesoderm (mesothelium).

There are differences of opinion on the relationship between the endothelium lining the vitellin vessels and that which is later found within the body of the embryo. (1) One view holds that the extraembryonic endothelium extends into the embryonic body and permeates its tissues to give origin to the whole of the endothelium of the embryonic haemo-lymph system. This is the so-called *angioblastic* theory which states that all the intra- and extraembryonic endothelium develops from precociously segregated angioblastic tissues. (2) The theory of *local* origin holds that the intraembryonic endothelium differentiates *in situ* from intraembryonic mesoderm and only secondarily becomes united with the extraembryonic vitelline network. This view holds that mesenchyme in any situation can become transformed into endothelium if the environmental conditions are suitable for it to do so, a view with a Lamarckian cast to it and one that might make some biologists skitterish but one that will command attention until definitive evidence proves it incorrect.

Although endothelium, as a membrane, can be discussed as a unit, implying that all endothelial cells are the same, there are some differences, as noted in many publications, all referred to in Luft's discussion (Volume II, Chapter 2) and the extensive review by Majno (1965) documenting the variety of capillaries. Flattened endothelial cells are joined together to form the innermost lining of both blood and lymphatic channels. On the luminal side of the cell surface, there may be an endocapillary layer, an acid muco-polysaccharide (Luft, 1965a,b, 1966, 1971a,b). Whatever one calls it, some material at this site seems to have an affinity for an electron-dense cationic dye, ruthenium red, suggesting that it is some sort of anionic substrate as yet unidentified.

There have been a spate of papers in recent years on the origin of blood vascular endothelium and speculations on its precursors (Poole *et al.*, 1958, 1959; Florey *et al.*, 1961; Stump *et al.*, 1963; O'Neal *et al.*, 1964; Mackenzie and Hackett, 1968) and on related matters having to do with the differentia-tion of white blood cells (Petrakis *et al.*, 1961; Ross and Lillywhite, 1965). De Bakey's group (Stump *et al.*, 1963; O'Neal *et al.*, 1964) offered the view that circulating blood in the growing pig contains cells capable of forming endothelium but in their experimental model—a midstream dacron hub in-side a large vessel prosthesis—the isolated luminal hub contained fibroblasts and smooth muscle cells as well as endothelial cells. Although it is quite an ingenious experimental model, the dacron hub that grew out tissue in mid-stream may have done so not because of the differentiation of cells from the blood but because injured and regenerating connective tissue cells, originating upstream at the prosthesis surgical margin, may have landed on the hub accidentally. Still, this model is worth examining carefully and some quite important *in vivo* evidence could possibly be constructed on it.

The endothelial cell may or may not have primacy in the mediation of intravascular inflammatory reactions [Grant and Epstein (1974) have evi-dence that it does], but it certainly is a critical concomitant of the reaction, and progress in understanding the character of this cell has been inhibited because of failure to isolate endothelium in purity and amounts that would permit its assay and manipulation. It is possible that this logjam has been broken. Maruyma (1963) reported that he was able to isolate cells of the human umbilical vein by trypsinizing them and then he was able to culture them. The cells in culture grew in sheets, he reported, "which were identified with endothelial cells." Recently, Jaffe *et al.* (1972) reported similar results. They incubated human umbilical veins with buffered collagenase solutions and the enzymatically removed intimal cells were cultured in medium 199. They claim to have distinguished the cultured cells from standard fibroblast cell lines, and they stained the cultured cells with fluoresceinated antithrombosthenin (F-AT), which also stains human endothelial cells and vascular and uterine smooth muscle in tissue sections. Thus they are in a position to study an *in vitro* model of the vascular wall. For other approaches to this problem, see Pomerat and Slick (1963), Tsutsumi and Gore (1969), Ellingson and Yao (1971), Sade and Folkman (1972), and Lewis *et al.* (1973). The various approaches to the culturing of endothelium, a formidable technological feat, could, if productive, break open an important frontier in the study of inflammatory reactions, making feasible biochemical studies of the vascular wall and, perhaps, a more sophisticated approach to the study of endothelial membranes and the factors that shift them back and forth between adhesive and non-adhesive states.

D. Healing

Sandison (1924, 1928) and Clark *et al.* (1931) in their papers dealing with the rabbit ear chamber have given a lucid description of the healing process as it occurs *in vivo*. This method provides a thin clot between a transparent platform and a coverslip into which new tissue grows and in which the dynamics of healing are easily observed. The first event is the appearance of macrophages which digest the fibrin clot and engulf the debris. Next a line of capillary loops becomes evident at the chamber edge, and capillary sprouts can be seen growing from the advancing edge of the loops. These capillary loops are quite fragile, and fresh hemorrhage along the advancing edge of the loops is always evident. Accompanying the loops are fibroblasts, and fibrous tissue is laid down along the line of advancing vessels. Lymphatics may also be seen growing into the newly formed tissue, and they tend to advance along the margin of blood vessels. In the course of 3–4 weeks the visible area is completely vascularized and a process of maturation occurs. A more adult pattern of vessel develops with well-differentiated arterioles, metarterioles, capillaries, and venules, and some of the vessels are resorbed.

This is healing in a sterile area, but the same process has been observed by us in the healing of an experimental tubercle in an animal receiving antimicrobial therapy. It is of interest that in the same minute tubercle there may be healing and fresh activity, with tissue destruction occurring simultaneously (see Volume III, Chapter 6 on chronic inflammation by Spector and Volume III, Chapter 10 on wound healing by Dumont).

VIII. Chemical Mediators of Inflammation

Just as bacteriology and immunology had a profound effect on the study of inflammation at the end of the Nineteenth Century so has biochemistry during the Twentieth Century. With the development of modern biochemical techniques, it is not surprising that the attention of many investigators should be directed toward the problem of chemical mediation of inflammation. Sir Thomas Lewis gave the original impetus to this field by emphasizing the role of histamine as an inflammatory agent.

A. Amines Having Inflammatory Activity

1. HISTAMINE

Sir Thomas Lewis (1927) was impressed by two observations: (a) the similarity between the triple response in the skin and (b) the variety of agents which could produce the triple response. It will be recalled that the triple response is the reaction which follows the heavy stroke of a sharp edge (such as a ruler edge) across the skin. First there is a dull red line which begins to appear in 20 seconds and is sharply demarcated and corresponds to the line of pressure. This is followed in about 30 seconds by a dull red halo (axon reflex) and lastly, after 70 seconds, by a wheal, which is at first dull red and subsequently becomes pale. Lewis noted that a variety of stimuli including pressure, heat, cold, and ultraviolet light could produce this reaction and therefore postulated the release in tissues of an "H" substance which caused the triple response. Learning of the work of Dale and Laidlaw (1910–1911) with histamine, he studied the response in the skin to intradermal histamine and found that it was not only identical in appearance to the triple response but the time relationships were the same. It was natural to assume that this was *the* chemical mediator of inflammation. Since the original description of histamine as such a mediator, a bewildering array of other presumed mediators have been identified. It is interesting, however, that Willoughby (see Volume II, Chapter 9) emphasizes that histamine still remains as the only chemical agent in the vast list of presumed mediators that fulfills all the criteria one would demand as scientific proof of its role in inflammation. This is to say, histamine is present at the site of injury at the appropriate time; its action is antagonized by antihistamine; histamine reproduces the events it is supposed to mediate; and if depleted from tissue the reaction is suppressed. Almost ironically, it turns out that histamine may constitute one of the molecular signals that helps to turn off the inflammatory response (Bourne *et al.*, 1972; see discussion in Chapter 5 on chemotaxis by Ramsey and Grant).

2. 5-HYDROXYTRYPTAMINE (SEROTONIN)

This vasoactive amine is known to be present in platelets, argentaffine cells of the gut, and mast cells of the rat and mouse. It is a vasodilator in man, but does not produce significant change in permeability. In the rat, however, it appears to be a potent inflammatory agent. As noted by Willoughby in Volume II, Chapter 9, the action of serotonin is transient and is usually associated with histamine release. Less is known of this amine than of histamine, but it is a frequently mentioned mediator. (For further discussion, see Volume II, Chapter 9, by Willoughby.)

B. Polypeptides (Plasma Kinins)

1. LEUKOTAXINE

Valey Menkin (1956) must be given a prominent place in the history of inflammation even though much of his biochemical work may have been inadequately controlled. None of the mediators he proposed, including leukotaxine, is accepted today as a chemically pure entity (Harris, 1953, 1954). Nonetheless, Menkin was one of the early champions of the concept of polypeptides as mediators of the inflammatory response, an idea whose time seems to have come and passed and come again in the long complex trail that winds through the literature from the days of von Haller (1757) and Dutrochet (1824).

2. BRADYKININ AND KALLIDIN

Another interesting episode in the history of inflammation is that of bradykinin and kallidin. Fortunately, recent advances in polypeptide chemistry have begun to bring order out of chaos. A composite picture is derived from the work of the following groups: Boissonnos et al. (1963), Elliott (1963), Rocha e Silva et al. (1949), Lewis (1960), Schacter (1963), and Webster and Pierce (1963).

In 1949, Rocha e Silva and co-workers described a substance released from the pseudoglobulin fraction of blood after incubation with snake venom (*Bothrops jararaca*) or trypsin which was capable of stimulating contraction of smooth muscle, lowering blood pressure, and causing increased capillary permeability. He called this active agent "bradykinin" because it caused a relatively slow contraction of muscle.

In 1928, Frey and Kraut discovered a vasodepressor principle in urine, and subsequently also in the pancreas, which they named kallikrein. Kallikrein has been shown to be an enzyme. They discovered that kallikrein existed in an inactive form in the blood that they called kallikreinogen. The inactive precursor (kallikreinogen) could be activated by acidification or by acetone in the test tube. Following the work of Rocha e Silva, Frey, Kraut, and Werle discovered that kallikrein liberated a plasma kinin from the blood that they called kallidin, which was capable of producing increased vascular permeability. (For a fuller discussion, see Volume II, Chapter 8.)

There followed considerable debate as to whether bradykinin and kallidin were the same polypeptide and whether one or both were important chemical mediators of inflammation. Fortunately the dispute was solved in the most direct way possible, by determining the chemical structures of both compounds. Bradykinin was synthesized by Boissonnos using a chemical structure proposed by Elliott as a starting point; and it was found to be a nonapeptide. Webster and Pierce as well as Werle worked out the structure of kallidin, and they found it to be a decapeptide that was a homolog of bradykinin containing an extra lysine residue. It is now supposed that kallidin-10 is converted to kallidin-9 (or bradykinin) by an aminopeptidase present in plasma.

3. PLASMA FACTORS AND THE RELEASE OF BRADYKININ

The story does not end there, for a number of other factors appear to be involved in the activation of the kallidin–10–bradykinin system. Armstrong and Keele (1954) found that fresh plasma after contact with glass liberated a substance which caused pain when applied to the base of a·blister. This action was similar to that of bradykinin and they called the substance pain-producing substance (PPS). Margolis (1959) suggested that a glass surface served to activate Hageman factor, previously implicated in the clotting mechanism (see Volume II, Chapters 8 and 9). Webster and Ratnoff (1961) subsequently demonstrated that the addition of activated Hageman factor to human plasma released kinins.

It would appear, therefore, that the release of bradykinin through enzymatic activation and subsequent cleavage of tissue or blood substrate in a fundamental way parallel the activation of the clotting process. Activated Hageman factor promotes the change of plasma kallikreinogen to kallikrein, which, in turn, activates kallidinogen to kallidin-10, and this is changed to kallidin-9 or bradykinin by a plasma aminopeptidase.

C. *Epinephrine and Norepinephrine: Potential Antimediators*

There has been a natural preoccupation of investigators with the identification of factors which produce cellular damage. However, it is important to appreciate that there may be other naturally occurring agents which tend to balance the injurious effect of mediators of inflammation, a subject that runs deep in the literature (see Opie, 1922) but is now resurfacing as a major experimental goal in this area (see discussion of this in Chapter 5 by Ramsey and Grant and in Volume III, Chapter 3 by Cochrane and Janoff). As Willoughby notes in Volume II, Chapter 9, it is possible to classify epinephrine and norepinephrine as antiinflammatory agents. He points out that if the rapid destruction of these agents is delayed by monamine oxidase inhibtion, there is some suppression of increased capillary permeability caused by thermal and chemical injury.

D. Other Factors

Much work has been done to clarify our knowledge of the complement system (see Volume III, Chapter 2 by Nelson; also discussions of this evidence in Volume III, Chapter 3 by Cochrane and Janoff and Chapter 5 by Ramsey and Grant) and its role in various aspects of the inflammatory process. C'1 esterase can be activated by the complement system, and Ratnoff and Lepow (1963) have found that C'1 esterase will cause increased capillary permeability. Recent studies have demonstrated that a deficiency in C'1 esterase inhibitor is present in the clinical syndrome of congenital angioneurotic edema (Donaldson et al., 1970). One difficulty that plagues the complement story is that inflammatory reactions seem to proceed unabated in the absence of complement (Lotz and Harris, 1956), and in vivo correlations of in vitro studies of complement are difficult to achieve, although, as Cochrane and Janoff point out, some clinical studies that seem to have merit have emerged in recent years.

The best defined mediators, namely, histamine and bradykinin, are inactivated rapidly and seem to be associated with the early stages of the inflammatory reaction. This has led to the search for other potential mediators, some of which may be involved in the later stages of inflammation, including permeability factors associated with plasma globulins (see Volume II, Chapter 8 by Wilhelm and review of this subject by Wilhelm, 1971), "slow reacting substance" or SRS (Feldberg and Kellaway, 1938; Orange and Austen, 1971), and endogenous pyrogen (Moses et al., 1964). More recent work has emphasized the role of lysosomal enzymes in the mediation of the inflammatory response (see discussion in Volume III, Chapter 3 by Cochrane and Janoff and in Chapter 5 by Ramsey and Grant) and the contribution of prostaglandins and cyclic AMP. In the burst of activity generated by these studies, it is too early to assign priorities, and speculative flow sheets, searching for perspective, have to be revised almost month to month. There is no doubt, however, that this area of activity will engage the interest of investigators for the foreseeable future, often with an aim toward finding a pure chemical that triggers the ultimate reaction on the final common pathway of the inflammatory response.

IX. The Electron Microscope and Changes in Ultrastructure

The introduction of the electron microscope has added still another dimension to the study of inflammation, and as the result of the studies by

Fawcett (1959), Palade (1953), Florey (1961), and others it has provided a much better understanding of the structure of normal endothelium, as well as offering some evidence concerning changes which occur in inflammatory reactions.

A. Normal Endothelium

The study of normal endothelium under high magnification does not reveal an intercellular cement substance, a point anticipated by Florey (Florey *et al.*, 1959). They junctions between cells are regular gaps about 30–50 Å wide, and frequently cell junctions are seen in which there is an electron-dense area (known in some tissues as an attachment belt or desmosome). A well-defined basement membrane is evident, but no layer of protein on the inner surface of the endothelium, as had been postulated by Zweifach, has been demonstrated. Yet, as noted earlier, Luft postulates a mucopolysacchride lining on the vessel wall and this could conceivably constitute a substrate for white cell sticking. Also readily apparent is the vesicular system first described by Palade (1953). These are invaginations of the internal surface of the cytoplasm called caveolae intracellulares. Within the cytoplasm are vesicles, and caveolae are visible on the external surface of the endothelium. Palade suggested that this represented a transport system for fluid and even particulate matter (Palade, 1960). He believed that colloidal substances such as ferritin and colloidal gold traverse the cytoplasm in vesicles.

Inasmuch as colloidal material could be transported via vesicles, Palade discarded this system as being responsible for semipermeability and suggested instead that the basement membrane was responsible for this property. Florey and colleagues have studied the same problem of transport by vesicles using perfused rabbit hearts. By using an isolated preparation, they were able to employ much higher concentrations of colloidal material, and they demonstrated as did Palade that vesicles did indeed appear to transport particulate matter, but they did not find that the basement membrane presented any significant barrier to the passage of such material. If colloidal particles can pass the basement membrane so can protein, and this raises the question of whether one can explain all the semipermeable characteristics of endothelium on the basis of the structure of the basement membrane. It would appear, however, that even though colloidal material does pass through the basement membrane it takes some time to do this and it may be true that the basement membrane does act as a semipermeable barrier, allowing only small amounts of protein to pass into the extravascular space.

B. Changes in Capillary Endothelium Associated with Increased Permeability

Another important contribution to our understanding of increased vascular permeability was the description of gaps between endothelial cells occurring in response to the injection of histamine or serotonin into the cremasteric muscle of the rat. Majno and Palade (1960) found that this occurred within 3–4 minutes after injection of the inflammatory agent, and they were able to visualize plasma seeping through the gaps by using colloidal mercuric sulfide as a marker. It was significant that gaps were first seen in venules 8–20 μm in diameter, suggesting that the venule was the principal reactive vessel in early inflammation, a point made by other observers using direct visual techniques. Further studies by Majno's group have shown that mediators such as histamine and bradykinin apparently cause endothelial contraction which creates gaps between the endothelial cells (Majno *et al.*, 1969, 1971).

C. Emigration of White Blood Cells

Studies on the emigration of white cells have been made by a number of investigators, but those of Marchesi and Florey (1960) are perhaps the most complete. These investigators could find no explanation morphologically for the "stickiness" of either leukocytes or endothelium. Leukocytes migrating through endothelial junctions were retained temporarily by the basement membrane, but were finally able to pass the basement membrane without leaving any obvious defect. Ultrastructure studies of inflammatory reactions have added a few bits of evidence to the play-by-play account of the gross movement of cells, but such studies have not, nor could they be expected to do so, created new insights into cell–cell interactions. These will come about when more is known of the chemistry of the cell and the properties of cell membranes.

X. Conclusions

Looking at the state of research in the field from the vantage point of a perspective of 150 years, it can be stated that much of what we know about the inflammatory process today was known in 1900 (see Harris, 1960, for a discussion of this point). Yet the stage seems to be set for an attack in depth on problems of critical importance and one has the impression of great vigor in the research enterprise as the study of the inflammatory process acquires molecular dimensions. In a field so vast and seemingly so chaotic (the inflammatory process itself is chaotic at times), predictions are dangerous. However, it is interesting to make them, if only to look back later to see how badly they misfired. In broad terms, then, we would like to hazard the guess that among the main endeavors of the next decade will be the following: (1) a concerted effort to isolate, characterize, and manipulate the endothelial cell, thus bringing studies of this critical entity into phase with other cell systems, about which a fair amount is known; (2) a continued preoccupation with chemical mediators, as pure as they come, but with this a strong balance to study the factors that wind down the process of inflammation, and this will probably stimulate a renewed interest in repair mechanisms. If the first 75 years of the century were dedicated to the processes that create inflammation, perhaps the last 25 years of the century will look more assiduously to processes that counteract it, these working in concert with the many intangibles that initiate and guide wound healing; and (3) an even more intense preoccupation with mechanisms of delayed hypersensitivity of the tuberculin type and the special role of the lymphocyte as a carrier of inflammatory signals. The suggestion by Thomas (1959) that homograft rejection may turn out to represent a mechanism for natural defense against neoplasia reopened the whole area of immunological surveillance (see discussion by Dvorak in Volume III, Chapter 7) and underscored again the interesting fact that both neoplasia and adaptive immunity evolved in the vertebrates. Perhaps it is not too much to suggest, even though there is little evidence at this time to support it, that even the degrading of protein by a degranulating leukocyte has the ultimate effect of changing self into nonself, and it is the nonself that the chemotactic cells are searching for. Yet since acute inflammatory reactions attract neutrophils, not lymphocytes, the formulation is too simple to accept, quite possibly is erroneous, and tends to confuse the properties of two members of the white cell series.

XI. Summary

1. Inflammation is a process that begins following a sublethal injury to tissue and ends with complete healing.
2. Between the injury and the healing a variety of cells are mobilized and undergo certain changes.
3. It is presumed that these changes are "good" for the organism, that is, the inflammatory process is a defense mechanism aimed at preserving the viability of living tissues.
4. However, sometimes the inflammatory signals seem to be scattered and disarranged, rather than proceeding stepwise through a symmetrical cascade to a noninflammatory endpoint.

5. It is possible that much of the inflammatory response is nonspecific and that the evolutionary process did not endow it with ultimate discrimination. When it gets turned on, therefore, by "accident" so to speak, and all the mechanisms start to operate at once, it is a quite damaging event, leading not to healing but to morbidity and death.

6. In the classic argument between Cohnheim and Metchnikoff, one that persists to this day, the chances are that both of the protagonists were correct on critical points: The endothelial cell is certainly a crucial intermediary in inflammatory reactions, as Cohnheim suggested, and chemotaxis is certainly an important inflammatory mechanism, as Metchnikoff insisted.

7. Many studies of the inflammatory process remain descriptive, but in recent years, notably in the last decade, research in the field is moving rapidly toward a molecular level. This will almost certainly dominate studies of the next decade.

8. One can make a bold, and possibly foolhardy, guess that for the foreseeable future, in areas where progress seems likely, there will be important contributions on the following three fronts: (1) on the study of isolated endothelial cells; (2) on the study of mediators not only of the inflammatory reaction but of mediators, cell products themselves, that shut off the system; and (3) on the study of delayed hypersensitivity of the tuberculin type and its possible relationship to neoplasia.

References

Adami, J. G. (1909). "Inflammation. An Introduction to the Study of Pathology." Macmillan, New York.

Addison, W. (1843). *Trans. Prov. Med. Surg. Ass.* **11**, 233.

Armstrong, D., and Keele, C. A. (1954). *Nature (London)* **174**, 791.

Arnold, J. (1873). *Arch. Pathol. Anat. Physiol. Klin. Med.* **58**, 203.

Arnold, J. (1876). *Arch. Pathol. Anat. Physiol. Klin. Med.* **66**, 77.

Arthus, M. (1903). *C. R. Soc. Bill.* **55**, 817.

Bauer, K. (1929). *Z. Zellforsch. Mikrosk. Anat.* **9**, 155.

Baumgarten (1884). *Berlin. Klin. Wochenschr.* (cited by Metchnikoff, 1892).

Berthet, J., and de Duve, C. (1951). *Biochem. J.* **50**, 174.

Berthet, J., Berthet, L., Appelmans, F., and de Duve, C. (1951). *Biochem. J.* **50**, 182.

Billingham, R. E., Brown, J. B., Defendi, V., Silvers, W. K., and Steinmuller, D. (1960). *Ann. N. Y. Acad. Sci.* **87**, 457.

Boissonnos, R. A., Guttmann, S., Jaquenoud, P. A., Pless, J., and Sandrin, E. (1963). *Ann. N. Y. Acad. Sci.* **104**, 5.

Born, G. V. R., and Cross, M. J. (1963). *J. Physiol. (London)* **168**, 178.

Bourne, H. R., Lichtenstein, L. M., and Melmon, K. L. (1972). *J. Immunol.* **108**, 695.

Boyden, S. (1962). *J. Exp. Med.* **115**, 453.

Breasted, J. R. (1930). "The Edwin Smith Surgical Papyrus," Vol. I. Univ. of Chicago Press, Chicago, Illinois.

Carrel, A., and Ebeling, A. H. (1922). *J. Exp. Med.* **36**, 365.

Carrier, E. B., and Rehberg, P. B. (1922). *Skand. Arch. Physiol.* **64**, 20.

Celsus, A. C. (1831). "De Medicina" (transl. from L. Targa's edition by A. Smith), p. 182. E. Cox, London.

Chambers, R., and Zweifach, B. W. (1940). *J. Cell. Comp. Physiol.* **15**, 255.

Clark, E. R., and Clark, E. L. (1930). *Amer. J. Anat.* **46**, 149.

Clark, E. R., Hitschler, W. J., Kirby-Smith, H., Rex, R. O., and Smith, J. W. (1931). *Anat. Rec.* **50**, 129.

Clayton, S., Born, G. V. R., and Cross, M. J. (1963). *Nature (London)* **200**, 138.

Cochrane, C. (1969). *Advan. Immunol.* **9**, 97.

Cohnheim, J. (1882). "Lectures on General Pathology, "Vol. I (transl. from the 2nd German ed. by A. B. McKee, New Sydenham Soc., London, 1889).

Collins, F. M., and Mackaness, G. B. (1971). *Cell. Immunol.* **1**, 266.

Cooper, E. L. (1969). *J. Exp. Zool.* **171**, 69.

Dale, H. H., and Laidlaw, P. P. (1910–1911). *J. Physiol. (London)* **41**, 318.

Day, N. K. B., Good, R. A., Finstad, J., Johannsen, R., Pickering, R. J., and Gewurz, H. (1970a). *Proc. Soc. Exp. Biol. Med.* **133**, 397.

Day, N. K. B., Gewurz, H., Johanssen, R., Finstad, J., and Good, R. A. (1970b). *J. Exp. Med.* **132**, 941.

Dominici, H. (1902). *Arch. Med. Exp.* **14**, 1.

Donaldson, V. H., Merler, E., Rosen, F. S., Willms-Kretschmer, K., and Lepow, I. H. (1970). *J. Lab. Clin. Med.* **76**, 986.

Downey, H. (1915). *Anat. Rec.* **9**, 73.

Downey, H. (1917). *Anat. Rec.* **12**, 429.

Drinker, C. K., and Yoffey, J. M. (1941). "Lymphatics, Lymph, and Lymphoid Tissue." Harvard Univ. Press, Cambridge, Massachusetts.

Dubos, R., and Dubos, J. (1952). "The White Plague Tuberculosis Man and Society." Little, Brown, Boston, Massachusetts.

Dubreil, G. (1913). *Arch. Anat. Microsc. Morphol. Exp.* **15**, 53.

Dutrochet, R. J. H. (1824). "Recherches anatomiques et physiologique sur la structure intime des animaux et des vegetaux et sur leur motilité." Bailliére et Fils, Paris.

Ebbecke, U. (1917). *Pfluegers Arch. Gesamte. Physiol. Menschen Tiere* **169**, 1.

Ebert, R. H. (1939). D. Ph. I. Thesis, University of Oxford, Oxford, England.

Ebert, R. H. (1952). *Amer. Rev. Tuberc.* **65**, 64.

Ebert, R. H., and Florey, H. W. (1939). *Brit. J. Exp. Pathol.* **20**, 342.

Ellingson, D. J., and Yao, K. T. S. (1971). *Exp. Cell Res.* **66**, 478.

Elliott, E. F. (1963). *Ann. N. Y. Acad. Sci.* **104**, 35.

Fawcett, D. W. (1959). *In* "The Microcirculation" (S. M. R. Reynolds and B. W. Zweifach, eds.), pp. 1–27. Univ. of Illinois Press, Urbana.

Feldberg, W., and Kellaway, C. H. (1938). *J. Physiol. (London)* **94**, 187.

Florey, H. W. (1961). *Proc. Roy. Soc., Ser.* A **265**, 1.

Florey, H. W. (1962). "General Pathology." Saunders, Philadelphia, Pennsylvania.

Florey, H. W., Poole, J. C. F., and Meek, G. A. (1959). *J. Pathol. Bacteriol.* **77**, 625.

Florey, H. W., Greer, S. J., Poole, J. C. F., and Werthessen, N. T. (1961). *Brit. J. Exp. Pathol.* **42**, 236.

Foot, N. C. (1919). *J. Med. Res.* **40**, 353.

Foot, N. C. (1925). *Anat. Rec.* **30**, 15.

Frey, E. K., and Kraut, H. (1928). *Naunyn-Schmiedebergs Arch. Exp. Pathol. Pharmakol.* **133**, 1.

Gaarder, A., Jonsen, J., Laland, S., Hellem, A., and Owren, P. A. (1961). *Nature (London)* **192**, 531.

Gewurz, H., Page, A. R., Pickering, R. J., and Good, R. A. (1967). *Int. Arch. Allergy Appl. Immunol.* **32**, 64.

Good, R. A., and Papermaster, B. W. (1964). *Advan. Immunol.* **4**, 1.

Gowans, J. L. (1957). *Brit. J. Exp. Path.* **38**, 67.

Gowans, J. L. (1959a). *Brit. Med. Bull.* **15**, 50.

Gowans, J. L. (1959b). *J. Physiol.* **146**, 54.

Gowans, J. L. (1961). *Ciba Found. Study Group* **10**, 107–108.

Gowans, J. L. (1962). *Ann. N. Y. Acad. Sci.* **99**, 432.

Gowans, J. L., and Knight, E. J. (1964). *Proc. Roy. Soc. (Biol.)* **159**, 257.

Gowans, J. L., and Uhr, J. W. (1966). *J. Exp. Med.* **124**, 1017.

Grant, L., and Epstein, F. (1974). In preparation.

Grant, L., Ross, M. H., Moses, J., Prose, P., Zweifach, B. W., and Ebert, R. H. (1967). *Z. Zellforsch. Mikrosk. Anat.* **77**, 554.

Grawitz, E. (1890). *Ver. Int. Med. Kongr., 10th Berlin* Abt. II, Vol. 3, p. 9.

Harris, H. (1953). *J. Pathol. Bacteriol.* **66**, 135.

Harris, H. (1954). *Physiol. Rev.* **34**, 529.

Harris, H. (1960). *Bacteriol. Rev.* **24**, 3.

Herzog, G. (1916). *Beitr. Pathol. Anat. Allg. Pathol.* **61**, 325.

Hovig, T. (1963). *Thromb. Diath. Haemorrh.* **9**, 264.

Hoyer, H. (1877). *Arch. Mikrosk. Anat.* **13**, 603.

Hudack, S., and McMaster, P. D. (1933). *J. Exp. Med.* **57**, 751.

Jaffe, E., Nachman, R. L., and Becker, C. G. (1972). *Abstr., 64th Annu. Meet. Amer. Soc. Clin. Invest., Atlantic City* 46a.

Jenner, E. (1800). "An Inquiry into the Cause and Effect of the Variolae Vaccinae, a Disease Discovered in Some of the Western Counties of England, Particularly Gloucestershire, and Known by the Name of Cowpox." Sampon Low, Berwick Street, Soho.

Kiyono, K. (1914). "Die vitale Karminspeicherung." Fischer, Jena.

Klebs, E. (1883). *Verh. Kongr. Inn. Med.* **2**, 139.

Knake, C. (1927). *Z. Zellforsch. Mikrosk. Anat.* **5**, 208.

Koch, R. (1882). *Berlin. Klin. Wochenschr.* **19**, 221.

Koch, R. (1890). *Deut. Med. Wochenschr.* **16**, 1029.

Koll, W. (1927). *Z. Zellforsch. Mikrosk. Anat.* **4**, 702.

Krogh, A. (1924). "The Anatomy and Physiology of Capillaries." Yale Univ. Press, New Haven, Connecticut.

Landis, E. M. (1934). *Physiol. Rev.* **14**, 404.

Landsteiner, K., and Chase, M. W. (1942). *Proc. Soc. Exp. Biol. Med.* **49**, 688.

Leber, T. (1888). *Fortschr. Med.* **6**, 460.

Lewis, G. P. (1960). *Physiol. Rev.* **40**, 647.

Lewis, J. L., Hoak, J. C., Maca, R. D., and Fry, G. L. (1973). *Science* **181**, 453.

Lewis, M. R., and Lewis, W. H. (1924). *Anat. Rec.* **29**, 391.

Lewis, T. (1927). "The Blood Vessels of the Human Skin and their Responses." Shaw, London.

Loeffler, R. (1884). *Mitt. Klin. Gesundh., Berlin* **2**, 421.

Lotz, M., and Harris, H. (1956). *Brit. J. Exp. Pathol.* **37**, 477.

Luft, J. H. (1965a). *In* "The Inflammatory Process" (B. Zweifach, L. Grant, and R. T. McCluskey, eds.), 1st ed., p. 121. Academic Press, New York.

Luft, J. H. (1965b). *J. Cell Biol.* **27**, 61A.

Luft, J. H. (1966). *Fed. Proc. Fed. Amer. Soc. Exp. Biol.* **25**, 1773.

Luft, J. H. (1971a). *Anat. Rec.* **171**, 347.

Luft, J. H. (1971b). *Anat. Rec.* **171**, 369.

McGregor, D. D., Koster, F. T., and Mackaness, G. B. (1971). *J. Exp. Med.* **133**, 389.

McJunkin, F. A. (1919). *Amer. J. Anat.* **25**, 27.

Mackenzie, J., and Hackett, M. (1968). *Arch. Surg. (Chicago)* **97**, 879.

Maino, G. (1965). *Handb. Physiol.* Sect. II, *Circulation* **3**, chapter 64, 2293.

Majno, G., Shea, S. M., and Leventhal, M. (1969) *J. Cell. Biol.* **42**, 647.

Majno, G., and Palade, G. E. (1960). *J. Biophys. Biochem. Cytol.* **11**, 607.

Majno, G., Gabbiani, G., Joris, I., and Ryan, G. B. (1971). *Abstr., 10th Annu. Meet., Amer. Soc. Cell Biol.* p. 127a.

Major, R. H. (1954). "A History of Medicine," Vols. I and II. Thomas, Springfield, Illinois.

Mallory, F. B. (1898). *J. Exp. Med.* **3**, 611.

Marchand, F. (1890). *Verh. Int. Med. Kongr.,* 10th Berlin Abt. II, Vol. 3, p. 6.

Marchesi, V. T., and Florey, H. W. (1960). *Quart J. Exp. Physiol. Cog. Med. Sci;* **45**, 343.

Margolis, J. (1959). *Aust. J. Exp. Biol. Med. Sci.* **37**, 239.

Maruyama, Y. (1963). *Z. Zellforsch. Mikrosk. Anat.* **60**, 69.

Maximow, A. (1902). *Beitr. Pathol. Anat. Allg. Pathol.* **5**, Suppl., 1.

Maximow, A. (1906). *Arch. Mikrosk. Anat. Entwicklungsmech.* **67**, 680.

Menkin, V. (1956). "Biochemical Mechanisms in Inflammation." Thomas, Springfield, Illinois.

Metchnikoff, E. (1885). *Quart. J. Microsc. Sci.* **24**, 112–117.

Metchnikoff, E. (1892). "Lectures on the Comparative Pathology of Inflammation" (Dover, New York, 1968).

Metchnikoff, E. (1905). "Immunity in Infective Diseases." Cambridge Univ. Press, London and New York.

Miller, J. F. A. P., and Sprent, J. (1971). *Nature (London)* **230**, 267.

Moe, N., and Jorgensen, L. (1967). *Acta Pathol. Microbiol. Scand., Suppl.* **187**, 70.

Moe, N., and Jorgensen, L. (1968). *Acta Pathol. Microbiol. Scand.* **72**, 519.

Moses, J. M., Ebert, R. H., Graham, R. D., and Brine, K. L. (1964). *J. Exp. Med.* **120**, 57.

Murray, E. G. D. (1948). *In* "Bacterial and Mycotic Infections of Man" (R. J. Dubos, ed.), pp. 1–13. Lippincott, Philadelphia, Pennsylvania.

Mustard, J. F., and Packham, M. A. (1971). *In* "Inflammation, Immunity and Hypersensitivity" (H.Z. Movat, ed.), p. 527. Harper, New York.

O'Neal, R., Jordan, G. L., Rabin, E., De Bakey, M., and Halpert, B. (1964). *Exp. Mol. Pathol.* **3**, 403.

Opie, E. L. (1922). *Physiol. Rev.* **2**, 552.

Orange, R. P., and Austen, K. F. (1971). *In* "Progress in Immunology" (B. Amos, ed.), p. 173. Academic Press, New York.

Page, A. R., Gewurz, H., Pickering, R. J., and Good, R. A. (1967). *In* "Immunopathology," 5th Int. Symp., Punta Ala, Italy. Grune & Stratton, New York, p. 221.

Palade, G. E. (1953). *J. Appl. Phys.* **24**, 1424.

Palade, G. E. (1960). *Anat. Rec.* **136**, 254.

Pappenheimer, J. R. (1953). *Physiol. Rev.* **33**, 387.

Parker, R. C. (1932). *J. Exp. Med.* **55**, 713.

Permar, H. H. (1920). *J. Med. Res.* **42**, 9.

Petrakis N., Davis, M., and Lucia, S. P. (1961). *Blood* **17**, 109.

Pfeiffer, R., and Bessau, G. (1910). *Zentralbl. Bakteriol., Parasitenk. Infektionskr. Hyg., Abt. l: Orig.* **56**, 344.

Pickrell, K. L. (1938). *Bull. Johns Hopkins Hosp.* **63**, 238.

Pomerat, C. M., and Slick, W. C. (1963). *Nature (London)* **198**, 859.

Poole, J. C. F., Sanders, A. G., and Florey, H. W. (1958). *J. Pathol. Bacteriol.* **75**, 133.

Poole, J. C. F., Sanders, A. G., and Florey, H. W. (1959). *J. Pathol. Bacteriol.* **77**, 637.

Porter, K. A., and Cooper, E. H. (1962a). *Lancet* **2**, 317.

Porter, K. A., and Cooper, E. M. (1962b). *J. Exp. Med.* **115**, 997.

Pullinger, B. H., and Florey, H. W. (1935). *Brit. J. Exp. Pathol.* **16**, 49.

Ranvier, M. L. (1890). *C. R. Acad. Sci.* **110**, 165.

Ratnoff, O. D., and Lepow, I. H. (1963). *J. Exp. Med.* **118**, 681.

Renaut, J. (1906). *Arch. Anat. Microsc. Morphol. Exp.* **9**, 495.
Renkin, E. M. (1959). *In* "The Microcirculation" (S. M. R. Reynolds and B. W. Zweifach, eds.), pp. 28–36. Univ. of Illinois Press, Urbana.
Rich, A. R. (1946). "The Pathogenesis of Tuberculosis." Thomas, Springfield, Illinois.
Rocha e Silva, M., Beraldo, W. T., and Rosenfeld, G. (1949). *Amer. J. Physiol.* **156**, 261.
Roux, E., and Yersin, A. (1888). *Ann. Inst. Pasteur, Paris* **2**, 629.
Sabin, F. R., Doan, C. A., and Cunningham, R. S. (1925). *Contrib. Embryol. Carnegie Inst.* **16**, 125.
Sade, R. M., and Folkman, J. (1972). *Micro. Res.* **4**, 77.
Sanderson, B. (1891). *Brit. Med. J.* **2**, 1085.
Sandison, J. C. (1924). *Anat. Rec.* **28**, 281.
Sandison, J. C. (1928). *Amer. J. Anat.* **41**, 447.
Schacter, M. (1963). *Ann. N. Y. Acad. Sci.* **104**, 108.
Schott, E. (1909). *Arch. Mikrosk. Anat. Entwicklungsmech.* **74**, 143.
Seeman, G. (1930). *Beitr. Pathol. Anat. Allg. Pathol.* **85**, 303.
Shwartzman, G. (1937). "Phenomenon of Local Tissue Reactivity." Harper (Hoeber), New York.
Spaet, T. H., and Zucker, M. B. (1964). *Amer. J. Physiol.* **206**, 1267.
Starling, E. H. (1896). *J. Physiol. (London)* **19**, 312.
Stemmerman, M., Baumgartner, H. R., and Spaet, T. H. (1971). *Lab. Invest.* **24**, 1979.
Stockinger, W. (1928). *Z. Gesamte Exp. Med.* **58**, 777.
Stump, M. M., Jordan, G., De Bakey, M., and Halpert, B. (1963). *Amer. J. Pathol.* **43**, 361.
Szecsi, S. (1912). *Folia Haematol. (Leipzig)* **13**, 1.
Thoma, R. (1878). *Arch. Pathol. Anat. Physiol. Klin. Med.* **74**, 360.
Thomas, L. (1959). *In* "Cellular and Humoral Aspects of the Hypersensitive States" (H. S. Lawrence, ed.), p. 529. Harper (Hoeber), New York.
Tripp, M. R. (1969). *In* "Immunity to Parasitic Animals" (G. J. Jackson, R. Herman, and I. Singer, eds.), p. 111. Appleton, New York.
Tsutsumi, H., and Gore, I. (1969). *Stain Technol.* **44**, 139.
van Heyningen, W. E. (1962). *In* "General Pathology" (H. W. Florey, ed.), Chapter 30, pp. 741–755. Saunders, Philadelphia, Pennsylvania.
von Behring, E., and Kitasato, S. (1890). *Deut. Med. Wochenschr.* **16**, 1113.
von Haller, A. (1757). "A Dissertation on the Motion of the Blood and on the Effects of Bleeding." Shiston & White, London.
von Möllendorf, W., and von Möllendorf, M. (1926). *Z. Zellforsch. Mikrosk. Anat.* **3**, 503.
von Pirquet, C. (1907). "Klinische Studien über Vakzination und Vakzinale Allergie." Deuticke, Leipzig.
von Recklinghausen, F. (1836). *Arch. Pathol. Anat. Physiol. Menschen Tiere* **28**, 157.
Waller, A. (1846). *Phil. Mag.* [4] **29**, 397.
Ward, P. A. (1967). *J. Exp. Med.* **126**, 189.
Ward, P. A., and Hill, J. (1970). *J. Immunol.* **104**, 534.
Webster, M. E., and Pierce, J. V. (1963). *Ann. N. Y. Acad. Sci.* **104**, 91.
Webster, M. E., and Ratnoff, O. D. (1961). *Nature (London)* **192**, 180.
Weidenreich, F. (1909). *Arch. Mikrosk. Anat. Entwicklungsmech.* **73**, 793.
Wilhelm, D. L. (1971). *Rev. Can. Biol.* **30**, 153.
Willoughby, D. A., Elizabeth, C., and Turk, J. L. (1969). *J. Pathol.* **97**, 295.
Ziegler, E. (1890). *Verh. Int. Med. Kongr.,* 10*th Berlin* Abt. II. Vol. 3, p. 1.
Zinsser, H. (1921). *J. Exp. Med.* **34**, 495.
Zweifach, B. W. (1961). "Functional Behavior of the Microcirculation." Thomas, Springfield, Illinois.

Chapter 2

BIOCHEMISTRY OF THE MAMMALIAN PLASMA MEMBRANE

EDWARD D. KORN

I. Introduction

A major development in modern biological thought has been the recognition that the animal cell is a bewildering maze of membranes and membranous organelles. Parallel with this revelation has been the realization that these membranes are not just the static barriers and demarcators of cellular space that they may appear to be in stark micrographs. Rather, membranes are dynamic structures in continual movement, both morphological and molecular. Moreover, major biochemical events of the cell occur in, on, or through membranes. The highly selective, often energy-coupled, transport of ions and molecules are not the only membrane phenomena but the complex processes of oxidative phosphorylation, photosynthesis, vision, and nerve conductance; the biosynthesis of lipid, proteins, and other macromolecules; hormone interactions; and processes such as pinocytosis and phagocytosis are also membrane phenomena. It is at the membrane that morphology and metabolism unite and that catalytic chaos is organized.

The ultimate experimental goal is the total elucidation of the structure, function, and biosynthesis of all cell membranes. This chapter, however, is restricted to the plasma membrane. Although discussions of membrane biochemistry frequently assume that all cell membranes are essentially identical, there is at this time little basis for such an assumption and some reason to believe to the contrary that the different functions of different membranes are reflected in significant differences, despite basic similarities, not only in their composition but also in their molecular organization (Korn, 1969a). For this reason, in discussing the organization of the plasma membranes of animal cells we will depend almost entirely on data obtained from studies of those membranes.

The experimental tasks are manifold: to determine the chemical and enzymatic composition of the membranes; to dissociate the membranes into their natural structural units and functional units; to develop techniques to recombine these minimal units into a membrane that is functionally and structurally identical to the original; and to discover the mechanism of membrane biosynthesis. In reality, all these appraoches are taken simultaneously, and progress in one area is a tremendous stimulus to success in others.

Unfortunately, the methodological and conceptual difficulties are immense. Morphological techniques are inherently static and do not reveal information at the molecular and atomic level. Physical and chemical methods are generally averaging techniques providing information on the mean properties of the membrane but not details of particular regions that may differ structurally and functionally one from the other. Model membranes and membrane models are useful but do not obviate the need to study the biological membrane. Enzymology has many weapons with which to fight in the sea of aqueous chemistry but possesses few tools with which to dig into the fertile fields of surface chemistry. But like the prospector of old the difficulties only convince us more that a rich bounty awaits those who persevere.

II. Morphological Background

A. *General Considerations*

Within the limits of light microscopy very little of cellular detail is discernible. One is aware of the nucleus; one can barely resolve a myriad of fascinating intracellular granules; one knows that certain regions of the cytoplasm stain differently with appropriate dyes. Membranes are not visible, of course, and it is only a few years since many would still argue intensely that there was no need to invoke the concept of a limiting cell membrane. Much of the physiological data invoked as evidence for the existence of such a structure could indeed be theoretically explained as properties to be expected at the interface between a gel-like cytoplasm and extracellular fluid. Yet still today this argument persists in another form, which, while not denying the existence of a plasma membrane, assigns many of the properties normally attributed to the membrane to specific adsorptive characteristics of structured cytoplasm (Ling, 1969a,b).

It was the electron microscope that revealed a new microcosmic world to challenge the biochemical cartographer. Consider, for example, the typical mammalian cell pictured at relatively low magnification in Fig. 1. Seeing this, no biochemist could continue to believe he understood cellular biochemistry because he could describe the products of an enzymatic reaction as it occurred in an extract of acetone-dried liver. The cell is not a rich soup but a highly structured array of surfaces, organelles, and particles.

The electron microscope is indeed a powerful tool. Instrumental magnification of several hundred thousand are attainable, and these can often be usefully enlarged photographically to total magnifications of 1 to 2 million. Moreover, resolution, the minimal distance by which two objects can be separated and still be distinguished, is of the order of 3 to 4 Å, i.e., atomic distances. Electron microscopy also has limitations, however. Difficulties encountered in attempting to interpret the image in molecular terms are discussed later (Section VI,B), but it is worth mentioning here one practical problem. The microscopist is severely limited in the quantity of material he can study. To examine completely one cell of diameter 40 μm, a microscopist would first dismember it into 1000 sections. To photograph the entire area of all these sections at the modest magnification of 25,000 would require

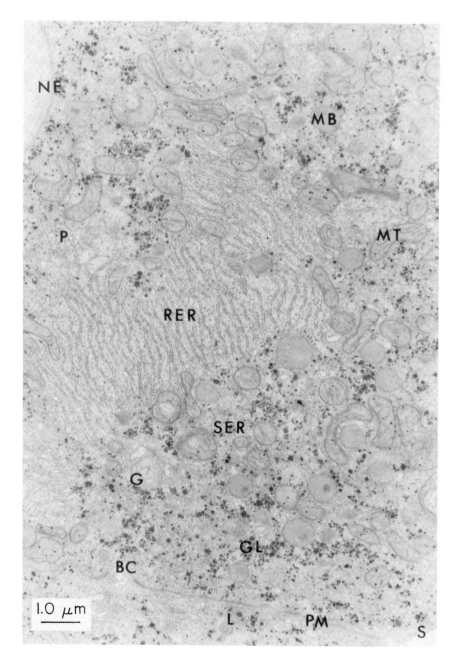

16,000 micrographs (8 × 10 in.). Obviously, a productive electron micros-copist must be diligent, patient, highly imaginative, and very cautious.

B. The Plasma Membrane

An essentially invariant image of the plasma membrane is obtained for most cells. Positively stained and sectioned membranes are seen in cross section as a trilaminar structure, 75 to 100 Å in width, which consists of two electron opaque bands separated by an electron translucent region. The three regions are of approximately equal width, but frequently the inner dark band is more electron dense than the outer one. Quite a lot of thought and effort have been expended in attempts to interpret this image in terms of the distribution of molecular species. We will have more to say later about the theoretical and experimental bases for such efforts (Section VI,B). For the present, it is sufficient to point out that in such preparations the tissue has been treated with glutaraldehyde and osmium tetroxide, extracted with ethanol, embedded in plastic, sectioned, and stained with uranyl acetate and lead citrate. The image is largely provided by the bound osmium, uranyl, and lead atoms, and its interpretation, therefore, is dependent not only on the adequacy of "fixation" at the molecular level but also on an understanding of the precise chemical groups which bind the heavy metals.

In organized tissue, cells are not physically independent of one another. There are at least four types of structures through which cells make apparent contact. These have been called *gap junctions* where the plasma membranes of adjacent cells lie very close but are separated by an electron translucent (but certainly not empty) space, *desmosomes* where the space between the plasma membranes of adjacent cells is filled with an electron dense material (after treatment for microscopy), *zonal occludentes* where the plasma mem-branes of adjacent cells are so closely apposed that the outer dense bands of their respective trilaminar images "fuse" into one band, thus providing a pentalaminar structural image, and *septate junctions* where the plasma mem-brane of adjacent cells appear to be connected by cross-linking septae which bridge the intercellular space and may or may not unite the two membranes into one. Views of these junctional regions *en face* also show interesting differences. Electron opaque particles in hexagonal array are seen on the outer surface of plasma membranes at gap junctions. Surface views of

---

Fig. 1. Normal rat liver parenchymal cell in thin section. BC, bile canaliculus; G, Golgi membranes; GL, glycogen; L, lysosomes; MB, microbodies; MT, mitochondria; NE, nuclear envelope; P, polysomes; PM, plasma membranes of two adjacent cells; RER, rough endoplasmic reticulum; SER, smooth endoplasmic reticulum; S, sinusoid. This micrograph was kindly provided by Dr. Carlo Bruni, University of Virginia Medical School.

desmosomes, on the other hand, reveal a hexagonal array of electron translucent regions separated by denser margins. In this case it is not yet defined whether the pattern is on the inner or outer surface. A similar pattern is seen in septate junctions.

The functional significance of these membrane junctions is not entirely clear. It would seem that the zonal occludentes do provide a barrier to the free diffusion of relatively low molecular weight molecules in the extracellular space around cells whereas the gap junctions may be regions of low-resistance electrical coupling between cells. It is not our purpose here to describe the morphology of these fascinating structural and functional specializations in detail but merely to indicate their existence and to emphasize that even at this level of analysis the plasma membrane is seen not to be homogeneous in structure.

Most tissue cells possess another layer of material usually considered to be external to the plasma membrane. It is seen in its most exaggerated form perhaps on the microvilli of the mucosal cells that line the villi of the small intestine. This extraneous coat, or glycocalyx, is rather ill defined chemically but presumably contains a high concentration of polysaccharides. To what extent the glycocalyx should be considered separate from, or continuous and integral with, the plasma membrane is not known.

Despite earlier claims to the contrary, there seem to be little if any stable connections between the plasma membrane and intracellular membranes such as the endoplasmic reticulum. It is certain, however, that there is a dynamic functional relationship between the plasma membrane and several intracellular membrane systems. Thus the plasma membrane can be internalized as vesicles in the ingestive processes of pinocytosis and phagocytosis, and the pinosomes and phagosomes which are formed can fuse with lysosomes which, in turn, are derived from the endoplasmic reticulum–Golgi complex. Conversely, secretion of many intracellular products such as zymogen granules by pancreatic cells, serum proteins by liver parenchymal cells, and a number of hormones is accomplished by fusion of membrane-enclosed vacuoles, often derived from the endoplasmic reticulum and Golgi membranes, with the plasma membrane. Appreciation of the magnitude and significance of these phenomena has led to the suggestion (de Duve, 1969) that the term "vacuome" be revived to describe all membrane-bound spaces of the cell except for the mitochondrion (and one might want to include the space enclosed by the outer mitochondrial membrane). The vacuome might be subdivided into exoplasmic space (pinosomes, phagosomes, and lysosomes) and endoplasmic space (rough and smooth endoplasmic reticulum and Golgi). Membranes-enclosing exoplasmic space fuse with each other but not with membranes enclosing endoplasmic space, although the latter ultimately fuse with the plasma membrane from which the former are derived. Such membrane "fusions" may, however, be much more complicated than would appear from the electron microscopic image of the process since the several membranes are very different in chemical and enzymatic composition and are, thus, not just one large membrane pool.

III. The Chemical and Enzymatic Composition of Plasma Membranes

A. *Introductory Comments*

Fundamental to the biochemical approach to membrane structure and organization is a complete description of the chemical and enzymatic composition of the membrane. Meaningful data can only be obtained from preparations of isolated plasma membranes proved to be free of significant contamination and known to include all true components of the membrane (DePierre and Karnovsky, 1973). In practice it has generally been found most convenient to disrupt the cell in such a way that maximal integrity of the plasma membrane is maintained and then to isolate that membrane by a combination of differential velocity and isopycnic centrifugations. As a routine guide to the isolation procedure, the plasma membrane can be followed by microscopic examination or by assay of an enzyme known to be a component of the membrane. Assessment of the purity of the final product more difficult. The following criteria are necessary but probably not sufficient.

The plasma membrane preparation should be free of contaminants recognizable by light and electron microscopy. The plasma membrane is often obtained as large membrane fragments whose only conceivable origin is the plasma membrane. Electron microscopy can also establish the absence of distinctive intracellular membranes and organelles such as fragments of the rough endoplasmic reticulum, mitochondria, and nuclei. Most preparations of plasma membrane, however, will contain small fragments of smooth membranes and vesicles whose origin cannot be unambiguously determined by electron microscopy since there are few if any features by which to distinguish plasma membrane from the smooth endoplasmic reticulum, lysosomal membranes, and the membranes of pinosomes and phagosomes.

Enzyme assays can help. Thus, succinic dehydrogenase is usually used as a sensitive indicator of the presence of mitochondria, and glucose-6-phosphatase and antimycin-insensitive NADH-cytochrome c reductase may serve (but perhaps somewhat less satisfactorily) as indicators of contamination by endoplasmic reticulum. Less often used are assays of various acid hydrolases which are contained in primary and secondary lysosomes. It should be emphasized that these methods are most useful when the specific activity of highly purified preparations of the membranes in question (mitochondria, endoplasmic reticulum, etc.) are also determined so that one can convert the specific enzymatic activity to percent contamination (by protein).

Determination of enzyme activity is somewhat less useful in a positive way, i.e., to determine the purity of the plasma membrane by assay of its inherent enzymatic activity. To measure the extent of purification of the plasma membrane by the degree of purification of a specific enzyme requires that the enzyme in question be a true component of the plasma membrane and only of the plasma membrane. For liver-cell plasma membranes, 5'-nucleotidase may satisfy these criteria. Enzymes other than 5'-nucleotidase are certainly present in the plasma membrane but similar activities may reside in other cell membranes. It will be apparent that each cell represents a special case.

Chemical analyses are also essential. It is uniquely characteristic of plasma membranes that the molar ratio of sterol to phospholipids is much higher than the ratio found for other cellular membranes and may approach 1:1. One assumes that the RNA and DNA contents of plasma membranes will be very low and that these two analyses can be used as a rough measure of contamination by ribosomes (rough endoplasmic reticulum) and nuclei. It must be considered, however, that either or both RNA and DNA might be specific components of the plasma membrane. Finally, glycoproteins and glycolipids are generally found to be enriched in the plasma membrane, and sialic acid may be specifically a component of the plasma membrane.

From the foregoing discussion it is apparent that an absolute measure of the extent of contamination of plasma membranes by other membranes is difficult to obtain and therefore it is essential that all possible criteria be employed. Yet more difficult is the determination that a preparation contains all the components of the plasma membrane and that "loosely" bound substituents have not been lost or inactivated during the isolation. We will not even attempt to evaluate the yet more theoretical question of what defines the limits of the plasma membrane. Where does the plasma membrane end and the cytoplasm, on one side, and the glycocalyx, on the other, begin. It is enough to attempt at this stage to delineate the major lipid and protein constituents of plasma membranes as they have been isolated.

B. Liver-Cell Plasma Membranes

1. ISOLATION PROCEDURES

The isolation procedure most generally used (Neville, 1960; Emmelot et al., 1964) produces relatively large fragments of plasma membrane by gentle homogenization in 1 mM NaHCO$_3$. The plasma membranes are separated from the soluble cytoplasm by low-speed centrifugation and, by careful partitioning of the stratified pellet, from nuclei, intact cells, and other heavy debris. The plasma membranes are then isolated by isopycnic centrifugation as the material which accumulates between layers of sucrose of densities 1.16 and 1.18. Most investigators (e.g., Emmelot *et al.*, 1964; Barclay *et al.*, 1967) feel that, as judged by electron microscopy, such preparations are free of nuclei, mitochondria, dense bodies, lysosomes, and rough endoplasmic reticulum although some Golgi membranes and an occasional collagen fiber may be present. Others (Lieberman *et al.*, 1967) find that as many as 25 % of the preparations have unacceptably high contamination by rough endoplasmic reticulum.

The addition of divalent cations to the buffer solutions has been advocated (Takeuchi and Terayama, 1965; Berman *et al.*, 1969) and contra-indicated (Neville, 1968; Emmelot and Bos, 1966), but the most recent evidence (Ray, 1970) is that the presence of 0.5 mM $CaCl_2$, and the use of more dilute homogenates, increases the yield of plasma membranes of higher enzymatic activity. Early adaptations of the procedure to utilize isotonic sucrose (Coleman *et al.*, 1967), even in the presence of divalent cations (Stein *et al.*, 1968), would seem not to have improved either the yield or purity of the preparation, but, more recently, procedures involving isotonic sucrose and NaCl have been more successful (Henning *et al.*, 1970; Touster *et al.*, 1970; Nigam *et al.*, 1971).

The basic method, which was developed for rat liver, can be applied to guinea pig liver but not to rabbit and cat liver (Lauter *et al.*, 1972). The method can be applied to bovine liver (Fleischer and Fleischer, 1969) to obtain more material than is obtainable from the more usual source of rat liver, and the use of zonal centrifugation shortens the time required for isolation and increases the final yield of membrane (El-Auser *et al.*, 1966; Pfleger *et al.*, 1968; Weaver and Boyle, 1969; Hinton *et al.*, 1970; Victoria *et al.*, 1971) with little if any sacrifice in purity.

In all these procedures the fact that the liver is not a homogeneous tissue composed of only one cell type has been ignored.

2. MORPHOLOGY OF ISOLATED MEMBRANES

By most procedures the liver-cell plasma membranes are obtained as flat sheets formed by open-ended fragments of membranes from several adjacent cells adherent through desmosomes and zonal occludentes (tight junctions) and are therefore recognizable as that portion of the membrane that forms the bile canaliculi. Within the bile canaliculi lie circular cross sections of membranes which may be profiles of microvilli as seen *in situ*. Smooth vesicles, both free and adherent to the membrane sheets, are also present. These are probably formed by rupture of the plasma membranes.

There are fewer vesicles when the preparation is made in the presence of $CaCl_2$ (Ray, 1970), and more vesicles are formed when more violent methods of cell rupture are employed (Graham *et al.*, 1968). By vigorous homogenization of the isolated membranes the membrane sheets are partially converted to smooth vesicles which can be separated from the residual sheets by density centrifugation (Evans, 1969, 1970). The lighter fraction is vesicular.

3. CHEMICAL COMPOSITION

The gross chemical compositions of plasma membranes preparations for which data are available are tabulated in Table I. Preparations 1 through 8 were obtained by similar procedures utilizing 1 mM $NaHCO_3$; preparation 9 was obtained using the recent modifications of $CaCl_2$ and a more dilute

TABLE I

Preparation	1	2	3[a]	4	5	6[b]	7
Reference	a	b	c	d	e	f	g
Density	1.16–1.18	1.16–1.18	1.16–1.18	1.16–1.22	1.16–1.18	—	1.18
Protein (mg/g liver)	0.25–0.63	—	—	—	—	0.6–1.0	—
Total lipid (mg/mg protein)	—	0.6	—	—e	0.67[d]	—	0.39
Glycerides (mg/mg protein)	—	0.1	—	—	0.03	—	0.1
Fatty acids (mg/mg protein)	—	—	—	—	0.046	—	0.035
Phospholipids (mg/mg protein)	0.28(0.4)[e]	0.35	—	0.42	0.26	0.43	0.255
Cholesterol (mg/mg protein)	0.06(0.08)[e]	0.1	—	0.056	0.017	—	0.052
DNA (mg/mg protein)	—	—	—	—	—	—	—
RNA (mg/mg protein)	—	—	—	—	—	—	—
Cholesterol phospholipid (mole/mole)	0.43	0.33	0.55	0.26	0.82	—	0.41

[a] Guinea pig liver.
[b] Ox liver.
[c] Mouse liver: I, plasma membrane; II, light subfraction; III, heavy subfraction.
[d] 26% of the total lipid was not accounted for.
[e] Approximately 30% of the protein was soluble in 0.15 M NaCl which would give these ratios for residual lipid and protein.

homogenate; preparations 10 through 14 were prepared in isotonic sucrose with or without the addition of divalent cations; and preparation 15 represents membranes obtained by the first procedure and two subfractions prepared from it.

Although in many cases the data are too fragmentary for adequate comparison, there would seem to be little agreement among them. Despite the apparent similarity in densities of the isolated membranes, the ratios of total lipid:protein vary from 0.25 to more than 0.95 and the molar ratios of cholesterol to phospholipid from 0.26 to at least 0.82. In only one case is cholesterol ester found. Similar variations are seen in the phospholipid composition in the relatively few instances where this has been analyzed (Table II). Whether these discrepancies represent differences in purity of

CHEMICAL COMPOSITION OF LIVER CELL PLASMA MEMBRANES

8	9	10	11	12	13	14	15^c		
							I	II	III
h	i	j	k	l	m	n	o		
1.185–1.194	1.16	1.13	1.16–1.20	1.16–1.18	<1.17	<1.17	1.17	1.12	1.18
0.88	1.3	1–2	0.25	0.44	0.46	2.9	—	—	—
0.44	—	0.53–0.97	—	—	0.43	—	—	—	—
0.01	—	—	—	—	0.08	—	—	—	—
0.01	—	—	—	—	—	—	—	—	—
0.27	0.65	0.42–0.75	0.61	—	0.22	0.74	0.95	1.61	0.85
0.1	—	0.11–0.23	0.13	—	0.09^f	0.30	0.20	0.37	0.18
—	—	—	0	0	—	0.01	0.004	0.004	0.003
—	0.01	—	0.07	0.032	—	0.07	0.001	0.003	0.003
0.74	—	0.49–0.6	0.42	—	0.9^g	0.81	0.42	0.46	0.42

^{f} Also contains cholesterol ester 0.04.

^{g} Includes cholesterol ester.

References: (a) Emmelot et al. (1964), (b) Dod and Gray (1968), (c) Coleman and Finean (1966), (d) Ashworth and Green (1966), (e) Skipski et al. (1965), (f) Fleischer and Fleischer (1969), (g) Stahl and Trams (1968), (h) Pfleger et al. (1968), (i) Ray (1970), (j) Coleman et al. (1967), (k) Takeuchi and Terayama (1965), (l) Berman et al. (1969), (m) Henning et al. (1970); Kaulen et al. (1970), (n) Touster et al. (1970), and (o) Evans (1970).

TABLE II

<small>PHOSPHOLIPID COMPOSITION OF RAT LIVER PLASMA MEMBRANES</small>

Preparation[a] (see Table I)	2	5	6[b]	8	11	13	16	17
Phosphatidylethanolamine	11	15	29.7	16	31.4	22.4	18.5	22
Phosphatidylserine	6	8	14.7	⎱11	3.6	⎱17.4	9.0	8
Phosphatidylinositol	6	7	6.5	⎰	0	⎰	7.3	⎱45
Phosphatidylcholine	41	37	43.1	33	40.8	34.8	34.9	⎰
Sphingomyelin	33	18	—	13	7.7	20.5	17.7	20
Phosphatidylglycerol phosphate	0	7	5.8	2.7	—	⎱2.3	—	—
Phosphatidylglycerol	—	—	—	—	—	⎰	4.8	—
Lysophosphatidylcholine	—	—	—	—	—	2.6	—	5

[a]Preparations are the same as in Table I except for preparations 16 (Ray *et al.*, 1969) and 17 (Morin *et al.*, 1972) which employ a Ficoll gradient in 0.5 mM Ca^{2+} (Kamat and Wallach, 1965).

[b]Ox liver.

the membranes or variations in analytic accuracy is difficult to judge. The possibility must also be considered seriously that the hepatic-cell plasma membrane may not have a unique composition; the molecular constituents may vary with age, nutritional status, strain, etc., even when the same species has been used. At least some of the differences, however, may be explained if, as generally suspected, the plasma membrane is a mosaic, different sections of which have different compositions. Some support for this view is found in preparation 15 (Table I, II, and IV) where the lipid:protein ratio and enzymatic content, but not the cholesterol:phospholipid ratio, are found to be different in the vesicular and membranous subfractions. Also, isolated gap junctions may have a composition very different from that of whole plasma membranes (Goodenough and Stoeckenius, 1972).

4. ENZYMATIC CRITERIA OF PURITY

It may be helpful in this connection to examine the available enzymatic, data as indicators of purity of the preparations analyzed. Thirteen of the preparations included in Tables I and II and at least seven other similar preparations have been analyzed for possible contamination by enzymes characteristic of mitochondria and endoplasmic reticulum (Table III). It is unfortunate that in only a few cases have the specific activities of the plasma membranes been compared directly to the specific activities of the purified mitochondria and endoplasmic reticulum. The range of specific activities of succinic dehydrogenase is fairly wide; in the few cases where the necessary data are provided the plasma membranes may have as much as

5 % of the specific activity of the mitochondria. Similarly, the glucose-6-phosphatase and antimycin-sensitive NADH-cytochrome c reductase specific activities of the plasma membranes are sometimes found to be as low as 5 % of the microsomal values but often are 20 % as high as the specific activities found for the microsomes, and in one case the plasma membranes and microsomes were of equal specific activity. There is reason, therefore, to suspect that, on a protein basis, many preparations of liver-cell plasma membranes are contaminated with 5 % mitochondria and perhaps 5 to 20 % microsomal membranes. This conclusion is compatible with the RNA analyses which are usually in the range of 10 to 30 μg/mg of protein [if one assumes that microsomes have an RNA:protein ratio of 0.25 to 0.3 (Ray et al., 1968)]. One must of course be aware of the possibility that enzymes thought to be specific for other cellular membranes may also be components of the plasma membrane, especially if the membranes are closely related physiologically. However, at this juncture one should probably err on the side of caution and assume that the plasma membranes are not pure.

5. Enzymes of the Plasma Membrane

It is generally agreed that at least three enzymes are genuine constituents of the liver-cell plasma membrane. A Mg-dependent ATPase, a Na, K, Mg-stimulated ATPase that is inhibited by ouabain, and a 5'-nucleotidase are all enriched in the plasma membrane relative to the whole cell homogenate and relative to the microsomal fraction (Table IV). Observed specific activities vary over a fairly wide range, but this may not only be due to variations in purity of the membrane fractions, since it appears that the presence of divalent cation is critical in order to obtain maximal recovery of at least the 5'-nucleotidase (Ray et al., 1970). Furthermore, these three enzymes may be differentially localized in subfractions prepared from isolated membranes (Evans, 1970) and the differences in Table IV may reflect differences in the portion of membrane that was isolated. The presence of the Na, K, Mg-stimulated ouabain-inhibited ATPase in the plasma membrane is reasonable in accordance with its presumed role in Na and K transport, and the localization of the 5'-nucleotidase to the membrane confirms one of the earliest cytochemical observations (Essner et al., 1958).

A number of other enzymes have been attributed to the plasma membrane by one or more investigators. In some cases the evidence is an enrichment of the enzyme relative to its concentration in the whole homogenate and the purified microsomal fraction. In other cases the evidence depends on the assumption of purity of the plasma membrane and a higher specific activity for the enzyme in the plasma membrane than in the microsomal fraction. [Recently evidence has been presented that the inorganic pyrophosphatase activity of plasma membranes is different from the more active microsomal

TABLE III

Preparation (see Table I)[a]	1	2	3	6	7	9	10	12	13	14
Succinic dehydrogenase or cytochrome oxidase										
Specific activity	0	0–10	—	0.2	0.28	—	0–0.15	1.2	0.04	—
Relative to homogenate	—	0–0.02	0.6	—	—	—	0–0.17	—	—	0.05–0.16
Relative to mitochondria	—	—	—	—	—	—	—	0.05	0.001	—
Glucose 6-phosphatase										
Specific activity	1.4	0.7–0.8	—	2.5	0.58	1.3	0.6–7.0	0.9	2.2	—
Relative to homogenate	—	1	0.4	—	—	—	0.2–2.0	0.3	—	0.7–1.1
Relative to microsomes	0.2	—	—	0.2	—	0.06	—	0.1	0.16	—
NADH-cytochrome c reductase										
Specific activity	7.7	—	—	5.2	—	—	—	—	—	—
Relative to homogenate	—	—	—	—	—	—	—	—	—	—
Relative to microsomes	0.2	—	—	0.03	—	—	—	—	—	—

[a] Preparations 1 through 17 are the same as listed in Tables I and II. Preparation 18 (Stein et al., 1968), 19 (Wattiaux-de Coninck and Wattiaux, 1969), and 20 (Pohl et al. 1969, 1971) are similar preparations for which chemical analyses were not presented. Preparations 21 (Hinton et al., 1970; Prospero et al., 1973) and 22 (Victoria et al., 1971) are by zonal methods. Preparation 23 (Nigam et al., 1971) employs isotonic

enzyme (Emmelot and Bos, 1970).] In several cases the only evidence is the occurrence of the activity in a fraction presumed, but not proved, to be relatively pure plasma membrane. In addition to the enzymes listed in Table IV, glycerylphosphorylcholine phosphodiesterase (Lloyd-Davies et al., 1972) nucleotide pyrophosphatase (Skidmore and Trams, 1970; Decker and Bischoff, 1972), sialidase (Schengrund et al., 1972), and acetylcholinesterase (Wheeler et al., 1972) may be present in liver plasma membranes.

In at least two instances cytochemical evidence supports the localization of an enzyme to the plasma membrane: nucleoside diphosphatase (Novikoff et al., 1962) and adenylcyclase (Reik et al., 1970).

It is obvious from Table IV that (a) the specific activities reported for the same enzyme in different preparations are frequently very different, (b) the purification of presumptive plasma membranes enzymes vary even within one preparation, and (c) in no case are there sufficient data to make a a complete and proper assessment of the purity of the plasma membrane preparation or its enzymatic content. As stated in Section III,A,it is imperative that specific activities of enzymes in the isolated plasma membranes be compared to the specific activities of those enzymes in highly purified preparations of other membranes likely to contaminate the plasma membrane preparation and, ideally, also to provide a flow sheet describing the distribution of the enzymes in the fractionation procedure. Coupled with the

ENZYMATIC ASSESSMENT OF PURITY OF LIVER CELL PLASMA MEMBRANE

	15										
I	II	III	16	17	18	19	20	21	22	23	24
0.03	0	0.05–0.22	—	0.01	1.3	0.72	0.18	0.19	0.03	3.0	2.5
—	—	—	0.003	0.02	0.12	0.07	0.12	0.12	0.02	0.16	0.1
—	—	—	0.0002	—	0.04	—	—	—	0.01	0.05	—
0.13	0–0.06	0.1–0.9	0.13	—	2.6	2.6	0.72	1.48	2.1	1.8	0.3
—	—	—	0.09	—	0.6	0.35	0.32	0.49	—	0.33	0.02
—	—	—	—	—	0.2	—	—	—	0.1	0.1	—
—	—	—	—	—	23.4	3.2	—	—	1.9	—	—
—	—	—	—	—	2.5	0.25	—	—	0.21	—	—
—	—	—	—	—	1.1	—	—	—	0.05	—	—

sucrose and NaCl. Preparation 24 (Graham *et al.*, 1968) is similar to preparation 4 (Table I). The specific activities of the three enzymes are given in μ moles of substrate reacted per milligram of protein per hour. Where available, the values for the activities of the plasma membrane relative to the specific activities of the whole homogenate and mitochondria or microsomes are also listed.

variations in chemical analyses (Tables I and II), the enzymatic data suggest that the isolation of liver-cell plasma membranes of high purity and defined composition is not yet a routine laboratory procedure.

Some of the variations among the data in Tables I–IV may be rationalized in light of the recent discovery (Evans, 1970) that vigorous homogenization of the isolated plasma membrane fragments it into at least two easily separable fractions. The heavier fraction (membrane sheets) and lighter fraction (membrane vesicles) differ in their enzymatic composition and lipid:protein ratio but not in the ratio of sterol:phospholipid (preparation 15, Tables I–IV). It is reasonable to suppose that in the original homogenization of the liver a similar fragmentation occurs so that the heterogeneous plasma membrane breaks into nonidentical pieces. The usual isolation procedures are designed to concentrate larger, heavier membrane sheets. Minor variations in technique among the several laboratories might lead to a significant variation in the percentage of lighter vesicles recovered with the heavier sheets, thus explaining at least some of the variable results. The addition of $CaCl_2$ to the usual buffers might lead to a greater recovery of the lighter fraction, which would explain the higher activity of 5′-nucleotidase, alkaline phosphatase, and Mg-ATPase in preparation 9 (Table IV), since these enzymes, but not the Na, K, Mg-ATPase, are particularly enriched in the vesicular fraction (preparation 15, Table IV).

TABLE IV

Enzymes of the Liver Cell Plasma Membrane[a]

Preparation[b]	1	2	3	6	7	9	10	12	13	14	15			16
---	---	---	---	---	---	---	---	---	---	---	I	II	III	
Mg-ATPase, specific activity	40	—	—	150	—	200	9–39	44	42	—	79	20–270	4–59	—
Relative to homogenate	—	—	—	—	—	—	4–10	6	—	—	—	—	—	—
Relative to microsomes	6	—	—	6	—	—	—	—	—	—	—	—	—	—
Na, K, Mg-ATPase, specific activity	12	—	—	—	—	—	—	8	23	—	33	0–0.8	18–42	58
Relative to homogenate	—	—	—	—	—	—	—	16	—	—	—	—	—	13
5'-Nucleotidase, specific activity	32	13–45	2	49	—	82	31–91	44	69	—	27	35–75	8–16	85
Relative to homogenate	—	—	6	—	—	—	13–24	12	21	—	—	—	—	5
Relative to microsomes	9	17–28	—	11	—	5	—	—	11	24	—	—	—	—
Phosphatidylinositolkinase, specific activity	—	—	—	—	—	—	—	—	—	—	—	—	—	—
Relative to homogenate	—	—	—	—	—	—	—	—	—	—	—	—	—	—
Relative to microsomes	—	—	—	—	—	—	—	—	—	—	—	—	—	—
Galactosidase, specific activity	—	—	—	0.4	—	—	—	—	—	—	—	—	—	—
Relative to homogenate	—	—	—	40	—	—	—	—	—	—	—	—	—	—
Relative to microsomes	—	—	—	7.5	—	—	—	—	—	—	—	—	—	—
L-α-Phosphatidephosphohydrolase, specific activity	—	—	—	—	0.28	—	—	—	—	—	—	—	—	—
Relative to homogenate	—	—	—	—	—	—	—	—	—	—	—	—	—	—

Enzyme												
p-Nitrophenylphosphatase, acid, specific activity	5.6	—	—	—	—	—	—	7.2	—	—	0.5–2.6	0.7–1.4
Relative to microsomes	—	—	—	—	—	—	—	2	—	—	—	—
p-Nitrophenylphosphatase, alkaline, specific activity	0.92	—	0	—	8	—	—	—	—	—	—	—
Relative to microsomes	—	—	—	—	—	—	—	—	—	—	—	—
Phosphodiesterase, acid, specific activity	0.68	—	—	—	16	1.1	—	—	—	—	—	—
Relative to microsomes	—	—	—	—	—	16	—	—	—	—	—	—
Phosphodiesterase, alkaline, specific activity	3.64	—	—	—	—	—	—	—	—	—	—	—
Relative to microsomes	—	—	—	—	—	—	—	—	24	6	20	3
Nucleoside diphosphatase, specific activity	—	—	—	—	—	—	—	—	—	—	—	—
Relative to homogenate	—	—	—	—	70	—	—	—	—	—	—	—
Nucleosidetriphosphatepyrophosphohydrolase, specific activity	—	—	—	—	—	—	—	—	—	—	—	—
Relative to microsomes	—	—	—	—	10	—	—	—	—	—	—	—
NAD-pyrophosphohydrolase, specific activity	5.7	—	—	—	—	—	—	—	—	—	—	—
AcylCoA-transferase, specific activity	—	—	—	0.27	—	—	—	—	—	—	—	—
Relative to microsomes	—	10	13	—	—	—	3.5	—	—	—	—	—
Leucyl-β-aminopeptidase, specific activity	—	11	13	—	—	—	0.3	—	—	—	—	—
Relative to microsomes	—	—	—	—	—	—	2.4	—	—	—	—	—
Hexokinase, specific activity	—	—	—	—	—	—	—	—	—	—	—	—
Adenylcyclase, specific activity	—	—	—	—	0.085	—	—	—	—	—	—	—
Relative to homogenate	—	—	—	—	—	—	—	—	—	—	—	—
Lipoprotein lipase, specific activity	—	—	—	—	—	—	—	—	—	—	—	—
Phospholipase A$_1$	—	—	—	—	—	—	—	—	—	—	—	—
Relative to microsomes	—	—	—	—	—	—	—	—	—	—	—	—
Phospholipase A$_2$	—	—	—	—	—	—	—	—	—	—	—	—
Relative to microsomes	—	—	—	—	—	—	—	—	—	—	—	—

TABLE IV (*continued*)

Preparation[b]	17	18	19	20	21	22	23	24	25	26	27	28	29	30	31
Mg-ATPase, specific activity	—	—	—	—	—	106	—	—	—	—	—	—	—	—	—
Relative to homogenate	—	—	—	—	—	7	—	—	—	—	—	—	—	—	—
Relative to microsomes	—	—	—	—	—	—	—	—	—	—	—	—	—	—	—
Na, K, Mg-ATPase, specific activity	35[c]	—	—	—	—	19	—	—	—	—	—	—	—	—	—
Relative to homogenate	4	—	—	—	—	12	—	—	—	—	—	—	—	—	—
5'-Nucleotidase, specific activity	28	61	47	38	103	36	46	7.7	7.2	—	—	—	—	—	57
Relative to homogenate	19	14	24	20	28	9.4	12	11	3.8	14	—	—	—	—	24
Relative to microsomes	3	7	—	—	—	6.5	—	—	3.1	6	—	—	—	—	20
Phosphatidylinositolkinase, specific activity	—	—	—	—	—	—	—	—	0.012	—	—	—	—	—	—
Relative to homogenate	—	—	—	—	—	—	—	—	0.5	—	—	—	—	—	—
Relative to microsomes	—	—	—	—	—	—	—	—	0.5	—	—	—	—	—	—
Galactosidase, specific activity	—	—	—	—	—	—	—	—	—	—	—	—	—	—	—
Relative to homogenate	—	—	—	—	—	—	—	—	—	—	—	—	—	—	—
Relative to microsomes	—	—	—	—	—	—	—	—	—	—	—	—	—	—	—
L-α-Phosphatidephosphohydrolase, specific activity	—	—	—	—	—	—	—	—	—	0.8–2.2	—	—	—	—	—
Relative to homogenate	—	—	—	—	—	—	—	—	—	6	—	—	—	—	—
p-Nitrophenylphosphatase, acid, specific activity	—	—	—	0.36	0.78	0.18	0.1	—	—	—	4.4	—	—	—	—
Relative to microsomes	—	—	—	—	—	—	—	—	—	—	4	—	—	—	—
p-Nitrophenylphosphatase, alkaline, specific activity	0.5	—	—	0.96	—	—	—	13	—	—	2.5	—	—	—	—
Relative to microsomes	10	—	—	—	—	—	—	—	—	—	36	—	—	—	—

Enzyme / activity									
Phosphodiesterase, acid specific activity	—	—	—	—	—	—	—	—	—
Relative to microsomes	—	—	—	—	—	1.5	—	—	25
Phosphodiesterase, alkaline specific activity	—	—	532	—	7.9	—	—	—	—
Relative to microsomes	—	—	23	—	—	15	—	—	17
Nucleoside diphosphatase, specific activity	47	—	—	—	—	—	—	—	—
Relative to homogenate	25	—	—	—	—	—	56	—	—
Nucleosidetriphosphatepyrophospho-hydrolase, specific activity	—	—	—	—	—	—	—	—	—
Relative to microsomes	—	—	—	—	—	—	60	—	—
NAD-pyrophosphohydrolase, specific activity	—	—	—	—	—	—	—	—	—
AcylCoA-transferase, specific activity	1	—	—	—	—	—	—	—	—
Relative to microsomes	—	—	—	—	11	—	—	—	—
Leucyl-β-aminopeptidase, specific activity	—	—	—	—	—	—	—	—	—
Relative to microsomes	—	—	—	—	—	—	2.9	—	—
Hexokinase, specific activity	—	—	—	—	—	—	—	—	—
Adenylcyclase, specific activity	0.001[d]	—	—	—	—	—	—	—	—
Relative to homogenate	5	—	—	—	—	—	—	—	—
Lipoprotein lipase, specific activity	—	—	—	—	—	—	—	0.07	—
Phospholipase A$_1$	—	0	—	—	—	—	—	—	0.5
Relative to microsomes	—	—	—	—	—	—	—	—	1.7
Phospholipase A$_2$	—	—	—	—	—	—	—	—	0.2
Relative to microsomes	—	0.1	—	—	—	—	—	—	1.0

[a] Specific activities are given in micromoles of product per milligram of protein in 1 hour of incubation.

[b] Preparations 1–24 are those described in Tables I and III; preparation 25 (Michell et al., 1967), 26 (Coleman, 1968), 27 (Lansing et al., 1967), 28 (Lieberman et al., 1967), 29 (Emmelot and Bos, 1966), 30 (Higgins and Green, 1966), and 31 (Newkirk and Waite, 1971, 1973) are similar preparations for which data to assess purity are sometimes but not always available.

[c] May not have been corrected for Mg^{2+}-ATPase.

[d] Stimulated 3 to 20-fold by glucagon and also modulated by insulin and epinephrine (Pohl et al., 1971; Emmelot and Bos, 1971a; Illiano and Cuatrecasas, 1972; Johnson et al., 1972; Birnbaumer et al., 1972; Ray et al., 1970).

In addition to differences in enzymatic activities between membranes isolated from liver and hepatomas (Hoeven and Emmelot, 1972; Emmelot and Bos, 1972), there are sex differences (Emmelot and Bos, 1971b) and differences in membranes isolated from isolated liver cells (Solyom et al., 1972), perhaps as a consequence of treatment with collagenase or hyaluronidase.

Finally, it should be remembered that liver consists of several cell types, and plasma membranes may be of mixed origins. It is generally assumed that all the enzymatic activities are derived from parenchymal cell membranes, but this has rarely been directly tested [adenylcyclase in parenchymal membranes does have six times the specific activity than in reticuloendothelial cell membranes (Sweat and Hupka, 1971)].

C. Intestinal-Cell Plasma Membranes

The brush border of the apical surface of the intestinal mucosal cell contains as many as 1000 microvilli (Palay and Karlin, 1959) each of which measures about 1×0.1 μm (Brandes et al., 1956). This extensive absorptive surface is covered by a deep layer of glycoprotein [the glycocalyx (Ito, 1969)]. The center of the microvillus is occupied by a supporting core of filaments that originate in the terminal web that lies just below the microvilli. On exposure to dilute solutions of EDTA the cell swells in the region of the brush border, so that the cell can be disrupted by blending, and the brush borders isolated by differential centrifugation (Miller and Crane, 1961b; Eichholz and Crane, 1965; Eichholz, 1967; Forstner et al., 1968b; Porteus, 1968; Hubscher et al., 1965). Such preparations are not plasma membranes. They are sheets of microvilli which contain cytoplasm, filaments (Overton et al., 1965; Boyd and Parsons, 1969), vesicles (Forstner et al., 1968a), sometimes nuclei (Porteous and Clark, 1965), and a varying residue of glycocalyx (Ito, 1969; Johnson, 1969), but probably not mitochondria. Further fractionation of these preparations allows the isolation of the plasma membrane (Eichholz, 1967; Forstner et al., 1968b) as a mixture of membranous sheets and vesicles with typical trilaminar structure in the electron microscope (Forstner et al., 1968a; Overton et al., 1965).

The membrane that has been isolated, then, represents one highly specialized region of the intestinal-cell plasma membrane. No significant contamination by other membranes has been revealed by electron microscopy, but the membranes seem not to have been analyzed for typical mitochondrial or microsomal enzymes. The brush border preparations from which the membranes are obtained, however, may have as much as 5 % contamination by mitochondria and 15 % contamination by microsomes by enzymatic criteria (Forstner et al., 1968ab). The ratio of total lipid to protein in the intestinal-cell plasma membrane was found to be in the same range as has been reported for liver-cell plasma membranes but much more glycolipid and less phospholipid were present (Table V). The molar ratio of cholesterol: phospholipid of 1.26 was much higher than for liver-cell plasma membranes, but this difference would disappear if the relevant ratio was cholesterol: polar lipids (phospholipids + glycolipids).

The intestinal mucosa is not only an active absorptive site but contains a number of digestive enzymes intimately associated with the microvillus. Biochemical studies have shown cellular hydrolysis of sucrose, maltose, and glucose-1-phosphate (Miller and Crane, 1961ab), and by histochemical and cytochemical techniques the microvillus has been shown to be the locus of acid phosphatase (Sheldon et al., 1955), alkaline phosphatase (Brandes et al., 1956), and leucine aminopeptidase (Nachlas et al., 1960). The isolated membrane has now been shown to have high specific activities for many hydrolytic enzymes (Table VI). The ATPase includes a Mg-ATPase and a Na,K,Mg-ATPase, both of which are of lower specific activity than in the liver-cell plasma membrane. The ouabain-sensitive ATPase (Na,K,Mg-ATPase) seems to be localized in a membrane fragment that can be separated from the microvillus portion (Fujita et al., 1972). In addition there is glucose-6-phosphatase activity which seems to be different from the microsomal enzyme (Hubscher and West, 1965) and from acid and alkaline phosphatases (Forstner et al., 1968a). Careful examination of Table VI reveals a generally satisfactory agreement between values obtained for the rat and hamster, but mouse may be different. It is also interesting that within one series of values the relative specific activities of the enzymes in the plasma membrane to the brush border are not constant.

D. Kidney-Cell Plasma Membranes

Two relatively uncharacterized preparations of kidney-cell brush border membranes have been described. Zonal centrifugation (Binckley et al., 1968) leads in one step to a preparation of undetermined purity which contains alkaline phosphatase, inorganic pyrophosphatase, glucose-6-phosphatase, Na,K,Mg-ATPase, and peptidase activity. The fraction has a very high ratio of phospholipid:protein (0.83) and molar ratio of cholesterol:phospholipid (1.1). Also, by repeated centrifugations of a kidney homogenate from 0.25 M sucrose (Fitzpatrick et al., 1969), a membrane fraction has been prepared which is enriched in Na,K,Mg-ATPase, Mg-ATPase, and adenyl cyclase and which, by electron microscopy, contains only a few disrupted mitochondria and vesicles derived from the endoplasmic reticulum. Assay of succinic dehydrogenase indicates less than 7% contamination by mitochondria, and cytochrome b5, a microsomal component, was not detectable.

TABLE V

CHEMICAL COMPOSITION OF RAT INTESTINAL BRUSH BORDER MEMBRANES

Reference	Total lipid	Glycerides	Cholesterol	Phospholipid	Glycolipid	Fatty acid	DNA	RNA	Chol/PL
Forstner et al. (1968a)	0.61	0.02	0.084	0.14	0.34	0.016	—	—	1.26
Forstner et al. (1968b)	—	—	0.085	0.126[a]	—	—	0.0046	0.013	1.35

[a]Recalculated assuming error in original table.

TABLE VI

ENZYMES OF THE INTESTINAL BRUSH BORDER PLASMA MEMBRANE[a]

	1^b	2^c	3^d	
			A	B
Sucrase	282(3.9)	118(1.7)	47(9)	1(0.2)
Maltase	756(4.5)	588(1.5)	—	—
Isomaltase	372(3.9)	186(1.6)	—	—
Lactase	17(4.3)	13(1.6)	—	—
Trehalase	17(11)	97(1.4)	—	—
Turanase	—	48(1.6)	—	—
Cellobiase	—	4(1.3)	—	—
β-Glucosidase	13(4.3)	—	—	—
Leucine aminopeptidase	—	13(1.3)	82(14)	1.8(0.3)
Leucyl-β-naphthylamidase	360	—	—	—
ATPase	6(3)	25(1.7)	—	—
Alkaline phosphatase	355(3.3)	407(1.1)	110(10)	2(0.2)
Oubain-sensitive ATPase	—	—	4(0.33)	78(6)

[a]Values are in μmoles product formed per mg protein in 1 hour for the membrane. The specific activity relative to the brush border is given in parentheses.

[b]Hamster; Eichholz (1967) and Malathi and Crane (1969).

[c]Rat; Forstner et al. (1968a).

[d]Mouse: A, microvillus membranes; B, basolateral membranes; Fujita et al. (1972).

Data from three somewhat better characterized preparations are summarized in Table VII. It is apparent that all are contaminated, at least by mitochondria, and that although the membranes do contain peptidases, saccharidases and alkaline phosphatase (also confirmed by cytochemistry (Molbert et al., 1960)) there is little agreement on the specific activities. Some of the differences may be caused by the presence of a mixture of membrane types (Heidrich et al., 1972), the above enzymes being present only in the brush border membranes.

E. Muscle-Cell Plasma Membranes

The interfibrillar space of the muscle cell contains two membrane systems: the sarcoplasmic reticulum (endoplasmic reticulum) and the T system (transverse tubular). The luminal space of the latter connects directly with the extracellular space (Huxley, 1959; Ryan et al., 1967), and thus, in effect, there are numerous inward projections of the sarcolemma (plasma membrane). Moreover, the muscle cell is encased in an extensive network of collagen. These factors, and the unusual nature of the cytoplasmic contents,

TABLE VII

Composition of Kidney Cell Brush Border Plasma Membranes

	1[a]	2[b]	3[c]
Phospholipid/protein, mg/mg	—	—	0.56
Cholesterol/phospholipid, mole/mole	—	—	0.59
Succinic dehydrogenase, μmole/hour/mg	0.03	0.02	2
Relative to homogenate	0.31	0.05	0.26
Glucose-6-phosphatase, μmole/hour/mg	0.01	0.78	0.21
Relative to homogenate	0.006	0.3	0.25
Acid phosphatase, μmole/hour/mg	0.01	—	0.28
Relative to homogenate	0.005	—	0.7
Alkaline phosphatase, μmole/hour/mg	108	3.48	1.98
Relative to homogenate	15.6	4.5	9.9
5'-Nucleotidase, μmole/hour/mg	—	—	56
Relative to homogenate	—	—	9.3
Total ATPase, μmole/hour/mg	58	28.2	—
Relative to homogenate	1.9	2.8	—
Maltase, μmole/hour/mg	—	23.7	—
Relative to homogenate	—	14	—
Trehalase, μmole/hour/mg	—	29.1	—
Relative to homogenate	—	12	—
L-Leucyl-β-naphthylamidase, μmole/hour/mg	—	—	20.7
Relative to homogenate	—	—	8.9

[a] Rat kidney; Wilfong and Neville (1970).
[b] Rabbit kidney; Berger and Sacktor (1970).
[c] Rat kidney; Price et al. (1972).

make isolation of the muscle-cell plasma membrane an unusually difficult task and, in fact, it has probably not been accomplished.

A rather harsh procedure developed for skeletal muscle (McCollester, 1962) has been applied in modified form to uterine smooth muscle (Carroll and Sereda, 1968). The partially characterized product is probably largely free of cytoplasm, and the molar ratio of cholesterol:phospholipid (0.47) suggests the presence of the plasma membrane. However, the low ratios of lipid:protein (0.12) and phospholipid:protein (0.062) suggest the presence of other protein constituents. A milder procedure employing differential centrifugation in sucrose gradients has produced a plasma membrane fraction from rat myometrium (Kidwai et al., 1971a) with a chemical composition more typical for plasma membranes from other sources: phospholipid:protein = 1.25 mg/mg and cholesterol: phospholipid = 0.82 moles/mole. The preparation may be as much as 10% contaminated by mitochondria but is enriched about five- to tenfold relative to the whole homogenate in 5'-nucleotidase, alkaline phosphatase, Mg^{2+}-ATPase, and leucyl-β-naphthylamidase.

A totally different procedure applied to rat skeletal muscle (Kono and Colowick, 1961) produced empty tubes, $300 \times 50 \ \mu m$, of high density (1.238–1.275) and low ratio of lipid:protein (0.18). These structures are destroyed by incubation with collagenase, and electron microscopy of a similar pre-preparation from frog skeletal muscle shows the presence of a thick layer of collagen in addition to the plasma membrane to which particles are attached (Koketsa and Tanaka, 1964). A more gentle procedure resulted in the isolation from rat skeletal muscle of a vesicular plasma membrane fraction (Kidwai *et al.*, 1973) with a much higher ratio of phospholipid: protein (1.2) but a molar ratio of cholesterol:phospholipid of only 0.11. This material was enriched about twofold in 5'-nucleotidase. Yet a third preparation of plasma membranes from rat skeletal muscle (Fiehn *et al.*, 1971) contains an intermediate ratio of phospholipid:protein, 0.51, and an approximately equimolar ratio of cholesterol:phospholipid, but half of the cholesterol was esterified. A membrane fraction has been isolated from rat cardiac muscle (Kidwai *et al.*, 1971b) which, although not free of mito-chondria, shows a fivefold enrichment in 5'-nucleotidase over the whole homogenate. In all preparations of muscle plasma membranes the specific activities of the presumed membrane enzymes are very much lower than for liver plasma membranes.

F. Nerve-End Plasma Membranes

When whole brain is homogenized in $0.32 \ M$ sucrose the presynaptic portion of the axonal membrane shears off to form a closed vesicle which surrounds cytoplasm, a few mitochondria, and numerous synaptic vesicles containing acetylcholine (Gray and Whittaker, 1962). The synaptosomes can be isolated by differential and isopycnic centrifugation and then ruptured by incubation under hypotonic conditions (Whittaker *et al.*, 1964; Hosie, 1964; Rodrigues de Lores Arnaiz *et al.*, 1967). This mixture can then be subfractionated to obtain a presynaptic plasma membrane to which a portion of the postsynaptic neuronal membrane is still attached (Cotman *et al.*, 1968a, 1969). Portions of membrane from two cells and the synaptic thickening are thus present. Assays of cytochrome oxidase and antimycin-insensitive NADH oxidase suggest that the preparation may contain as much as 15% mitochondrial contamination and 7% microsomal con-tamination. Despite this the specific activity of the Na,K,Mg-ATPase is some 50 times higher than for liver-cell plasma membranes (although purified only sevenfold over the whole homogenate), emphasizing the high content of this enzyme in nervous tissue. A different preparation (Morgan *et al.*, 1971; Breckenridge *et al.*, 1972) is estimated to be 85–90% pure, the major contaminant being outer mitochondrial membrane. The two preparations have similar lipid compositions (Table VIII) but very different

TABLE VIII

COMPOSITION OF RAT BRAIN SYNAPTOSOMAL MEMBRANE

	1^a	2^b	3^c
Phospholipid/protein, mg/mg	0.7–0.9	0.7	—
Ganglioside/protein, mg/mg	0.08–0.1	—	—
Cholesterol/phospholipid, mole/mole	0.44–0.49	0.44	—
Phospholipid composition, %			
Diphosphatidyl glycerol	0.7	—	—
Phosphatidic acid	0.6	—	—
Phosphatidylethanalamine	34	36	—
Phosphatidylcholine	40	44	—
Phosphatidylserine	14	} 15	—
Phosphatidylinositol	4		—
Sphingomelin	5	4	—
Lysophosphatidylcholine	0.7	1	—
Na, K-ATPase, μmole/hour/mg	80	762	12
Relative to homogenate	10	7	2.6
5′-Nucleotidase, μmole/hour/mg	~4	—	2.2
Relative to homogenate	4	—	1.6
Acetylcholinesterase, μmole/hour/ mg	~4	—	21.3
Relative to homogenate	~0.7	—	1.4

[a]Morgan et al. (1971); Breckenridge et al. (1972).
[b]Cotman et al. (1968a, 1969).
[c]Cotman and Matthews (1971).

enzymatic specific activities. A third preparation (Cotman and Matthews, 1971) has yet a different enzymatic composition. Finally, yet another preparation from rat brain (Levitan et al., 1972) gives much higher yields of membrane, the Na,K-ATPase of which although only sevenfold purified has the highest specific activity of all. These data suggest that all these preparations contain varying amounts of two or more different membranes. In fact, research with the electroplax organ of electric eel has clearly shown that the acetylcholinesterase is present in a membrane fragment from the innervated surface which can be cleanly separated from the membrane fragments derived from the noninnervated surface which contains the Na,K-ATPase (Bauman et al., 1970; Bourgeois et al., 1972; Cohen et al., 1972; Olsen et al., 1972; de Plazas and De Robertis, 1972; De Robertis, 1971). A preparation from squirrel monkey brain has a similar phospholipid composition but a higher ratio of cholesterol:phospholipid, 0.74 (Sun and Sun, 1972), than those from rat.

G. Lymphocyte Plasma Membranes

The importance of lymphocytes and, in particular, the lymphocytic plasma membrane in immunological and inflammatory responses will not be discussed here since it is undoubtedly discussed thoroughly elsewhere in these volumes. Although immunochemical characteristics of the cell surface might be studied without isolation of the plasma membrane, it is apparent that a complete understanding of the physiological function of the membrane will be immensely facilitated by thorough characterization of the purified plasma membrane.

Smooth membrane vesicles identified as plasma membranes have been isolated by two procedures from homogenates of pig mesenteric lymph nodes (Allan and Crumpton, 1970; Ferber et al., 1972) and from human tonsils (Demus, 1973). The absence or near absence of detectable succinic dehydrogenase indicates little mitochondrial contamination, but the acid phosphatase and glucose-6-phosphatase activities are high in all preparations (Table IX). The high ratios of cholesterol to phospholipid, however, suggests

TABLE IX

COMPOSITION OF LYMPHOCYTE PLASMA MEMBRANE

	Pig [a]	Pig [b]	Man [c]	Calf [d]	Man[e]
Phospholipid, mg/mg protein	0.44	0.57	0.6–0.7	1.3	0.54
Cholesterol, mg/mg protein	0.22	0.29	0.21–0.26	0.39	0.20
RNA, mg/mg protein	0.03	0.03	0.02	0.03	0.03
DNA, mg/mg protein	0	0.01	0.01	0	0
Cholesterol/phospholipid (mole/mole)	1.01	1.03	0.69–0.75	0.61	0.75
5'-Nucleotidase, μmoles/hour/mg	10.1	7.5	14	2.6	3.9
Relative to homogenate	12	25	14	8	—
Succinic dehydrogenase, μmoles/ hour/mg	0	0	0.01–0.04	0	—
Relative to homogenate	—	0	0.05–0.2	0	—
Acid phosphatase, μmoles/hour/mg	0.51	—	4–6	10.4	0.22
Relative to homogenate	0.7	—	2–3	4	—
Glucose-6-phosphatase, μmoles/ hour/mg	0.3	—	1	0.56	0.02
Relative to homogenate	1	—	1.2	1.8	—

[a] Mesenteric lymph nodes; Allan and Crumpton (1970).

[b] Mesenteric lymph nodes; Ferber et al. (1972).

[c] Tonsils; Demus (1973).

[d] Calf thymocytes; Van Blitterswijk et al. (1973).

[e] Human thymocytes; Allan and Crumpton (1972).

that the plasma membranes may be reasonably pure (perhaps the tonsil preparation less so) and that possibly the two phosphatases are components of the membrane. The plasma membrane fraction is enriched in 5'-nucleotidase, but the specific activity of this enzyme is not as high as has been obtained for other plasma membranes. A threefold enrichment (relative to the homogenate) of lysolecithin acyltransferase is also reported (Ferber et al., 1972).

In view of their different physiological responses it might be expected that T- and B-lymphocyte plasma membranes will differ in composition, and there is at least one report that their intramembranous structures, as revealed by freeze-cleavage electron microscopy (Section VI,B), are distinguishable (Mandel, 1972). Also, plasma membranes from three types of chicken lymphocytes each contain from one to four proteins that are not present in all three cell types (Ragland et al., 1973).

Plasma membranes have recently been isolated from calf (Van Blitterswijk et al., 1973) and human (Allan and Crumpton, 1972) thymocytes (Table IX). The preparation from calf thymocytes has a suspiciously high ratio of phospholipid to protein, suggesting that protein may have been lost during isolation. The thymocyte plasma membrane may have less 5'-nucleotidase than the lymphocyte membrane. From their relatively low levels of acid phosphatase and glucose-6-phosphatase, it might be surmized that the lymphocyte and thymocyte plasma membrane preparations of Allan and Crumpton (1970, 1972) are better than some of the others.

TABLE X

PLATELET PLASMA MEMBRANES[a]

	Membrane fraction	
	d, 1.090	d, 1.120
Phospholipid, mg/mg protein	1.4	1
RNA, mg/mg protein	0.01	0.01
Cholesterol/phospholipid	0.49	0.45
Succinic dehydrogenase, relative to homogenate	0.07	0.14
Esterase, relative to homogenate	0.37	0.66
Alkaline phosphatase, relative to homogenate	0.91	1.05
Leucine aminopeptidase, relative to homogenate	0.81	0.90
Mg ATPase, relative to homogenate	4.1	4.4
Na, K, Mg ATPase, relative to homogenate	2.2	2.4
Phosphodiesterase, relative to homogenate	8.4	7.5
Acid phosphatase, relative to homogenate	3.8	4.4

[a] Allan and Crumpton (1970).

H. *Platelet Plasma Membrane*

Sucrose gradient centrifugation of washed human platelet homogenates has led to the isolation of two fractions both believed to originate from the plasma membrane (Barber and Jamieson, 1970, 1971). The less dense fraction contains vesicles of average diameter 1750 Å and the more dense fraction vesicles of average diameter 700 Å. The chemical composition of these membranes is unusually high in phospholipid (Table X) and somewhat low in cholesterol when compared to other plasma membranes, and their enzymatic composition (Table X) provides some reason for questioning their purity. On the other hand, the human platelet is formed by fragmentation of the megakaryocyte in the bone marrow, and there is some difference of opinion about the precise origin of the platelet outer membrane (Behnke, 1968; Schultz, 1966), so it may be atypical.

I. *L-Cell Plasma Membranes*

Several reagents have been employed (Warren *et al.*, 1966) for stabilizing the plasma membrane of the L cell so that large membrane "ghosts" are obtained on homogenization. The purified membranes obtained by differential centrifugation are apparently quite free of other structures as judged by electron microscopy but do have more amorphous material attached to the cytoplasmic surface than is generally seen in preparations of plasma membranes from other cells. The membranes have been assayed for Mg-ATPase and Na,K,Mg-ATPase. Both are present (Table XI) but only

TABLE XI

COMPOSITION OF THE PLASMA MEMBRANE[a]

	Whole cells	Membranes		
		FMA	Zinc	Tris
Protein, mg	100	—	2.3	2.6
RNA, mg/mg protein	0.05	—	0.05	0.04
Total lipid, mg/mg protein	0.23	0.66	—	0.68
Glycerides, mg/mg protein	0.019	0.11	—	0.13
Phospholipid, mg/mg protein	0.19	0.38	—	0.39
Cholesterol, mg/mg protein	0.024	0.14	—	0.15
Fatty acids, mg/mg protein	0.003	0.018	—	0.012
Cholesterol/phospholipid, mole/mole	0.26	0.69	—	0.74
Mg-ATPase, μmole/mg/hour	1.9	—	1.1–2.6	2.3–3.0
Na, K, Mg-ATPase, μmole/mg/ hour	1.1	—	0.7–1.4	1.4–3.0

[a]Warren *et al.* (1967); Weinstein *et al.* (1969).

TABLE XII

PHOSPHOLIPID COMPOSITION OF L-CELL PLASMA MEMBRANE[a]

	Whole cells	Membranes	
		FMA	Tris
Phosphatidylcholine	43.0	30.6	32.2
Phosphatidylethanolamine	23.3	11.3	10.4
Phosphatidylserine	6.9	4.4	4.0
Phosphatidylinositol	3.8	5.4	5.1
Sphingmyelin	9.3	23.1	24.4
Phosphatidic acid	4.5	11.2	12.8
Diphosphatidylglycerol	0.7	—	—
Lysophosphatidylcholine	2.1	5.7	5.0
Lysophosphatidylethanolamine	3.9	2.6	2.6
Lysophosphatidic acid	0.8	1.8	1.3
Plasmalogen	12.3	7.9	8.1

[a]Weinstein *et al.* (1969).

minimally enriched over the whole homogenate and of much lower specific activity than has been found for plasma membranes from other sources. The relatively high amount of RNA (Table XI) is thought to be a true membrane component (Glick and Warren, 1969). The ratios of lipid:protein, phospholipid:protein, and cholesterol:phospholipid are similar to the higher values found for liver-cell plasma membranes. The phospholipid composition also resembles that of liver-cell plasma membranes, especially in the high content of sphingomyelin (Table XII). The glycolipids of this preparation have also been described in thorough detail (Weinstein *et al.*, 1970).

Much less well-characterized plasma membranes have been isolated by a rapid method employing a two-phase aqueous system (Brunette and Till, 1971). The membranes also have appreciable amorphous material on their cytoplasmic surface and an ATPase specific activity equal to those isolated by Warren *et al.* (1966, 1967). A third method (Heine and Schnaitman, 1971) isolates phagocytic vesicles from L cells that have phagocytosed latex particles (Wetzel and Korn, 1969), but it is not proper to consider the phagosome membrane identical to the plasma membrane since intracellular fusions occur rapidly (Wetzel and Korn, 1969).

J. HeLa-Cell Plasma Membranes

Plasma membranes of the HeLa cell have been isolated as large ghosts which in electron micrographs seem to be free of other structures (Bosman *et al.*, 1968). They are also judged to be free of mitochondria, endoplasmic reticulum, and Golgi membranes by the absence of detectable succinic dehydrogenase, esterase, and UDPase, respectively (Table XIII). The membranes contain a Na,K,Mg-ATPase, alkaline phosphatase, and phosphodiesterase of relatively high specific activity, all which are enriched, but not equally, over their concentrations in the whole cell homogenate (Table XIII). In particular, 5'-nucleotidase and a collagen : glucosyl transferase are of very high specific activity in the plasma membrane, and these have been found in no other membrane fraction. The chemical analysis of this preparation shows no RNA, a lipid:protein ratio typical of that for other plasma membranes, and a high ratio of cholesterol:phospholipid (Table XIV).

A plasma membrane fraction isolated from HeLa cells by a very different

TABLE XIII

ENZYMATIC COMPOSITION OF HeLa CELL PLASMA MEMBRANES

	Plasma membrane	
Reference	1[a]	2[b]
Mg-ATPase		
Specifiic activity	—	1.5
Relative to homogenate	—	—
Na, K, ATPase		
Specific activity	35.8	1.6
Relative to homogenate	28	—
Alkaline phosphatase		
Specific activity	0.67	—
Relative to homogenate	21	—
Phosphodiesterase		
Specific activity	0.24	—
Relative to homogenate	6	—
5'-Nucleotidase		
Specific activity	35	—
Relative to homogenate	115	—
Collagen: glucosyl transferase		
Specific activity	—	—
Relative to homogenate	145	—
Succinic dehydrogenase		
Specific activity	0	—
Esterase		
Specific activity	0	—

[a]Bosman *et al.* (1968); Hagopian *et al.* (1968).
[b]Boone *et al.* (1969).

TABLE XIV

CHEMICAL COMPOSITION OF HeLa CELL PLASMA
MEMBRANES[a]

Protein, mg/100 mg homogenate	3.6
Total lipid, mg/mg protein	0.67
Phospholipid	0.31
Cholesterol	0.17
RNA	0
Cholesterol/phospholipid	1.05

[a]Bosman *et al.* (1968).

procedure (Boone *et al.*, 1969) has a low activity for NADH-cytochrome c reductase, less than 3% RNA, and is essentially free of contaminants as judged by electron microscopy. This preparation has a very low ATPase activity (perhaps because it was subjected to sonication) and has not otherwise been analyzed. A third preparation of HeLa-cell plasma membranes has been characterized only by electron microscopy, which is insufficient (Atkinson and Summers, 1971).

K. *Plasma Membranes from Other Cells*

Plasma membranes have been isolated from several other cell types of vertebrate origin including Ehrlich ascites tumor cells (Kamat and Wallach, 1965), chick embryo liver (Rosenberg, 1969), and chick and mammalian embryo fibroblast (Perdue and Sneider, 1970; Perdue, 1970; Perdue *et al.*, 1971, 1972; Gahmberg, 1971; Renkonen *et al.*, 1972; Lelievre, 1973). Membranes from adipose tissue (McKeel and Jarett, 1970) have been fractionated to give fractions enriched in 5'-nucleotidase and a hormone-stimulated adenyl cyclase (Laudat *et al.*, 1972; Combret and Laudat, 1972), as is also true for thyroid cells (Yamashita and Field, 1970; Wolff and Jones, 1971). Plasma membranes have been isolated from bovine mammary gland (Keenan *et al.*, 1970), and crude preparations have been obtained from lung (Ryan and Smith, 1971), bovine taste buds (Lo, 1973), and olfactory epithelium (Koyama *et al.*, 1971). In addition, there is an extensive literature on plasma membranes from erythrocytes and spheroplast membranes from bacteria and reports on isolation of plasma membrane from yeast and amoebae, none of which will be discussed in this article.

L. *Concluding Comments*

It is apparent that the preparations of plasma membranes from tissue cells do not represent the entire plasma membrane but rather specific segments which may well not be representative of the membrane as a whole. Thus, the brush border surface of the intestinal mucosal cell, the region from which the isolated plasma membranes comes, would be expected to have a different enzymatic content, and perhaps also gross chemical and morphological differences, from other regions of the cell surface. The same would apply to the liver cell where the isolated plasma membrane seems largely to be derived from the bile front surface. It may be that plasma membrane preparations from isolated cells grown in culture (HeLa and L cells) are more representative of the entire surface.

The purity of most preparations of plasma membranes is far from absolute. Within this limitation, however, it is certain that the plasma membrane has a greater concentration of cholesterol and of sphingomyelin than other cell membranes. Whether the observed variations in the cholesterol:phospholipid ratio among membranes from different tissues are real differences among cell types, as has been suggested (Weinstein et al., 1969), is open to question since values reported for the same membrane by different laboratories often vary. If the plasma membrane is a chemical mosaic so that the cholesterol were not evenly distributed, for example, segments isolated from different regions of the membrane might have different ratios of cholesterol to phospholipid.

The obvious differences in chemical composition of plasma membranes isolated from the same source but by different methods and in different laboratories should be taken seriously. It is a warning that all preparations are not of equal purity. Some or all are significantly contaminated by other membranes; some or all have lost lipid or protein constituents during isolation. In evaluating the data to be discussed in the next sections and in examining future papers where the protein constituents or biosynthetic capabilities of membranes are assessed or compared (especially when membranes are from physiologically abnormal cells), it is essential to determine that the membranes are of adequate purity and have maintained their integrity.

IV. Isolation of Plasma Membrane Proteins

A. Liver-Cell Plasma Membranes

Approximately 30% of the proteins of liver-cell plasma membranes isolated by the most commonly used procedure are soluble in 0.15 M NaCl (Emmelot et al., 1964; Barclay et al., 1967) which inevitably raises the question of whether they should be considered an integral part of the membrane. Unfortunately, these proteins have not been characterized in any way, so there is no basis for judging either their origins or their functions.

The remainder of the membrane can be disintegrated by sonication to particles that are too small to be sedimented at 100,000 g for 30 minutes. When centrifuged in solutions of high density, flotation occurs so that the lipoprotein aggregates can be divided into at least three density classes, each of which appears to give a fairly sharp peak in analytical ultracentrifugation (Bont *et al.*, 1969; Barclay *et al.*, 1967, 1972). Undoubtedly, sonication disrupts the membrane into lipoprotein aggregates, but the possible heterogeneity of such fractions would not be revealed by the analytical techniques used and there is no evidence that the fractions obtained represent membrane units. It is quite likely that nonspecific associations occur among lipids and proteins that are dissociated from membranes by sonication.

Similarly, plasma membranes can be dissociated in 1% deoxycholate (Emmelot *et al.*, 1970), producing a myelinlike membrane fragment (thought to be artifact) enriched 15-fold in ATPase activity and a dense pellet enriched in tight junctional fragments. There is a preliminary report of the purification of mouse-hepatocyte gap junctions which may contain only one major protein (20,000 daltons) and one major phospholipid (phosphatidylcholine) (Goodenough and Stoeckenius, 1972).

The true complexity of membrane protein is probably most correctly indicated by polyacrylamide gel electrophoresis. At least 20 protein bands are found in electrophoretic patterns of membranes solubilized by mixture of 1% deoxycholate and 2% Triton-X 100 (Widnell and Unkeless, 1968), and as many bands also from membranes solubilized in 8 M urea (Neville, 1968). Both of these solubilizing procedures have been used to obtain fractions from which a highly purified protein has been obtained. By far the best resolution, however, is obtained by polyacrylamide gel electrophoresis in sodium dodecylsulfate. This technique separates proteins on the basis of molecular weight, utilizing the sieving properties of the gel, all the proteins having been rendered equally charged by virtue of the interaction with SDS. It is always possible, however, that a single band contains more than one protein of similar molecular weights.

Rat liver plasma membranes can be separated by SDS-gel electrophoresis into 35 to 40 polypeptides (Neville and Glossmann, 1971) of 16,000 to more than 360,000 MW. No bands that account for at least 1% of the protein were common to plasma membranes, mitochondria, and endoplasmic reticulum. Only three bands were common to liver and kidney membranes, the most prominent of which has a molecular weight of 48,000. Of these proteins, some six were glycoproteins (Glossmann and Neville, 1971) ranging in approximate molecular weights from 96,000 to greater than 250,000 and four of these have mobilities similar to glycoproteins of kidney plasma membranes.

5'-Nucleotidase has been purified some 90-fold from detergent-solubilized membranes to a fraction which shows only one major and several minor bands on gel electrophoresis (Widnell and Unkeless, 1968). The major band is estimated to account for perhaps 3 % of the total protein of the plasma membrane and, as isolated, is the fraction which contains 1.5 μmoles of sphingomyelin (and no other lipid) per milligram of protein. Association of the sphingomyelin with the enzyme has not yet been demonstrated.

Another protein, not known to have enzymatic activity, which accounts for about 10 % of the total protein of liver-cell plasma membranes has been isolated free of lipid and sugar (Neville, 1969). It can be extracted from membranes by as mild a treatment as dialysis for 24 hours at 4°C against a solution of 1 mM EDTA, pH 7. The protein is found (by immunochemical techniques) to be specifically a component of liver and of plasma membranes. This well-characterized protein has a molecular weight of 70,000, contains a relatively high content of polar amino acids and little proline, is 100 % α-helix, and appears to be a rigid rod of a length of 700 to 1000 Å consisting of two or three chains. In all these respects it is similar to paramyosin of muscle, but the suggestion, on that basis, that the protein may be involved in cell movement is highly speculative (but intriguing). Although no enzymatic activity is attributed to the isolated protein, one cannot, of course, be certain that the native protein is without catalytic function.

Liver cells and isolated parenchymal plasma membranes specifically bind insulin (Freychet et al., 1971ab; Cuatrecasas et al., 1971) with a K_d of about 7×10^{-11} M and degrade insulin in an independent process (Freychet et al., 1972). It has recently proved possible to solubilize a lipid-free insulin receptor of apparent molecular weight of about 300,000 from liver membranes (Cuatrecasas, 1972a,b). At least one function of membrane-bound insulin may be to regulate the activity of an insulin-sensitive cyclic-AMP phosphodiesterase of plasma membranes (House et al., 1972).

Liver-cell plasma membranes also have specific binding sites for epinephrine (Tomasi et al., 1970) and glucagon (Tomasi et al., 1970; Rodbell et al., 1971c) and can specifically inactivate glucagon (Pohl et al., 1972). The membrane-bound glucagon activates membrane-bound adenylcyclase (Birnbaumer et al., 1971; Rodbell et al., 1971a,b) in a process dependent on guanyl nucleotides (Rodbell et al., 1971c,d). Activation of adenylcyclase by glucagon is dependent on membrane phospholipids (Pohl et al., 1971) apart from the phospholipid requirement of adenylcyclase (Rethy et al., 1971). Liver-cell plasma membranes can be specifically adsorbed to, and eluted from, glucagon–agarose columns (Krug et al., 1971). Since this affinity chromatography binds about 75 % of the glucagon receptors and 60 % of the membrane protein, glucagon receptors are probably present in most membrane fragments. The glucagon-receptor protein has not been purified.

Thus, only two proteins of the liver-cell plasma membrane have been isolated in a reasonably highly purified state. There is no indication of what percentage of the total membrane proteins are accounted for by all the other known enzymatic activities. The electrophoretic data do indicate that there will be no single protein present in a concentration that accounts for more than perhaps 10 % of the total membrane proteins.

B. Proteins from Plasma Membranes of Other Cells

1. Fat Cells

Insulin binds to fat cells (Freychet et al., 1971b) and to fat-cell plasma membranes in a manner (Hammond et al., 1972) suggesting the presence of both high ($K_d = 5 \times 10^{-10} M$) and low ($K_d = 3 \times 10^{-9} M$) affinity receptors. The insulin receptors of intact fat cells can be modified and inactivated by proteolytic enzymes (Cuatrecasas, 1971a). More identical insulin receptors are exposed at the surface on the removal of phospholipids (Cuatrecasas, 1971b), and, as with liver cells, at least the high affinity insulin receptor can be solubilized by neutral detergents (Cuatrecasas, 1972a,b).

2. Kidney

By SDS–polyacrylamide gel electrophoresis at least 30 to 40 polypeptides can be shown to be present in isolated rat kidney plasma membranes (Neville and Glossmann, 1971) of which perhaps three are common to rat liver plasma membranes including one of 48,000 daltons. Kidney plasma membranes probably contain about eleven glycoproteins from about 50,000 to more than 300,000 daltons (Glossmann and Neville, 1971).

3. HeLa and L- Cells

Membranes of HeLa cells and of L cells isolated by the Tris method (Warren et al., 1966) have been examined by gel electrophoresis in urea–sodium dodecylsulfate solutions after rendering them radioactive by chemical methylation (Kiehn and Holland, 1969). Indications were obtained for multiple components, perhaps as many as 100, in the broad range of molecular weights of 15,000 to 100,000 with most components between 45,000 and 75,000. Data obtained by this labeling technique are not readily interpretable. No single major component was present in either preparation. The marked heterogeneity of proteins of isolated L-cell plasma membranes has been confirmed by SDS–polyacylamide gel electrophoresis (Greenberg and Glick, 1972); at least six glycoproteins are present among the many polypeptides of 15,000 to 230,000 MW.

4. Lymphocytes

About 95 % of the proteins of pig-lymphocyte plasma membranes can be solubilized in 2 % deoxycholate with retention of many enzymatic activities (Allan and Crumpton, 1971). These membranes and also human- and pig-thymocyte plasma membranes show at least 20 polypeptide bands in rather poorly resolved SDS–polyacrylamide electrophoretic gels (Allan and Crumpton, 1972).

5. Platelets

Plasma membrane from human platelets contain at least 20 polypeptides of between 10,000 and 250,000 MW including three glycoproteins (Nachman and Ferris, 1972; Barber and Jamieson, 1971; Phillips, 1972).

6. Nerve-End Membranes

When isolated synaptosome membranes are treated with Triton X-100, about 40 % of the protein and 75 % of the acetylcholinesterase is solubilized while all the 5′-nucleotidase and alkaline phosphatase remains with an insoluble fraction that resembles the synaptic complex (Cotman *et al.,* 1971). Both the soluble and insoluble fractions contain 30 to 40 polypeptides (Levitan *et al.,* 1972). Perhaps five glycoproteins are contained in the intact membranes (Breckenridge and Morgan, 1972).

C. *Comments*

The importance of proteins in the function of membranes is obvious and unquestioned. Furthermore, several recent theories of membrane organization propose a major role for the proteins as integral components of the membrane continuum sometimes with the postulation of a specific "structural" protein; and many studies of membrane biosynthesis are dependent on measuring the incorporation of radioactive precursors into membrane proteins. For all these reasons it is essential that more effort be made in assessing the number and nature of membrane proteins and in isolating and identifying pure proteins.

V. Biosynthesis of the Plasma Membrane

This very important phase of membrane biochemistry has received relatively little attention, and for good reason. In order to perform biosynthetic experiments in the most meaningful way it is necessary to be able to isolate and identify specific proteins and little progress has been made in that area. It is possible however to pose a number of questions which one would like to have answered. Are the lipids or the proteins of the plasma membrane synthesized in the plasma membrane or elsewhere in the cell? If the constituents of the plasma membrane are synthesized elsewhere in the cell, how do they get to the plasma membrane? Are the lipids and proteins synthesized separately and incorporated into the membrane essentially independently or are they synthesized as a lipoprotein? Can membranes be synthesized *de novo* or is it necessary to have an existing membrane to act as template? This topic has recently been thoroughly reviewed (Siekevitz, 1972).

A. Incorporation of Radioactive Precursors

The rate of incorporation of radioactive leucine into the rat liver-cell plasma membrane *in vivo* seems to be very much slower than the rate of its incorporation into the endoplasmic reticulum (Ray *et al.*, 1968), especially for proteins greater than 50,000 daltons (Barancik and Lieberman, 1971). Moreover, whereas the injection of cycloheximide inhibits the incorporation of leucine into total cell proteins within 10 seconds, the rate of its incorporation into plasma membrane proteins continues undiminished for several hours. The suggested interpretation is that the plasma membrane proteins are synthesized in the endoplasmic reticulum and transported to the plasma membrane through a large pool that turns over slowly. Glucosamine is also incorporated more slowly into the glycoproteins of liver-cell plasma membranes than into microsomal glycoproteins (Kawasaki and Yamashina, 1971; Evans and Gurd, 1971), suggesting that the latter is the precursor of the former, and plasma membrane proteins and glycoproteins seem to have the same half-life of about 37 hours (Kawasaki and Yamashina, 1971). On the other hand, although the half-lives of different phospholipids of the plasma membrane differ from each other, they are, except for sphingomyelin, similar to the half-lives of the same phospholipid of the endoplasmic reticulum (Lee *et al.*, 1973). It seems reasonable to conclude, tentatively at this stage of ignorance, that proteins, glycoproteins, and lipids of the liver-cell plasma membrane are synthesized in the endoplasmic reticulum and are inserted separately into the plasma membrane by mechanisms not now understood. The plasma membrane has the enzymatic ability to modify the fatty acid composition of phospholipids but not to synthesize them *de novo*.

In growing L- cells no evidence could be found for a differential rate of turnover of the protein, lipid, and carbohydrate portions of the plasma membrane (Warren and Glick, 1968), and the rates of synthesis of membrane in growing and stationary cultures seemed to be the same. In stationary cultures the rate of membrane degradation equalled the synthetic rate.

Evidence for protein synthesis by isolated plasma membranes has been obtained for the L-cell plasma membrane (Glick and Warren, 1969). The synthesis has essentially all the properties and requirements of protein synthesis by mammalian microsomal preparations but the radioactive proteins give a very different pattern on gel electrophoresis than the proteins synthesized by suitable microsomal controls. It will be remembered from earlier in this review (Section III, I) that this preparation of plasma membrane is particularly enriched in RNA containing 8 to 11 % of the total cell RNA (and 10 to 12 % of the total cell protein). These are exciting observations and one looks with great interest for continuation of these experiments and more definitive proof that microsomal ribosomes are not involved and that the radioactivity is incorporated into proteins of the plasma membrane.

Similarly, one must be cautious in interpreting reports of incorporation of radioactive amino acids into proteins of purified synaptosomal membranes as evidence for their ability to synthesize proteins independently. In one report many proteins are labeled by a cycloheximide-inhibited chloramphenicol-insensitive process (Gilbert, 1972), and in a contradictory report only three proteins are labeled by a chloramphenicol-inhibited process (Ramirez *et al.*, 1972). It must be rigorously shown that these biosynthetic processes represent protein synthesis *de novo*, independent of microsomes.

B. Relationship between the Plasma Membrane and Other Cell Membranes

Endocytosis (pinocytosis and phagocytosis) is accomplished by the formation of a vesicle whose membrane is derived from the plasma membrane. This vesicle then migrates internally. Thus one must assume that in some cells a number of intracellular vesicles are more or less immediately derived from the plasma membrane. To what extent the protein and lipid compositions of the membrane may be altered in this process is not known but it has been shown for amoebae that the phagosome membrane resembles very closely the plasma membrane (Wetzel and Korn, 1969; Ulsamer *et al.*, 1971). Moreover, lysosomes fuse with the pinosomes and phagosomes and one must assume a closer similarity among these membranes than exists between two membrane systems that are incapable of fusion.

The reverse situation (exocytosis) also exists wherein intracellular membranes fused with the plasma membranes. Exocytosis includes, for example, the secretion of zymogens by the pancreas and serum proteins by the liver.

Available data show very clearly that the enzymatic and chemical composition of the total pool of rough endoplasmic reticulum, smooth endoplasmic reticulum, and plasma membranes are very different (Korn, 1966a, 1969a). What is not known is whether within the heterogenous groups of membranes designated as rough and smooth endoplasmic reticulum there may be segments of membranes with composition similar to the plasma membrane. Preliminary evidence suggests, for example, that the Golgi membranes may have a sphingomyelin and cholesterol content intermediate between that of the smooth endoplasmic reticulum and the plasma membrane in rat liver (Keenan and Morre, 1969).

VI. Molecular Organization of the Plasma Membrane

A. Introduction

The many hypotheses for membrane structure can be grouped into four categories: (1) the phospholipid bilayer, (2) the lipid micelle, (3) the globular lipoprotein, and (4) the mosaic lipid-globular protein. In this arbitrary classification it is not to be assumed that any hypothesis is all-or-none; no one would dispute the possibility that there may exist local regions organized differently from the bulk of the membrane and that such hypothetical areas may be of great functional importance. Moreover, the four models are not so unrelated as to preclude the possibility of many intermediate states so that in reality one may have a membrane structure that is not distinctively any of the four proposed above. Nonetheless, it is useful to keep these four simplified examples in mind when one considers the possible ways to arrange lipids and proteins into membranes.

It is necessary to emphasize in the present context that these theoretical membrane structures are derived by the integration of data obtained by many different techniques applied to membranes of widely different origins and functions. Few of the data come from studies on plasma membranes if one excludes, as we have done in the present review, the erythrocyte ghost and the bacterial membrane.

The following paragraphs will give only the briefest outlines of the four models and of the evidence on which they are based. Several recent reviews are available in which these matters are discussed in great detail (Korn, 1969a,b; Branton, 1969; Stoeckenius and Engleman, 1969; Lucy, 1968; Singer, 1971; Hendler, 1971; Singer and Nicholson, 1972; Urry, 1972; Oldfield and Chapman, 1972) and the reader is urged to consult them. In this discussion the aim is to present enough information to determine to what extent the available data on animal plasma membranes allow a decision among the four hypotheses.

B. *The Phospholipid Bilayer Theory and Model Membranes*

When anhydrous phospholipids are placed in an aqueous environment the phospholipids arrange themselves spontaneously into bilayers separated by water. Each bilayer consists of two monolayers of phospholipid molecules. In the "monolayer" the phospholipid molecules lie side by side with their fatty acid chains fully extended and parallel. In the bilayer the two "monolayers" are oriented so that their fatty acyl chains face each other, forming an interior paraffinic region while their polar head groups are at the aqueous interfaces. Although there may be appreciable London-van der Waals interactions between adjacent hydrocarbon chains in each monolayer (since this would be the sum of the interactions between two chains of 16 to 20 methylene groups which might be in parallel alignment) such forces would be less between the acyl chains of the phospholipids in the two sides of the bilayer (since, unless there were appreciable interdigitation of acyl chains, such interactions would be restricted largely to the terminal methyl groups). An alternative view of the formation of bilayers is that the hydrophobicity of the hydrocarbon chains forces them away from the water.

Finally, one can consider the effects of the hydrocarbon chains on the structure of water itself. Water is a highly structured liquid. The insertion of paraffinic chains into the water would result in tremendous disorder of water molecules, and since the lowest energy state is where the maximal interaction of water obtains, the hydrocarbon chains must be isolated from the aqueous phase. The specific arrangement as bilayers is probably favored because the structure of the phospholipid molecule is such that the cross-sectional area of the two fatty acyl groups is approximately equal to the area of the polar head group. This means that a planar arrangement of adjacent phospholipid molecules is favored since it minimizes their packing volume and because other arrangements (spherical for example) would necessitate that the polar groups be much further apart, separated by water, and thereby create the energetically unfavored aqueous–hydrocarbon interface.

When phospholipids are dispersed in water with gentle agitation, "liposomes" are formed which consist of multiple bilayers in an onionlike arrangement (Bangham, 1968). The bilayers close in on themselves to form concentric shells separated by water. (If closed shells were not formed, hydrocarbon chains would be exposed to water at the edges of the planar bilayer.) On sonication, such large aggregates can be disintegrated into small vesicles (250 to 500 Å in diameter) bounded by a single phospholipid bilayer (Huang, 1969). (The minimal size of such vesicles is probably dictated by the same considerations discussed above. If the radius of curvature were too small, large gaps would separate the polar heads groups and water would be disordered at the hydrocarbon interface.) Artificial single bilayer membranes can also be made by applying a solution of lipid in a suitable organic solvent to a hole in a plastic barrier separating two aqueous phases (Tien and Diana, 1968). These model phospholipid bilayer membranes (Henn and Thompson, 1969) share some of the properties of the plasma membrane, for example, high electrical resistance, high water permeability, low surface tension; and they can be altered to mimic others, cation selectivity, for example. However, there are still numerous properties of the plasma membrane such as active transport and group translocation that have not yet been developed in the experimental models.

One argument for the structure of the plasma membrane as that of a phospholipid bilayer is based on the similarity of the X-ray diffraction patterns of certain artifical bilayer systems and naturally occurring myelin and the extrapolation of this structure to the plasma membrane because of the continuity between myelin and the plasma membrane of the Schwann cell (Korn, 1966a). The important link in this argument is the validity of the extrapolation of the structure of myelin to that of the plasma membrane. This is largely dependent on the assumption that the typical trilaminar image of a plasma membrane as seen after osmium tetroxide fixation is caused by the accumulation of heavy metal specifically at the polar groups of phospholipids. It is reasoned that the electron dense lines represent the polar head groups of a phospholipid bilayer and the electron lucent region is the hydrocarbon interior. Indeed the artifical bilayer systems do give just such an image under suitable conditions but such preparations are often very difficult, if not impossible, to fix under conditions used for natural membranes.

There are several more important weaknesses in this argument, however. Although the chemical basis of the fixation reactions is not well established it appears very probable that during fixation with osmium tetroxide much of the osmium is covalently linked to polyunsaturated fatty acids of phospholipids (Korn, 1966b,c, 1967). This places at least some of the heavy metal in the hydrocarbon region (contrary to the above assumption) but, more important, it would be expected to result in significant alterations of lipid (and protein) structure (Korn, 1967; Dreher *et al.*, 1967; Lenard and Singer, 1968).

Perhaps a more serious weakness is the fact that the electron microscopic image of some biological membranes is unaltered when fixation is carried out after solvent extraction of essentially all the lipids (Fleischer *et al.*, 1967; Napolitano *et al.*, 1967) and that other membranes remain intact, and with largely unaltered images, after enzymatic hydrolysis of about 70 % of the phospholipid polar head groups (Ottolenghi and Bowman, 1970; Glazer *et al.*, 1970). Thus the trilaminar electron microscopic image is not dependent on the presence of lipid and, therefore, cannot be assumed to be diagnostic of the specific arrangement of phospholipid molecules. It has been argued (Hendler, 1971) to the contrary that since the electron microscopic image shows the location of protein it therefore must be distributed primarily on two surfaces of a structure not revealed by microscopy. This is taken as evidence in support of a phospholipid bilayer as the underlying structure. Another interpretation (Korn, 1967) would be that the electron microscopic image is caused by heavy metals (OsO_2) accumulated at the membrane–water interface with little or no dependence on what specific groups lie at that interface and is, therefore, uninterprable in molecular terms.

Recent experimental evidence derived from bacterial membranes demonstrates that the thermal transitions of lipids in the intact membranes are those to be expected of phospholipid bilayers (Reinert and Steim, 1970; Steim et al., 1969; Engleman, 1970). A bilayer structure is also readily compatible with the orientation of marker molecules in membranes as measured by electron-spin and nuclear-magnetic-resonance studies, which have also been carried out mainly, but not exclusively, with bacterial mem-membranes (Kaufman et al., 1970; Tourtellotte et al., 1970; Hubbell and McConnell, 1969). These studies provide probably the strongest evidence at this time for phospholipid bilayers in biological membranes, although strictly interpreted they are probably not incompatible with regions of monolayers of phospholipids within which a phospholipid molecule would be oriented in much the same way as in a bilayer.

If plasma membranes are composed of lipid bilayers, then the quantity of lipid in the membrane must be the correct amount to form bilayer sufficient to cover the surface of the cell. With certain assumptions as to the degree of packing of the lipid molecules, this is so for the erythrocyte membrane (Korn, 1966a; Bar et al., 1966), but similar data are not available for any other membrane system.

One major weakness of the lipid bilayer theory is that it leaves unexplained the role of proteins. In its most simplified form, the bilayer model relegates the proteins to the surfaces of the lipid bilayer where they would be bound, in theory if not by necessity, largely through polar (ionic) linkages. Although very little is known about the interactions of lipids and proteins in the membrane, it is fair to say that evidence for significant ionic linkages does not exist. Membrane lipids and proteins are dissociated by reagents that would not be expected to disrupt ionic bonds, and proteins are not lost from membranes when the phospholipids are extensively degraded by enzymatic digestion. Increasing evidence (Kaback, 1970) that active transport of ions, sugars, and amino acids occurs through the mediation of specific proteins implies that a single protein molecule may be exposed to both membranes surfaces and thus serve as a "carrier.". This would necessitate at least some interruption of the lipid bilayer structure.

C. The Lipid Micelle Theory

Although the simpler bilayer is often the favored structure for phospholipids in the presence of excess water, it is not the only possible stable structure (Luzzatti and Husson, 1962; Luzzatti, 1968). Especially in the presence of other molecules, phospholipids will organize themselves into a variety of three-dimensional arrays (Lucy and Glauert, 1964) including globular micelles in which the hydrocarbon chains occupy the center of a sphere whose surface is formed by the polar head groups. From the considerations discussed above, in simple systems, structures such as these will be favored by the presence of wedge-shaped molecules such as lysophospholipids where the polar head groups have a greater cross-sectional area than the paraffinic chains (Lucy, 1970). In more complex systems, similar results might be a consequence of interactions with proteins or carbohydrates. Evidence for such structure in plasma membranes (or any biological membranes) is meager although there is electron microscopic evidence which has been interpreted to indicate the presence in membranes of globular structures of an appropriate diameter (Korn, 1969a). One should be aware, however, of the real possibility of electron optical artifacts (Zingsheim, 1972).

Theoretical arguments have been put forth that the temporary local formation of such lipid micellar regions in the plasma membrane might be the mechanism underlying membrane fusion (Lucy, 1970). If two membranes, as they approached one another, underwent a bilayer to micellar transition, there might be formed a region of disordered micelles derived from both membranes which could then arrange themselves into one continuous bilayer when order was reestablished. The proposed events at the biochemical level would be the enzymatic formation of local concentrations of lysophospholipids which would lead to micelles and the subsequent reacylation of the lysophospholipids which would induce bilayer formation. This possibility has been given some experimental support by the demonstration that the addition of large amounts of lysolecithin to a suspension of avian erythrocytes results in the fusion of the erythrocyte membranes to form large sincytia composed of a number of fused cells (Poole et al., 1970).

D. The Globular Lipoprotein Theory

From thermodynamic considerations alone the most stable configuration for many proteins is a globular structure such that the polar amino acids face the aqueous environment and the nonpolar amino acids are oriented inwardly. This arrangement maximizes water–water interactions and hydrogen bonding between water molecules and polar amino acids while facilitating at the same time internal interactions among the amino acids of the protein. The absence of appreciable β-structure detectable by infrared spectroscopy in most membranes (Wallach and Zahler, 1966; Green and Salton, 1970) and the indication of α-helical and random coil arrangements from optical rotatory dispersion and circular dichroism spectra are compatible with this idea (Wallach and Zahler, 1966; Lenard and Singer, 1966; Steim, 1968). Similarly, the appearance of globular structures in at least some positively stained electron micrographs (Sjöstrand, 1968; Sjöstrand and Barajas, 1970) of membranes and in negatively stained preparations (Fernández-Morán *et al.*, 1964) is subject to this interpretation. These data have led to the proposal, in several related forms, of a membrane structure based on globular proteins in which the lipids are supposed to be interacted around the surface of the protein largely through their fatty acyl groups (Benson, 1966). Direct evidence for such structures is lacking at this stage and it would largely depend on evidence for lipoprotein subunits of suitable dimensions that could be isolated, characterized, and reassembled into membranes. The structure seems unlikely to the extent that the lipid layer would shield the protein polar groups from water.

E. The Mosaic Lipid–Globular Protein Theory

This most recent proposal attempts to meet all the theoretical and experimental data for membrane structure by suggesting that the protein constituents of membranes are globular, largely α-helical units which make up certain areas of the membrane whereas other regions, perhaps overlapping, would consist of shorter regions of lipid bilayer (Singer and Nicholson, 1972; Singer, 1971; Lenard and Singer, 1966; Glazer *et al.*, 1970; Wallach and Zahler, 1966; Vanderkoii and Green, 1970). In its many possible varieties of details this concept allows for proteins to be integral constituents of the membrane continuum where they could act as structural elements (thus perhaps explaining the integrity of the membrane after removal of lipid) and as carrier proteins, for example. It also allows for the phospholipid to be present as bilayer (or monolayer) so as to satisfy the more imperative evidence that such structures exist, but does not require that the lipid bilayer be the major cohesive force in the membrane continuum. At the same time it permits perhaps the lowest energy state for all membrane constituents by allowing the polar groups of both lipids and proteins to lie at the aqueous interface and for the nonpolar portions of both to be buried in the interior. There may be specific interactions between the polar groups and between the nonpolar portions of the lipids and proteins (Tanford, 1972). This theory may also be a reasonable explanation for the images of membranes obtained by the newest electron microscopic technique of freeze cleavage. This method apparently splits the membrane along an internal fracture plane largely caused by the weakness of the hydrophobic interactions (Branton, 1966, 1967; Pinto da Silva and Branton, 1970; Tillack and Marchesi, 1970). The final image (Koehler, 1968) is of two internal membrane surfaces with globular projections (fewer for the plasma membrane and very many for mitochondrial, chloroplast, and retinal membranes), which might be the globular proteins, and with some pits corresponding to the particles on the opposite cleaved surface.

F. *Spectroscopic Data for Plasma Membranes*

The theoretical considerations have been discussed in general terms mainly because for the plasma membrane there are very few data with which to evaluate them. Only two isolated plasma membranes seem to have been analyzed by physical techniques. One is from Ehrlich ascites carcinoma cells (Wallach and Zahler, 1968; Wallach and Gordon, 1968) for which the infrared spectral data suggest the absence of protein in the β-structure (as suggested in one version of the original phospholipid bilayer theory), and optical rotatory dispersion and circular dichroism measurements indicate that most of the proteins is α-helical. On the other hand, it is claimed (Avruch and Wallach, 1971) that the rat adipocyte plasma membrane contains significant protein in the β-conformation. These data, and similar data for erythrocyte and bacterial membranes, were once interpreted to indicate the existence of significant protein–protein interactions or interactions between the acyl chains of lipids and proteins as proposed by advocates of globular lipoprotein and mosaic theories of membrane structure. Such interpretations were probably premature. The interactions were invoked to explain the small but real red shift of the ORD and CD spectra of membrane proteins when compared to soluble proteins. It now seems certain that the red shift is, in fact, an optical artifact derived from the particulate nature of the membrane systems (Urry and Ji, 1968; Urry and Krivacic, 1970; Urry et al., Urry, 1972). Nonetheless it is probably still correct to say that no data exist for ionic interactions between lipids and proteins while there are many indications that the predominant interactions are hydrophobic.

G. *Electron Microscopy of Plasma Membranes*

1. INTRODUCTION

The image of the plasma membrane obtained by the thin-sectioning technique cannot, in the opinion of some, be related definitively to the molecular organization of the membrane because of uncertainties about the effects of "fixation" and dehydration and because the specific localization of the electron dense metals has not been established (Section II, B). Nevertheless, the trilaminar image that is characteristically observed for plasma membranes in sections of glutaraldehyde–osmium tetroxide-fixed material has usually been cited as evidence for the phospholipid bilayer theory for membrane structure and reasonable, if not conclusive, arguments can be presented to support this interpretation (Section VI, B). Two other electron microscopic techniques, negative staining and freeze cleavage, provide alternative methods of viewing membranes. The results of such procedures when applied to plasma membranes will be briefly reviewed in this section.

When biological material is suspended in a solution of any one of several inorganic salts (potassium phosphotungstate, uranyl acetate, and ammonium molybdate are commonly used), deposited on a microscopic grid, and the water allowed to evaporate, the organic material is revealed as an electron translucent island in a lake of electron dense salt (hence "negative stain"). The technique is particularly useful in delineating surface structures. These may be revealed as projections into the dense stain or as surface patterns produced by unequal distribution of the stain. Such membrane differentiations are usually not seen in thin sections either because they are not preserved or because their detection requires the fortuitous coincidence of a section that is tangential to the plane of the membrane and that is oriented normal to the electron beam. However, there are also limitations to the negative staining technique. For one, the method is not applicable to intact tissue and only rarely can it be used with isolated cells. In general, only isolated plasma membranes can be viewed by negative staining. It is also necessary to be concerned about the possibility of artifacts introduced during the drying procedure since the ionic strength and osmolality of the solutions must increase to high levels as water evaporates. It is possible, however, that before these effects develop to harmful proportions the negative stain "sets" to an amorphous glass which fixes the membrane.

The much newer method of freeze cleavage may be, for membranes, the most informative electron microscopic method. In this method the specimen is rapidly frozen at $-150°C$ with or without prior fixation in glutaraldehyde. The frozen block is then fractured, not cut, along natural cleavage planes of low resistance. Additional noncleaved surfaces can be exposed by sublimation of the surrounding ice at very low pressure at $-100°C$. The exposed surfaces are then shadowed with a coating of platinum and carbon and the biological material is removed. The replica is recovered and examined in the electron microscope. The advantages of this method are that the rapid freezing seems to cause little damage (since frozen cells are viable when thawed) and that the fracture seems frequently to occur through an inner plane of the membrane, thus allowing visualization of the interior of the membrane that is not otherwise observable (Branton, 1966; Tillack and Marchesi, 1970; Pinto da Silva and Branton, 1970; Branton, 1967).

2. OBSERVATIONS

Benedetti and Emmelot (1968) have thoroughly reviewed their extensive electron microscopic studies of plasma membranes isolated from rat liver cells. Only a brief outline of their observations will be presented here. The isolated plasma membranes are predominantly large sheets of portions of plasma membranes from two or more adjacent cells held togeher by tight junctions. The membrane profiles in thin section are trilaminar structures 80 Å wide as are observed in sections of intact liver. Treatment of the isolated membranes with EDTA transmutes the trilaminar structure into one of globular appearance because of creation of transverse densities across the electron translucent middle layer. In the regions of the tight junctions the central dense line shows a globular appearance after treatment with EDTA and is linked to the inner dense lines by ladderlike transverse densities that cross the translucent regions.

In contrast to mitochondrial inner membranes (Fleischer *et al.*, 1967), the plasma membranes do not seem to survive extraction of lipids unless they are previously fixed with glutaraldehyde after which at least 75% of the phospholipid can be extracted with organic solvents with little change in the electron microscopic image of the membranes in thin sections. Ultimately, such observations must be very valuable for the interpretation of membrane structure.

When these isolated liver-cell plasma membranes are negatively stained with phosphotungstate either one of two profiles is seen. Many membranes have a fine granular surface with smooth edges. Others have edges, and to some extent the surface, covered with a uniform array of globular particles 50–60 Å in diameter (Fig. 2). These particles may appear to be separated from the membrane by a gap of 20 Å, to be attached to the membrane through 20 Å fibers, or to be attached directly to the membrane surface (Benedetti and Emmelot, 1965).

A different image is obtained when the negative staining is carried out at 37°C. In this case some areas of the surface are covered with an hexagonal array of subunits with a central dense pit (phosphotungstate) with center-

Fig. 2. Isolated rat liver plasma membranes negatively stained with phosphotungstate at low temperature (Benedetti and Emmelot, 1968). The membrane surface is covered with globular particles of average diameter 50–60 Å. The particles are most clearly seen at the edges of the membrane where sometimes a stalk appears to attach them to the membrane surface (inset). This micrograph was kindly provided by Dr. Benedetti and is reprinted with permission of Academic Press.

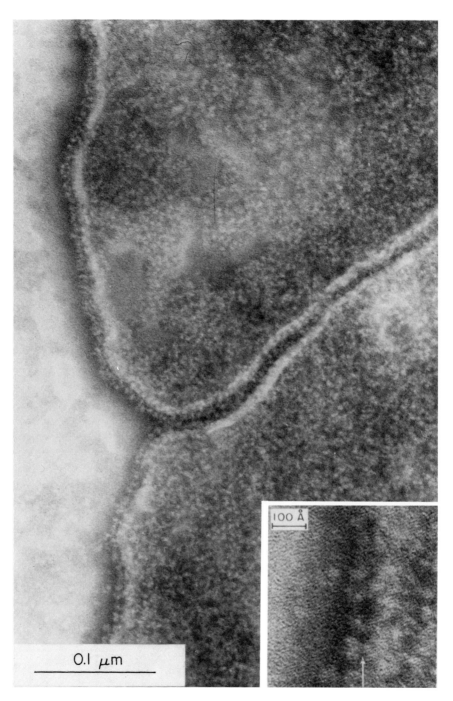

to-center spacing of 80–90 Å (Fig. 3). When the isolated membranes are treated with 1% deoxycholate only the regions held together by tight junctions are preserved and these seem consistently to be the site of the hexagonal surface patterns. Similar hexagonal patterns have been seen in surface views of thin sections of other tissues (Robertson, 1963; Revel and Karnovsky, 1967) where they have usually been interpreted as surface structures (proteins?) which do not penetrate to the interior of the membrane. Benedetti and Emmelot suggest to the contrary that in the tight junctions these structures may be caused by specific arrangements of phospholipids rather than proteins.

For several years it has been known that when liver is freeze cleaved two different surfaces are seen. One is covered with particles and the other with depressions the frequency of which varies for general membrane, gap junctions, and tight junctions (Weinstein and Someda, 1967; Branton, 1969; Meyer and Winkelmann, 1969). Some have thought that these surfaces represent the true outer surface of the membrane and the true inner (cytoplasmic) surface of the plasma membrane, respectively. However, as mentioned in Section VI,G,1, it now seems definitely established that the cleavage plane lies within the interior of the membrane and that the replicated surfaces are artificial ones created within the membrane by the procedure. This interpretation has recently been convincingly confirmed for mouse liver plasma membranes (Chalcroft and Bullivant, 1970) by recovering replicas of both surfaces produced by a single cleavage (Fig. 4). Three different regions of plasma membrane are recognizable, and their general structure can be interpreted in a way that is quite compatible with the negatively stained image of isolated plasma membranes.

The general plasma membrane of the cell shows one cleavage surface covered with 100–150 Å particles while the other surface is smoother with depressions that in some instances match the particles. (The fact that there are fewer depressions on one surface than particles on the other is thought to be due to technical difficulties in detecting depressions by the shadowing procedure.)

Gap junctions are seen in matched pairs (Fig. 4) to give rise to one surface of closely packed particles and a matched surface of closely packed depressions which often are in an hexagonal array with center-to-center spacing of 90 Å. Thus, in contrast to the randomly scattered particles within the general plasma membrane, the gap junctions seem to contain tightly packed

Fig. 3. Isolated rat liver plasma membrane negatively stained with phosphotungstate at 37°C (Benedetti and Emmelot, 1968). The membrane surface shows an hexagonal array of tightly packed hexagonal units with center-to-center spacing of 90 Å. This micrograph was kindly provided by Dr. Benedetti and is reprinted with permission of Academic Press.

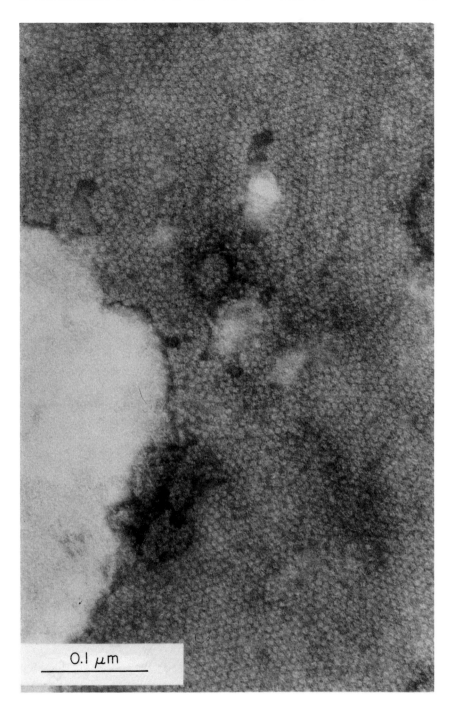

0.1 μm

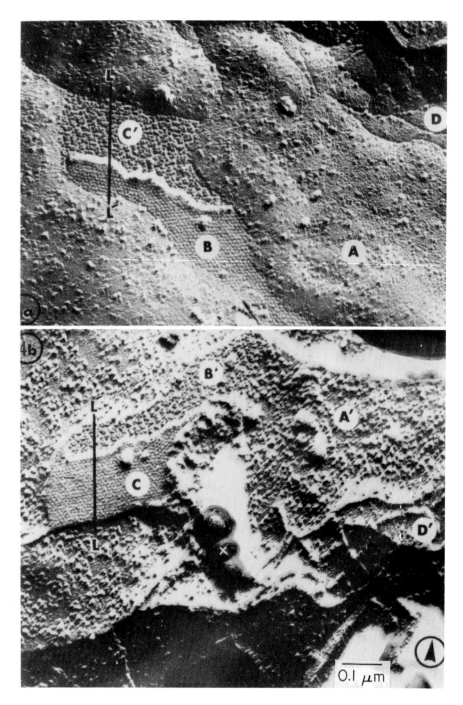

0.1 µm

particles within the interior of the membrane. These observations agree with the negatively stained image of hexagonal arrays in membrane surfaces except that the latter were thought to be in the region of tight junctions.

Yet another arrangement is seen at tight junctions which form continuous seals between cells. Here (Fig. 4) ridges are seen on one face of the cleavage and these are matched by furrows on the other surface. Valleys which lie between the ridges on one surface are also exactly matched by hills which rise between the furrows on the other surface so that the tight junction shows a quilted appearance in its freeze-cleaved replica.

The nature of the particles that are revealed by freeze cleavage is not known and there is no reason to assume similarity among the particles seen in the general plasma membrane, those at the gap junctions, and the ridges of the tight junctions. The evidence is becoming very strong, however, that all these structures lie within the interior space of the membrane, are frequently almost as deep as the membrane, and, within the gap junctions, lie very close to one another. Such evidence requires some modification of the pure phospholipid bilayer theory of membrane structure.

H. Enzyme Localization within the Plazma Membrane

Independent of the more general question of the molecular architecture of the membrane one can seek the localization of specific enzymes within the plasma membrane. This was perhaps first done with the plasma membrane of the intestinal brush border, the surface of which is covered with 60 Å particles (Johnson, 1967, 1969). These particles are still present on the isolated plasma membranes (Overton et al., 1965).

When crude intestinal preparations were allowed to autolyze or were digested with papain (Semenza et al., 1965), two maltases, two lactases, and isomaltase were solubilized. The release of enzymes is temporally associated with the release of surface glycoproteins (Forstner, 1971). With brief exposure of isolated plasma membranes to papain (Eichholz, 1968, 1969), all the sucrase, maltase, isomaltase, and lactase activities are released and these are obtained in a fraction of 60 Å particles which are indistinguishable (Johnson, 1967, 1969) from the particles seen to be attached to the

---

Fig. 4. Complementary replicas of both sides of a freeze-cleaved mouse liver parenchymal-cell plasma membrane (Chalcroft and Bullivant, 1970). Three distinct regions are distinguishable. The general plasma membrane gives rise to a more particulate (A′) and less particulate (A) face; the gap junction is seen as an hexagonal array of particles (B′ and C′) and a matching array of depressions (B and C); the tight junction is identified by one surface of interconnecting ridges (D′) and a complementary surface of interconnecting furrows. (D) Ice crystals are seen at X. This micrograph was kindly provided by Dr. Bullivant and is reprinted with permission of The Rockefeller University Press.

original membrane. On the other hand, by mild trypsin digestion it is claimed that 90–100 % of the sucrase, maltase, and isomaltase can be released while most of the particles are still attached (Benson *et al.*, 1971), thus making less certain the identification of the saccharidases with the particles.

In similar experiments it has been found that digestion of isolated rat liver-cell plasma membranes with papain releases both the membrane-attached globular particles (Section VI, G) and the aminopeptidase(s), suggesting that the enzyme(s) is a component of the particles (Emmelot *et al.*, 1968; Emmelot and Visser, 1971). This is in circumstantial agreement with the known localization by histochemical techniques of that enzyme to the bile canaliculi (Monis, 1965) which is the site of the globular particles revealed by negative-staining electron microscopy.

These and similar experiments lend support to the idea of a mosaic membrane at least with regard to the distribution of enzymes. If such experiments are to be informative for the structure of the membrane *per se*, it must be shown that the enzymes are an integral part of the membrane continuum. To the extent that they exist as particulate appendages to the membrane, the localization of enzymes is intrinsically of interest but not germane to the major problem of the structure of the membrane.

I. Glycoproteins of the Outer Cell Surface

It is by now fairly well established that all the glycoproteins of plasma membranes are on the outer surface of the cell where the carbohydrate moieties are exposed. In the human erythrocyte there is considerable evidence, in fact, that the glycoprotein is almost the only membrane protein accessible from outside the cell to proteolytic enzymes, enzymatic iodination, and chemical labeling (Phillips and Morrison, 1970, 1971a,b,c; Bretscher, 1971a,b, c; Steck *et al.*, 1971; Marchesi *et al.*, 1972). It, as well as all the other red cell membrane proteins, is accessible from inside the erythrocyte ghost. These data suggest that the glycoprotein spans the erythrocyte membrane with the N-terminal amino acid end of the polypeptide, bearing the carbohydrate, exposed on the outer surface and the C-terminal end of the polypeptide at the inner surface. The polypeptide would then have a region that spans the hydrophobic interior of the phospholipid bilayer. Evidence for an internal sequence of approximately 30 hydrophobic amino acids in the glycoprotein supports this concept (Segrest *et al.*, 1972, 1973).

Such detailed evidence is not yet available for plasma membranes of the cells considered in this article. Nonetheless, it is clear that most, if not all, of the carbohydrate moieties of glycoproteins are on the outer cell surface where they are active antigenic sites and receptors for plant lectins.

However, it may not be only glycoproteins that are accessible from the outside of many mammalian cells. Whereas only the three glycoproteins of the plasma membranes of human platelets are digested by trypsin (Phillips, 1972; Nachman and Ferris, 1972), these and four additional proteins can be enzymatically iodinated (Phillips, 1972).

Among the many functions of glycoproteins on the cell surface, at least one seems to be associated with the differential state of the cell. Thus, the glycoproteins of virus-transformed cultured cells are significantly different from the glycoproteins of stationary cells (Buck et al., 1971a,b) but similar to the surface glycoproteins of cells in metaphase (Glick and Buck, 1973). Similarly, the relatively undifferentiated intestinal epithelial crypt cell has a much lower rate of glycoprotein turnover than the highly differentiated cell of the upper villus (Weiser, 1973a).

There may be a correlation between mitotic cell growth and virally transformed cells and cell surface glycoproteins with altered (incomplete) polysaccharide chains. Glycosyl transferases are present on cell surface membranes (Roth et al., 1971; Weiser, 1973b; Jamieson et al., 1971) and completion of the polysaccharide may correlate with cessation of cell growth or differentiation (Weiser, 1973b). These glycosyl transferases may also play a role in cell recognition and adhesion to other cells (Roth et al., 1971) and adhesion of platelets to collagen (Jamieson et al., 1971), the incomplete polysaccharide of glycoproteins on one cell surface (or collagen) perhaps serving as the acceptor for the glycosyl transferase of another cell (Roth and White, 1972).

J. Concluding Comments

A concensus is beginning to form around the generalized concept that the phospholipids and sterols of plasma membranes are in a bimolecular structure. This bilayer need not be symmetrical and, in fact, there are specific data for erythrocytes indicating that the outer half of the bilayer is enriched in sphingomyelin, phosphatidylcholine, and cholesterol while almost all the phosphatidylethanolamine and phosphotidylserine may be on the inner half of the bilayer (Gordesky and Marinetti, 1973; Bretscher, 1972).

There may be proteins lying on the surfaces of this bilayer and there are almost certainly proteins that lie within the bilayer, some of which undoubtedly span the entire membrane and are associated with the intramembranous particles revealed by freeze-cleavage electron microscopy. In many regions the proteins may be sufficiently concentrated so that they interact with one another. In that case it would be moot to argue whether the membrane is a protein matrix with the interprotein gaps filled with phospholipid–sterol bilayer or a lipid bilayer with many interspersed proteins.

The lipid bilayer is "fluid" in the sense that the membrane exists at a temperature above the transition temperature (melting point) of the phospholipid acyl chains. It is often suggested, but not proved, that proteins are free to move as mobile, floating islands within this lipid sea. In fact, such mobility has been observed only for certain surface antigens (Frye and Ediden, 1970; Ediden and Fambrough, 1973), plant hemagglutin receptors in transformed cells (Singer and Nicholson, 1972), and in the "capping" phenomenon of lymphocytes (Raff and de Petris, 1973; Karnovsky and Unanue, 1973). In none of these cases has it been demonstrated that the receptor proteins are integral proteins of the membrane lying partially within the lipid bilayer.

Protein mobility within a fluid membrane, however important it may be for certain specific phenomena, should not be overemphasized. It is certain that plasma membranes of tissue cells contain highly stable differentiated regions that are morphologically and functionally distinct and, therefore, contain specific proteins and, probably, specific lipids in specific associations.

References

Allan, D., and Crumpton, M. J. (1970). *Biochem. J.* **120**, 133.

Allan, D., and Crumpton, M. J. (1971). *Biochem. J.* **123**, 967.

Allan, D., and Crumpton, M. J. (1972). *Biochim. Biophys. Acta* **274**, 22.

Avruch, J., and Wallach, D. F. H. (1971). *Biochim. Biophys. Acta* **241**, 249.

Ashworth, L. A. E., and Green, C. (1966). *Science* **151**, 210.

Atkinson, P. H., and Summers, D. F. (1971). *J. Biol. Chem.* **246**, 5162.

Bangham, A. D. (1968). *Prog. Biophys. Mol. Biol.* **18**, 29.

Bar, R. S., Deamer, D. W., and Cornwell, D. G. (1966). *Science* **153**, 1010.

Barancik, L. C., and Lieberman, I. (1971). *Biochem. Biophys. Res. Commun.* **44**, 1084.

Barber, A. J., and Jamieson, G. A. (1970). *J. Biol. Chem.* **245**, 6357.

Barber, A. J., and Jamieson, G. A. (1971). *Biochemistry* **10**, 4711.

Barclay, M., Barclay, R. K., Essner, E. S., Skipski, V. P., and Terebus-Kekish, O. (1967). *Science* **156**, 665.

Barclay, M., Barclay, R. K., Skipski, V. P., Essner, E. S., and Terebus-Kekish, O. (1972). *Biochim. Biophys. Acta* **255**, 931.

Bauman, A., Changeux, J.-P., and Benda, P. (1970). *FEBS Lett.* **8**, 145.

Behnke, O. (1968). *J. Ultrastruct. Res.* **24**, 412.

Benedetti, E. L., and Emmelot, P. (1965). *J. Cell Biol.* **26**, 299.

Benedetti, E. L., and Emmelot, P. (1968). *In* "The Membranes" (A. J. Dalton and F. Haguenau, eds.), pp. 33–120. Academic Press, New York.

Benson, A. A. (1966). *J. Amer. Oil Chem. Soc.* **43**, 265.

Benson, R. L., Sacktor, B., and Greenawalt, J. W. (1971). *J. Cell Biol.* **48**, 711.

Berger, S. J., and Sacktor, B. (1970). *J. Cell Biol.* **47**, 637.

Berman, H. M., Gram, W., and Spirtes, M. A. (1969). *Biochim. Biophys. Acta* **183**, 10.

Binckley, F., King, N., Milikin, E., Wright, R. K., O'Neal, C. H., and Wundram, I. J. (1968). *Science* **162**, 1009.

Birnbaumer, L., Pohl, S. L., and Rodbell, M. (1971). *J. Biol. Chem.* **246**, 1857.

Birnbaumer, L., Pohl, S. L., and Rodbell, M. (1972). *J. Biol. Chem.* **247**, 2038.

Bont, W. S., Emmelot, P., and VazDias, H. (1969). *Biochim. Biophys. Acta* **173**, 389.

Boone, C. W., Ford, L. E., Bond, H. E., Stuart, D. C., and Lorenz, D. (1969). *J. Cell. Biol.* **41**, 378.

Bosman, H. B., Hagopian, A., and Eylar, E. H. (1968). *Arch. Biochem. Biophys.* **128**, 51.

Bourgeois, J.-P., Ryter, A., Menez, A., Fromageot, P., Boquet, P., and Changeaux, J.-P. (1972). *FEBS Lett.* **25**, 127.

Boyd, C. A. R., and Parsons, J. S. (1969). *J. Cell Biol.* **41**, 646.

Brandes, D., Zetterqvist, H., and Shelden, H. (1956). *Nature (London)* **177**, 382.

Branton, D. (1966). *Proc. Nat. Acad. Sci. U.S.* **55**, 1048.

Branton, D. (1967). *Science* **158**, 655.

Branton, D. (1969). *Annu. Rev. Plant Physiol.* **20**, 209.

Breckenridge, W. C., and Morgan, I. G. (1972). *FEBS Lett.* **22**, 253.

Breckenridge, W. C., Gombos, G., and Morgan, I. G. (1972). *Biochim. Biophys. Acta* **266**, 695.

Bretscher, M. S. (1971a). *Nature (London)* **231**, 229.

Bretscher, M. S. (1971b). *J. Mol. Biol.* **58**, 775.

Bretscher, M. S. (1971c). *J. Mol. Biol.* **59**, 351.

Bretscher, M. S. (1972). *J. Mol. Biol.* **71**, 523.

Brunette, D. M., and Till, J. E. (1971). *J. Membrane Biol.* **5**, 215.

Buck, C. A., Glick, M. C., and Warren, L. (1971a). *Science* **172**, 169.

Buck, C. A., Glick, M. C., and Warren, L. (1971b). *Biochemistry* **10**, 2176.

Carroll, P. M., and Sereda, D. D. (1968). *Nature (London)* **217**, 66.

Chalcroft, J. P., and Bullivant, S. (1970). *J. Cell Biol.* **47**, 49.

Cohen, J. B., Weber, M., Huchet, M., and Changeaux, J.-P. (1972). *FEBS Lett.* **26**, 43.

Coleman, R. (1968). *Biochim. Biophys. Acta* **163**, 111.

Coleman, R., and Finean, J. B. (1966). *Biochim. Biophys. Acta* **125**, 197.

Coleman, R., Michell, R. H., Finean, J. B., and Hawthorne, J. N. (1967). *Biochim. Biophys Acta* **135**, 573.

Combret, Y., and Laudat, P. (1972). *FEBS Lett.* **21**, 45.

Cotman, C., Mahler, H. R., and Anderson, N. G. (1968a). *Biochim. Biophys. Acta* **163**, 272.

Cotman, C., Blank, M. C., Moehl, A., and Snyder, F. (1969). *Biochemistry* **8**, 4606.

Cotman, C. W., and Matthews, D. A. (1971). *Biochim. Biophys. Acta* **249**, 380.

Cotman, C. W., Levy, W., Barker, G., and Taylor, D. (1971). *Biochim. Biophys. Acta* **249**, 406.

Cuatrecasas, P. (1971a). *J. Biol. Chem.* **246**, 6522.

Cuatrecasas, P. (1971b). *J. Biol. Chem.* **246**, 6532.

Cuatrecasas, P. (1972a). *Proc. Nat. Acad. Sci. U.S.* **69**, 318.

Cuatrecasas, P. (1972b). *J. Biol. Chem.* **247**, 1980.

Cuatrecasas, P., Desbuquois, B., and Krug, F. (1971). *Biochem. Biophys. Res. Commun.* **44**, 333.

Decker, K., and Bischoff, E. (1972). *FEBS Lett.* **21**, 95.

de Duve, C. (1969). *In* "Lysosomes in Biology and Pathology" (J. T. Dingle and H. B. Fell, eds.), Vol. 1, pp. 3–40. North-Holland Publ., Amsterdam.

Demus, H. (1973). *Biochim. Biophys. Acta* **291**, 93.

de Pierre, J. W., and Karnovsky, M. L. (1973). *J. Cell Biol.* **56**, 275.

de Plazas, S. F., and de Robertis, E. (1972). *Biochim. Biophys. Acta* **274**, 253.

de Robertis, E. (1971). *Science* **171**, 963.

Dod, B. J., and Gray, G. M. (1968). *Biochim. Biophys. Acta* **150**, 397.

Dreher, K. D., Schulman, J. H., Anderson, O. R., and Roels, O. A. (1967). *J. Ultrastruct. Res.* **19**, 586.

Ediden, M., and Fambrough, D. (1973). *J. Cell Biol.* **57**, 27.

Eicholz, A. (1967). *Biochim. Biophys. Acta* **135**, 475.

Eichholz, A. (1968). *Biochim. Biophys. Acta* **163**, 101.

Eichholz, A. (1969). *Fed. Proc., Fed. Amer. Soc. Exp. Biol.* **28**, 3034.

Eichholz, A., and Crane, R. K. (1965). *J. Cell Biol.* **26**, 687.

El-Auser, A. A., Fitzsimmons, J. T. E., Hinton, R. H., Reid, E., Klucis, E., and Alexander, P. (1966). *Biochim. Biophys. Acta* **127**, 556.

Emmelot, P., and Bos, C. J. (1966). *Biochim. Biophys. Acta* **121**, 434.

Emmelot, P., and Bos, C. J. (1970). *Biochim. Biophys. Acta* **211**, 169.

Emmelot, P., and Bos, C. J. (1971a). *Biochim. Biophys. Acta* **249**, 285.

Emmelot, P., and Bos, C. J. (1971b). *Biochim. Biophys. Acta* **249**, 293.

Emmelot, P., and Bos, C. J. (1972). *J. Membrane Biol.* **9**, 83.

Emmelot, P., and Visser, A. (1971). *Biochim. Biophys. Acta* **241**, 273.

Emmelot, P., Bos, C. J. Benedetti, E. L., and Rumke, P. H. (1964). *Biochim. Biophys. Acta* **90**, 126.

Emmelot, P., Bos, C. J. and Benedetti, E. L. (1968). *Biochim. Biophys. Acta* **150**, 364.

Emmelot, P., Feltkamp, C. A., and Dias, H. U. (1970). *Biochim. Biophys. Acta* **211**, 43.

Engleman, D. M. (1970). *J. Mol. Biol.* **47**, 115.

Essner, E., Novikoff, A. B., and Masek, B. (1958). *J. Biophys. Biochem. Cytol.* **4**, 711.

Evans, W. H. (1969). *FEBS Lett.* **3**, 237.

Evans, W. H. (1970). *Biochem. J.* **166**, 833.

Evans, W. H., and Gurd, J. W. (1971). *Biochem. J.* **125**, 615.

Ferber, E., Resch, K., Wallach, D. F. H., and Imm, W. (1972). *Biochim. Biophys. Acta* **266**, 494.

Fernández-Morán, H., Oda, T., Blair, P. O., and Green, D. E. (1964). *J. Cell Biol.* **22**, 63.

Fiehn, W., Peter, J. B., Mead, J. F., and Gan-Elepano, M. (1971). *J. Biol. Chem.* **246**, 5617.

Fitzpatrick, D. F., Davenport, G. R., Forte, L., and Landon, E. J. (1969). *J. Biol. Chem.* **244**, 3561.

Fleischer, B., and Fleischer, S. (1969). *Biochim. Biophys. Acta* **183**, 265.

Fleischer, S., Fleischer, B., and Stoeckenius, W. (1967). *J. Cell Biol.* **32**, 193.

Forstner, G. G. (1971). *Biochem. J.* **121**, 781.

Forstner, G. G., Sabesin, S. M., and Isselbacher, K. J. (1968a). *Biochem. J.* **106**, 381.

Forstner, G. G., Tanaka, K., and Isselbacher, K. J. (1968b). *Biochem. J.* **109**, 51.

Freychet, P., Roth, J., and Neville, D. M. (1971a). *Proc. Nat. Acad. Sci. U.S.* **68**, 1833.

Freychet, P., Roth, J., and Neville, D. M. (1971b). *Biochim. Biophys. Res. Commun.* **43**, 400.

Freychet, P., Kahn, R., Roth, J., and Neville, D. M. (1972). *J. Biol. Chem.* **247**, 3953.

Frye, L. D., and Ediden, M. (1970). *J. Cell Sci.* **7**, 319.

Fujita, M., Ohta, H., Kawal, K., Matsui, H., and Nakao, M. (1972). *Biochim. Biophys. Acta* **274**, 336.

Gahmberg, C. G. (1971). *Biochim. Biophys. Acta* **249**, 81.

Gilbert, J. M. (1972). *J. Biol. Chem.* **247**, 6541.

Glazer, M., Simpkins, H., Singer, S. J., Sheetz, M., and Chan, S. I. (1970). *Proc. Nat. Acad. Sci. U.S.* **65**, 721.

Glick, M. C., and Buck, C. A. (1973). *Biochemistry* **12**, 85.

Glick, M. C., and Warren, L. (1969). *Proc. Nat. Acad. Sci. U.S.* **63**, 563.

Glossmann, H., and Neville, D. M. (1971). *J. Biol. Chem.* **246**, 6339.

Goodenough, D. A., and Stoeckenius, W. (1972). *J. Cell. Biol.* **54**, 646.

Gordesky, S. T., and Marinetti, G. V. (1973). *Biochem. Biophys. Res. Commun.* **50**, 1027.

Graham, J. M., Higgins, J. A., and Green, C. (1968). *Biochim. Biophys. Acta* **150**, 303.

Gray, E. G., and Whittaker, V. P. (1962). *J. Anat.* **96**, 79.

Green, D. H., and Salton, M. R. J. (1970). *Biochim. Biophys. Acta* **211**, 139.

Greenberg, C. S., and Glick, M. C. (1972). *Biochemistry* **11**, 3680.

Hagopian, A., Bosmann, H. B., and Eylar, E. H. (1968). *Arch. Biochem. Biophys.* **128**, 387.

Hammond, J. M., Jarett, L., Mariz, I. K., and Daughaday, W. H. (1972). *Biochem. Biophys. Res. Commun.* **49**, 1127.

Heidrich, H.-G., Kinne, R., Kinne-Saffran, E., and Hannig, K. (1972). *J. Cell Biol.* **54**, 232.

Heine, J. W., and Schnaitman, C. A. (1971). *J. Cell Biol.* **48**, 703.

Hendler, R. W. (1971). *Physiol. Rev.* **51**, 66.

Henn, F. A., and Thompson, T. E. (1969). *Annu. Rev. Biochem.* **38**, 241.

Henning, R., Kaulen, H. D., and Stoffel, W. (1970). *Hoppe-Seyler's Z. Physiol. Chem.* **351**, 1191.

Higgins, J. A., and Green, C. (1966). *Biochem. J.* **99**, 631.

Hinton, R. H. Dubrota, M., Fitzsimmons, J. T. R., and Reid, E. (1970). *Eur. J. Biochem.* **12**, 349.

Hoeven, R. P., and Emmelot, P. (1972). *J. Membrane Biol.* **9**, 105.

Hosie, R. J. A. (1964). *Biochem. J.* **96**, 404.

House, P. D. R., Paulis, P., and Weidemann, M. J. (1972). *Eur. J. Biochem.* **24**, 429.

Huang, C. (1969). *Biochemistry* **8**, 344.

Hubbell, N. L., and McConnell, H. M. (1969). *Proc. Nat. Acad. Sci. U.S.* **64**, 20.

Hubscher, G., and West, G. R. (1965). *Nature (London)* **205**, 799.

Hubscher, G., West, G. R., and Brindley, D. N. (1965). *Biochem. J.* **97**, 629.

Huxley, A. (1959). *Ann. N.Y. Acad. Sci.* **81**, 446.

Illiano, G., and Cuatrecasas, P. (1972). *Science* **175**, 906.

Ito, S. (1969). *Fed. Proc., Fed. Amer. Soc. Exp. Biol.* **28**, 12.

Jamieson, G. A., Urban, C. L., and Barber, A. J. (1971). *Nature (London)* **234**, 5.

Johnson, C. B., Blecher, M., and Giorgio, N. A. (1972). *Biochem. Biophys. Res. Commun.* **46**, 1035.

Johnson, C. F. (1967). *Science* **155**, 1670.

Johnson, C. F. (1969). *Fed. Proc., Fed. Amer. Soc. Exp. Biol.* **28**, 26.

Kaback, H. R. (1970). *Annu. Rev. Biochem.* **39**, 561.

Kamat, V. D., and Wallach, D. F. H. (1965). *Science* **148**, 1343.

Karnovsky, M. J., and Unanue, E. R. (1973). *Fed. Proc., Fed. Amer. Soc. Exp. Biol.* **32**, 55.

Kaufman, S., Steim, J. M., and Gibbs, J. H. (1970). *Nature (London)* **225**, 743.

Kaulen, H. D., Henning, R., and Stoffel, W. (1970). *Hoppe-Seyler's Z. Physiol. Chem.* **351**, 1555.

Kawasaki, T., and Yamashina, I., (1971). *Biochim. Biophys. Acta* **225**, 234.

Keenan, T. W., and Morre, D. J. (1969). *Biochemistry* **9**, 19.

Keenan, T. W., Morre, D. J., Olson, D. E., Yunghans, W. N., and Patton, J. (1970). *J. Cell Biol.* **44**, 80.

Kidwai, A. M., Radcliffe, M. A., and Daniel, E. E. (1971a). *Biochim. Biophys. Acta* **233**, 538.

Kidwai, A. M., Radcliffe, M. A., Duchon, G., and Daniel, E. E. (1971b). *Biochem. Biophys. Res. Commun.* **45**, 901.

Kidwai, A. M., Radcliffe, M. A., Lee, E. Y., and Daniel, E. E. (1973). *Biochim. Biophys. Acta* **298**, 593.

Kiehn, E. D., and Holland, J. J. (1969). *Proc. Nat. Acad. Sci. U.S.* **61**, 1370.

Koehler, J. K. (1968). *Advan. Biol. Med. Phys.* **12**, 1.

Koketsa, K., and Tanaka, R. (1964). *Amer. J. Physiol.* **207**, 509.

Kono, T., and Colowick, S. (1961). *Arch. Biochem. Biophys.* **93**, 520.

Korn, E. D. (1966a). *Science* **153**, 1491.

Korn, E. D. (1966b). *Biochim. Biophys. Acta* **116**, 317.

Korn, E. D. (1966c). *Biochim. Biophys. Acta* **116**, 325.

Korn, E. D. (1967). *J. Cell Biol.* **34**, 627.

Korn, E. D. (1969a). *Theor. Exp. Biophys.* **2**, 1.

Korn, E. D. (1969b). *Annu. Rev. Biochem.* **38**, 263.

Koyama, N., Sawada, K, and Kurihra, K. (1971). *Biochim. Biophys. Acta* **241**, 42.

Krug, F., Desbuquois, B., and Cuatrecases, P. (1971). *Nature (London), New Biol.* **234**, 268.

Lansing, A. I., Belkhode, M. L., Lynch, W. E., and Lieberman, I. (1967). *J. Biol. Chem.* **242**, 1772.

Laudat, M. H., Pairault, J., Bayer, P., Martin, M., and Laudat, P. (1972). *Biochim. Biophys. Acta* **255**, 1005.

Lauter, C. J., Solyom, A., and Trams, E. G. (1972). *Biochim. Biophys. Acta* **266**, 511.

Lee, T. C., Stephens, N., Moehl, A., and Snyder, F. (1973). *Biochim. Biophys. Acta* **291**, 86.

Lelievre, L. (1973). *Biochim. Biophys. Acta* **291**, 662.

Lenard, J., and Singer, S. J. (1966). *Proc. Nat. Acad. Sci. U.S.* **56**, 1828.

Lenard, J., and Singer, S. J. (1968). *J. Cell Biol.* **37**, 117.

Levitan, I. B., Mushynski, W. E., and Ramirez, G. (1972). *J. Biol. Chem.* **247**, 5376.

Lieberman, I., Lansing, A. I., and Lynch, W. E. (1967). *J. Biol. Chem.* **242**, 736.

Ling, G. N. (1969a). *Science* **163**, 1335.

Ling, G. N. (1969b). *Nature (London)* **221**, 386.

Lloyd-Davies, K. A., Michell, R. H., and Coleman, R. (1972). *Biochem. J.* **127**, 357.

Lo, C-H. (1973). *Biochim. Biophys. Acta* **291**, 650.

Lucy, J. A. (1968). *In* "Biological Membranes" (D. Chapman, ed.), pp. 233–288. Academic Press, New York.

Lucy, J. A. (1970). *Nature (London)* **227**, 815.

Lucy, J. A., and Glauert, A. M. (1964). *J. Mol. Biol.* **8**, 727.

Luzzatti, V. (1968). *In* "Biological Membranes" (D. Chapman, ed.), pp. 71–123. Academic Press, London.

Luzzatti, V., and Husson, F. (1962). *J. Cell Biol.* **12**, 207.

McCollester, D. (1962). *Biochim. Biophys. Acta* **57**, 427.

McKeel, D. W., and Jarett, L. (1970). *J. Cell Biol.* **44**, 417.

Malathi, P., and Crane, R. K. (1969). *Biochim. Biophys. Acta* **173**, 245.

Mandel, T. E. (1972). *Nature (London), New Biol.* **239**, 112.

Marchesi, V. T., Tillack, T. W., Jackson, R. L., Segrest, J. P., and Scott, R. E. (1972). *Proc. Nat. Acad. Sci. U.S.* **69**, 1445.

Meyer, H. W., and Winkelmann, H. (1969). *Protoplasma* **68**, 253.

Michell, R. H., Harwood, J. L., Coleman, R., and Hawthorne, J. N. (1967). *Biochim. Biophys. Acta* **144**, 649.]

Miller, D., and Crane, R. K. (1961a). *Biochim. Biophys. Acta* **52**, 281.

Miller, D., and Crane, R. K. (1961b). *Biochim. Biophys. Acta* **52**, 293.

Molbert, R. G., Duspiva, F., and von Deimling, O. H. (1960). *J. Biophys. Biochem. Cytol.* **7**, 387.

Monis, B. (1965). *Nature (London)* **208**, 587.

Morgan, I. G., Wolfe, L. S., Mandel, P., and Gombos, G. (1971). *Biochim. Biophys. Acta* **241**, 737.

Morin, F., Tay, S., and Simpkins, H. (1972). *Biochem. J.* **129**, 781.

Nachlas, M. M., Monis, B., Rosenblatt, D., and Seligman, A. M. (1960). *J. Biophys. Biochem. Cytol.* **7**, 261.

Nachman, R. L., and Ferris, B. (1972). *J. Biol. Chem.* **247**, 4468.

Napolitano, L., LeBaron, F., and Scaletti, J. (1967). *J. Cell Biol.* **34**, 817.

Neville, D. (1960). *J. Biophys. Biochem. Cytol.* **8**, 413.

Neville, D. (1968). *Biochim. Biophys. Acta* **154**, 540.

Neville, D. (1969). *Biochem. Biophys. Res. Commun.* **34**, 60.

Neville, D. M., and Glossmann, H. (1971). *J. Biol. Chem.* **246**, 6335.

Newkirk, J. D., and Waite, M. (1971). *Biochim. Biophys. Acta* **225**, 224.

Newkirk, J. D., and Waite, M. (1973). *Biochim. Biophys. Acta* **298**, 562.

Nigam, V. N., Morais, R., and Karasaki, S. (1971). *Biochim. Biophys. Acta* **249**, 34.

Novikoff, A. B., Essner, E., Goldfischer, S., and Hues, M. (1962). *Symp. Int. Soc. Cell Biol.* **1**, 149.

Oldfield, E., and Chapman, D. (1972). *FEBS Lett.* **23**, 285.

Olsen, R. W., Meunier, J.-C., and Changeaux, J.-P. (1972). *FEBS Lett.* **28**, 96.

Ottolenghi, A. C., and Bowman, M. H. (1970). *J. Membrane Biol.* **2**, 180.

Overton, J., Eichholz, A., and Crane, R. K. (1965). *J. Cell Biol.* **26**, 693.

Palay, S. L., and Karlin, L. J. (1959). *J. Biophys. Biochem. Cytol.* **5**, 363.

Perdue, J. F. (1970). *Biochim. Biophys. Acta* **211**, 184.

Perdue, J. F., and Sneider, J. (1970). *Biochim. Biophys. Acta* **196**, 125.

Perdue, J. F., Kletzien, R., and Miller, K. (1971). *Biochim. Biophys. Acta* **249**, 419.

Perdue, J. F., Kletzien, R., and Wray, V. L. (1972). *Biochim. Biophys. Acta* **266**, 505.

Pfleger, R. C., Anderson, N. G., and Snyder, F. (1968). *Biochemistry* **7**, 2826.

Phillips, D. R. (1972). *Biochemistry* **11**, 4582.

Phillips, D. R., and Morrison, M. (1970). *Biochem. Biophys. Res. Commun.* **40**, 284.

Phillips, D. R., and Morrison, M. (1971a). *FEBS Lett.* **18**, 95.

Phillips, D. R., and Morrison, M. (1971b). *Biochemistry* **10**, 1766.

Phillips, D. R., and Morrison, M. (1971c). *Biochem. Biophys. Res. Commun.* **45**, 1103.

Pinto da Silva, P., and Branton, D. (1970). *J. Cell Biol.* **45**, 598.

Pohl, S. L., Birnbaumer, L., and Rodbell, M. (1969). *Science* **164**, 566.

Pohl, S. L., Birnbaumer, L., and Rodbell, M. (1971). *J. Biol. Chem.* **246**, 1849.

Pohl, S. L., Krans, H. M. J., Birnbaumer, L., and Rodbell, M. (1972). *J. Biol. Chem.* **247**, 2295.

Poole, A. R., Howell, J. I., and Lucy, J. A. (1970). *Nature (London)* **227**, 810.

Porteous, J. W. (1968). *FEBS Lett.* **1**, 46.

Porteous, J. W., and Clark, B. (1965). *Biochem. J.* **96**, 159.

Price, R. G., Taylor, D. G., and Robinson, D. (1972). *Biochem. J.* **129**, 919.

Prospero, T. D., Burge, M. L. E., Norris, K. A., Hinton, R. H., and Ried, E. (1973). *Biochem. J.* **132**, 449.

Raff, M. C., and de Petris, S. (1973). *Fed. Proc., Fed. Amer. Soc. Exp. Biol.* **32**, 48.

Ragland, W. L., Pace, J. L., and Doak, R. L. (1973). *Biochem. Biophys. Res. Commun.* **50**, 118.

Ramirez, H., Levitan, I. B., and Mushynski, W. E. (1972). *J. Biol. Chem.* **247**, 5382.

Ray, T. K. (1970). *Biochim. Biophys. Acta* **196**, 1.

Ray, T. K., Lieberman, I., and Lansing, A. I. (1968). *Biochem. Biophys. Res. Commun.* **31**, 54.

Ray, T. K., Skipski, V. P., Barclay, M., Essner, E., and Archibald, F. M. (1969). *J. Biol. Chem.* **244**, 5528.

Ray, T. K., Tomasi, V., and Marinetti, G. V. (1970). *Biochim. Biophys. Acta* **211**, 20.

Reik, L., Petzold, G. L., Higgins, J. A., Greengard, P., and Barnett, R. J. (1970). *Science* **168**, 382.

Reinert, J. C., and Steim, J. M. (1970). *Science* **168**, 1580.

Renkonen, O., Gahmberg, C. G., Simons, K., and Kaariainen, L. (1972). *Biochim. Biophys. Acta* **255**, 66.

Rethy, A., Tomasi, V., and Trevisani, A. (1971). *Arch. Biochem. Biophys.* **147**, 36.

Revel, J. P., and Karnovsky, M. J. (1967). *J. Cell Biol.* **33**, C7.

Robertson, J. D. (1963). *J. Cell Biol.* **19**, 201.

Rodbell, M., Krans, H. M. J., Pohl, S. L., and Birnbaumer, L. (1971a). *J. Biol. Chem.* **246**, 1861.

Rodbell, M., Krans, H. M. J., Pohl, S. L., and Birnbaumer, L. (1971b). *J. Biol. Chem.* **246**, 1872.

Rodbell, M., Birnbaumer, L., Pohl, S. L., and Krans, H. M. J. (1971c). *J. Biol. Chem.* **246**, 1877.

Rodbell, M., Birnbaumer, L., Pohl, S. L., and Sundby, F. (1971d). *Proc. Nat. Acad. Sci. U.S.* **68**, 909.

Rodrigues de Lores Arnaiz, G., Alberti, M., and de Robertis, E. (1967). *J. Neurochem.* **14**, 215.

Rosenberg, M. D. (1969). *Biochim. Biophys. Acta* **173**, 11.

Roth, S., and White, D. (1972). *Proc. Nat. Acad. Sci. U.S.* **69**, 1485.

Roth, S., McGuire, E. J., and Roseman, S. (1971). *J. Cell Biol.* **51**, 536.

Ryan, D. G., Simpson, F. O., and Bertaud, W. S. (1967). *Science* **156**, 656.

Ryan, J. W., and Smith, V. (1971). *Biochim. Biophys. Acta* **249**, 177.

Schengrund, C.-L., Jensen, D. S., and Rosenberg, A. (1972). *J. Biol. Chem.* **247**, 2742.

Schultz, H. (1966). *Verh. Deut. Ges. Pathol.* **50**, 239.

Segrest, J. P., Jackson, R. L., Marchesi, V. T., Guyer, R. B., and Terry, W. (1972). *Biochem. Biophys. Res. Commun.* **49**, 964.

Segrest, J. P., Hakane, I., Jackson, R. L., and Marchesi, V. T. (1973). *Arch. Biochem. Biophys.* **155**, 167.

Semenza, G., Auricchio, S., and Rubino, A. (1965). *Biochim. Biophys. Acta* **96**, 487.

Shelden, H., Zetterqvist, H., and Brandes, D. (1955). *Exp. Cell Res.* **9**, 592.

Siekevitz, P. (1972). *Annu. Rev. Physiol.* **34**, 117.

Singer, S. J. (1971). *In* "Membrane Structure and Function" (L. I. Rothfield, ed.), pp. 146–222. Academic Press, New York.

Singer, S. J., and Nicholson, G. L. (1972). *Science* **175**, 720.

Sjöstrand, F. S. (1968). *In* "The Membranes" (A. J. Dalton and F. Hagenau, eds.), pp. 151–210. Academic Press, New York.

Sjöstrand, F. S., and Barajas, L. (1970). *J. Ultrastruct. Res.* **32**, 293.

Skidmore, J. R., and Trams, E. G. (1970). *Biochim. Biophys. Acta* **219**, 93.

Skipski, V. P., Barclay, M., Archibald, F. M., Terebus-Kekish, O., Reichman, E. S., and Good, J. J. (1965). *Life Sci.* **4**, 1673.

Solyom, A., Lauter, C. J., and Trams, E. C. (1972). *Biochim. Biophys. Acta* **274**, 631.

Stahl, W. L., and Trams, E. G. (1968). *Biochim. Biophys. Acta* **163**, 459.

Steck, T. C., Fairbanks, G., and Wallach, D. F. H. (1971). *Biochemistry* **10**, 2617.

Steim, J. M. (1968). *In* "Molecular Association in Biological and Related Systems" (F. Gould and E. D. Goddard, eds.), pp. 259–302. Amer. Chem. Soc., Washington, D. C.

Steim, J. M., Tourtellotte, M. C., Reinert, J. C., McElhaney, R. N., and Rader, R. L. (1969). *Proc. Nat. Acad. Sci. U.S.* **63**, 104.

Stein, Y., Widnell, C., and Stein, O. (1968). *J. Cell Biol.* **39**, 185.

Stoeckenius, W., and Engleman, D. M. (1969). *J. Cell Biol.* **42**, 613.

Sun, G. Y., and Sun, A. Y., (1972). *Biochim. Biophys. Acta* **280**, 306.

Sweat, F. W., and Hupka, A. (1971). *Biochem. Biophys. Res. Commun.* **44**, 1436.

Takeuchi, M., and Terayama, H. (1965). *Exp. Cell Res.* **40**, 321.

Tanford, C. (1972). *J. Mol. Biol.* **67**, 59.

Tien, H. T., and Diana, A. L. (1968). *Chem. Phys. Lipids* **2**, 55.

Tillack, T. W., and Marchesi, V. T. (1970). *J. Cell Biol.* **45**, 649.

Tomasi, V., Koretz, S., Ray, T. K., Dunnick, J., and Marinetti, G. V. (1970). *Biochim. Biophys. Acta* **211**, 31.

Tourtellotte, M. E., Branton, D., and Kieth, A. (1970). *Proc. Nat. Acad. Sci. U.S.* **66**, 909.

Touster, O., Aronson, N. N., Jr., Dulaney, J. T., and Hendrickson, H. (1970). *J. Cell Biol.* **47**, 604.

Ulsamer, A. G., Wright, P. L., Wetzel, M. G., and Korn, E. D. (1971). *J. Cell Biol.* **51**, 193.

Urry, D. W. (1972). *Biochim. Biophys. Acta* **265**, 115.

Urry, D. W., and Ji, T. H. (1968). *Arch. Biochem. Biophys.* **128**, 802.

Urry, D. W., and Krivacic, J. (1970). *Proc. Nat. Acad. Sci. U.S.* **65**, 845.

Urry, D. W., Masotti, L., and Krivacic, J. (1970). *Biochem. Biophys. Res. Commun.* **41**, 521.

Van Blitterswijk, W. J., Emmelot, P., and Feltkamp, C. A. (1973). *Biochim. Biophys. Acta* **298**, 577.

Vanderkooi, G., and Green, D. E. (1970). *Proc. Nat. Acad. Sci. U.S.* **66**, 615.

Victoria, E. J., VanGolde, L. M. G., Hostetter, K. Y., Scherphof, G. L., and Van Deenen, L. C. M. (1971). *Biochim. Biophys. Acta* **239**, 443.

Wallach, D. F. H., and Gordon, A. (1968). *Protides Biol. Fluids, Proc. Colloq.* **00**, 47–53.

Wallach, D. F. H., and Zahler, P. H. (1966). *Proc. Nat. Acad. Sci. U.S.* **65**, 1552.

Wallach, D. F. H., and Zahler, P. H. (1968). *Biochim. Biophys. Acta* **150**, 186.

Warren, L., and Glick, M. C. (1968). *J. Cell Biol.* **37**, 729.

Warren, L., Glick, M. C., and Nass, M. K. (1966). *J. Cell Comp. Physiol.* **68**, 269.

Warren, L., Glick, M. C., and Nass, M. K. (1967). *In* "The Specificity of Cell Surfaces" (B. D. Davis and L. Warren, eds.), pp. 109–127. Prentice-Hall, Englewood Cliffs, New Jersey.

Wattiaux-de Coninck, S., and Wattiaux, R. (1969). *Biochim. Biophys. Acta* **183**, 118.

Weaver, R. A., and Boyle, W. (1969). *Biochim. Biophys. Acta* **173**, 377.

Weinstein, D. B., Marsh, J. B., Glick, M. C., and Warren, L. (1969). *J. Biol. Chem.* **244**, 4103.

Weinstein, D. B., Marsh, J. B., Glick, M. C., and Warren, L. (1970). *J. Biol. Chem.* **245**, 3928.

Weinstein, R. S., and Someda, K. (1967). *Cryobiology* **4**, 116.

Weiser, M. M. (1973a). *J. Biol. Chem.* **248**, 2536.

Weiser, M. M. (1973b). *J. Biol. Chem.* **248**, 2542.

Wetzel, M. G., and Korn, E. D. (1969). *J. Cell Biol.* **43**, 90.

Wheeler, G. E., Coleman, R., and Finean, J. B. (1972). *Biochim. Biophys. Acta* **255**, 817.

Whittaker, V. P., Michaelson, I. A., and Kirkland, R. J. A. (1964). *Biochem. J.* **96**, 293.

Widnell, C. C., and Unkeless, J. C. (1968). *Proc. Nat. Acad. Sci. U.S.* **61**, 1050.

Wilfong, R. F., and Neville, D. M. (1970). *J. Biol. Chem.* **245**, 6106.

Wolff, J., and Jones, A. B. (1971). *J. Biol. Chem.* **246**, 3939.

Yamashita, K., and Field, J. B. (1970). *Biochem. Biophys. Res. Commun.* **40**, 171.

Zingsheim, H. P. (1972). *Biochim. Biophys. Acta* **265**, 339.

Chapter 3

CELL INJURY

B. F. TRUMP AND W. J. MERGNER

I. Introduction

A. Concepts of Cell Injury

Since the work of Rudolph Virchow (1858), the dominant concept of pathology regards disease processes as the result of the reactions of cells to injury (see Rather, 1966). The purpose of the present chapter is to present our current concepts of the consequences and progression of the cellular response to injury. For previous reviews of various aspects of cell injury see the following: Cameron (1951), De Reuck and Knight (1964), Farber and Magee (1966), Trump (1972), Trump and Arstila (1971), Trump and Ericsson (1965), Trump and Ginn (1969), and Trump *et al.* (1969, 1971a, 1972b, 1973a).

1. DEFINITIONS

An injury can be defined as any physical or chemical stimulus that perturbs cellular homeostasis (Trump and Ginn, 1969). Such a perturbation may be transient and rapidly adapted to by the cell with no subsequent effect on homeostatic ability or it may be a more prolonged effect to which the cell may adapt only by a series of structural and functional modifications or to which it succumbs, resulting in cell death. The effects of injury on a cell can be visualized as follows. We might, for example, consider an injury such as complete ischemia. It is clear that when ischemia occurs the cell first enters a reversible stage before it finally passes a "point-of-no-return," after which it is said to be "dead" in the sense that it can no longer recover even if the injurious agent is removed in this case, even if the blood supply is restored (Judah and Rees, 1959; Majno et al., 1960). We can define then, at least in theory, a reversible phase and an irreversible phase. The reversible phase extends from the point of injury to the point-of-no-return. This period of reversibility in ischemia has been estimated to be approximately 20 minutes in the case of heart muscle (Jennings et al., 1969; Sommers and Jennings, 1964) and approximately 25–40 minutes in the case of liver or kidney at 37°C (Baker, 1956; Vogt and Farber, 1968). It is, however, difficult to estimate with certainty in such clamp–reflow studies. Following this point the cells no longer show reversibility or recoverability even if the injurious agent is removed, and the cells therefore enter the phase of necrosis. Necrosis is visualized as a series of predominantly hydrolytic reactions which convert the dead cell to a mass of debris.

Cell death may be defined as the irreversible loss of integrated cell activity resulting in an inability to maintain homeostatic mechanisms. It is, thus, to be clearly distinguished from cell necrosis. Necrosis refers to the subsequent degeneration of a dead cell into component molecules which gradually approach physicochemical equilibrium with the environment (Trump, 1972). Many of the reactions accounting for necrosis are autolytic, that is they are the result of the action of endogenous hydrolytic enzymes, predominantly those within lysosomes. Reactions that occur as part of the necrotic process also include denaturation of protein, alteration of cell pH, and massive ion and water shifts (Trump et al., 1971a). It is to be further noted that cells do not undergo necrosis following all forms of cell death; for example, if cells are killed by lethal agents that inactivate enzyme systems such as a formaldehyde fixative, the cell is essentially stabilized in the prelethal structural state. Of course, such methods form the basis of structural studies of cells since they preserve cells for study by methods such as embedding and sectioning which would otherwise be structurally quite damaging to the cell and its parts. It is also important in this context to define the term *autolysis* since great confusion has been associated with the use of this term over the years (Majno *et al.*, 1960). It is common in pathology to define auto-lysis as the sequence of changes that occur in various internal organs following the death of the animal (Robbins, 1967), and it is often assumed that in some mysterious way such changes differ from necrosis occurring in an organ during the life of an animal, i.e., an ischemic infarct. Detailed studies of the two situations, however, reveal no essential difference in the processes. Some differences, however, do indeed exist in various parts of infarcts. They are largely confined to cells at the infarct margin where collateral circulation makes more extensive ion and water movements to and from the cells possible (Herdson *et al.*, 1965). Cells, therefore, show an accumulation of excessive amounts of calcium by mitochondria. Cells in the center of the infarct do not appear to differ from changes in cells occurring in necrosis *in vitro* unless the former is complicated by such extraneous events as bacterial infection. Strictly speaking, the term autolysis refers to self-digestion. Much of it results from the effects of acid hydrolases derived from lysosomes but other enzy-mes, e.g., those from microorganisms, often contribute. Lysosomes, as will be pointed out later, are ordinarily quite stable even under the conditions of high hydrogen ion concentration, characteristic of necrotic cells (Hawkins *et al.*, 1972). However, in the necrotic phase the enzymes probably finally escape into the cell sap as evidenced by digestion of cell components such as DNA, RNA, and proteins (Berenbom *et al.*, 1955a,b).

2. Effects of Injury on Cells

A general conceptualization of the life of cells and the effects of injury on them is shown in Fig. 1.* In this figure we have shown two principal types of cells termed dividing cells and nondividing cells (see Baserga and Wiebel, 1969, for review). Dividing cells are cells that are in the mitotic cycle and include such cells as primitive cells in the bone marrow, primitive germ cells, and the precursor cells in the intestinal tract. Nondividing cells are cells that are not in the mitotic cycle and are normally assumed to be in prolonged G_1 phase, although some of these cells, such as adult neurons, are so-called "sterile" cells and apparently do not have the capability of reentering the mitotic cycle.

We will first consider the effects of injury on nondividing cells. Following injury, a nondividing cell either dies or does not die. If it dies, it may or may not undergo necrosis, depending on the type of injury (see above). Injured, nondividing cells that do not die may either reenter the cycle and become dividing cells or may not enter the cycle, whereupon the effects of the injury may continue or may disappear, as in the case of reversible injuries. Consider the case of dividing cells. During normal development and during the normal

*See pages 201–257 for all figures.

adult life of a mammal, certain dividing cells leave the mitotic cycle and become nondividing cells, whereupon they are subject to the rules applying to nondividing cells as just mentioned (see reviews by Gelfant and Smith, 1972; and Mueller, 1969). Such situations include, for example the maturation of epidermal cells of the skin, the formation of adult polymorphonuclear leukocytes, and the formation of the mature sperm cells or oocytes (Prescott, 1972). Once this has happened they become subject to the considerations applying to nondividing cells. When an injury is applied to dividing cells, this can either result in death with or without necrosis or may not result in death. If death does not result, the mitotic cycle may become arrested, whereupon the cells become subject to the rules of nondividing cells or cycle arrest does not occur. If cycle arrest does not occur, several possibilities again exist, these include malignant transformation, where the cells continue indefinitely as dividing cells; mitotic death, where the cells undergo death at a subsequent mitotic division; or continued division without transformation, where they become subject to the usual rules applying to dividing cells. Note that in the diagram (Fig. 1) this entire interaction is depicted as a closed system where the only way cells can leave the cycle is by dying.

Perhaps a few examples will serve to clarify this point. First, consider the simple case of killing cells rapidly by chemical fixatives such as osmium tetroxide. In this case, if we apply it either to a dividing or nondividing cell, the cell dies rapidly and does not undergo necrosis. Next consider the case of lethal ischemic damage to a nondividing cell such as a myocardial muscle cell. Following application of the injury to this cell, it does not enter the cycle, but its lifetime is greatly reduced to 30 minutes to 1 hour, whereupon it dies and undergo necrosis. That is, it passes through the diagram as follows: "nondividing" $\longrightarrow$ "does not die" $\longrightarrow$ "does not cycle" $\longrightarrow$ "nondividing" $\longrightarrow$ "dies" $\longrightarrow$ "undergoes necrosis." During this time interval the cell undergoes a multitude of changes which represent the reaction of the cellular regulatory mechanisms to the injurious stimulus. Following death, other reactions occur that are termed necrosis as mentioned above. It is believed that dividing, nontransformed cells normally have a limited number of divisions which are related to the life span of the animal (Krohn, 1966; Hayflick, 1966, 1968; Hayflick and Moorhead, 1961). That is, these cells, though injured by the stress of life, do not die, do not undergo cycle arrest, and keep rotating through the dividing cell box; ultimately, however, they do undergo cycle arrest and become nondividing cells, age, die, and undergo necrosis.

Radiation injury is an example of an injury to a dividing cell that does not result in immediate death, does not result in cycle arrest, but does result in mitotic death at a subsequent division. Malignant transformation of a nondividing cell such as an hepatocyte would involve an injury that does not kill the cell, but which does cause the cell to enter the mitotic cycle and to be affected by a sublethal injury that does not result in cycle arrest and is followed by transformation, whereupon the cell continues indefinitely in the mitotic cycle.

3. PROGRESSION OF CHANGES

A different way of looking at the effects of injury on cells is shown in Fig. 2. For our purposes, cells may be considered as automata, that have the capability of self-replication and self-repair. Thermodynamically, they can be considered as "open" systems that are constantly interacting with their environment (Katchalsky and Curran, 1965). They are not at equilibrium with the environment and accordingly are undergoing constant perturbations because of large chemical, electrical, and other gradients. For example, potassium is continually leaking from the cell and sodium is continually leaking into the cell, and it is only through appropriate active regulatory mechanisms that the cell is able to maintain internal homeostasis in the face of a hostile extracellular environment (Tosteson, 1963). It also seems evident that once a cell leaves the mitotic cycle, which it seems to always do during G_1 phase, either through normal or abnormal stimuli, its lifetime is limited, it begins to age, and ultimately will die unless it succeeds in reentering the mitotic cycle. This ageing is reflected cytologically in cells by the gradual accumulation of pigmented residual bodies which presumably form by autophagy with retention of increasing amounts of membranous and other debris.

In the diagram (Fig. 2) time is plotted along the abscissa, the units of time varying depending on the particular situation under consideration. Levels of homeostatic ability and organizational degradation are plotted along the ordinate. The two are separated by a dotted line which represents the limit of degradation that can be tolerated without the cell passing a "point-of-no-return" and dying.

Higher magnification views illustrating the normal perturbations of homeostasis are shown in two places along the ageing line. The cell is continually adapting to these and we do not normally speak of them as injuries. Note that the perturbations are greater as the cell ages, reflecting the lesser capability with age of regulatory mechanisms to adapt to normal perturbations. Among the hypotheses to explain the slope is progressive protein cross-linking (Björksten, 1971), perhaps due to thermal denaturation (Johnson and Pavelec, 1972). Finally, a line is shown indicating the approach to physicochemical equilibrium with the environment.

Along the top of the graph the events of the mitotic cycle are shown. Note that the slope of this line is parallel with the abscissa, indicating the infinite "life" of cells that stay in the mitotic cycle. In situation 1, a cell in the mitotic cycle is lethally injured at the arrow. The cell rapidly changes its homeostatic ability along line A, passes the point-of-no-return, and undergoes necrosis, attaining physicochemical equilibrium. In situation 2, a cell leaves the G_1 part of the cycle, either through a normal or abnormal stimulus, and begins differentiation. This is accompanied by an increasing slope which is normally termed the "ageing" of the cell, approaching the point of cell death at point 7. This line would, for example, correspond to the life of a typical nondividing cell such as a myocardial muscle cell, a kidney tubule cell, or a liver cell. Situation 3 refers to an injury applied to this cell. In the case of an acute lethal injury such as acute ischemia, the cell descends along "B" and finally passes the point-of-no-return, undergoing necrosis. During the time from event 3 to the time it crosses the point-of-no-return, the cell is undergoing a series of reactions to injury which attempt to restore homeostasis. If the injurious stimulus is removed prior to the point-of-no-return, recovery can occur, along pathways such as B1 or B2 and cells again return to the normal ageing line.

Situation 4 refers to an injury of a nondividing cell which causes the cell to reenter the cell cycle along curve C. Reentry usually occurs in the G_1 phase. In certain types of injury, the cell may undergo mitotic death and leave from M phase along C2 and undergo necrosis; in others, it may continue along curve 5 for a normal span of cell divisions. This is obviously of great importance to repair by regeneration which occurs in the liver and kidney. It should also be noted that injuries to cells in the mitotic cycle may also be followed by mitotic death along C2 at the next or a subsequent mitotic division. Event 5 refers to an injury of the cell in the mitotic cycle which is followed by transformation, indicated by line E. Line D refers to a cell leaving the cycle, ageing, and dying, following its normal span of cell divisions. Event 6 refers to subacute or chronic injury to an ageing, nondividing cell which may be followed by two possibilities, either an increase in the life span along line G or a decreased life span along line F. There are probably many more examples of line F, which probably includes such changes as hypertrophy, atrophy, increased autophagy, and fatty changes, although information regarding the precise effect of these on life span is lacking. There are fewer examples of event G, although the work of Johnson and Pavelec (1972) on effects of slight reductions, of temperature on prolonging cell life in culture may represent such a case.

It should be pointed out that physicochemical meaning for the types of curves shown in Fig. 2 can be adduced. In our studies of cell injury in model systems, where we have monitored intracellular electrolytes, water, and cofactors such as adenine nucleotides, the course of change in these in relation to the time of cell death often follow curves similar to those shown in the figure. A good example is the loss of potassium following an acute injury which follows approximately the type of time course, including the change in slope after the point of cell death, shown by curve B. Recovery, which can be indicated by extrusion of water from swollen slices and recovery of respiration, can be shown to follow a curve approximating B1 or B2 (Trump, 1970).

B. Cellular Control Mechanisms

The structural–functional relationship of cellular transducing systems is emphasized in the following diagram (Fig. 3). It demonstrates several types of energy transduction processes occurring in biological systems such as electron-transport energy, high energy phosphate bond energy, and ion-gradient energy. These are shown as interconvertible through intermediate types of transducing systems indicated by X. Arrows indicate the transformation of energy. For example, transduction of energy derived from electron transport ($\sim e$) into high energy phosphate bond energy ($\sim P$) or ion-gradient energy ($\sim I$) is shown. The transduction proceeds in either direction. Structural changes at some level precede or accompany these transitions. These are indicated by three conformational states $C–C_3$. Regardless of how one considers the hierarchy of structural and functional relations, no one would deny that the structural change is a close concomitant of such interconversions. Various membrane systems possess one or more of these systems and a fairly good case can be made that mitochondria possess all these abilities (Mueller and Rudin, 1969).

The following diagram (Fig. 4) places the mitochondrion in a cellular environment and represents a simplified way of looking at the effects of injury on the whole cell system. The internal environment, on which all metabolic activities are dependent, is maintained, in large part, by the activities of the cell membrane. For example, the action of ion pumps extrudes sodium and calcium and accumulates potassium and magnesium. A large portion of the cellular production of ATP seems to be involved in such ion-regulatory mechanisms, which also are intimately involved with the maintenance of normal cell volume (Tosteson, 1963; Leaf 1959, 1970). In general, these mechanisms are driven by high energy compounds such as ATP which is usually supplied by combinations of mitochondrial and glycolytic phosphorylation. The transport of sodium at the cell surface provides one example of a feedback loop on mitochondrial function because, if the sodium pump is stimulated, more ADP is generated which, in turn, stimulates mitochondrial respiration (Lehninger, 1964). These ion pumps must balance the corresponding leaks into the cell in order to maintain intracellular composition and volume. If these leaks are increased by injury, for example, with antibody and complement (Croker *et al.*, 1970; Hawkins *et al.*, 1972), with mercurials (Sahaphong and Trump, 1971) or with certain antibiotics (Saladino *et al.*,

1969) such as amphotericin, more sodium enters and the pumps must work faster to maintain cell composition. In general, this is associated with stimulation of mitochondrial phosphorylation and with characteristic morphological changes in the mitochondria (Saladino *et al.*, 1969). In the case of hypoxia or ischemia (ischemia being a combination of hypoxia, substrate deficiency, and lack of perfusion), mitochondrial function stops rapidly. The anaerobic glycolytic pathway may maintain the concentration of ATP for a time. The glycolytic pathway is initially believed to be activated through feedback mechanisms such as stimulation of phosphofructokinase (PFK) (Kübler and Spieckermann, 1970). It has been shown that in some systems, especially neoplasias (Williamson *et al.*, 1970), the glycolytic pathway can be stimulated in such a way as to almost replace mitochondrial energy production. *In vivo*, however, the compensation provided by glycolytic ATP production exists only for a limited period of time, and it provides only a limited amount of total energized phosphate compounds. It seems that one common denominator injurious to both aerobic and anaerobic pathways is the rise in hydrogen ion concentration through inhibition of enzymes such as PFK (see review by Sobel, 1972). For example, Kübler and Spiekermann (1970) found that the ATP values in heart muscle fell from their normal of 7 μmoles/gm to 2.5 μmoles/gm within 20 minutes, the approximate time that the point-of-no-return was reached (Braasch *et al.*, 1968). Simultaneously the ADP/ATP ratio increased and a series of changes was noted in the various organelles. Opie (1972) noted also increased PFK activity in the nonschemic myocardium.

In order to consider the effects of acute injury on cells, it is first necessary to consider in more detail the normal relationships between the activities of the cell membrane and cell energy metabolism. This is shown in diagrammatic form in Fig. 5. In this figure, the relationship between glycolysis, the citric acid cycle, the mitochondrial electron-transport, chain and membrane permeability is indicated. Bars are shown for ATP, ADP, inorganic phosphate, NAD, and NADH with indications of feedback, stimulation, or inhibition.

In mammalian cells, cellular volume and ionic composition are regulated by the activity of membrane pumps (usually regarded as ATPases) which must counteract the tendency toward the Donnan equilibrium which occurs because of the presence of negatively charged, nondiffusible intracellular macromolecules, predominantly protein (Netter, 1970). The pump must balance the effects of the leaks of these ions down their concentration gradients; if the pump is inhibited for any reason, the cells will tend to increase in total cation and water content, water being generally assumed to be in equilibrium across the membrane (Tosteson, 1963; Robinson, 1968; Williams and Wacker, 1967).

Consider the case of complement lysis (Hawkins *et al.*, 1972) which renders the membrane more permeable to ions. This causes an influx of sodium and an efflux of potassium, which presumably immediately stimulates the sodium-potassium ATPase. This, in turn, is believed to consume ATP and to generate ADP and inorganic phosphate. The ADP and phosphate act to stimulate mitochondrial phosphorylation, which is heralded by a burst of oxygen consumption. The increased content of intracellular sodium ultimately appears to be inhibitory to mitochondrial function and, thus, its regulatory mechanism cannot be maintained indefinitely. Moreover, if the leak is greater than the pump can handle, which in the case of complement lysis it would be, cell volume control is lost and the cells swell. Further increases in membrane permeability occur later with loss of magnesium and uptake of calcium.

The damaging effects of entering calcium on the cells is partly illustrated in recent paper by Zimmerman et al. (1967) in which reinstitution of calcium perfusion following calcium-free perfusion in the rat heart results in extensive electron microscopic changes identical with those described in stage 5 (see below).

In the presence of phosphate, calcium entering the cell is rapidly accumulated by the mitochondria and forms precipitates of calcium phosphate, usually in the form of apatites within the mitochondrial inner compartment (Figs. 30 and 31) (Saladino et al., 1969; Carafoli et al., 1971; Hawkins et al., 1972; Riley and Schraer, 1972). The pump can also be affected by direct inhibitors of the ATPase such as ouabain or by conditions such as anoxia or metabolic inhibitors that inhibit oxidative phosphorylation and, therefore, limit the supply of ATP to the pump (Trump et al., 1971a; Ginn et al., 1968; Saladino and Trump, 1968; Trump and Ginn, 1969). In this case, changes occur more slowly because the normal leak rates are maintained, at least initially. In the case of anoxia or of inhibitors of the electron-transport system, supply of ATP is shut off acutely. As ATP utilization continues, ADP and inorganic phosphate accumulate. Moreover, as the glycerol phosphate shuttle is shut down in the absence of oxygen, the lactate dehydrogenase begins to effectively compete for NADH (Pasteur effect), and lactate begins to accumulate (Lehninger, 1970). Moreover, the loss of the ATP inhibition at the phosphofructokinase step, together with ADP stimulation, begins to increase the flow along the glycolytic pathway. At the same time, however, accumulation of lactate, phosphate, and other acids including fatty acids lead to accumulations of protons which themselves begin to inhibit the phosphofructokinase reaction. Even though calcium efflux is inhibited and leak occurs, in this case mitochondrial accumulation of calcium does not occur, probably because of limitations of high energy phosphate in the mitochondria as well as the inhibitory effects that protons have on this process (Trump et al., 1971a).

II. Progression of Changes in Lethal Injury

A. Ischemia

1. GENERAL COMMENTS

We will first consider the reactions of cells to lethal injury arbitrarily separating the sequence of changes into stages which have been defined by the study of various experimental models in animal or human systems studied by biopsy or immediate autopsy (see Ginn et al., 1968; Trump et al., 1973a; and reviews by Scarpelli and Trump, 1971; Trump and Arstila, 1971). We will then return to a detailed consideration of the significance of organelle changes at each stage and comment on the interactions between various organelle systems.

There have been various hypotheses advanced to explain why cells lose the ability to survive or why they die following acute lethal injuries such as ischemia, chemical toxins, or microbiological agents. Prominent among these hypotheses have been the "suicide-bag" hypothesis of lysosomes, originally rather cautiously advanced (de Duve and Beaufay, 1959), but which has more recently been regarded as, perhaps, a generalized explanation for lethal injury. Evidence, however, is by no means definitive. Moreover, experiments in out laboratory have constantly failed to reveal such evidence (Trump et al., 1962, 1965b; Goldblatt et al., 1965; Hawkins et al., 1972). Similar arguments have been advanced in the case of protein synthesis, proposing that alterations of this function are limiting for cell survival. It now seems clear that such injury in cells not in the cell cycle (i.e., G_0 or "sterile") is not followed by acute cell death; indeed, it is not associated with significant subcellular alterations, at least acutely.

It is evident from study of model systems conducted in our laboratory that cells lethally injured by a variety of injurious agents, for example, chemical agents, microbiologic agents, physical agents, though varying in the initial interactions and response, ultimately appear to reach a common pattern of change in the necrotic phase which is relatively independent of the cell and injury type (Trump et al., 1971a). This commonality of appearance is presumably related to similarities of organelle function and interaction in various cell types. It is also related to the mechanisms ultimately responsible for loss of cell viability which may be relatively few in number.

On the other hand, it does seem from our studies that there are at least two types of events that will promote acute cell death in a pattern that mimics to a remarkable degree the types of changes that are seen in vivo in mammals, including man. These are: (1) interruption of the functional properties of the cell membrane and (2) primary attack on the bioenergetic system of the cell by either anoxia or ischemia or by models thereof, for example, metabolic inhibitors. Obviously, these two events affect related reactions (Laiho *et al.*, 1971).

2. STAGES OF CELL INJURY

Figure 8 shows our hypothesis of the progression of organelle changes following acute lethal injury. Stage 1 is a normal cell (Figs. 9 and 10). Following lethal injury, progression through the stages 2–7 occurs. The following represents our working hypothesis of the pathogenetic sequence. Following the cessation of vascular perfusion the initial cellular effects include decreased pO_2, decreased removal of cell by-products, and limitation of extrinsic substrate. This is quickly followed by decrease and then absence of respiration which is, in turn, rapidly followed by decrease in the levels of intracellular ATP and increase in the levels of ADP and inorganic phosphate (Williamson *et al.*, 1970). Among the consequences of this is stimulation of phosphofructokinase activity (Kübler and Spieckermann, 1970), an increased rate of glycolysis, increased lactate and decreased glycogen, and a decrease in cell pH (stage 1A). One of the effects of the decrease in cell pH is clumping of nuclear chromatin (Fig. 14) (Trump *et al.*, 1965c) which, in turn, is followed by inactivity of nuclear RNA synthesis (Hay and Revel, 1963; Littau *et al.*, 1964). This is clearly a reversible change (Trump and Bulger, 1968a; (Fig. 16). Among the consequences of the fall in ATP concentration is a decrease in the activity of ion pumps at the cell membrane that lead to leaks of sodium, potassium, calcium, and magnesium down their concentration gradients. However, these changes are, so far as we know, not expressed until a somewhat later stage. Very early after ischemic injury the mitochondria lose their matrix granules (Trump *et al.*, 1965a).

One of the earliest changes that can be seen in cells after a variety of acute lethal injuries is enlargement of the volume of the endoplasmic reticulum that is reflected in dilatation of the endoplasmic reticulum (stage 2) (Fig. 12) (Smuckler *et al.*, 1962; Smuckler and Trump, 1968; Trump *et al.*, 1965d). This initial change can be correlated with increased sodium and decreased potassium content of the cell and often with increased water content (Trump, 1970), although recent studies by Laiho and Trump (1973) indicate that significant dilatation of the endoplasmic reticulum can occur with decreased total cell volume. The implied mechanism is intracellular redistribution of fluid. This stage also is clearly reversible and occurs before the point-of-no-return (Trump and Bulger, 1968b; Bassi and Bernelli-Zazzera, 1964).

At this time the contours of cell membrane structures such as microvilli begin to be distorted (Figs. 13 and 26) and alterations in the membrane-associated magnesium-dependent ATPase can be seen (Goldblatt *et al.*, 1965; Trump *et al.*, 1962). As the pH continues to fall in the cell sap, it is probable that inhibition of PFK occurs, with a gradual decrease in the rate of glycolysis, tending to stabilize with the glycogen levels at low but significantly greater than zero values and resulting in continuation of the fall in cellular ATP concentration. This fallen ATP begins to be reflected by decreased functions of the various active systems such as protein synthesis, continued cessation of ion pumps at the cell surface, and most probably by cessation of ion accumulation by mitochondria which begin to undergo shrinkage of the inner compartment.

This shrinkage heralds the onset of stage 3 (Fig. 17) which can be re-produced *in vitro* by conditions that inhibit respiration (Laiho *et al.*, 1971; Saladino and Trump, 1968; Croker *et al.*, 1970) or that result in stimulation of respiration by formation of ADP (Saladino *et al.*, 1969), both of which are accompanied by loss of ions such as potassium from the inner compartment. As long as the mitochondria remain condensed, intactness of the inner membrane is implied and probably this also implies preservation of function by the inner membranes (Trump, 1973) since the structural proteins of the membrane are essentially synonymous, so far as is known, with the active enzyme proteins such as the coupling factors and electron-transport proteins (Vanderkooi, 1972). At this stage the condensation of mitochondria is associated with dilatation of endoplasmic reticulum (ER) and cell sap, both of which correlate with gradual increases in sodium and water contents as well as with decreases in potassium and magnesium. Decreased potassium content is another factor which is associated with inhibited protein synthesis (Lubin, 1967), although at this stage the membrane-bound polysomes appear unaltered and maintain both their ordered arrangements and their membrane attachments (Trump *et al.*, 1965d). The increased water content at this stage is often reflected by the presence of blebs or "blisters" on the cell surface. Within the blebs the viscosity of the protoplasm is low as inferred from increased Brownian motion of cytoplasmic particles, by its loosened appear-ance in electron micrographs, and by its lack of density with phase and interference microscopy. Blebs on the cell surface are especially dramatic in time lapse movies where they are seen to appear and disappear rather rapidly (Zollinger, 1948). They appear as if fluid of low viscosity had accumulated in the ectoplasmic zone, resulting in blistering and blebbing of the cell surface. By now the chromatin clumping has become more marked and it is probable that the pH of the cytoplasm is still decreasing.

Although stages 1A, 2, and 3 seem to be clearly reversible (Trump and Bulger, 1968b), the changes soon become irreversible and manifested in the cell by the appearance of stage 4. Among the factors which appear to be in-volved in this transformation are a series of membrane permeability changes involving the mitochondria and the cell membrane, both of which probably reflect basic chemical as well as structural changes in the molecular architec-ture of these respective membranes.

These events are most dramatically reflected by increased inner membrane permeability in mitochondria and the beginning of high amplitude swelling in many mitochondrial profiles which characterize stage 4 (Fig. 18) (Mergner *et al.*, 1972a). Swelling is associated with increased contents of sodium, potassium, and calcium in the inner compartments, although the precise nature of the ions present in the mitochondria probably depends on the composition of the cytoplasm. Among the factors which may result in this structural damage to the mitochondrial inner membrane is the continued magnesium deficiency (Mergner *et al.*, 1972a) and possibly the release of fatty acids and phospholipids resulting from phospholipase action on membranes (Boime *et al.*, 1968). Moreover, the mitochondrion possesses endogenous phospholipases which can be activated by factors such as increased levels of calcium known to be present at this time. Functionally, the structural changes are reflected by alteration in the function of F_1 particles, measurable as a change in the magnesium-stimulated ATPase activity in the inner membrane and by a decreased respiratory control index (Trump *et al.*, 1971). Some of this is also reflected by a decrease in the P/O ratio (Fonnesu and Severi, 1956). In the endoplasmic reticulum, although the ribosomes remain attached to the membrane surface, their capacity to incorporate amino acids in isolated microsomes incubated *in vitro* is reduced and the organization of ribosomes into polysomes seems to be altered (Smuckler and Trump, 1968). Since the defective amino acid incorporation can be repaired at this stage by addition of artificial messengers such as poly U, a messenger ribosome- association defect was postulated. This appears to coincide with the recent result of Sarma *et al.* (1972) on carbon tetrachloride poisoning in livers. This study also suggested that factors other than the messenger-ribosome association appear to be important in maintaining the ribosome membrane interaction. Change in membrane stability is also manifested by whorl formations involving the cell membrane, especially in areas of redundancy such as invaginations, for example, at the base of renal tubular cells, and villi (Trump and Ginn, 1969).

In the next stage the cells become clearly irreversibly altered and enter the phase of necrosis (Figs. 19 and 20). This is characterized by massive swelling of all mitochondria (Trump *et al.*, 1962, 1965c; Caesar, 1961; Caulfield and Klionsky, 1959; Huebner and Bernhard, 1961), which show a marked increase in membrane permeability associated with leak of proteins, including matrix enzymes and cofactors (Griffin *et al.*, 1965a,b; Jennings, 1965; Jennings *et al.*, 1969) to the cell sap and ultimately through the cell membrane to the extracellular space (Goldblatt *et al.*, 1965). Cell sap enzymes are probably lost before mitochondrial or other organelle enzymes (Farrell *et al.*, 1972). In the case of CPK, the mitochondrial CPK appears not to contribute to the serum elevation. The question of the usefulness of mitochondrial marker enzymes for evaluation of mitochondria intactness was examined by

Pycock and Nahorski (1971). The authors concluded that the most satisfactory mitochondrial indicator enzyme in rat heart was succinate dehydrogenase and isocitrate dehydrogenase. The inner membrane shows denaturation of the F_1 particles and continued inactivation of the inner membrane magnesium-stimulated ATPase.

It should be noted that although the inner membrane spheres on small stalks are easily visible by negative staining if mitochondria are treated in hypotonic solutions, either prior to or during negative staining; they may not exhibit this configuration in the normal *in vivo* state (Mergner *et al.*, 1972b). Experiments in our laboratory have recently indicated that in the native state they may be embedded in or on the membrane, possibly representing a closely associated intrinsic membrane protein. However, the hypotonic negative-staining treatment provides a satisfactory way to visualize these on tubular membrane derivatives (Sjöstrand *et al.*, 1964) and to correlate structure and function in normal and abnormal mitochondria, and their disappearance or change in the negative-stained images does appear to correlate with the magnesium-stimulated ATPase activity as determined chemically. Also at this time prominent flocculent densities appear in the inner compartment (Trump *et al.*, 1965a), presumably the result of denaturation of matrix proteins (Trump *et al.*, 1965a). Among the factors that may be responsible is the entry of protons into the inner compartment from the cell sap which is maximally acidic at this time. Change in the cell membrane at this stage is characterized by marked increases in permeability, as measured by penetration of large particles such as vital dyes and decrease in membrane electrical resistance. Black and Berenbom (1964) proposed several mechanisms for the increased uptake of vital dyes. Factors which, according to the authors, influence the reliability of the positive dye exclusion test are serum concentration, cell concentration, and staining time. This is also reflected by leak of cell sap enzymes such as lactate dehydrogenase into the medium. Further changes in the cell surface membrane include greater development and compaction of the whorls, especially in areas with membrane redundancy, and separation of cell junctions. The latter might be attributable to the increase in intracellular calcium reported by Loewenstein (1973) to foster the separation of cells in the region of junctional complexes. At this stage, the lysosomes begin to swell as evidenced by increased size and clarification of the matrix (Trump *et al.*, 1965b) and condensation of the contents. Although this is probably reflected by increased free and unsedimentable activity in tissue homogenates or in isolated lysosome fractions (Griffin *et al.*, 1965a,b), there is no evidence of release of marker proteins such as ferritin from the lysosomes into the cell sap at this stage (Hawkins *et al.*, 1972). Although in models of cell injury we reported a leak of acridine orange into the cytoplasm, it appears that this can be explained on the basis of the loss of the pH gradient between the lysosome and the cell exterior with structural changes in the inner membrane spheres by negative staining (Mergner *et al.*, 1972b; Hawkins *et al.*, 1972). It is estimated that lysosomes maintain a gradient of 1 to 2 pH units below the cytoplasm, which means they might be estimated to have an internal pH of 5 to 4.5. As the cell pH decreases, this gradient is lost, and dye molecules such as acridine orange, which are more lipid soluble in nonassociated form, probably redistribute. Acridine orange staining of lysosomes can probably be used as an indicator of cell pH in the sense that once the lysosome–cytoplasm gradient is lost, the acridine leaks into the cell sap, where it appears green instead of orange because it is dispersed in a larger volume.

In phase 6 the changes are mainly characterized by a rapid acceleration in the rate of digestion of intracellular constituents as measured by increases in free amino acids, acid-soluble phosphorus, and decreases in protein, DNA, and RNA (Berenbom *et al.*, 1955a,b). This is reflected morphologically by beginning karyolysis and changes in the staining pattern of the cytoplasm, including increased affinity for anionic dyes such as eosin (Trump *et al.*, 1965c). At this stage there is evidence that lysosomal contents can escape into the cell and, indeed, the disappearance of the macromolecular components of the cell, as well as the persistence of lysosomal hydrolases as compared with many other enzymes, strongly indicates that lysosomal leakage is followed by digestion. Other membrane systems show great rearrangements including vesiculation, wrappings, formation of tubular forms in the inner compartment of mitochondria, disappearance of ribosomes from the ER membrane surface, alterations in the nucleolus, disappearance of microbody matrices, and frequent visualization of breaks in the plasma membrane contour.

The final stage (stage 7) (Fig. 22) is characterized by the appearance of new structures in the cytoplasm which occur as large, dense inclusions, often larger than the nucleus, composed of dense, homogeneous, osmiophilic material with lamellar regions in lacunae within the bodies or at the margins of the bodies (Trump *et al.*, 1965d). These periodic regions resemble stacks of membranes, although the fine structure within the bodies has not been discerned. These bodies seemingly correspond to the myelin of Virchow, so-named because of the resemblance to bodies which Virchow observed during autolysis in various cell types and their similarity to the bodies which form by aqueous interaction with the white matter of the central nervous system. The precise chemical nature of these bodies has not been defined. They probably contain mixtures of lipid, including cholesterol, phospholipid, and fatty acids, and some may represent metal soaps of fatty acids. In general, at this stage most enzyme activities, including the lysosomal hydrolases, have approached zero, and by light microscopy the cells have the familiar appearance of cells at the center of an old infarct with eosinophilia, karyolysis, and indistinct cell outlines. Cells in a typical infarct become more or less stabilized in this condition, probably through the fixation effect of denaturation unless other factors are present such as occur in caseous or gummatous necrosis. In part, this is probably explainable on the basis that hydrolases and other enzymes are inactivated, and unless other sources of enzymes such as those produced by microorganisms are present the cells are stabilized for long periods of time in this state. Furthermore, equilibration once again occurs during phase 7 when the extracellular fluid pH approaches physiological levels. Greater and greater calcium binding by these cells is observed, possibly related to the change in pH as well as to changes in reactive protein sites. How much of the calcium binding is mitochondrial is not known, and it is not likely that much of it is since typical calcifications are not seen and since a source of energy for its accumulation is not present. (See also Trump *et al.*, 1972a.)

B. *Other Types of Lethal Injury*

Although we know most about lethal and acute injury from ischemia and related conditions such as inhibition of mitochondrial function with or without inhibition of glycolysis, certain differences between this and other forms of acute injury have recently been defined. Aside from ischemia, the next best understood example is lethal injury resulting from direct attack on the cell membrane. This can be induced in cells by several means including antibody and complement (Green *et al.*, 1959), nonpenetrating organic mercurials such as PCMBS (Fig. 11), polyene antibiotics such as amphotericin, ultraviolet irradiation, and surfactants (Saladino *et al.*, 1971), and direct mechanical injury to the cell membrane (Trump and Bulger, 1968b). Cells injured by the above-mentioned agents at the appropriate concentrations develop rapid cell death and lysis which can be most readily studied and measured in isolated cells either in monolayer or suspension culture. The principal difference between this and cell injury following ischemic damage is the rate of response and the magnitude of the cell volume alteration (Fig. 6). Once a lethal injury is applied to the cell membrane, cells rapidly swell because of the so-called colloid osmotic lysis, first recognized in erythorocyte lysis. Ehrlich ascites cells treated with PCMBS show increases in volume of up to 200 to 300 % of the zero time control within 1 hour (Laiho *et al.*, 1971). Within the first 5 minutes the cells pass from stage 1 to stage 3 and within the first 30 minutes to stage 5. This is presumably initiated by rapid entry of the extracellular fluid and leak into the various intracellular compartments with rapid progression from stage 1 to stage 5. One of the factors, namely, decreased cytoplasmic pH, may well be absent since equilibration occurs rapidly with the extracellular fluid. This, in turn, is probably related to a difference in behavior of cationic intralysosomal dyes such as acridine orange, which in this form of injury maintain their intralysosomal localization right through stage 5 and into stage 6, probably because rapid equilibration with the extracellular fluid at physiological pH permits maintenance of the normal pH gradient across the lysosomal membrane. Other data such as retention of markers including ferritin indicate that lysosomal membrane integrity is maintained well into the phase of necrosis. In injury directed at the plasma membrane, mitochondrial calcification (Fig. 21) readily occurs (Gritzka and Trump, 1968; Reynolds, 1965).

The two examples, then, represent two basic reasonably well-understood models of acute lethal cell injury; that is, conditions that interfere with mitochondrial supply of high energy compounds and injuries that directly attack the cell membrane. In regard to the cell membrane, a sequence essentially identical to that seen after ischemia can be reproduced in cells treated with ouabain, a specific inhibitor of the cell membrane ATPase (Ginn *et al.*, 1968). Other commonly studied systems of acute injury are less well understood either because of the complexities of the studies related to the type of model or because of insufficient studies. A good example is carbon tetrachloride-induced liver necrosis. In this model centrilobular necrosis of the liver occurs 12 to 24 hours after the oral administration of the compound. Although available evidence favors the notion that cell injury is mediated by membrane peroxidation induced by free radical resulting from cell metabolism of carbon tetrachloride (Recknagel, 1967; Glende and Recknagel, 1969), the pathogenetic sequence at the subcellular level is not understood. Dilatation of the ER and dispersions of polysomes represent early and probably reversible changes, although this cannot be well tested with carbon tetrachloride, (Reynolds, 1963, 1965; Stowell and Lee, 1950). It is presently debated whether, in fact, these ribosomes initially detach from the membrane (Smuckler and Arcasoy, 1969; Smuckler and Benditt, 1965). Cell membrane injury is soon associated with a decreased transmembrane potential difference and rapid falls in cellular ATP levels. Similar conclusions were reached by Enwonwu (1972). By 8 and 12 hours, mitochondria undergo condensation, typical of stage 3, and beginning within a few minutes after giving carbon tetrachloride, changes resembling peroxidation lesions of microsomes *in vitro* can be seen. Experience with model-type experiments mentioned above would suggest that the important interactions involve either the cell membrane, the mitochondrial membrane, or both; however, because of the difficulties in timing the onset of lethal change in this *in vivo* system, it is difficult at the moment to define the pathogenesis with certainty. The carbon tetrachloride studies do serve to emphasize the context of the final common pathway following diverse types of injury, although the initial interactions with the injurious agents certainly vary. It also seems to provide an example that demonstration of the earliest observable morphological and biochemical changes following administration of a compound to an animal does not assure importance in terms of pathogenesis of lethal injury since defects in protein synthesis occur within an hour (Bernelli-Zazzera *et al.*, 1960; Smuckler *et al.*, 1962) and, although initially it was suggested that this might lead to cell death, many recent experiments employing other inhibitors of protein synthesis on G_0 cells including rat liver parenchymal cells (Shelburne *et al.*, 1973; Verbin *et al.*, 1971; Shelburne and Trump, 1968) indicate that virtually complete inhibition of protein synthesis is not followed by acute cell death of the type seen after carbon tetrachloride. Although earlier experiments utilizing puromycin seem to indicate that the inhibition of protein synthesis was related to puromycin cytotoxicity, recent studies by Longnecker (1972) seem to indicate that these cytotoxic effects may be caused by puromycin-induced toxic peptides, since retreatment by cycloheximide prevents the cytotoxic effects on the pancreas of puromycin. Furthermore, cycloheximide alone in doses giving comparable inhibition of protein synthesis does not produce toxicity equivalent to puromycin. The long-term effects of inhibition of protein synthesis in G_0 cells have not been established although it seems probably that ultimately cell death would, in fact, result. In this vein it is established that enucleation of cells such as amoeba is also not followed by acute death but is compatible with survival for several days. Thus, neither the genetic nor the protein synthetic apparatus seems to be critical for survival over short time periods measured, at least in some cells, in days.

Figure 7 shows three parameters of ischemic liver homogenates: adenosine triphosphatase (ATPase) activity, indicating integrity of the machinery for oxidative phosphorylation; free amino acids, indicating the function of released hydrolytic enzymes; and hydrogen ion concentration, indicating the changes in the internal environment of cells caused by partially inhibited metabolism. The striking difference in the time relationship indicates that alteration of the bioenergetic machinery and metabolic events have come to an end within 30 minutes to 1 hour; that is long before acid hydrolases have any significant effect, which is 6 hours after injury, and also long before their maximum activity is reached (24 hours).

C. The Suicide-Bag Hypothesis

During the past 10 years, the concept has frequently been advanced that lysosomes may burst open within injured but still living cells and that the subsequent release of hydrolytic enzymes into the cell sap and inappropriate self-digestion may be significant factors in causing the death of the cell (Hawkins *et al.*, 1972). This hypothesis has two parts: first, that release of enzymes from lysosomes should occur, following a specific injury, prior to the cell death; and second, that this extent of antemortem enzyme release should be sufficient to cause the death of injured cells in some cases.

A great deal of biochemical evidence, taken from many different models of cell injury, has been presented in support of the concept of lysosomes as threats to the survival of injured cells (Van Lancker and Holtzer, 1959). In most cases, the data are insufficient to firmly establish this concept, however, since it is difficult, if not impossible, to distinguish the enzyme release from lysosomes which might occur in intact injured cells from the enzyme solubilization which occurs during the processes of homogenizing the cells and preparing subcellular fractions. This induced solubilization may well be greater when injured cells are homogenized. Some histochemical studies have been interpreted as suggesting rupture of lysosomes before cell death (Bitensky, 1963; Bitensky et al., 1963), and some have yielded evidence inconsistent with this interpretation (Trump and Bulger, 1968a; Ericsson et al., 1967; Trump et al., 1965b; Goldblatt et al., 1965). Electron microscopic studies of well-controlled models of cell injury have generally failed to provide evidence for antemortem lysosome rupture, but this negative evidence is inconclusive, because of the vagaries of fixation in injured cells and the uncertainty as to the expected appearance of cells whose lysosomes have discharged their enzymes. Previous studies have failed to disclose evidence of perilysosomal deterioration; however, even if lysosomal enzymes were released, it has been suggested that they would diffuse rapidly throughout the cell.

In experiments utilizing two types of cell injury in a tissue culture system, the possibility was tested that lysosome rupture may be a lethal cellular reaction to injury and thus an important general cause of irreversibility of damage in injured tissue. Prior labeling of secondary lysosomes with the fluorochrome acridine orange (Robbins and Marcus, 1963; Allison and Young, 1961; Canonico and Bird, 1969) and with ferritin was used to trace changes in lysosomes after applying an injury. The metabolic inhibitors were used to block the cell's energy supply. Antiserum and subsequent complement attack were applied to damage the surface membrane, producing rapid loss of cell volume control. The cytolytic action of complement was lethal to sensitized cells within 2 hours, but results showed that lysosomes did not rupture for approximately 4 hours and in fact did not release the fluorescent dye until after reaching the postmortem necrotic phase of injury. Cells treated with metabolic inhibitors also showed irreversible alterations, while lysosomes remained intact and retained the ferritin marker. The fluorochrome marker, acridine orange, escaped from lysosomes early after metabolic injury.

Recent studies on the existance of a pH gradient of between 1 and 2 between the lysosomal interior and exterior suggests a mechanism whereby release of acridine orange after inhibition of energy metabolism could occur. Since acridine orange is a cationic dye which is lipid soluble, existence of a decreased pH inside the lysosome would favor its accumulation in lysosomes.

Acridine orange has the interesting property of showing metachromatic red fluorescence when it is bound in high concentrations and a green fluorescence when it is present in low concentration. When it is concentrated in the lysosomes it fluoresces red-orange, but after release and binding to other cell components it fluoresces green (Bradley, 1961).

Since the pH of the cytoplasm is known to decrease markedly after inhibition of energy metabolism, this would disperse the gradient and be expected to redistribute the acridine orange. The fact that this does not occur after complement lysis can be explained on the basis of rapid equilibration of extracellular with intracellular pH after induced leak in the cell membrane, thus maintaining the gradient across the lysosome membrane. The results are interpreted as evidence against the concept that lysosome rupture threatens the survival of injured cells. Lysosomes appear to be relatively stable organelles which, following injury of the types studied, burst only after cell death, acting then as scavengers which help to clear cellular debris (Hawkins *et al.*, 1972).

Additional possible conditions resulting in cell death following the proposed mechanism of the suicide-bag hypothesis of de Duve have recently been presented. Weissmann and co-workers (for review, see Weissmann, 1971; Schumacher and Phelps, 1971) have presented evidence that crystals of sodium urate behave in a fashion somewhat similar to that proposed for silica after engulfment and containment within the digestive vacuoles (Allison, 1968). It has been proposed that both of these crystal types appear to be membrane lytic for both natural and artificial membrane systems affecting membrane hydrogen bonds and resulting in perforation of the limiting membrane of the digestive vacuole and release of hydrolases into the cytoplasm. Additional evidence presented in favor of this hypothesis is simultaneous release of both cytoplasmic and lysosomal enzymes to the extracellular space. Unfortunately, however, in neither of these cases has ultrastructural evidence of membrane defects or leakage of intralysosomal probe molecules into the cytoplasm prior to cell death been presented. It has recently been suspected that factors other than the lysosome-limiting membrane may be important in lysosomal enzyme binding or release (Hawiger *et al.*, 1972). Somewhat similar arguments have been adduced for silica (Allison *et al.*, 1966a,b). Preliminary experiments in our laboratory using asbestos and silica indicate that marker probes such as horseradish peroxidase are retained within the lysosome at a time when the cell has undergone necrosis by the criteria defined above (M. L. Shin and B. F. Trump, unpublished observation). It should also be pointed out that data are lacking by which sequential release of enzymes from various intracellular compartments can be timed and correlated with the onset of cell death. For example, we do not presently know whether release of cytoplasmic enzymes such as lactate dehydrogenase can occur prior to the point of cell death. Furthermore, it has not been established in either the silica case or the monosodium urate case whether the lysosome is still in continuity with the extracellular space. Continuity of phagolysosomes with the extracellular space has been recognized in the case of bacterial phagocytosis and presumably is responsible for the leak of hydrolases into the surrounding medium following phagocytosis (Henson, 1972). In the case of simple phagocytosis this may not be accompanied by seepage of cytoplasmic marker enzymes. In the case of silica and monosodium urate it is conceivable that damage to the phagolysosomal membrane occurs while continuity still exists with the cell surface, permitting rapid influx of extracellular fluid into the cell sap and rapid efflux of both lysosomal and cell sap enzymes to the extracellular space. If this is the case, then it becomes merely a variant of damage to the cell membrane itself, which has been well characterized for the case of complement lysis or nonpenetrating mercurials.

It has been previously proposed that photosensitization in which lysosomes are loaded with compounds such as acridine orange followed by irradiation with blue light which induces so-called membrane photo-oxidation was evidence of the suicide-bag mechanism since dispersion of acridine orange in the cytoplasm was seen after ultraviolet irradiation (Allison et al., 1966a,b). We recently repeated these experiments in which we loaded Chang cell lysosomes both with ferritin and with acridine orange and then irradiated with blue light. Rapid cytolysis and dispersion of acridine orange were noted. Electron microscopic study of thin sections revealed dispersal of ferritin from the lysosomes into the cell sap and, also, into the nucleoplasm concometantly with typical stage V type changes. This experiment is important in that it shows that if particles are released from the lysosomes they can, indeed, be visualized in the cell sap and are not washed out during the fixation and embedding process; furthermore, it emphasizes that distribution of lysosomal contents within the cell cytoplasm can occur very rapidly. On the other hand, they do not definitively establish the suicide-bag mechanism, since interaction of the blue light with acridine orange molecules bound to the cell surface could result in the cell membrane-type of progression through the cell injury sequence rapidly, as described above. In a recent study of viral infection, Allison and Mallucci (1965) suggested that the suicide-bag mechanism might play a role in lysosomal and cell injury and death following lytic virus infection. We repeated these experiments in which the lytic virus polio was inoculated in HeLa cell cultures. The process of cell lysis was followed over a 24-hour period. Lysis began to occur around 8 to 10 hours after inaculation. When the lysosomes of the HeLa cells had been preloaded with acridine and ferritin prior to polio virus interaction, the sequence proceeded as usual, however, dispersal of ferritin into the cell sap did not occur nor did the acridine dissipate from the lysosomes (Daniels *et al.*, 1973; Allison and Sandelin, 1963).

D. *Notes on Other Types of Acute Lethal Injury*

The foregoing mainly represents our interpretation of the events following two types of acute lethal injury, inhibition of ATP synthesis and direct attack on the cell membrane. Obviously there are many other situations in which acute lethal injury occurs, however, at the present time these have not been sufficiently elucidated to warrant inclusion in this chapter. For example, an important cause of lethal injury in several fields of biomedical science is the damage resulting from freezing and thawing. Precise mechanisms have not been completely worked out, however, most recent investigators in the area favor the notion that damage by intracellular ice crystals, either direct or through changes in the local microenvironment induced by reduced salt concentration, results in lethal injury primarily through the effects on cell membranes (Trump *et al.*, 1964). A possible role of lysosomal hydrolases has also been postulated. Acute lethal injury by membrane peroxidation was mentioned above in context with carbon tetrachloride interactions, however, there may well be many other substantial examples of such damage including damage by primiquin or other peroxidizing agents in glucose 6-phosphate dehydrogenase–deficient erythrocytes. Damage caused by mechanical trauma has been incompletely investigated however, some parameters of membrane deformation in erythrocytes have been studied (Rand, 1964; Rand and Burton, 1964; Lundquist *et al.*, 1971; Weed and LaCelle, 1969; Weed *et al.*, 1969). The overall role of cell volume regulation by cells in the pathogenesis of acute lethal injury, though highly suggestive, needs much further exploration before each of these findings can be related to this overall theory. Damage by irradiation and antimitotic agents has hardly been explored; the concept of mitotic cell death needs much further study to rationalize it with our other concepts of acute cell injury (de Estable-Puig and Estable-Puig, 1971; de Estable-Puig *et al.*, 1971).

III. Chronic Cell Injury

Many types of cell injury do not result in acute cell death but result in prolonged changes which represent new or altered steady states which may be reversible or irreversible and associated in theory with retardation of prolongation of the cell's life span. Such reactions may involve any of the cell's organelles and often are reflected by characteristic patterns of organelle change. At the present time the only satisfactory way to consider these alterations is by presenting the primary alterations of each cellular system. After doing this, however, we will attempt to show how interactions between various systems can result in the classic patterns of chronic cell injury.

A. Alterations Predominantly Involving the Cell Membrane

1. ALTERATIONS IN TRANSPORT AND PERMEABILITY

A variety of conditions change membrane characteristics and can be associated with modifications in membrane transport and permeability phenomena. These include disorders related to cation and water movements as well as specific transport defects for substrates such as amino acids. It appears that these conditions can be either congenital or acquired. The acquired forms often result from toxic interactions with the cell surface.

The best studied of this type is aminoaciduria which changes in the excretion of specific groups of amino acids in the urine resulting from defects in transport of amino acids by the proximal tubular cells (Christensen, 1968, 1973). This can be a genetic abnormality or it can result from toxicity, for example, administration of lead (Goyer, 1968). In the latter case, the defect may be less of a primary defect in the cell membrane since it may result from interaction of lead with mitochondria. More examples are known of defects in cation transport and permeability, especially in the erythrocyte. A variety of types of hemolytic anemias are associated with alterations in sodium/potassium transport often accompanied by increased cation permeability of the cell membrane (Parker and Welt, 1972). Examples of this include malaria, congenital hemolytic anemia, sickle cell anemia, and lead toxicity. Direct modification of the cell membrane cation pump following therapy with digitalis can also be demonstrated with subsequent effects on red cell ionic composition. In a disease which involves widespread cellular disturbances in ion transport such as cystic fibrosis, abnormalities in red cell transport have also been described. In the syndrome associated with shock, burns, uremia, and related diseases, termed the "sick-cell" syndrome by Welt (1967), there seems to be an acquired abnormality in transport resulting in increased sodium and decreased potassium content of red cells (see Parker and Welt, 1972, for review). Genetic defects in cation transport have been well characterized in the so-called high and low potassium sheep red cells, and recently it has been shown that incubation of successive generations of cells with ouabain will select a population of resistant cells which possess no sensitivity toward ouabain. Changes in the transport ability at various stages of differentiation have also been described by Christensen (1968, 1973), and it is probable that the neoplastic transformation of cells is also associated with altered transport properties at the cell surface membrane. The potential importance of protein lipid interactions in cell membrane properties is emphasized by so-called Zieve syndrome (Westerman *et al.*, 1968), which exists in alcoholics and involves abnormalities of plasma and red cell membrane lipids with correlated changes in red cell osmotic fragility. For reviews of this subject, see Sciver (1970), Lessin *et al.*, (1972), McKay *et al.* (1969), and Siekevitz (1972).

Prominent cell shape changes occur in the injured renal corpuscle where the visceral epithelial cells undergo so-called "loss" of foot processes or foot process "fusion" in the nephrotic syndrome. The mechanism of this has been argued over the years and, on the basis of thin sections, it was inferred that it could not result from fusion but probably from a shape change (Trump and Benditt, 1962). This concept was recently confirmed by scanning electron microscopy. Arakawa and Tokunaga (1972) concluded that so-called fusion is not caused by syncytial formation but rather by swelling and retraction of the process. As noted in the earlier paper based on thin sections, this is much more compatible with reversal as determined by levels of protein in the urine.

Electron microscopic evidence of "pores" induced in the plasma membrane during complement lysis has been described by Dourmashkin and Rosse (1966).

2. NEOPLASIA

Changes in the characteristics of the cell surface and especially the glycocalyx (Bennett, 1963) represent striking and probably important expressions of the neoplastic transformation (Emmelot and Benedetti, 1967; Warren *et al.*, 1973; Sakiyama and Robbins, 1973; Burger, 1973) (Fig. 25). This is a rapidly developing field but already it is clear that many properties of the neoplastic cell including disordered patterns of growth, invasion, metastasis, and defective intercellular communications are likely to be related to changes in the properties of the cell surface. Among the properties that have been elucidated are changes in the organization of cell junctions, changes in surface charge, appearance of new surface antigens and agglutinin-binding sites such as Conconavalin A-binding sites and carcinoembryonic antigen (Gold and Freedman, 1965), and changes in the glycocalyx.

Inbar *et al.* (1972) have recently reviewed changes in binding sites and proposed that changes in the surface structure and transformation can be explained by three types of changes in binding sites: an exposure of cryptic sites, a concentration of exposed sites by decreased cell size, and a rearrangement of exposed sites without a decrease in cell size resulting in clustering of sites. All three changes result in an increased density of sites in the surface areas that contain sites. These changes probably illustrate the importance of cell surface modifications in cell behavior and cell–cell interactions, although it is not presently known whether they are to be considered as primary or secondary events of malignant transformation.

3. VIRAL-INDUCED CHANGES IN THE CELL SURFACE

The general field of cellular virology provides numerous and often dramatic examples of chronic alterations in cell surface properties (Warren *et al.*, 1973; Brady *et al.*, 1973; Sakiyama and Robbins, 1973). The cell surface membrane is important in both the uptake and release phase of viral–cell interactions and the membrane may undergo a number of dramatic structural and functional changes during these events. Examples include fusions of encapsulated virus envelopes with the cell membrane during the uptake phase and budding of naked virions out of the cell through or by being enveloped by the cell membrane in the release process as in the case of myxo- and para-myxoviruses (Donnelly and Yunis, 1971). The persistence of viral antigens which are newly formed during the virus infectious cycle seems to be related to the cell fusion that can be induced by viruses, including Sendai and herpes-like virions (Bachi and Howe, 1972). It thus seems evident that addition of viral proteins or other antigens to the cell membrane results in a chronic change in the property of the membrane that is probably related to some of the neoplastic changes mentioned above. Vaccinia virus infection has provided an interesting model of abnormal membrane biogenesis (Dales and Mosbach, 1968; Rafferty, 1973).

4. CELL JUNCTIONS

Still relatively little is known about modifications of junctions in chronic cell injury, though changes have been seen in regeneration (Yee, 1972) and neoplasias. Decrease in the level of extracellular calcium clearly modifies the structure and properties of the cell junctions even in the so-called tight junction regions; this results, also, in marked changes in cell shape (Bulger and Trump, 1969b; Trump and Bulger, 1971; Bennett, 1973). In the kidney tubule when dissociation by treatment in Ca-free medium is induced, the cells tend to round up and general tissue disorganization occurs (Fig. 27). Some of this may be attributable to loss of support sites for intracellular filaments, but other parts of it may be related to defective functions of intracellular filaments and tubules in the absence of extracellular calcium. Changes in junctions in neoplastic cells were mentioned above. A possible role of vesicle-junction interaction in cell–cell communication was recently presented by Peracchia (1972). Changes in cell junctions following trauma have been described (Rhodes and Karnovsky, 1971).

5. Alterations in Movements

Movements of the cell membrane, including pseudopod extension and withdrawal and phagosome and secretory granule fusions and fissions, constitute important activities of this region. Some of these activities seem to be related to activities of cytoplasmic filaments in the large ruffling movements in certain cells that can be modified or prevented by treatment with cytochalasin. Hormone-induced changes in the cell surface have been studied in the thyroid. Mechanisms of formation of various types of ridges, flaps, and septa may occur in the thyroid after stimulation with thyrotropic hormone. In some instances pseudopod-like extensions may break off, forming detached buds of the cytoplasm. This is well known in mitosis but occurs on a smaller scale as well and appears to be important in differentiation of subcell types such as sperm, which at a certain stage elaborates and eliminates part of the cytoplasm through this means. Changes in cell surface contour during the mitotic cycle are dramatic, especially at the time of mitosis when marked blebbing occurs (R. W. Rubin *et al.*, 1972). Red cell degradation in the spleen may involve elaboration of membrane buds, and similar budding has been noted in trauma-induced hemolysis, for example, in patients with ball valve prostheses. In one type of hemolysis, esotropy of the red cell membrane occurs (Fig. 24) (Ginn *et al.*, 1969).

6. Changes in Membrane Turnover; Cell Shape Change

One example of the rapid exotropic type of shape change in the red cell is the formation of so-called echinocyte, which is a spicule bearing, crenated-appearing cell which greatly contrasts with the normal biconcave disk form or discocyte. The echinocyte can easily be produced by saline wash of red cells, especially if they are mounted under a cover slip, and is also seen in a variety of disease states where it has various terms; in uremia it is called burr cells; in liver disease, spur cells; in microangiopathic hemolytic anemia, helmet cells (McKay *et al.*, 1969). It is interesting that the discocyte–echinocyte equilibrium which is reversible is apparently dependent on a number of factors, most of which are extrinsic to the red cell itself, including serum factors. It has also been inferred that intrinsic alterations involving the glycolytic energy pathway hexokinase and phosphofructokinase alter the cation pump mechanisms and also may lead to transformation of the cell into the kinocytic form where the surface–volume ratio is significantly increased by loss of water and electrolytes into the surroundings. Exactly what might be removed to result in the change is not known; however, scanning microscopy has shown adherence of a shaggy-type of material adherent to the external sursurface which may be nonspecifically absorbed protein which could be removed by a simple washing (Weinstein, 1969).

Development of elaborate folds and villi also occurs in response to other stimuli (Fig. 26). In the renal glomerulus, for example, complex folds and villi develop in the nephrotic syndrome, possibly related to the presence of protein in the glomerular filtrate (Trump and Benditt, 1962). Presence of circulating antigen–antibody complexes may also induce the formation of similar processes in endothelial cells. Development of structures abnormal for the cell in question was described by Steiner and Carruthers (1962) in the liver in which cilia formed following adminstration of α-naphthyliso-thiocyanate. Induction of phagosomes is a related process which can occur in some cells following exposure to inducers which include proteins, and at least in the blood monocyte such induction of phagocytosis seems to act as a part of a control mechanism on acid hydrolase synthesis. In a recent study of Werb and Cohn (1972), they noted the decrease of 5′-nucleotidase after stimulated phagocytosis and observed that recovery of cell surface nucleo-tidase required about 10 to 12 hours following phagocytosis, the new synthesis requiring the presence of exogenous cholesterol molecules and being inhibited by inhibitors of protein or RNA synthesis.

7. MYELIN

Alterations in myelin can be regarded as a special case of cell membrane alterations, and changes in myelin are important in many diseases of the central and peripheral nervous system such as multiple sclerosis and experi-mental allergic encephalitis (Raine *et al.*, 1969) and experimental neuritis (Lampert, 1969) and in the axonal reaction, which appears after surgical and traumatic interruption of peripheral or central axons. Changes described in myelin include separation of lamellae with splitting of both minor and major dense lines in cerebral edema, transformation of myelin lamellae into granular debris and vesicles in certain chemical toxicities of the peripheral nervous system such as lead poisoning (Lampert and Schochet, 1968), pre-sumably the result of primary injury to Schwann cells or oligodendrocytes, and binding of antigen antibody and complement to the oligodendroglia and/or myelin with release of lipases and esterases and consequent destruction. Another example of development of abnormal cilia occurs in the olfactory sensory epithelial cells where numerous basal bodies and cilia can be induced, presumably involving disorders of ciliary replication. Development of lamellar bodies in Schwann cell cytoplasm induced by alcoholic injury has been described by Sun *et al.* (1972).

8. MEMBRANE REPAIR

New membrane formation after injury involving the cell surface has been described by Griffin *et al.* (1969) following laser microbeam irradiation, and in a recent paper it has been shown that the properties of the cell sap can assist repair of cell membrane defects by forming a small clot at the site of microelectrode penetration which effectively seals a plasma membrane defect (Szubinska, 1971, 1972). In recent investigations, Szubinska (1971) proposed that *Amoeba proteus* forms a new membrane after injury outside the limits of the old membrane. The "new membrane" is separated from the plasma membrane complex by less than 1 μm. The author furthermore proposed a role of small, dense droplets of 100–1200 Å in diameter which are normally present in the cytoplasm of the amoeba in the formation and expansion of the plasma membrane.

9. OTHER CHANGES

Other examples of abnormalities in structure and function of the plasma membrane are the hypoxic vacuoles, the intracellular canaliculi of parietal cells in atrophic gastritis, effect of proton irradiation, and lamellar bodies in Schwann cells after alcohol injection for pain relief (Sun *et al.*, 1972).

The so-called intracellular canaliculi of parietal cells represent invaginations of the cell surface; numerous microvilli abutting on the extracellular space are so enclosed. This structure is poorly developed in cases of atrophic gastritis. Injection of betazole causes changes in the appearance of the villi with closure of the lumen, dilatation of the villi, and depletion of apical vesicles. So-called "metaplasia" with development of cilia in abnormal loci has been described after chemical toxicity (Steiner and Carruthers, 1962).

So-called hypoxic vacuoles (Fig. 23) seen in the liver after acute hypoxia represent large vacuoles several microns in diameter along either the bile canalicular or sinusoidal margin. This new type of cytoplasmic vesicle has been traced to invagination of the plasma membrane by Schofield and Grossman (1968). These authors examined liver cell vacuolization produced in five goats by electrocution, by means of histochemical adenosine triphosphate activity associated with plasma membrane. The authors determined that the lining of these large vacuoles developing in livers under these circumstances are of plasma membrane origin. The authors proposed hypoxia and alteration of the membrane charge as the etiologic factor in combination with the electric current. Occasionally these can be seen to connect with the cell surface (Oudea, 1963), and their origin is also indicated by their magnesium ATPase activity. The prime stimulus for formation of these vacuoles is presently unknown. They resemble somewhat the long vacuoles forming from the apical membrane of proximal tubules of the flounder kidney, which seem to participate in a type of rapid transport system for colloidal particles (Bulger and Trump, 1969a).

Changes in the outer segments of the retina following irradiation with protons, laser beams, or other particles such as nitrogen beams from a betatron have been described (Silver and Lawwill, 1972). These give swelling of the membrane stacks with disarray and disruption of the disks or flattened membrane sacks. The appearance of very striking lamellar bodies in Schwann cell cytoplasm following injection of alcohol for pain relief has been noted and related to possible changes in cell membrane and myelin. Effects of Australian spider venoms on the motor end plate have been described by Hamilton (1972). Red-back spider venom results in depletion of synaptic vesicles and appearance of numerous filaments with clustering of remaining vesicles and deformation of mitochondria which tend to appear condensed.

10. CHANGES IN MEMBRANE FINE STRUCTURE

Many studies utilizing freeze etching and cleaving have established the presence of membrane-associated particles localized inside the membrane which may in some instances be associated with the surface glycocalyx (Marchesi, 1971). Although changes in these particles in association with disease has not been established, there are reports suggesting that they may be modified under certain conditions such as changing the membrane lipid composition (James *et al.*, 1972), changes in pH (Pinto da Silva, 1972), and treatment of membranes with phospholipase.

B. Mitochondria

1. CHANGES IN REPLICATION AND TURNOVER

The details of mitochondrial turnover are still incompletely worked out, although in the liver it has been estimated that they may have a half-life of approximately 7–10 days (Fletcher and Sanadi, 1961). Whether the mitochondrial components turn over individually or whether the mitochondria turn over as a unit, for example, in autophagic vacuoles, is also not clear. It has been suggested that the total mass of mitochondria per cell is controlled (Bahr and Zeitler, 1962; Glas and Bahr, 1966), and that under some conditions may consist of larger numbers of smaller mitochondria and in others of fewer numbers of larger mitochondria. Evidence has also been presented that mitochondria are normally limited to a certain size prior to replication. The details of mitochondrial replication are being rapidly worked out, and it now seems established that certain mitochondrial proteins such as cytochrome c and the F_1 particle (or inner membrane ATPase) are produced in the cytoplasm (Tzagaloff, 1971), whereas others such as the juncture protein of the ATPase complex are produced by mitochondrial protein synthesis. Tzagaloff (1971) and Schatz (1970) furthermore postulated that both the mitochondrial and the cytoplasmic system are required for assembly of respiratory enzymes (for review, see Schatz, 1970).

A variety of abnormal conditions result in dramatic changes involving mitochondrial division and turnover, often resulting in the formation of very large mitochondria (or megamitochondria) (Fig. 28) commonly associated with a decrease in total number of mitochondria. These large mitochondria may be bizarre in shape with disorganized appearing cristae and often in man associated with paracrystalline inclusions in the inner compartment. Among conditions associated with the formation of megamitochondria are ageing (Sohal *et al.*, 1972; Tauchi and Sato, 1968), vitamin E and selenium deficiency, thiamine deficiency (Wu *et al.*, 1971), deficiency of essential fatty acids (Bailey *et al.*, 1967), alcoholism, choline (Sugioka *et al.*, 1969), iron and copper deficiency (Wohlrab and Jacobs, 1967; Dallman and Goodman, 1970), riboflavin deficiency (Luse *et al.*, 1962; Tandler *et al.*, 1969), and hypertrophy of the kidney (Johnson and Amendola, 1969). The exact significance of this to mitochondrial function is not known, however, it is known that at least in some instances isolated megamitochondria may exhibit normal function (Wu *et al.*, 1971), whereas in other instances a partially decreased metabolism of certain substrates is observed; abnormally small mitochondria were observed after prolonged treatment with ethidum bromide (Soslau and Nass, 1971).

Reduction in mitochondrial number in the liver can be produced by simple starvation for 7 days as shown by Scarpelli *et al.*, (1971), who utilized this as a means of studying mitochondrial growth control by using subsequent treatment during the refeeding phase with chloramphenicol or cycloheximide. Comparison of the inhibitory effect of amino acid incorporation exhibited by cycloheximide with that of chloramphenicol indicated to these authors that the outer membrane and matrical proteins were synthesized by systems localized in the ER, whereas those of the inner membrane were synthesized both in the mitochondrion and in the ER. They noted that 10 days were required to return from about half to normal levels, which compared favorably with half-life estimates of between 8.5 and 12.4 days obtained by Fletcher and Sanadi. An important model for the study of mitochondria genesis has been yeast cells (Criddle and Schatz, 1969), which as facultative aerobes respond to anoxia by repression of mitochondrial biogenesis and depletion of the mitochondrial population. This can be reversed when aerobic conditions are reestablished. In considering these studies of mitochondrial size changes, it is important to distinguish between increase in size owing to swelling and increase in size owing to increased structural components. Unfortunately many papers in the literature have not made such distinctions and it is difficult or impossible to derive many definitive conclusions from them. Furthermore, the principals of stereological morphometry have also to be kept in mind since marked shape changes can be interpreted as number changes if they are not taken into account. Evaluation of numbers of mitochondria by the use of electronic particle counts of mitochondrial fractions also has serious problems since increased lability may result in changes in the degree of fragmentation during homogenization, giving more or less particles per mitochondrion depending on the situation (Gear and Bednarck, 1972). Redundancies of the outer membrane following chloramphenicol treatment after refeeding are interesting and have been interpreted as indicating greater growth of the outer membrane because of a uniform requirement for cytoplasmic protein synthesis in that structure. Close associations of mitochondria to ER in the liver have been often commented on, and evidence of glucose 6-phosphatase activity in the outer membrane has been reported. It seems reasonable that the outer membrane is a derivative of the ER although the complete story here remains to be shown. King *et al.* (1972) noted increased cytoplasmic smooth membranes after chronic exposure to tissue culture cells to chroramphenicol and ethidium bromide. The present concept would regard the mitochondrion as the result of coordinated activities between cytoplasmic DNA, RNA, and protein metabolism and the same factors going on in the mitochondrion. How this control is achieved is not presently clear, although evidence indicates that a variety of injurious factors may disturb this balance and result in changes of various types in number, size, and function of the mitochondria.

The increase in size of mitochondria is often associated with a decrease in number, at least in fly muscle, although the total percentage area occupied in the sarcoplasm decreased (Sohal *et al.*, 1972). This may be associated with decreased phosphorylating ability (Bulos *et al.*, 1972). Tribe and Ashhurst (1972) attribute the increase in mitochondrial size in the ageing fly to marked repair and replacement of mitochondrial proteins and in this way infer that this may be related to the effects of oxidative phosphorylation. Hagopian *et al.* (1972) noted the appearance of megamitochondria in the hibernating bat heart following treatment with reserpine. Precipitations of silica in the mitochondrial matrix of uncertain pathogenesis were described by Policard *et al.* (1961). F. Rubin *et al.* (1970, 1972a,b) postulated that ethanol has structural and functional effects on mitochondria by the mechanism of interfering with hepatic mitochondrial biogenesis with a reduction of certain components of the electron-transport chain. Functionally, such mitochondria exhibit decreased rates of respiration and fatty acid oxidation (Orci and Stauffacher, 1971).

2. ALTERED MITOCHONDRIAL METABOLISM

An increasing number of examples of altered mitochondrial metabolism that are not associated with acute cell death is being reported. These may have striking consequences on the cell as well as on the mitochondria, including changes in number and size as well as accumulation of by-products or precursors proximal to the site of a metabolic block within the mitochondrion itself. In many cases the pathogenetic basis of mitochondrial lesions is not known.

In chronic lead toxicity, for example, there is inhibition of the enzyme ferrochelatase which is found only within the mitochondrion and represents the final step in heme biosynthesis (Grinstein *et al.*, 1959; Remington, 1937). Inhibition of this enzyme by lead in the erythrocyte precursors in the bone marrow results in accumulation of iron pigments resembling hemosiderin within the inner mitochondrial compartment (Bessis and Breton-Gorius, 1959) (Fig. 29). The mitochondria have decreased elements of the electron-transport chain in chronic lead poisoning. Lead toxicity also appears to cause a chronic mitochondrial lesion in kidney tubules which has been correlated with the Fanconi syndrome of lead poisoning, although the cells do not undergo acute cell death (for review, see Albahary, 1972). These mitochondria also respond differently to induced conformational changes *in vitro*, i.e., transitions from state IV to state III. Along the same lines, the cardiac myopathy caused by cobalt ingestion has been related to a chronic defect in mitochondrial function involving the pyruvate decarboxylase complex. Mitochondria are reported to appear swollen, although the cells do not undergo acute necrosis.

The occurrence of inclusions within the intracrystal spaces has been well documented in the oocyte where yolk crystals can be demonstrated in the outer compartment of mitochondria which at the same time is quite deformed and forms long protrusions extending far into the cytoplasm. The authors (see Massover, 1971) also suggest that ultimately the mitochondrion can be freed of the inclusions by extrusion of parts of the outer compartment by budding, leaving membrane bound crystals in the cytoplasm and mitochondria devoid of crystals.

A particular type of electron dense granule has been described in the swollen mitochondria of apparently necrotic cells of cobalt cardiomyopathy. These granules are dense and homogeneous with more sharp margins than the usual flocculent densities and have been interpreted as representing cobalt lipoid acid complexes (Alexander, 1972). Lipoic acid, a coenzyme of the citric acid cycle, forms an irreversible complex with cobalt (Webb, 1962; Sekhri *et al.*, 1972).

Chronic hypoxic treatment of cultured mammalian cells has recently been demonstrated to result in mitochondrial changes. This includes changes in the isoenzyme patterns of mitochondrial enzymes and change in the morphology whereby the mitochondria become smaller with less numerous cristae and with clarification of the matrix (Henderson, 1972). Concomitant changes include accumulation of triglyceride droplets resulting from inability of fatty acid oxidation (Gordon, 1972). These lipid droplets may be in close proximity to or even indenting the mitochondrial profiles. This is a common pattern of lipid accumulation in the heart, where, again, it is probable owing to inhibition of fatty acid oxidation. Administration of ethanol to non-alcoholic subjects results in mitochondrial abnormalities which may relate to the controversial pathogenesis of cell injury in alcoholism. Recently, Ruebner *et al.* (1972) have reported defects of mitochondrial membrane biogenesis and reduction of concentration of components of the electron-transport chain, including cytochrome b and cytochrome a–a₃ in chronic alcoholism. Interference with oxidative phosphorylation and fatty acid oxidation was also noted, which, in turn, correlated with increased fragility and swelling of mitochondria *in vitro*. Interference with mitochondrial protein synthesis was also noted, and because of its metabolism through the alcohol dehydrogenase reaction, changes in the redox potential to which the mitochondria are exposed may further modify mitochondrial function. The relationship of all these changes to the megamitochondria which occur in alcoholics is not clear.

A relationship between structural and functional impairment in lead poisoning has been postulated by Goyer and Krall (1969), who observed that a large portion of kidney mitochondria obtained from lead-poisoned rats do not transform from condensed to orthodox conformation during stage IV respiration. Some did transform into the orthodox form but they rapidly degenerated (Goyer *et al.*, 1968; Goyer, 1968).

King and King (1971) have studied the effects of prolonged oxygen deprivation on mitochondrial morphology of L cells and noted that a reduction in specific activity of cytochrome oxidase is followed by reduction in size of mitochondria with apparent condensation in the mitochondrial inner compartments after 9 days of oxygen depletion.

Changes in oxidative phosphorylation, possibly related to lipid deposition and accompanied by increase in hexokinase, glucose 6-phosphate dehydrogenase, and α-glycerol phosphate dehydrogenases with parallel decreases in phosphofructokinase, were described by Paterson *et al.* (1972) in the spontaneous cardiomyopathy occurring in the B10 14.6 strain of Syrian hamster. This is an interesting model for studying the development of cardiac insufficiency in congestive failure caused by overload as well as by cardiomyopathy which it resembles.

Formation of so-called atypical mitochondria with disordered cristae often forming stacks of membranes was studied and reviewed by Riede and Rohr (1971) after following a variety of treatments including cycloheximide, acetyl salicylic acid, vitamin E, sodium hydrocholic acid, and malonic acid. Mitochondria appeared to have a clarified matrix in some regions with stacks of cristae in the inner compartment. For full review of this entire problem and reference to the literature see their paper.

Gonzalez-Licea (1972) observed that mitochondria of absorptive cells of the small intestine underwent marked qualitative and quantitative changes when the animals were either suckling or fasting. In nonfasted suckling rats, mitochondria had numerous cristae and denser matrix then the surrounding cytoplasm and frequent contact with fat droplets, nucleus, or other mitochondria. In 24-hour-fasted rats, the matrix was light and the cristae were less or decreased in numbers and were adherent to each other. These changes were related to changes in ion and water transport in different metabolic states.

The nonthyrotoxic hypermetabolic syndrome originally reported by Luft *et al.*1962; Ernster and Luft, 1963; Ernster *et al.*, 1959; Afifi *et al.*, 1972) presents a striking example of altered mitochondrial structure and function in which the mitochondria are very loosely coupled; the patients exhibit hyperpyrexia but have no evidence of thyroid gland dysfunction. Isolated mitochondria from such patients show considerably higher rates of oxygen consumption with poor coupling activity, and on electron microscopic study they have very closely packed cristae often in a zigzag configuration, resembling those in mitochondria from cells with hypermetabolic states such as canary mycoardium and occasionally crystal or paracrystal formations apparently resulting from reorganization of cristae.

In a variety of chronic modifications of cell function, the mitochondria go into the condensed configuration. In general these seem to correlate with conditions that promote changes in the ATP and ADP levels in the cell and that are associated with stimulated metabolic activity. These include stimulation of sodium transport by induction of plasmalemma leak with amphotericin B and stimulation of amino acid transport by rat jejunal segments (Jasper and Bronk, 1972). In both cases, respiration by the cell is stimulated and the mitochondria become condensed. It has recently been shown that the condensation lags behind the respiratory stimulation, thus indicating that it is not primary in this regard and is more likely a secondary effect. As discussed above under the section on acute lethal injury, the explanation of this phenomenon may be the competition between ADP phosphorylation and accumulation of potassium ion. Leak of ions and water from the mitochondria following increased stimulation with ADP results in the shrunken mitochondria, especially when severe, undergoing a further transformation, resulting in ring or doughnut-like forms which give doughnut profiles in thin sections.

Studies by Schafer (1972) on glycerin-extracted mitochondria indicate aggregation of a substance in the mitochondrial matrix following addition of ATP, which is related to the presence of contractile proteins in the matrix by the author.

3. MISCELLANEOUS CHANGES

A variety of miscellaneous changes have been described in mitochondria under various conditions of cell injury, which will be mentioned briefly, although their significance is not known. Many of these represent accumulations of material in the matrix. Occasionally, such condensations are apparently the result of clumping of intramitochondrial DNA, resembling the patterns seen in mitochondria of lower forms.

For example, polio virus infection of Hela cells after 6 to 8 hours result in mitchondrial DNA aggregates in the inner compartment. Paracrystalline arrays are well known in human hepatic mitochondria, and although they have been associated in the past with various diseases (Ekholm and Edlund, 1960), they also clearly appear in healthy individuals (Wills, 1965); their significance remains unkown. The same is true of a variety of fibrillar and helical filamentous profiles that have been seen in the matrix or intracristal space in various conditions. The occurrence of dense homogeneous bodies in the intracristal space termed sometimes "corpra intra-cristam" (Frei and Sheldon, 1961) has been reported in a variety of circumstances including hyperplasia of the mouse epidermis, in the corneal epithelium in vitamin A deficiency (Sheldon and Zetterqvist, 1956), and in the mitochondria of endamoeba (Vickerman, 1960) during encystation. Mitochondrial vacuolation and densification of the "limiting" membrane has been seen in thallium neuropathy (Spencer et al., 1972).

The production of C-type virus particles within the inner mitochondrial compartment has been described (Savage and Hackett, 1972). The mitochondria involved are typically enlarged or swollen with a considerable degree of cristae disorganization. Particles are usually situated in the periphery of the mitochondria, sometimes between the inner and outer mitochondrial membranes and are associated with budding-type configurations along the inner membrane. Formation of septate fusions between outer mitchondrial membranes has been described in damaged mitochondria (Bulger and Trump, 1968).

Max (1972) observed that mitochondria isolated from rat gastrocnemius muscle subjected to disuse atrophy displayed a marked loss of respiratory control at a very early stage in the wasting phenomenon. This abnormality could be reversed by bovine serum albumin. It was postulated by Max that the effect was caused by free fatty acids. It was, furthermore, stressed that mitochondrial dysfunction may be of significance in the initiation of disuse atrophy.

C. The Cytocavitary Network

1. GENERAL CONSIDERATIONS

The cytoplasm of eukaryotic cells contains a variety of membrane-bound cavities, sacs, vesicles, and other profiles. It is thought that they are functionally in continuity with each other as well as in specified types of continuity with the cell surface. This system contains a series of internal spaces containing various materials, but often apparently watery in nature, separated by a membrane from the cell sap. This membrane differs in various parts of the system. The system differs from the complex spaces that can occur within deep infoldings of the cell membrane; though the latter may also exist as deeply within the cell, the invaginations still surround spaces that are in direct continuity with the extracellular space as evidenced by electron dense tracer penetration. Though the space within the cytocavitary network is topologically equivalent to the extracellular space, the continuity is often functional, resulting from temporal sequences of membrane fissions and fusions in so-called transport vesicles. The increased knowledge of the relationships between various parts of this system in the last several years has revealed many of the rules concerning transport and the presence of functional continuities between various parts of this system. As a result of this, it seems that all intracellular membrane-bound structures, with the exception of the mitochondria and chloroplasts, can be considered as parts of this system which exist in continuity from time to time. There is even some question concerning plastids since recent, though fragmentary, evidence indicates that the outer membranes of these structures may in fact be part of the system, and the inner membrane containing the active parts of these structures as well as their DNA may reside within its cavities. A recent attempt to demonstrate connections between the outer mitochondrial membranes in fungi and the ER was made by Bracker and Grove (1971).

To emphasize the functional relationships between the various portions of this system of membranes, it is useful to conceptualize these structures as forming various parts of a complex functionally interrelated system that permeates the cytoplasm. Recently, various names have been proposed for this complex such as the cytocavitary network, the vacuolar apparatus, and the vacuome. Since the terms vacuolar apparatus and vacuome were used in the earlier days of cytology to refer to structures which, though perhaps a part of the system that we presently know, could not have been known in the present form, we prefer the term cytocavitary network which emphasizes the idea of a functional network throughout the cell and the idea that the network consists of cavities in the cytoplasm separated from the cell sap by a membrane. The cavities within the cytocavitary network seem to be concerned with activities such as transport, digestion, and storage. The membranes also clearly have other functions related to active transport, some relationship to protein synthesis, and many other metabolic activities, for example, those involved in drug metabolism and detoxification and metabolism of steroids. In order to gain access to the system from the cell sap, it is necessary for materials to cross the membrane lining the cytocavitary network. This can occur in bulk form by the formation of buds resembling those that occur at the cell surface, but in this case budding into the lumens of the network or by poorly understood transport processes perhaps involving active transport enzymes in the case of small molecules, and as yet undisclosed mechanisms in the case of polypeptides which must pass from their site of synthesis on membrane-bound polysomes across the membrane to the lumen of the ER. Transport between the various parts of this system evidently is direct in the case of morphologically continuous parts of this system; otherwise it can occur by membrane vesiculation, on the one hand, with fusion, on the other hand, resulting in transport vesicles similar to those occurring in pinocytosis and secretion at the cell surface.

The outline of this system is summarized in the Fig. 32 which also emphasizes relationships of the two principal types of membrane involved. Those parts most related to the cell membrane and which have a membrane of similar thickness ($\sim$ 100 Å) include the phagosomes, the primary and secondary lysosomes, the residual bodies, the secretory granules, and parts of the maturing face of the Golgi apparatus. Those parts with thinner membranes on the order of 60 Å in thickness include the forming face of the Golgi apparatus, the smooth and the rough ER, the peroxisomes, both parts of the nuclear envelope, the annulate lamellae, and, if they are to be included, the outer membrane of plastids and mitochondria.

The functional activities of this system including those of its membranes differ markedly in various subdivisions though much is still to be learned about these complex interrelationships. Moreover, it is apparent that there is a considerable intracellular traffic conveying materials between various parts of this system—evident in experiments involving time-lapse movies and in kinetic experiments employing radioautography or visible tracer particles. It is also seemingly evident that although this system is functionally interconnected in the sense that one can trace continuities between all its parts at one time or another by means of various experiments, there is, in the steady state of a normal cell, directed traffic in the sense that the system behaves as if valves or sphincter-like mechanisms exist (Fig. 44). For example, material brought into the cell by phagocytosis is first taken into phagosomes or pinocytotic vesicles which receive hydrolases by fusion with primary lysosomes or preexisting secondary lysosomes and followed by intracellular digestion in the resultant digestive vacuole or secondary lysosome. Simultaneously, budding of cytoplasm into these structures may occur, which is one way that multivesicular bodies are formed. These digestive vacuoles also receive contents derived from autophagocytosis through other fusions. Ultimately, nondigestible debris appear to be converted to pigmented material, known as lipofuscin pigment. Such residual bodies may fuse with the surface by a process resembling the reverse of pinocytosis with extrusion of the contents to the extracellular space. It is, however, apparent that particles taken in by pinocytosis do not pass retrograde into the Golgi or into the ER, nuclear envelope, or microbodies. On the other hand, materials within the ER such as proteins or lipoproteins resulting from synthetic activities associated with the membrane of the ER can be transported through this system to the Golgi apparatus, the final step apparently involving transition vesicles in an ATP-dependent step. The materials, perhaps after modification in the Golgi region, are packaged in secretory vesicles, which can fuse either with the cell surface or with the digestive vacuoles or phagocytic vacuoles.

In some cells such as the proximal convoluted tubule of the kidney, it appears that the amount of lysosomal protein synthesized may be remarkable. A study by Nayyar and Koenig (1972) has recently shown that in the proximal tubule of the rat kidney a major portion of protein and glycoprotein synthesis is devoted to the production of lysosomal constituents. After administration of label, the labeling was primarily over the rough ER in 5 minutes, the Golgi in 15, and by 30–60 minutes appeared in the lysosomes. In the case of N-acetylmanosamine, labeling appeared to proceed initially in the Golgi apparatus, correlating with the glycosil additions known in other systems in that organelle. Once again, directed traffic occurs, and in the phenomenon that has come to be known as crinophagy materials that under normal conditions are released to the cell surface may in other instances be released into digestive vacuoles. The mechanisms involved in these oriented movements are presently unknown, but may well be related to differences such as those reflected in membrane thickness and staining.

Once visualizing the cytocavitary network in this way it becomes possible to broaden one's concept of the diverse parts of this system which from time to time have been given various names on various arbitrary criteria. A good example of this is the former rigid definition of the lysosome as a single membrane-bound body containing acid hydrolases. Such a rigid definition does not conform to our present knowledge of the dynamic properties of the cytocavitary network, and if applied rigidly lend to erroneous conclusions. Such particles cannot therefore be rigidly defined only on the basis of content of acid hydrolases or other single criteria because they exhibit functional differences from time to time and functional interconnections with other parts of the system.

2. Membrane Movements

The fundamental characteristics of movements in various parts of the cytocavitary network and between the cell sap space, the space within the cytocavitary network, and the extracellular space can be considered as forward or reverse movements of two simple geometric processes termed *exotropy* and *esotropy*. These are geometrically opposite processes. Esotropy (*Greek*: turning in) refers to a turning in of the membrane toward the cell sap followed by fission to form a new membrane-bound cavity; the cavity is topologically equivalent to the extracellular space or the space within the cytocavitary network. When this phenomenon occurs in the reverse direction (reverse esotropy), the vesicle fuses with the membrane, bringing the content of the vesicle into continuity with the space within the cytocavitary network or the extracellular space. Exotropy (*Greek*: turning out) refers to a turning out of the membrane toward the extracellular space or toward the space of cyto-cavitary network followed by fusion and formation of a new membrane-bound structure containing cell sap and materials within it such as organelles. This phenomenon can also occur in the opposite direction (reverse exotropy) in which case the cell sap of the two compartments is brought into continuity following fusion.

It should be noted that the polarity of the membrane is opposite in the two cases. In an exotropic vesicle the glycocalyx side of the membrane is directed outwardly, that is, toward the extracellular space or space within the cyto-cavitary network, and the cytoplasmic side of the membrane is directed outwardly toward the cell sap which it contains. In an esotropic vesicle the glycocalyx side of the membrane is directed toward the center of the vesicle and the cytoplasmic side of the membrane is directed toward the outside of the vesicle.

Examples of esotropy in the forward direction include pinocytosis, the elaboration of transport vesicles from the ER to the forming side of the Golgi apparatus, the elaboration of secretory vesicles from the maturing face of the Golgi apparatus, and the formation of microbodies. Examples of reverse esotropy include fusion of secretory granules with the cell membrane, fusion of Golgi vesicles with phagosomes, and fusion between various granules such as different populations of secondary lysosomes. These movements can apparently be very rapid indeed. Steinman and Silver (1972) recently esti-mated that $\sim 50\%$ of macrophage–plasmalemma area can be interiorized per hour.

Rohlich *et al.* (1971) observed the degranulation of mast cells after addition of the histamine liberator 48/80. Degranulation in this system of rat mast cells occurred at different intervals ranging from 10 to 60 seconds after addition of the liberator. After a latent period in this system, degranulation started in the most peripherally located granules. The membrane of the granule fused with the plasma membrane, resulting in a pore bridged by a thin diaphragm. This was followed by rupture of the diaphragm and extrusion of the granular matrix. The same process advanced toward the cell interior. During this extrusion process, extracellular tracers showed that the intra-cellular cavities were in unbroken communication with the extracellular space from the very beginning of their formation, while no tracer was found in nondegranulating mast cells. It was postulated by the authors that release of histamine occurs by action of the extracellular ionic milieu from the granular matrix.

As mentioned above, forward exotropy results in eliminating part of the cell substance into the cytocavitary network or into the extracellular space. Examples of this include the formation of vesicles in multivesicular bodies (Arstila *et al.*, 1971), the well-known autophagy in which portions of cytoplasm containing organelles as large as mitochondria are budded into the cavities of the ER (Arstila and Trump, 1968), cell division itself, lipid secretion in mammary gland, and the budding of many viruses which have envelopes, such as herpes virus, influenza virus, and mammary tumor virus, either into the cytocavitary network or directly to the extracellular space at the cell surface. Elimination of parts of the cytoplasm and/or nuclei during cell maturation also appears to occur by this basic process; for example, in the maturation of spermatocytes in which part of the cytoplasm is thrown off and in the elimination of nuclei from maturing erythrocytes in mammals.

Reverse exotropy results in the fusion of a membrane-bounded body with another one, bringing the two portions of the cell sap into continuity and as such is seen in intercellular fusions, for example, formation of multinucleated giant cells in various virus infections or in chronic granulomas, in the formation of cell hybrids with Sendai virus, and in the various fusions that occur during embryonic development such as the fusion of myoblasts to form myotubes. Fertilization of the ovum in mammals can also be regarded as an example of reverse exotropy, since after breakdown of the acrosomal vesicle the sperm membrane fuses with that of the oocyte. Recently it has been suggested that certain membrane-bounded viruses enter cells by fusing their membrane with the membrane of the cell surface (Coward *et al.*, 1970).

The fundamental differences between exotropy and esotropy are still not known though Danielli has put forth an hypothesis suggesting that the direction in which membrane buds form can vary depending on changes in surface pressure on either the cytoplasmic or the extracellular side of the membrane (Danielli, 1967). The existence of membrane polarity seems well established, and marked differences have been noted between the surface or glycocalyx side of the membrane and the cytoplasmic side which may have various juxtamembranal cytoplasmic components bound to it. Recent studies employing cytochalasin B or compounds such as vinblastine, vincristine, or cholchicine indicate some relationship between cell membrane movements, microtubules, and cytoplasmic filaments. The nature of this relationship awaits elucidation. There are also suggestions that levels of intracellular calcium and cyclic AMP may be involved, and recent studies in our laboratory in which autophagy can be induced in the liver of rats or in liver slices *in vitro* by cyclic AMP or dibutyryl cyclic AMP seem to implicate cyclic AMP in the process. Also of interest are experiments in which esotropy can be induced in red blood cells by suspending the cells in media containing membrane-active agents such as vitamin A or primaquine, suggesting that polarized interactions may at least in part contribute to these membrane movement. These may involve intrinsic or extrinsic membrane proteins; indeed, orientation of membrane particles in relation to caveolae has been recently seen in freeze-etched endothelium (Smith and Ryan, 1972).

The use of the two terms esotropy and exotropy, both of which can occur in either the forward or the reverse direction, emphasizes the difference in polarity between the two types of processes and the similarity between the processes in each category. These geometric relationships and reversibilities seem not to have been clearly recognized in the past and a variety of terms, some of which are used interchangeably for both exotropy and esotropy, such as exocytosis, eccytosis, and encytosis seem to be less desirable in this regard.

Figure 32 summarizes dynamic relationships within and between cytoplasmic membrane systems.

Note that the several compartments of the cytocavitary network are not in direct continuity; continuity is provided by forward and reverse esotropic vesiculation. Note also that only some pathways are bidirectional, such as that between the phagolysosome system and the extracellular space. Movements between the Golgi compartment and the cell surface or the phagolysosome compartment appear to be in one direction only; similarly, movements from the ER to the Golgi compartment also seem to be only unidirectional. These vesiculation movements, which evidently transport materials from one compartment to another, seem to depend often on the presence of high energy compounds such as ATP. Note also that the nucleus is topologically equivalent to an exotropic bud within the cytocavitary lumen, although in this case periodic fusions of the membrane at the sites of nuclear pores probably permit interchanges between the contents of the nucleoplasm and the cell sap. It is also likely that the nuclear envelope reforms after mitosis not by exotropic budding but by segregation type vesicles which surround the mitotic material and fuse, resulting in enclosure within the network. Such a process is also apparently involved with cell plate formation in dividing plant cells. Also note that certain granules such as microbodies bud off of the ER by forward esotropy and then appear to exist as membrane-bounded structures in the cytoplasm. Also shown are two Golgi "by-pass" pathways. In the one case, which has mainly been suggested for collagen secretion, vesicular movements appear to convey collagen precursors directly from the ER to the cell surface without passing through the Golgi. In the other pathway, termed the GERL complex by Novikoff, direct communication between ER and some lysosome compartments has been postulated in the Golgi region. Question marks also indicate possible connections, possibly during formation of the outer mitochondrial membrane with the membrane of the ER. Exotropic budding is shown into each compartment were it has been seen and also into the extracellular space at the cell surface.

3. ENDOPLASMIC RETICULUM

Manifestations of chronic cell injury in the ER are both diverse and numerous (Goldblatt, 1969; Smuckler and Arcasoy, 1969). Modifications in this organelle constitute an important site of alteration in chronic injury related to the manifold metabolic activities of these membrane systems.

a. RIBOSOME MEMBRANE RELATIONSHIPS.   Changes in the association of ribosomes and ER membranes are commonly observed after administration of cell toxins which do not necessarily result in acute cell death. Since these are often associated with inhibition of protein synthesis, this emphasizes that such inhibition does not result in acute cell death. For example, administration of ethionine to rats results in defective protein synthesis and fatty liver within a few hours. Associated with this is detachment of polysomes from the ER and scattering of free ribosomes into the cell sap (Fig. 33). The lesion is readily reversible following administration of adenine whereupon the ribosomes appear to reaggregate and regain their membrane association. Loss of Ca and Mg following irradiation has been related to ribosome release from membranes (Goldfeder and Mukerjee, 1972).

Detachment of polysomes from the membrane is usually associated with their breakdown and appearance of monosomes in the cell sap. At least in some instances the sedimentation properties of the monosomes may be markedly altered as well. This detachment from the membrane is apparently always associated with defective protein synthesis *in vivo* or *in vitro*, although in some cases it has been possible, at least partially, to repair the defect through the use of artificial messengers such as polyuridylic acid (Smuckler and Trump, 1968). The precise mechanisms involved in the membrane detachment have not been worked out; it was mentioned above, however, that conditions known to modify membrane structure are especially prone to promote such detachment. It is highly probable that the membrane attachment is of great significance to polysome function. There are, for example, indications that the membrane may contain some type of message itself and that the ER electron-transport system may be involved in the generation of high energy intermediates for driving protein synthesis. At the same time, it should be noted that membrane detachment is not a prerequisite for protein synthesis inhibition. The antibiotic cycloheximide, for example, which inhibits, at the ribosome level, does not promote dissociation and in fact tends to stabilize polysomes against the dissociation that can be induced by other protein synthesis inhibitors such as puromycin.

In scurvy, changes in ribosomal patterns paralled the defects in collagen synthesis. The potential reversibility of polyribosome dissociation is illustrated in a recent paper by Wengler and Wengler (1972). These authors noted that increased tonicity of the medium with either sodium chloride or sucrose resulted in reversible polysome dissociation in HeLa cells. They noted that the process was reversible at least three times and inferred that it was probably caused by a specific block of initiation of protein synthesis. Recently, Sarma *et al.* (1972) have questioned the so-called detachments of membrane-bound ribosomes from membranes such as that described by Smuckler and co-workers, asserting that following carbon tetrachloride poisoning, although the polysome organization is lost, the ribosomes remain in some way attached to the membrane.

b. ALTERATIONS IN TRANSPORT. Under a number of conditions the transport of materials through the ER seems to be modified and protein-rich materials accumulate within the ER cisternae. One striking example of this is the formation of so-called Russell bodies in the plasma cells in areas of chronic inflammation.

A probable defect in the transport of lipoproteins which accumulate in the ER rather than in the Golgi, giving small dense homogeneous droplets in the ER cisternae, has been reported in ethionine hepatotoxicity (Arstila and Trump, 1972). A role of *N*-acetyl neuramimic acid binding in the transport of lysosomal enzymes through the ER has recently been postulated (Goldstone and Koenig, 1972).

Transport defects across the ER membrane are less well characterized; however, there is evidence in the myocardium of defective calcium binding, transport, and release by the sarcoplasmic reticulum in heart failure. According to this hypothesis, this defect results in mitochondrial accumulation of calcium rather than accumulation in the ER with subsequent disturbances in contraction excitation coupling (Gertz *et al.*, 1967; Suko *et al.*, 1970).

c. STIMULATION OF ER MEMBRANE SYNTHESIS. This category includes a widespread and important series of ER reactions to drugs and hormones, including carcinogenic compounds, resulting in induction of ER membrane and enzyme synthesis. This rapidly burgeoning field has not only greatly increased the understanding of drug detoxification and drug–drug and drug–hormone interactions, but it has also contributed considerable basic information on the structure and function, formation, and turnover of the ER as an organelle. This system, which was first discovered by Brodie and associates (1955, 1958), involves a hydroxylating electron-transport system involving at least two catalytic components; a cytochrome called P450 and the flavo protein catalyzing a reduction of the cytochrome by NADPH, which is termed NADPH cytochrome P450 reductase (Fig. 36) (Orrenius and Ernster,

1971; Fouts, 1962; Orrenius, 1968; Remmer *et al.*, 1966; Orrenius *et al.*, 1965; Ikeda and Otsuji, 1971). The system also involves ferrous iron and requires NADPH. The components are intimately associated with the membranes of the ER, and the system is involved in a variety of drug metabolizing reactions, which, depending on the nature of the drug, may lead to oxidation of an aromatic ring or hydrocarbon side chain, an oxidative dealkylation or deamination, or the formation of a sulfoxide. Lately it has been found that microsomes from liver, cerebral cortex, testis, ovary and placenta, and other organs catalyze NADPH and oxygen-dependent hydroxylation of various steroids and that a similar system is also present in adrenal cortex mitochondria. Moreover, a similar or identical system can also be involved in hydroxylation of aliphatic hydrocarbons and the omega oxidation of fatty acids, especially in the kidney. Considering the manifold activities of this system involving both endogenous and exogenous compounds, it is not surprising that it is involved in a variety of pathological processes.

This is expressed in terms of cell structure and function by initiation of synthesis of ER membranes and enzymes which first involves the rough and later the smooth ER and within a few days by vast accumulations of ER (Staubli *et al.*, 1969) within hepatic parenchymal cells (Figs. 36 and 37) (Orrenius *et al.*, 1965; Stäubli *et al.*, 1969; Weibel *et al.*, 1969; Burger and Herdson, 1966; Glaumann and Jakobsson, 1969). This is most marked in the centrilobular area. The induction involves increased rates of both protein and RNA synthesis as well as a decrease in the rate of breakdown or turnover of at least the flavoprotein which may also contribute. Whether this induction proceeds by way of direct interaction of the drug with the genetic system or by way of some mediator of cell origin is not known. There are also indications that steroid hormone metabolism, by way of the hydroxylating system, and steroid hormones might, in turn, act as mediators in the drug-induced enzyme synthesis. Certainly marked cross reactions between diverse types of drugs have been observed, which would be expected if these are mediated through a common enzyme system, and this mutual inducibility has in fact constituted an important argument in favor of the idea of a final common pathway. One exception recognized by Conney (1967) concerns carcinogenic compounds such as the polycyclic hydrocarbons including 3,4-benzanthracene and 3 methylocholanthrene. In this case the enhanced liver hydroxylating activity is directed only toward polycyclic hydrocarbons, whereas activities toward other compounds increased only slightly or not at all. Polycyclic hydrocarbons are also associated with a shift in the absorption of P450 to 448 nm that exhibits an increased affinity for the polycyclic hydrocarbons and a decreased affinity for other drugs and hormones.

The proliferation of the ER is accompanied by increased rates of phospholipid synthesis although here again a simultaneous slowing down of lipid catabolism may be a contributory factor. Mechanisms of altered turnover await elucidation, and it has been difficult or impossible to implicate lysosomes by way of autophagic vacuoles in this process.

Glaumann (1971b) showed functional and structural heterogeneity of the ER. He distinguished three microsomal subfraction isolated on ion-containing sucrose gradients. These subfractions differed in their sensitivity toward ions in enzyme distribution, in incorporation rates of lipid precursors as well as in neutral lipid content, and in response to phenobarbital and methylcholanthrene administration (Glaumann, 1970; Glaumann and Dallner, 1970).

Such work indicating diversity within the smooth ER emphasizes the importance of keeping an open mind concerning this organelle since at the moment it is a "no man's land." Increased application of refined methods of cytochemistry and cell fractionation are needed to further define subsystems within it.

The cross reactivities of the system provide the opportunity for drug interactions involving antagonisms or synergisms which can result in toxic metabolism. The best studied example of this is carbon tetrachloride hepatotoxicity. Carbon tetrachloride is metabolized by the ER to form a free radical CCl_3, which, in turn, is believed to initiate lethal membrane peroxidation in hepatic parenchymal cells. Since the membrane hydroxylating system is involved with peroxidation, possibly involving the ferrous iron moiety, and since the ER metabolism is responsible for the toxic action of carbon tetrachloride, it would be anticipated that prior stimulation of the system with phenobarbital would result in increased toxicity of a given dose of carbon tetrachloride. Such, indeed, appears to be the case and doses of carbon tetrachloride which alone do not result in necrosis can be made to do so by pretreating the animal with phenobarbital. Similar interactions which include many chlorinated hydrocarbons used as insecticides coupled with the activity of the system in steroid metabolism have given rise to many speculations concerning possible modifications of endogenous hormone metabolism by exposure of animals to insecticides. Such a case is the example of the soft eggshell produced by insecticides in peregrine falcons. The eggs are believed by some to have resulted from hydrocarbon induction followed by altered steroid metabolism and defective eggshell calcification. There are many examples of electron microscopic studies in which proliferations of ER can be seen in cells, sometimes very rapidly after administration of the compound in which a relationship to the drug metabolizing system has not as yet been established. Such a case is the large clusters of smooth ER seen in locust muscle after denervation in which large clusters of SER, often forming whorls, appear to distend the sarcoplasm. Some of these may well be related to the degenerative phase as mentioned below.

A protective action of phenobarbital against other agents is suggested by studies such as those of Ikeda and Ohtsuji (1971), who noted a protection against toluene and benzene toxicity in the rat following pretreatment with phenobarbital. Administration of fructose stimulates proliferation of ER in both the liver and intestine which is associated with increased formation of glucose 6-phosphatase (Hugon *et al.*, 1972).

d. DEGENERATION.   For want of a better term, we are calling as "degeneration" a variety of phenomena described in the ER in which it forms various clusters and whorls termed by various names including myelin forms, fingerprint changes (Steiner *et al.*, 1964; Stenger, 1963; Amick and Stenger, 1964; Bruni, 1960; Herdson *et al.*, 1964; Porter and Bruni, 1959), glycogen bodies, etc. (Figs. 15 and 16). These have been described in a variety of cells following various compounds and their mechanism is generally unknown. In the case of Dieldrin, an insecticide which induces the drug-metabolizing sequence in the liver, the situation has been studied in more detail, and the results indicate that following an induction period with proliferations and increased drug metabolizing activity a toxic or other effect supervenes and large numbers of cisternae appear to collapse, forming whorls and fingerprints, at the same time the enzyme activities appear to decrease. It is known that formation of tightly packed whorls is a phenomenon which occurs in damaged or labilized membranes, and it may well be that these suffer from defects which make them more sensitive and cause a labilization.

A striking conversion of ER membrane to cylindrical structures was described in the interstitial cells of dehydrated rats (Bulger *et al.*, 1966). The cylinder walls were composed of helically arranged pentagonal tubules seemingly representing a molecular rearrangement of the membranes (Barber and Bernheim, 1967).

Membrane lipid peroxidation represents another case of toxic effects on the ER membrane in which the membranes also aggregate and undergo characteristic changes associated with liberation of dense material which appears to "glue" the profiles together to form a characteristic appearing mass (Arstila *et al.*, 1972b). One of the best examples of this can be seen in the livers of carbon tetrachloride-poisoned animals where large aggregates filled with smudgy dense material can be seen (Fig. 34). This system has been studied *in vitro*, stimulated initially by the work of Hochstein and Ernster (1964) and Ernster *et al.* (1968), and showed that addition of ferrous iron, NADPH, and ADP together with suspension of rat liver microsomes *in vitro* were followed by a burst of oxygen consumption and liberation of peroxidation end products such as malonyl dialdehyde. Studies of such a system at the EM level have revealed the appearance of clusters of ER vesicles associated with dense material of uncertain origin (Fig. 35), possibly involving ribosome uncoiling and denaturation and accompanied by rapid inactivation of glucose 6-phosphatase activity (Arstila *et al.*, 1972b; Shinozuka, 1971). The lesion cannot be readily repaired by addition of phospholipid in contrast to phospholipase C treatment, and it is paralleled by liberation of products which form color reactions with thiobarbituric acid, presumably malonyl dialdehyde. An alternative hypothesis of the carbon tetrachloride effect has been proposed by Farber *et al.* (1971).

An example of a reversible alteration in isolated ER fragments is provided by studies with purified phospholipase C which produces a reversible inactivation of the enzyme glucose 6-phosphatase (Trump *et al.*, 1970). Shortly following treatment the glucose 6-phosphatase activity goes to zero; however, the defect can be repaired by readdition of phospholipids, either a mixture of phospholipids or purified phospholipid such as phosphatidyl ethanolamine. Phospholipase C treatment of this type is associated with liberation of roughly 70 to 80% of the phospholipid, the diglyceride being retained by the membrane. When this was studied structurally, there is indeed a reversible structural alteration involving an increase in thickness of the membrane and focal accumulations of eccentric densities resembling neutral lipid droplets between the inner and outer dense laminae of the microsomal membrane. Following readdition of phospholipid the alteration appears to be reconstituted and the membrane is returned to normal thickness.

A detailed study of membrane denaturation following carbon tetrachloride was presented by Reynolds and Ree (1971). The authors examined the involvement of the ER in periods following immediately after poisoning with carbon tetrachloride. The authors stated that the distribution of low molatile ^{14}C derived from carbon tetrachloride in subcellular fractions and chemical constituents of liver cells did not change within periods ranging from 15 minutes following poisoning to 2 hours. The following changes were seen. Diene conjugation in microsomal lipids nearly doubles during the first 15 minutes, raising to a peak value at that time while oxidative dimethylase activity and cytochrome P450 decreases. Increase in cell sap RNA and decrease in amino acid incorporation into microsomal protein are not apparent at the end of the first hour. The extent of radioactive carbon tetrachloride binding and lipid diene conjugation are relatively constant and do not increase in proportion to does or injury. Permanent aggregation of smooth surfaced ER profiles appear in centrilobular parnechymal cells within 30 minutes following poisoning in livers fixed by perfusion with osmium tetroxide.

Lipoperoxidation in the pathogenesis of renal necrosis of weanling rats fed a choline deficient diet was investigated by Monserrat *et al.* (1969), who also showed the preventive effects of diphenyl-*p*-phenylene diamine and α-tocopheral acetate.

e. MEMBRANE MOVEMENTS.   Alterations in the movements of ER membranes constitute important factors in the formation of lysosomes by the process of autophagy. Similar processes are involved in viral envelope formation, and in the case of both herpes-like virus and vaccinia virus, budding of virions into cisternae derived from ER has been described. More common, however, is the envelopment of organelles such as mitochondria by ER cisternae through the process of exotropy, resulting in the double membrane-limited stages of autophagic vacuoles. Although all portions of the cytocavitary network may be involved in this process, it seems to be the ER, especially smooth cisternae, that is most commonly involved in it.

Various types of tubular structures have been found in the ER of endothelial and other cells in many conditions including lupus erythematosus and a variety of malignant tumors including sarcomas, lymphomas, and leukemias. The structures have a convoluted tubular form in common, suggesting myxoviruses. Baringer and Swoveland (1972) observed similar particles in the ER of endothelial cells in the brain after herpes simplex virus. Within 8 days after inoculation, tubular structures in tight arrays were seen associated with the ER of endothelial cells. It has been suggested that they represent a host reaction rather than virus particles *per se* and may represent a reaction of rather widespread occurrence.

Specialized forms of parallel arrangement and clustering of SER, termed "myeloid bodies," can occur following administration of choline chloride to light-adapted frogs. Some of these myeloid bodies, composed of parallel arrays of ER disposed in clusters of tubular profiles, were extremely large and have been considered to function in relationship to photoreception or vitamin A storage. It has been suggested that the myeloid body together with SER is involved in choline metabolism and that increased membrane synthesis may be involved.

4. NOTES ON THE GOLGI APPARATUS AND PEROXISOMES

Relatively little is known about changes in the Golgi apparatus in cell injury apart from dilatation, fragmentation, and wrapping, as described above under Acute Cell Injury, Section II,A. One recent study in which amoebae were treated with the compound emetine suggested first a marked increase in the number of Golgi stacks followed by a decrease (Flickinger, 1971). Inhibition of lipoprotein transport following ethionine hepatotoxicity was reported (Figs. 38 and 39). This resulted in absence of lipoprotein droplets in the Golgi with appearance of these droplets in the ER. A similar change was seen with acid phosphatase, which in treated livers was located in smooth cisternae and lysosomes rather than in the lamellae, either in Golgi or GERL, depending on the interpretation on the maturing surface. Golgi components are probably also involved in reactions involving cell membrane formation and formation of the glycocalyx. Recent evidence for a vitamin A-dependent step involving glycosyl transferase activity has been presented and has been related to the effect of vitamin A on cell maturation and its reversal of pre-malignant changes. Induction of a glycosyl transferase activity in the Golgi was noted in salt water stress of salt glands of domestic ducklings (Higgins *et al.*, 1972). This stress is associated with a marked increase in cell membranes of the lateral and basilar surface of these ion transporting epithelia. Following induction, acyl transferase activity was localized only within the lamellae of the Golgi complex, and it has been suggested that the phospholipid component of the cell membrane is assembled in the Golgi region. Similar conclusions were reached in phenobarbital stimulated livers, however, here the increased acyl transferase reaction product was largely found in the smooth microsomes (Higgins and Barrnett, 1972). Another example of appearance of unusual materials within the Golgi is provided by iron stimulation of liver cells in experimental hemosiderosis in which ferritin and hemo-siderin particles may be localized within Golgi lamellae, presumably prior to their elaboration into the lysosome system (Arstila *et al.*, 1970).

Marked increase in the activity of ATPase as well as acid phosphatase in motor neurons were noted both with forced physical activity and administration of tetanus toxin.

Studies by Jonek *et al.* (1971), suggest the possibility of induced changes in the Golgi apparatus in cells such as neurons following severe physical exercise in mice promoted by forced swimming. The authors noted increase in the extent and reactivity of thiamin paraphosphatase in the Golgi apparatus of motoneurons.

An increase in number and size of lysosomes and hypertrophy of the Golgi has been described in denervated muscles although myofibrils were not found within the enlarged lysosomes suggesting to the authors that this may be turnover initiated by extralysosomal factors. On the other hand, breakdown products in the cytoplasm might be responsible for the induced stimulation.

5. ABNORMALITIES IN PEROXISOMES

Peroxisomes represent a distinct group of storage vacuoles which form as diverticula of the cytocavitary network (de Duve and Baudhuin 1966). These vacuoles have been found in a variety of different cell types, especially in the hepatocytes and renal proximal tubular cells of vertebrates and in some protozoa (Hruban and Rechcigl, 1969), although particles belonging to the general class of peroxisomes are currently found in almost all tissues. Structurally, microbodies are typified by their thin (65–70 Å), single, limiting membrane, their finely granular inner matrix, and in some species by an electron dense core and/or a so-called marginal plate. The core may be either amorphous or paracrystalline. They also frequently contain a marginal plate, a term which refers to an electron dense plate about 85 Å thick. It is separated from the limiting membrane by a narrow space. Microbodies are known to contain a number of peroxidative enzymes such as catalase, urate oxidase, D-amino acid oxidase, and in some instances enzymes associated with glycogen metabolism such as malate synthetase. Although their biological function has not yet been completely elucidated, these enzymes are known to participate in the metabolism of uric acid, and there are strong indications that they are involved in carbohydrate oxidation, in gluconeogenesis, in energy production, and in the oxidation of reduced NAD. They may also participate in the metabolism of lipids, bile acids, and prostaglandins. Recently, microbodies have been found to represent but one type of peroxisomes. See also Fig. 68.

Relatively little is known about the role of peroxisomes in the pathogenesis of cellular injury (Hruban and Rechcigl, 1969). The structure and number of microbodies are known to change after the administration of a wide variety of chemical compounds such as salicylates, chlorophenoxyisobutyrate (CPIB), lithocholic acid, and taurocholic acid (Fig. 40). Since all these compounds are known to decrease serum cholesterol levels, it has been postulated that microbodies may participate in the breakdown of cholesterol and may, therefore, play a role in the susceptibility to atherosclerosis. An interesting hypothesis regarding a possible role of catalase in cellular injury was proposed by de Duve (1969), who suggested that this enzyme may form a safety device for oxidation of hydrogen peroxide in case of accelerated production. Since free hydrogen peroxide is a potent inducer of lipid peroxidation, the excess of catalase within microbodies could thus serve as an important inhibitor of intracellular lipid peroxidation. Focal accumulations in portions of the ER have been seen in endocrine cells although the significance of this is not clear. Increased formation of microbodies which begins as localized accumulations of microbody enzymes such as catalase, urate oxidase, and D-amino acid oxidase within portions of the ER following by pinching-off, is observed following administration of hypolipidemic drugs such as CPIB (Reddy et al., 1969).

6. ABNORMALITIES IN INTRACELLULAR DIGESTION

The term lysosome was originally used by de Duve and his associates (de Duve, 1959) to refer to a class of cytoplasmic particles limited by a membrane and containing acid hydrolytic enzymes which are capable of rapidly digesting many components of the cell (see reviews by de Duve, 1964; de Duve and Wattiaux, 1966; Dingle and Fell, 1969) (Figs. 41–43). The enzymes exhibit the property of structure-linked latency. This term describes a situation during which the particles are intact, the substrate cannot gain access to the enzyme, and measured enzyme activities are low. If the membrane is damaged, substrate gains access to enzyme and the enzyme activity can be measured. In a homogenate the extent of this damage can be measured as an increase in free enzyme activity and can be regarded as an estimate of lysosomal integrity. If the damage is more severe, the enzymes may escape completely from the lysosomes, and enzyme activity can be measured in the supernatant after centrifugation at 100,000 g for 30 minutes.

Although the concept of the lysosome as defined by its content of acid hydrolases has been an extremely useful one, it is now apparent that lysosomes represent special cases of secretory and digestive vacuoles which bend imperceptibly between acid hydrolase-containing and nonacid hydrolase-containing structures and, indeed, transform from the one type into the other. In the present chapter, therefore, they are considered the part of the cytocavitary network that is chiefly concerned with intracellular digestion. Intracellular digestion is a process of importance in a wide variety of normal and pathological cellular reactions.

In addition to acid hydrolases, digestive vacuoles contain an unknown number of certain non-enzymatic components. These include iron in the form of ferritin or hemosiderin, polysaccharides, complex glycoproteins, glycogen, plasminogen activator, an anti-bacterial substance known as phagocytin, and some heat-stable hemolysins. In Wilson's disease, copper is stored in hepatic lysosomes (Goldfischer, 1963).

Defective formation of lysosomes occurs in the group of syndromes that occur in several mammals variously termed Chediak-Higashi syndrome in aleutian mink, gray cattle, beige mice, etc., as described by Lutzner et al. (1965) These large granules, the pathogenesis of which is still uncertain, probably are also functionally abnormal. Prieuer et al. (1972) recently noted that the abnormal lysosomes of the proximal tubule of CHS mice had a defect in degradation of protein or other matter obtained by endocytosis that is possibly related to the abnormal leukocyte.

a. HETEROPHAGY. Heterophagocytosis refers to the esotropic uptake of particles such as macromolecules or macromolecular complexes from the surface of the plasma membrane. Often this uptake is referred to as endocytosis or pinocytosis (Cohn, 1971). This results in the appearance of the heterophagosome, which carries ingested particles toward the cell center. The heterophagosome acquires acid hydrolases by fusion with Golgi-derived vesicles or by fusion with preexisting digestive vacuoles to form a new digestive vacuole (Hirsch and Cohn, 1960; Zucker-Franklin and Hirsch, 1964). The material within may then be hydrolyzed to either indigestible debris or soluble intermediates such as small dipeptides or amino acids, which can be reutilized or released from the cell.

The role of heterophagy in nutrition is, of course, exemplified in unicellular forms such as amoeba which derive their nutrition solely in this way. In contrast the significance of heterophagy in the nutrition of mammalian cells is poorly understood; its mechanisms are clearly present in many cells and are often important to the animal as a whole. For example, cells lining the proximal convoluted tubules of the kidney have well-developed systems for heterophagy and are continually reabsorbing proteins from the lumen that have passed through the glomerulus (Oliver *et al.*, 1954) (Fig. 45). This is of possible importance in the conservation of body protein. When the glomerulus is diseased, as in glomerulonephritis, much more protein leaks through and much more is reabsorbed by the tubules (Ericsson, 1965). Heterophagocytosis of microorganisms by leukocytes constitutes an important defense mechanism against infection. In this instance, the specific granules of the leukocyte fuse with the phagosome, releasing digestive enzymes and other antibacterial substances into it. It has recently been suggested that antigen processing via heterophagy in macrophages is an essential preliminary step in the stimulation of immunoglobulin synthesis by antibody-producing cells. A more controversial area is the possible role of heterophagic uptake in memory transfer and in the uptake of interfon. Certain endocrine secretory cells such as thyroid epithelium take up colloid via heterophagy before processing and then releasing it into the bloodstream. Heterophagy is also apparently at work in the newborn intestine during suckling to reabsorb maternal immunoglobulins present in milk. A general mechanism for the turnover of necrobiotic cells is heterophagy by scavenging phagocytes or parenchymal cells.

Abnormal uptake of soluble materials is often reflected by the appearance (Fig. 46) of intracellular vacuoles which represent distended phagosomes and digestive vacuoles. A striking example is the watery vacuolization of the proximal tubule following the administration of mannitol or sucrose to patients. This condition has been termed osmotic nephrosis (Janigan *et al.*, 1960; Trump and Janigan, 1962; Trump, 1961). Insoluble and/or indigestible material is often retained within the digestive vacuoles of phagocytes. This is the basis of tatooing and of anthracosis. In tattooing, these pigments are retained for a lifetime in the digestive vacuoles of cutaneous macrophages, and in anthracosis, inhaled carbon is retained for years in pulmonary phagocytes (Fig. 47).

Watery enlargment of lysosomes can also be produced by ethionine (Goldblatt and Williams, 1969). Changes in permeability are believed to be induced by the marked loss or reduction of ATP produced by ethionine, resulting in osmotic swelling.

Norseth and Brendeford (1971) found that the intercellular distribution of inorganic and organic mercury in the liver differed with various mercury compounds. The results demonstrated that inorganic mercury, defined as mercury not bound covalently to carbon atoms, is accumulated by the lyso-somal apparatus of the liver. The carbon mercury compounds were most efficiently concentrated in microsomal systems. Brunk and Brun (1972) demonstrated the uptake of lead into lysosomal systems and postulated the existence of membrane stability by the action of heavy metals.

The precise kinetics of digestion within the lysosome have not been defined. An interesting note on the intracellular lysing time of phagosome and resul-ting digestive vacuole in the thyroid gland was provided in a recent study by Petrovic (1972) in which the uptake of colloid, processing by the follicle cell, and release were studied by time-lapse cinematography. It was noted that the droplet remains visible for periods ranging between 20 and 89 minutes and that the lyse then was related to the number of droplets, their life span usually being longer when the number is higher than when it is lower.

The role of phagocytosis in protection against infection was recently studied in macrophages, and in the case of mycobacterium the organism has been found to exert a marked effect on the normal process of lysosomal uptake and diffusion. In the case of *Mycobacterium tuberculosis*, which is a facultative intracellular parasite, fusion of primary by lysosomes with the phagosome has been shown to be inhibited with living organisms in contrast to organisms that have been heat killed (Armstrong and Hart, 1971). The mechanism of fusion inhibition if not known, although it is believed that it may involve the membrane surface coat. The possible fusion lack has been noted with histoplasmosis and toxoplasma. Miller and Garbus (1971) in studies of phagocytosis of *Salmonella* noted the difference in the burst of oxygen consumption that normally accompanies phagocytosis with pathogenic versus non-pathogenic strains. The influence of chemical compounds on fusion was studied by Sidransky et al. (1972), who noticed that cortisone blocked fusion of lysosomes with phagosomes containing aspergillus (Merkow et al., 1971).

The role of intralysosomal uptake of staphylococcal enterotoxin B was described by Normann and Stone (1972). Presumably, intravenously admin-istered enterotoxin localized in the kidney after glomerular filtration, and Norman and Stone's data indicate that degradation of the toxin with release of low molecular weight substances can occur in kidney lysosomes.

A role for lysosomal digestion in antigen processing on the part of macro-phages has been suggested. This process implies uptake of antigens with partial digestion and release of a digestive product to the macrophage that may be released from cells or may stimulate release of a macrophage factor which, in turn, modifies lymphocytes.

Smooth muscle digestive vacuoles have been studied in relation to athero-sclerosis (May and Paule, 1972) and changes in the sedimentation characteristics of lysosomal enzymes noted in atherosclerotic regions. Whether this is primary or secondary has not been determined although one possibility is that atherosclerosis represents an acquired storage disease (Peters *et al.*, 1972).

b. INTRACELLULAR TRANSPORT. An example of increased transport of material to the lysosomes for storage is provided by ferritin and hemosiderin storage in the liver cell. Apoferritin is synthesized, in part, on the rough ER and transported through that system to the Golgi apparatus and then to the lysosomes where storage and turnover occur. Much ferritin is probably also added by autophagy of that in the cell sap. In conditions associated with increased levels of iron in the bloodstream, iron taken up by the liver cell may be added to the apoferritin, which is in the cytocavitary network, to form ferritin, which is relatively immune to attack by lysosomal enzymes and hence accumulated within all hepatic lysosomes (Fig. 48). If this continues, the liver becomes loaded with iron and much of the ferritin becomes converted to an insoluble, rather poorly characterized iron-containing protein called hemosiderin. In periods of iron depletion, iron is released from ferritin within the lysosomes and reenters the bloodstream. In two disease states, hemochromatosis and hemosiderosis, abnormal amounts of ferritin and hemosiderin are stored within hepatic lysosomes (Arstila *et al.*, 1972a). Since ATP is necessary for transport within the ER and through the Golgi system, ATP deficiency results in defective transport of lysosomal enzymes and nonenzymatic components. In lead toxicity, localization of lead in lysosomes has been seen (Swartzendruber and Mateer, 1972).

c. AUTOPHAGOCYTOSIS. The phenomenon of autophagocytosis (Ashford and Porter, 1962) is similar to heterophagocytosis. In this instance the vacuole appears to form by exotropy into a cisterna of ER (Figs. 49–52) or other portion of the cytocavitary network (Ericsson and Trump, 1964; Arstila and Trump, 1968). This results in the enclosure of a portion of cytoplasm, such as a mitochondrion, in a double-walled sac. Enzyme is added by fusion of endosecretory vesicles or digestive vacuoles with the outer membrane of the sac in the double-walled stage (Arstila and Trump, 1969). The inner membrane then apparently thickens to resemble the membrane of other digestive vacuoles. Both autophagy and heterophagy are apparently energy-requiring processes which utilize ATP or other high energy intermediates, but the forces involved in these membrane movements are not fully understood.

Recent evidence strongly indicates that this phenomenon, at least in the liver cell, may be mediated by cyclic AMP in a process that involves cell microtubules (Shelburne *et al.*, 1973). Cyclic AMP or dibutyryl AMP *in vitro* will also induce conformational changes in ER, forming multilaminated bodies surrounding organelles such as mitochondria (Shelburne *et al.*, 1973).

Certain endocrine cells, such as those of the anterior pituitary, secrete hormones to the extracellular space. In conditions where secretion is shut off, the hormone is transferred to the lysosome system where it is destroyed. Thus, the direction of this secretory step can provide control over release of secretory material.

In a study of autophagy in plant cells, Cresti *et al.* (1972) described autophagic vacuole formation during a suspended growth period and development of *Eranthis hiemalis* endosperm. The authors note that the methods of formation of autophagic vacuoles resemble those in animal cells, but describe two methods of formation, the one caused by closing of ER cisternae which close around portions of cytoplasm, forming a sequestrium; the authors note that one or more cisternae can be involved in the case of stacks of cisternae, forming more complex bodies. The other method is described as fusion of membrane-bound tubular structures which are arranged so as to surround a mass of cytoplasm. The authors also noted a proximity between the autophagic vacuoles and elements of the Golgi apparatus.

Inadequate autophagic digestion may result from enzyme deficiencies or deletions. Certain toxic compounds such as trypan blue (Lloyd *et al.*, 1968) Triton WR-1339, chloroquine, and neutral red are concentrated within lysosomes and may result in inactivation of one or more enzymes (Beck *et al.*, 1967). This can lead to functional alterations of particular importance in developing embryos, where administration of such compounds may result in congenital malformations. Evidence of the altered digestive capabilities with these compounds is apparently provided by accumulation of increased amounts of membrane debris within the lysosomes and sometimes lysosome enlargement (Fig. 54). Decreased cell protein turnover may occur (Poole and Wibo, 1972) and normal turnover of cell protein may well involve lysosomal hydrolases.

d. PHYSIOLOGICAL AND PATHOLOGICAL FUNCTION OF AUTOPHAGY.   Autophagy provides an obvious means for organelle turnover. In the liver cell, for example, it is estimated that the rate of mitochondrial turnover (half-life ~ 10 days) could be accounted for by autophagocytosis and that at least some of the hepatic glycogen turnover occurs within autophagic vacuoles (Hers, 1965). Autophagocytosis may also serve as a mechanism of nutrition under favorable conditions such as general starvation, specific dietary deficiencies (Charvat *et al.*, 1972), or inhibition of protein synthesis in some organs. Accepting the reduction in number of organelles, the cell seems to behave as if it will utilize its own substance in order to maintain homeostasis. Recently, Arstila *et al.* (1972a) studied the progress of change in the included mitochondria.

Some of the most dramatic examples of increased autophagy occur in association with involutionary processes such as the atrophy of the mammary gland after lactation, the atrophy of the secondary sex organs in elderly persons, or after castration (Brandes *et al.*, 1962; Helminen and Ericsson, 1970, 1971a,b, 1972) and the atrophy of functional units in organs such as the liver or kidney that accompanies progressive ischemia. In all such cases, organ remodeling is accompanied by the appearance of large autophagic vacuoles which ultimately become pigmented residual bodies (Weber, 1964; Jordan, 1964). Romen and Bannasch (1972) observed accumulation of lipoid bodies and mucopolysaccharides in tubular epithelium of the rat kidney in experimental thrombosis of the renal vein. The authors stated that these findings resemble the lysosomal bodies observed in human gangliosidoses and certain mucopolysaccharidoses.

Autophagy also seems to have important relations to differentiation and cell division (Behnke, 1963; Fisher and Fisher, 1963). Phytohemagglutinin-stimulated lymphocytes exhibit numerous autophagic vacuoles. Large numbers of autophagic vacuoles are observed in the regenerating liver after hepatectomy. It has been suggested that autophagocytosis could be related to cell division functioning in the destruction of antimitotic materials.

One of the interesting points about autophagy is that the newly formed autophagic phagosomes and lysosomes have much different physical properties than do the normal preexisting secondary lysosomes. Since they are larger and less dense, they exhibit increased fragility during homogenization. Thus, in cells in which autophagy has been induced, for example, by glucagon, one sees biochemically an increase in both free and unsedimentable activity, which reflects clearly in this case not release of enzyme but the fact that the enzyme-containing autophagic vacuoles have an increased fragility, and with usual homogenizing procedures they are damaged. Thus, many of the early papers claiming to show increased free and unsedimentable activity and the conclusions concerning enzyme release after cell injury reflected not enzyme release but the fact that these injurious agents induced autophagocytosis (Deter and de Duve, 1967).

After ligation of the mammary duct, Helminen and Ericcson (1971a,b) observed that in response to isolated milk stasis, degenerative alteration of the mammary gland epithelium was produced. This was accompanied by an increase in the concentration and total activity of lysosomal enzymes in the mammary gland and was noxious enough to give rise to a gross envolution of the gland.

e. ABNORMAL FUSIONS. An abnormality possibly related to abnormal fusion comprises a group of diseases in various animals including Aleutian trait in the mink, partial albino cattle, and the Chediak-Higashi syndrome in man. Aleutian mink trait, the best studied of these syndromes, results from an alteration of one gene and possibly one enzyme. In many cells, primary and secondary lysosomes, secretory granules, and pigment granules are bizarre in shape.

The mechanism of granulomatous disease remains unknown. It has been suggested that some of the methodology used to measure fusion, degranulation kinetics, and kinetics of ingestion may not be sufficiently sensitive to reveal defects even if they do exist. One of the problems in studying the pathogenesis of these diseases involving abnormal phagocytosis is that alternate pathways of bacterial killing may exist and make it very difficult to identify the definitive defect in a given disease. Evidence of differences in bactericidal mechanisms between cells has recently been provided when it was noted that the peroxidase activity of bacteria-containing phagolysosomes in the liver markedly differed between Kupffer cells and neutrophilic polymorphonuclear leukocytes. It is inferred that different bactericidal mechanisms exist between the two cells.

f. Changes in Lysosomal Enzymes. In some cells, stimulation of pinocytic uptake of digestible materials induces the synthesis of increased amounts of acid hydrolases. This apparently represents genetic induction and can be inhibited by inhibitors of RNA or protein synthesis.

On the other hand, since there are many enzymes present in the digestive vacuoles, one could postulate a series of diseases in which each of the enzymes is deficient or absent (Hers, 1965) (Fig. 55). Some such diseases have been identified. In general, these diseases result in accumulation of materials within ambidigestive vacuoles in various cells throughout the body; often the accumulation results in rather clear vacuoles since the stored materials are relatively soluble (Haust *et al.*, 1969). In other instances, storage diseases may result from synthesis of abnormal materials which cannot be digested by the normal enzymes. Many of these storage diseases exert their most serious effects on neurons. These diseases may be susceptible in therapy by replacement of the missing enzyme in at least some organs, applying the principle which allows the mixing of contents between heterophagic and autophagic vacuoles. It has been shown in Pompe's disease (type II glycogen storage disease), for example, that parenterally administered α-glucosidase will be taken into the liver cell and result in removal of glycogen from the vacuoles. Acquired relative deficiency of α-glucosidase in renal tubule lysosomes may occur after giving streptozotoan (Orci and Stauffacher, 1971).

It is beyond the scope of this chapter to completely review the lysosomal storage diseases, however, it should be pointed out that storage diseases are being discovered for virtually all lysosomal enzymes. In addition to Pompe's disease, these include defects, for example: in β-D-glucosidase (Gaucher's disease), of N-acetyl-D-glucosamminidase (San Filipo disease), of α-D-galactosidase (Fabry's disease), N-acetyl-β-D-hexosaminidase (Tay-Sachs disease), of sphingomyelinase (Niemann-Pick)s disease), myeloperoxidase (myeloperoxidase deficiency), of β-D-galactosidase (Kabbe's disease), and of N-acetyl-β-hexosaminidase A and B (Sandhoff's disease). The prototype of defective bactericidal function is chronic granulomatous disease. Recent research has made it clear that the classic form is but one of the many inherited disorders in which phagocytosis proceeds normally, but cells cannot kill the ingested bacteria (Douglas *et al.*, 1969a,b). In some patients with severe infections and normal immunoglobulins, a phase of missing bactericidal capability may open the way to effective therapy (Douglas and Fudenberg, 1969).

A new familial metabolic disorder that has been described by Nadler and Egan (1970) is characterized by deficiency of lysosomal acid phosphatase. Infants afflicted by this disease show failure to thrive, intermittent attacks of hypotonia, lethargy, opisthotonus, and internal bleeding (see also Scott *et al.*, 1967; Moser, 1970).

g. RESIDUAL BODIES AND STORAGE. Although most material within digestive vacuoles is digested in normal cells, some debris remains (Brunk and Ericsson, 1972). This debris is largely lipid, a fact probably related to the relative lipase deficiency of the digestive vacuoles. The debris often becomes auto-oxidized and forms pigmented autofluorescent materials which are termed lipofuscin or ageing pigment. The debris-filled bodies are called residual bodies (Figs. 56 and 57). In some cells, the residual bodies are known to fuse with the plasma membrane and discharge the debris (Bradford *et al.*, 1969); in others, however, this probably cannot occur and lipofuscin-filled residual bodies tend to accumulate. The neuron is such a cell; neuronal lipofuscin or ageing pigment increases in a linear fashion with age. Neurons become, as it were, filled with the debris of a lifetime.

h. ROLE OF DIGESTION IN INJURED CELLS. A variety of chronic sublethal injuries results in the formation of increased numbers of autophagic vacuoles (Hruban *et al.*, 1962, 1963, 1972; Napolitano, 1963; Novikoff, 1959; Novikoff and Essner, 1962; Horie *et al.*, 1971). Pathogenetic factors include damage to membranes in organelles, decreased nutrition, regeneration of cells, aging, neoplasia, and damage by bacterial products. It appears that damage to organelle membranes, which occurs as a nonspecific feature of many diseases, is especially effective in promoting the formation of autophagic vacuoles. One known pathogenetic factor involved in membrane damage is the lipid peroxidation which occurs experimentally in animals deficient in antioxidants such as vitamin E (Howes *et al.*, 1964); numerous autophagic vacuoles result promptly from such deficiencies. Allison (1968) proposed a hypothesis of carcinogenesis based on autophagic destruction or alteration of chromosomes to produce mutations. It is true that certain chemical carcinogens, especially the polybenzenoid hydrocarbons, are concentrated in lysosomes, but this theory of carcinogenesis is yet to be established.

Lethal digestion has been proposed as a process involving conversion of an innocuous to a harmful substance by digestion. A possible example of the process would be esotropic uptake of virus. Uncoating of the virus in lysosomes may release the infectious nucleic acid which would then be free to infect the host.

i. HYDROLASE RELEASE FROM CELLS. Damage of cells by release of hydrolases by lysosomes was first studied in connection with vitamin A, which has been shown to stimulate release of proteases from cartilage lysosomes, resulting in injury to the cartilage matrix (Lucy *et al.*, 1961; Fell and Thomas, 1960; Dingle, 1963). The mechanisms whereby this might occur, that is, by cell disintegration as opposed to secretion of lysosomal enzymes by reverse esotropy, has still not been clearly defined. Another mechanism resulting in lysosomal enzyme release is cytolysis. For example, that resulting from antibody and complement attack or attack on the cell membrane by a variety of compounds including bacterial toxins and chemical substances, including surfactants or proteolytic enzymes which result in breakdown of all cell membrane systems including lysosomal membranes. Simultaneous with lysosomal enzyme release under these circumstances is release of virtually all cell constituents such as cell sap enzymes, enzymes within the mitochondrial matrix, potassium, and a variety of cell metabolites including adenine nucleotides.

Lysosomal enzymes are released from cells in the acute inflammatory reaction and appear to be responsible for some of the changes in capillary permeability at the site of inflammation (Fig. 53). Leukocyte granules also contain leucocidin, which can act on other leukocytes to produce degranulation and loss of digestive enzymes. Inadequate release of lysosome contents can result in accumulation of residual bodies or lipofuscin pigment.

Extrusion of lysosomal enzymes to the extracellular space in what has become known as frustrated phagocytosis has been described by Henson (1972) and studied in detail by Weissmann *et al.* (1972). According to this concept, antigen–antibody complexes, if attached to surfaces such as the basement membrane, attract leukocytes, which instead of engulfing the particles, release lysosomal constituents by reverse esotropy, fusing with the partially internalized cell membrane of the frustrated phagosome. This release is apparently an active secretory process requiring environmental calcium, energy metabolism, inhibition by agents thought to increase cyclic AMP, and stimulation by cytochalasin B. The effect of cyclic AMP has not been explained although biphasic effects have been suggested, and it has been noted that high concentration of cyclic AMP might result in random aggregations of microtubules, preemptively causing organization of tubulin into tubules directed in abnormal areas, not necessarily toward the cell surface or toward phagocytic vacuoles. The possible relationship of this to immunological disease is evident and includes attack on the glomerular basement membrane in nephrotoxic nephritis.

An imaginative method for lysosomal enzyme release was suggested by Miller *et al.* (1973) and related to possible interactions between *Endamoeba histiolytica* and the host, which involved budding of the cell membrane above a closely approximated acid phosphatase positive vesicle, which then formed extensions from which vesicles bud and detach toward the host–parasite interface, delivering lytic enzymes through an apocrine-type process. If this interesting observation can be confirmed it would provide another type of secretion of lysosomal enzymes. Although release of lysosomal enzymes in hemorrhages and other types of shock has been described, its mechanism remains obscure (Barankay *et al.*, 1969; Janoff, 1964).

In the model system involving cell injury and alteration of the permeability of the lysosomal membranes by administration of the surface-active agent triton WR-1339, Iturriaga *et al.* (1969) observed that marked aggravation of cell injury occurred if carbon tetrachloride was combined with Triton WR-1339.

Detailed study of ageing in the rat myocardium by Travis and Travis (1972) indicated marked age-associated changes from 18 to 33 months including residual bodies, autophagic vacuoles containing glycogen, as well as mitochondria and ultimately formation of lipofuscin-type pigment. Inclusions of ER have been observed by Kovacs (1971).

Abnormalities of the lysosomal system in Dublin-Johnson syndrome were postulated by Baba and Ruppert (1972). The authors found pigment which corresponded to dense bodies which consisted of aggregates of osmiophilic dense material intermixed with fine granular, globular material. Histochemical tests showed acid phosphatase activity in portions of these dense bodies. These findings indicated to the authors that the lysosomal dysfunction was present as a possible pathogenetic factor of this disorder.

D. *Cytoplasmic Ground Substance*

1. General Considerations

The cytoplasmic ground substance comprises the continuous phase of cytoplasm and consists of a gel-like material in which are suspended structures such as microtubules, microfilaments, glycogen deposits, free ribosomes, proteins such as hemoglobin, and lipid droplets. It has been difficult to study because of its lack of formed materials in the electron micrographs.

Rapid changes in viscosity of this compartment have been noted in movies of injured cells, for example, in the sap within membranous blebs at the cell surface. Increased Brownian motion of cytoplasmic particles, such as mito-chondria, denotes changes in protoplasmic viscosity. The proteins of the cell sap may play a role in cell volume regulation through ion binding, contraction, or other conformational change.

2. ALCOHOLIC HYALINE

The term alcoholic hyaline designates a type of degeneration within hepatic cells originally described by Mallory (1914) in patients with alcoholic cirrhosis. It consists of cytoplasmic clumps of eosinophilic material that form multiple droplets and irregular meshworks distributed predominantly in the perinuclear cytoplasm of hepatic cells. Using light microscopy, masses of alcoholic hyaline appear acidophilic and irregular in outline; they stain with dyes reacting with phospholipid. With the electron microscope, hyaline is characteristically found in areas which normally contain large amounts of rough ER and is associated with disarray, fragmentation, and disappearance of the rough ER (Biava, 1964; Flax and Tisdale, 1964). It is composed largely of a meshwork of fibrils approximately 80–100 Å thick (Fig. 59). The patho-genesis of alcoholic hyaline is not clear; one current hypothesis states that it is derived from membranes of the ER. It should be differentiated from megamitochondria, which are also seen in the liver cells of alcoholics (see also Schaffner et al., 1963; Klion and Schaffner, 1968). Another hypothesis asserts that it is a reflection of a disturbance in microfilament formation or turnover. It should also be noted that it is somewhat akin to the so-called neurofibrillary tangles in damaged neurons.

3. CHANGES IN MYOFILAMENTS

Changes in the size and number of myofilaments have been observed in both atrophy and hypertrophy of muscle. Especially striking is the toxicity of plasmocid for muscle (Price et al., 1962); this quinoline derivative causes complete dissolution of I-band components including actin filaments; Z lines also disappear (Fig. 60). In the human muscle disease known as Zenker's hyaline degeneration, changes in the ground substance consisting of de-creased density and loss of fibrils seem to account for the characteristic light microscopic appearance. Smooth muscle myosin can aggregate following injury to form clusters of thick filaments (Rosenbluth, 1972) (see also Yunis and Samaha, 1971; Nordlander and Singer, 1972).

4. OTHER CYTOPLASMIC FILAMENTS

The presence of various types of cytoplasmic filaments, some of which are not affected by cytochalasin, has been suggested from studies on the eye of the snail, Helix aspersa. These filaments appeared in bundles in pigment cells. Abnormalities of cell movements may involve changes in cytochalasin-sensitive cytoplasmic filaments. Evidence was recently presented for a role of such changes in altered water movements in toad bladder (Davis *et al.*, 1972). Precipitation of actinomyosin complexes in damaged smooth muscle cells has been described and may present a very striking morphological alteration in the smooth muscle cell cytoplasm.

The introduction of cytochalasin B as an experimental tool for the study of microfilaments has yielded some new insights into changes in the cell sap in damaged cells. Recently, Miranda and Godman (1972) noted the formation of fibril aggregates in CD-treated muscle cells, which at later intervals aggregated, were sequestered by SR and later expelled from the cells. The formation of so-called "leptomeric" bodies, which represent striated organelles, presumably resulting from fibril aggregation was also noted. To some extent, especially at early intervals, these changes were reversible. Such studies with cytochalasin A and B also emphasize the relation between filaments and cell shape and even possibly surface blebbing (Springer and Perdue, 1972; Goldman, 1972). In platelets the filaments may be related to the shape change and not to the degranulation (White and Estensen, 1972).

5. MICROTUBULES

Microtubules are generally defined as cylindrical structures of approximately 250 Å in diameter with electron dense walls and a less dense interior. A relationship between microtubules and cellular shape (red blood cells) and intracellular movements seems well established; chromosomal movements during mitosis and the motion of spermatozoa are examples. Microtubules have also been postulated to take part in the transport of water and small ions and in the formation of a skeletal support in epithelial cells. It is not known how microtubules develop.

Effects of microtubules on directed nerve fiber growth in culture was studied by Handel (1971). It was noted that an interference with microtubules with either colchicine or cold treatment resulted in inhibition of fiber outgrowth and suggested that microtubules may be involved in both outgrowth and elongation. However, since nerve fibers exposed to colchicine did not retract, it was suggested that maintenance of the fiber processes may not be entirely a function of colchicine but that contacts with other cells and supporting matrix could also play a role.

The role of microtubules in cellular injury is for the present poorly understood. They are rather labile structures, which completely disappear after the use of certain fixatives or at low temperatures. On the basis of their association with cellular movements, one might speculate that abnormalities in their growth or function could seriously hamper cell function in general.

Similarly, disappearance of the microtubules in axons could seriously impair transport of materials along the axon. A role for microtubules in constraining so-called saltatory movements of cell particles has been defined. Saltatory movement refers to rapid back-and-forth linear movements of cytoplasmic particles such as mitochondria or lysosomes. In the presence of colchicine, which induces fragmentation of microtubules, these cytoplasmic movements become disordered. Colchicine and vinblastine also affect the microtubules of the mitotic spindle, and its application results in mitotic arrest at metaphase. An increasing role of microtubules and filaments is being found in the control of lysosomal enzyme secretion (Hoffstein *et al.*, 1972). A recent study of axons (Hinkley and Samson, 1972) reported transformation of axonal microtubules by halothane, which they attempted to relate to the anesthetic properties of this compound.

The presence of cytoplasmic crystals in human hepatocytes has been described although its significance remains unknown. It has been reported in a variety of pathological conditions.

The appearance of paracrystalline inclusions following treatment with vinblastine has been well established (Fig. 61) (see, for example, Tyson and Bulger, 1972). These can measure several microns in diameter and may be composed of closely packed tubules measuring approximately 250 Å in diameter, each composed of globular 150-Å subunits (Goode and Maugel, 1972). In the case of neurons, the vinblastine-induced crystals are somehow related to the induced blockage of the processes or rapid exoplasmic transport which is thought to function normally in the supply of materials to the synapses.

Jockusch and Blessing (1971) demonstrated that vinblastine alkaloids form precipitates with proteins other than microtubular proteins. These proteins which precipitate with vinblastine have actinlike properties. The authors compared ultra-structural appearance of vinblastine precipitates of microtubular proteins and actin in three different organisms. They stated that while precipitates derived from slime mold extract showed exclusively amorphous densely stained aggregates which looked similar to those obtained with purified actin, the precipitates from brain extracts were heterogeneous and contained hexagonal material and helical structures in addition to amorphous material. The older aggregates were thought to be composed of microtubular protein while the amorphous material was thought to contain actin as well as possible other proteins. A role of salts concentration on microfilament formation and contraction has been suggested for epithelial cells. Exposing the basal ends of epithelial cells to extracellular fluid appears to induce microfilament formation, which appears to be independent of calcium ions and is prevented by chtochalasin B. Recently it has been proposed that the presence of a double helix in microtubules derived from paracrystals suggests another role of microtubules in cell movements involving contraction (see also Seil *et al.*, 1969).

6. CHANGES IN CELL SAP OF ERYTHROCYTES

A striking series of examples of cell sap change is provided by observations of erythrocyte abnormalities, often in association with hemolytic disease.

Changes in cell viscosity have received attention in red blood cells since the visco-elastic properties of the red cell are involved in its normal passage through tissue capillaries and through microsecretory sieves of the spleen and other portions of the reticuloendothelial systems. Changes in its visco-elastic properties such as plasticity, deformability, internal viscosity, etc., affects the red cell's ability to traverse the microcirculation and may result in hemolysis and other changes based primarily on physical-chemical changes in the cell sap.

Mammalian erythrocytes may exhibit several types of pathological change in components of the cell sap. In certain types of hemolytic anemia, especially those induced by phenylhydrazine or other drugs associated with oxidative denaturation of hemoglobin, precipitates called Heinz bodies occur within the red blood cell (Jacob, 1970). These consist of relatively insoluble products of hemoglobin denaturation. It has also been suggested that these precipitates may form during the normal process of red cell senescence, leading to red cell destruction. The initial morphological lesion in Heinz body development is the formation of an apparently crystalline structure, which usually appears in the region of mitochondria and grows by coalescence and condensation, finally coming to lie just beneath the cell membrane. These structures result in considerable distortion of cell shape and deformation of the plasma membrane. It is though that such changes within the cytoplasm of red cells render the cells relatively rigid, increasing the chances of injury as cells pass through limited spaces such as the splenic cords. The resulting injury to the cell membrane presumably predisposes to hemolysis by accelerating erythrophagocytosis.

A striking conformational change in the cell sap occurs during red blood cell sickling in sickle cell anemia (Murayama, 1966). In well-oxygenated blood from patients with this disease, the red cells are morphologically indistinguishable from normal erythrocytes. When the oxygen tension is reduced, however, the cells shrink and crumple into sickle or holly leaf shapes. The only chemical difference between normal and sickle hemoglobin lies in the substitution of valine for glutamic acid at the sixth position in the two β chains (Pauling *et al.*, 1949; Perutz *et al.*, 1965) This single amino acid substitution has two major effects; first, it causes deoxygenated hemoglobin, or S, to be much less soluble than deoxygenated normal hemoglobin or either form of oxyhemoglobin; second, a new molecular conformation ensues which predisposes to neat molecular packing. Other physical characteristics confirm the parallel alignment of hemoglobin molecules. Electron microscopic study reveals microtubular paracrystalline structures which, on further study, are found to represent hollow cables, each formed of six hemoglobin monofilaments.

7. CHANGES IN DENSITY

Cell sap has been observed to exhibit marked changes in electron density after cell injury. A diffuse increase in density producing so-called dark cells and suggesting selective dehydration of individual cells has been observed in many nonspecific types of injury where it is often associated with dilatation of the ER. Decrease in density of the cell sap may occur in conditions causing acute dilatation of the cisternae of the ER. Changes in cell sap streaming and gelation, though common and possibly important in cell injury, are poorly understood. Some of these changes may depend on divalent cation concentration (Kessler, 1972), and changes in the gel nature could relate to Ling's (Ling *et al.*, 1973) concepts of cell compositional control (Lewis, 1923). Another form of coagulation of cell sap can occur when there is denaturation of the cytoplasm as in thermal burns or laser irradiation.

In a paper regarding sublethal ischemia of the myocardium, De La Iglesia and Lumb (1972) noted large vacuoles which represent modified blebs containing predominantly glycogen but interdigitating with recesses of other cells in the myocardium. Occasional mitochondria were noted in the blebs, but by and large they were relatively clear and contained mainly glycogen and fine protein mercurials.

8. FATTY CHANGE

Although certain accumulations of triglyceride seem to occur within the ER, it cannot be excluded that triglycerides may also accumulate in another compartment, possibly within the cytoplasmic ground substance. A definitive limiting membrane cannot be identified around most large lipid droplets (Fig. 62). (See below for additional information.)

E. Changes in the Nucleus

Changes in the nucleus constitute important manifestations following both acute and chronic injury cell injury, though effects on nuclear function do not appear to be capable of explaining the pathogenesis of acute lethal injury. The system obviously works in concert with other parts of the cell concerned with transcription and translation such as the nucleolus and the cytoplasmic polysomes. The significance of nuclear changes in injury are probably related to the stage of the mitotic cycle in which the cells exist at the time of injury. Unfortunately, the detailed studies of such relationships are not available, however immediate lethality does not appear to be explained on the basis of nuclear events (cf. enucleation in cells such as amoeba is not followed by immediate death), yet at the same time some of the lethal effects of radiation and radiomimetic drugs appear to be related to nuclear effects in cells in the cell cycle.

Changes in Aggregation and Distribution of Chromatin

Shortly following a variety of injury types the nuclear chromatin becomes clumped along the nuclear envelope and around the nucleolus (Figs. 63 and 64). This change was alluded to in Section II,A. This change is initially reversible and may involve physicochemical changes involving the binding forces of the surfaces of nucleohistone fibrils. Along with the clumping, interchromatin granules are segregated and often appear as aggregates along the interface between the chromatin and other parts of the nucleoplasm. At later stages following lethal injury, the clumps of chromatin gradually disappear, presumably the result of attack by cathepsins and nucleases. In some instances the nucleus shrinks and the chromatin remains. The change is known as pyknosis. Rapid reversibility of chromatin clumping has been observed during the early stages, and Lewis (1923) noted that chromatin can be clumped and reversed numerous times without apparently interference with the subsequent mitotic history of the cell.

A variety of types of nuclear inclusions have been seen in various types of cell injury. The first are known as pseudoinclusions (Fig. 66) because they represent deep invaginations of cytoplasm with its contents into the nucleus rather than true inclusions within the nucleoplasm. These can easily be identified by noting the double-walled nuclear envelope between the nucleoplasm and the inclusion. Irregularities of the nucleus appear to predispose to pseudoinclusions and they are especially prominent in cells that are in the mitotic cycle.

True inclusions (Fig. 67), on the other hand, represent inclusions within the nucleoplasm and occur in a variety of chronic cell injuries including heavy metal poisoning with lead or bismuth and a variety of virus infections, especially DNA viruses. In the latter, the virions may produce striking paracrystalline arrays within the nucleoplasm. Many other kinds of accumulations forming nuclear inclusions have been noted including fibrils, glycogen, vesicles, triglycerides, and vacuoles, and tubular structures have been seen.

F. The Role of Nucleus and Protein Synthesis in Chronic Cell Injury

Although various steps of protein synthesis and genetic transcription take place in different parts of the cell, these are considered as a system because of the important interrelationships which they exhibit. The system comprises the nucleus, the nucleolus, the membrane-bound polysomes within the cytoplasm, and the free polysomes within the cell sap.

1. ALTERATIONS IN THE NUCLEUS

There are marked variations in the structural and functional activities of the nucleus during different phases of the mitotic cycle. During interphase, some regions of the chromatin called heterochromatin appear to remain condensed (Mirsky and Osawa, 1961). They are essentially inactive in RNA synthesis, which presumably takes place on the expanded portions of the chromatin (euchromatin). Chromatin fibrils are attached to the nuclear envelope adjacent to the nuclear pores and may have some effect on inducing formation of the latter structures.

The nucleus also contains a variety of other granules called interchromatin granules, perichromatin granules, perichromatin fibrils, and coiled bodies. The functional significance of all the granules is still poorly understood, although they may function as carriers of RNA.

The nucleoplasm is separated from the cytoplasm by a nuclear envelope which is continuous with the ER from which it appears to form after mitosis is completed. The two membranes come together at the nuclear pores with obliteration of the perinuclear cisterna. This cisterna often markedly enlarge in injured cells. It seems clear that the pores serve as semipermeable barriers between nucleus and cytoplasm and may be the pathway for transfer of RNA or other macromolecules to the cytoplasm.

The significance of nuclear change in cell injury probably depends on the stage of the cell cycle at the time of injury. In postmitotic cells, interference with nuclear function does not seem to be immediately lethal for the cell. Accordingly, it cannot apparently explain the progression to cell necrosis after acute injuries such as ischemia. In fact, there are numerous experiments employing suitable cell types that indicate that the entire nucleus may be removed from a cell by microdissection without killing the cell until several days have passed.

There is also, on the other hand, a series of nuclear changes in lethal and sublethal reactions to injury, which is of importance not only in recognizing the effects of cell injury but also in understanding their pathogenesis.

2. NUCLEAR INCLUSIONS

Various types of nuclear inclusions have been described in injured cells. The structures known as pseudoinclusions (Fig. 65) represent deep cytoplasmic indentions into the nucleus that, because of the plane of section, appear to reside within the nucleoplasm (Kleinfeld *et al.*, 1956; Leduc and Wilson, 1959). These can be easily identified by the nuclear pores in the envelope surrounding them. Pseudoinclusions increase in number as the nuclei become irregular and are often observed to occur in cells undergoing rapid turnover.

True inclusions (Fig. 66) represent accumulations which are actually located in the nucleoplasm. Among the most characteristic of these are aggregates of virus particles which may be striking because of their crystalline array. Intranuclear inclusions may also occur in the nuclei of renal tubules in heavy metal poisoning with bismuth or lead (Beaver and Burr, 1963; Beaver, 1961). Many other kinds of accumulation of vesicles, glycogen, concentric lamellar bodies, fibrillar structures, vacuoles, and tubular or filamentous inclusions have been described but are of unknown significance. The presence of large bundles of intranuclear fibrillary aggregates was noted by de Estable-Puig and Estable-Puig (1971) and de Estable-Puig *et al.* (1971) after aluminum hydroxide exposure.

Another example of filamentous inclusions in the nucleus that can be very striking is seen in so-called inclusion body myositis, a chronic progressive wasting and weakness of muscles, idiopathic in origin. The filamentous material in the inclusions has a striking resemblance to thick myofibrils.

3. ALTERATIONS IN THE NUCLEOLUS

In general, nucleoli have three distinct constituents: (1) dense ribosome-like particles 150–200 Å in diameter, (2) filaments 80–100 Å in diameter, and (3) intranucleolar chromatin fibrils identical with the fibrils in the nucleoplasm (Bernard and Granboulan, 1968). The ribosome-like particles and the 80–100 Å filaments seem to represent both RNA and protein. The fibrils are arranged in an open skeinlike structure sometimes termed the nucleolonema, whose open regions (nucleolar vacuoles) contain the chromatin fibrils of the intranucleolar chromatin which, with the condensed chromatin in the periphery of the nucleolus (nucleolus-associated chromatin), may represent the so-called nucleolar organizer. Nucleoli have a constant relationship to specific chromosomes and tend to be constant in number and position for a given species.

In recent years it has been established that both the 28 S and the 18 S components of ribosomal RNA are synthesized in the nucleolus. This synthesis proceeds via the RNA polymerase reaction and is sensitive to actinomycin D.

Numerous carcinogenic and antimetabolic agents have been noted to induce changes in the structure and function of the nucleolus, which may be related to their metabolic effects. Among these are actinomycin D, aflatoxin, and ultraviolet irradiation, all which interfere with DNA-dependent RNA synthesis (Goldblatt *et al.*, 1969; Stevens, 1964; Shofe, 1964). These agents cause segregation of stratification of the nucleolar components into regions composed of particles, RNA–protein fibrils, and chromatin fibrils, respectively, plus an altered RNA–protein component or dense plaque. They also apparently arrest the production of RNA subunits within the nucleolus (and elsewhere in the nucleus). Similar changes in the nucleolus have been observed by Weiss and Meyer (1972) in coxsackie virus A9 infection in the monkey kidney.

Ethionine, which traps adenine in the formation of *s*-adenosylethionine, inhibits RNA and protein synthesis. Components of the nucleolus are widely dispersed, but can be reaggregated after the administration of adenine (Shinozuka *et al.*, 1968).

4. VARIATION IN SUSCEPTIBILITY TO INJURY IN DIFFERENT PHASES OF THE CELL CYCLE

It is important to study variations in sensitivity to toxic or other injurious agents throughout the division cycle (Baserga and Weibel, 1969). This variation is extremely important in pathobiology because it constitutes a possible basis of current cancer chemotherapy and radiotherapy and helps substantially to explain the side effects of these compounds.

Variations in sensitivity to injury in different mitotic phases is especially evident following injury by ionizing irradiation or radiomimetic agents such as the nitrogen mustrads, which are so-called alkylating agents. It seems that cells in early G1 and G2 phases are the least sensitive, and cells in M, late G1, or early S phase are the most sensitive. In many cells, irradiation extends the interphase period and retards entry into mitosis by extension of the time in G2. Cytologic changes observed in the nucleus during cell division include (chromosome breaks) bridge formation between chromosomes at anaphase and chromosomal fragmentation. In contrast, some cells such as spermatogonia and lymphocytes evidently exhibit an immediate cytolytic type of death after irradiation.

In another category are agents exhibiting differential effects during the cell cycle, the so-called spindle poisons, which include colchicine, griseofulvin, vincristine, and vinblastine. All these agents presumably interfere with the formation of the mitotic spindle, possibly by binding with specific microtubule proteins, thus stabilizing or blocking the process of mitosis in metaphase. Evidence indicates that microtubule subunit synthesis parallels mitosis but that subunits are stable and may persist in cells for several days (Bucher and Berkley, 1972). Another type of interference is apparently produced by N_2O which seems to interfere with the chromosome spindle fiber interaction (Brinkley and Rao, 1972).

G. Special Examples of Chronic Injury

1. HYPERTROPHY AND ATROPHY

A common total cellular manifestation of chronic injury is changes in the size and growth of the cell, either an increase or a decrease. These are commonly referred to by the names hypertrophy and atrophy which refer to increases or decreases, respectively, in cellular dry mass, normally mass caused by changes in cell components. Some examples of hypertrophy have been well studied, perhaps the best studied is the case of phenobarbital-stimulated hypertrophy of the liver, referred to above in Section III,C,3. However, studies have also been performed on kidney and heart muscle. In general, these studies indicate induction of DNA and protein synthesis, although usually the induction of DNA synthesis is a reflection of cell division as well. Increased protein synthesis is, however, usually associated with the formation of increased cytoplasmic components such as mitochondria, cytoplasmic filaments, endoplasmic reticulum, etc. Partial passage of cells through the mitotic cycle without telophase and cytokinesis has often been postulated as one of the causes of cell hypertrophy. Recently, Jago (1969) has described the development of hepatic megalocytosis following chronic pyrrolizidine alkaloid poisoning. However, a recently proposed mechanism for formation of multinucleated giant cells has been provided by studies utilizing cytochalasin B (Krishan and Whitlock, 1972), which seems to prevent migration due to its effects on microfilaments of the daughter cells which then tend to form multinucleated cells.

A relationship of acute demand such as severe stress and increase of mitochondria mass in heart muscle cells has been postulated by Laguens and Gomez-Dumm (1967). A similar study by McCallister and Brown (1965) showed that mitochondria in hypertrophic heart increase in size and show distinct morphological characteristics.

In studies on lysosomal enzyme activity in normal and hypertrophied mammalian myocardium, Tolnai and Beznak (1971) found that in hypertrophic myocardium p-nitrophenylphosphatase and other lysosomal enzyme activities were increased, but the relative distribution and localization subcellularly were essentially the same as in normal myocardium.

2. FATTY CHANGES

Lipid metabolism involves a great number of lipid substances and structures which are metabolically interrelated with each other. Lipids perform a variety of special functions in cell structure and metabolism. There are the triglycerides (TG) functioning mainly in storage, phospholipids (PL), important structural units of cellular membranes and cholesterol, which function as an important constituent of membranes and as a hormone precussor. It comes as no surprise, therefore, that multiple events affecting cellular integrety also affect lipid metabolism. Inspite of the great variety of disturbances of lipid metabolism, however, the reactions visible in cells in chronic cell injury are fairly uniform. They are usually observable as accumulations of lipid substances either as triglyceride droplets in the cytoplasm of cells or as lipid material in the endoplasmic reticulum or Golgi apparatus and secretory vesicles. The lipid metabolism in cells of organs such as the liver is further-more affected by metabolic changes of peripheral tissues such as skin or muscle which cause increased demand on the metabolic or secretory activity of the liver cells. In the normal adult, triglyceride stores in adipose tissue amount to about 12 kg as compared to 0.5 kg glycogen (Havel, 1972). The glycogen stores in contrast are mainly located in skeletal muscle (400 gm glycogen). The distribution of lipids is regulated by hormonal action, e.g., insulin.

Insulin counteracts the liberation of triglycerides from adipose tissue and promotes the storage of triglycerides by stimulation of the hormone-sensitive lipase in the adipose tissue or by inhibition of the lipase which liberates trigylcerides from the adipose tissue and by promotion of glucose meta-bolism. Interactions of FA and TG can also occur by hormonal action such as epinephrine.

Fat is absorbed through the intestinal cells by partial hydrolysis and recombination and delivered to the bloodstream as chylomicrons, trigly-cerides, and a small amount of phospholipid and cholesterol surrounded by a carrier protein. It is transferred into adipose cells in the periphery of the cir culation where, prior to storage, it is hydrolyzed again. Recently, Mahley *et al.* (1971) proposed that the intestinal cells produce also approximately 17% of the very low density lipoproteins (VLDL). VLDL as particles of 250 to 800 A size and chylomicrons as particles above 800 A are found within the tubular network of the Golgi apparatus of intestinal epithelial cells and furthermore in secretory vesicles derived from the Golgi apparatus. VLDL isolated from rat intestinal epithelial cells were shown to contain the same protein characteristics as plasma VLDL and low density lipoproteins.

The liver secretes several fractions of lipoprotein, one fraction is a VLDL, fraction two is the low density lipoprotein, and fraction three is a high density lipoprotein (HDL). In general, toxic insults to the liver mainly affect the sec-retion of the VLDL and have much less influence on the high density lipo-protein. The following diagram (Fig. 69) demonstrates the main features of intracellular lipid metabolism of the 'liver cell. From the periphery, tri-glycerides are mobilized cells through the action of hormones such as epinephrine or growth hormone labeled as "c". The hormonal action in the opposite direction is labeled as "i." Fatty acids are present in the plasma either as saturated fatty acids or as unsaturated fatty acids, usually bound to serum albumin. The fatty acids from adipose tissue are absorbed by the liver cells. This process can be inhibited by the detergent Triton X-100 (j). In the liver the free fatty acids are esterified: Some esterified fatty acids are unsaturated. If fatty acids are unsaturated they are first converted by isomerases. Fatty acids can be liberated from cytoplasmic fat droplets (Lipase c), from membranes (Lipase m), or resorbed from chylomicron (Lipase c). In each case they gain access to the same pool. The liberation from cytoplasmic fat droplets can be inhibited by insulin. Fatty acids are esterified in the outer membrane of mitochondria, a process inhibited by alcohol "d." The fatty acid co-enzyme A is then converted to carnitine esters which are then able to tra-verse the mitochondrial membrane. Inside the membrane, coenzyme A esters [CoA (m) esters] with mitochondrial coenzyme A are formed which then are further metabolized either by the formation of acetyl coenzyme A acetyl CoA (m) or by the formation of acetyl coenzyme A. Acetyl coenzyme A gives rise to two alternative pathways; one pathway with acetyl coenzyme A can lead over hydroxyl methylgluteryl coenzyme A to the formation of ketone bodies or it can pass from intermediary products of mevalonic acid and squalenes which, furthermore, are transformed to cholesterol. Acetyl coenzyme A can, furthermore, be combined with oxaloacetic acid which is metabolized in the Kreb's cycle. An alternate pathway leads over propionic coenzyme A which is transformed to succinic coenzyme A which then enters the Krebs cycle. The synthesis of fatty acids begins with citrate which is transported across the membrane and combined with coenzyme A (C), from cytoplasm which results in the formation of oxaloacetic acid and acetyl coenzyme A. Malonyl coenzyme A is formed by binding Co_2 which then, by the protein complex of the fatty acid Synthetase, is transformed to fatty acid coenzyme A. Elong-ation of fatty acids can occur in mitochondria as well as at the ER. Neutral fat is formed by combination of 1-glycerol-3-phosphate with fatty acids as-sociated with the liberation of coenzyme A and inorganic phosphate. Fatty acid coenzyme A, however, can also be combined with 1-glycerol-3-phos-phate to form phosphatidic acid which is the key substance in the formation of phospholipids. Phospholipids are resynthesized by the performance of several intermediary steps. Phospholipids then are secreted into the lumen of the ER where they are combined with the protein moiety to form phos-pholipo proteins (Glaumann, 1971a). Cholesterol is secreted into the lumen of the ER are triglycerides. They form the lipid substances present in the ER of cells, the triglycerides mainly join the fraction of very low density lipo-protein and are secreted into the cytoplasm.

Pathogenetic mechanisms leading to the accumulation of lipids in the cytoplasm of liver cells can be described under four headings. The first is a situation in which the rate of synthesis of hepatic triglyceride is normal but there is a block in the utilization. The second is a situation where there is no impairment in utilization of hepatic triglycerides but where the rate of their synthesis is increased. The third is a situation in which there is both an increase in the rate of hepatic triglyceride synthesis and a block in their utilization. The fourth is a situation in which synthesis of hepatic triglyceride takes place in a compartment of the cell other than the ER where such synthesis normally occurs. (Lombardi, 1965).

a. NORMAL RATE OF SYNTHESIS, BLOCK IN UTILIZATION. A number of substances such as carbon tetrachloride ethionine and puromycine are capable of producing a block in the secretion of triglycerides into the plasma and these substances have been found indeed to produce fatty liver. Deficiency such as choline deficiency also leads to fatty liver through the inhibition of the normal phospholipid biosynthesis process ("a", "b", "c") (Aiyar et al., 1964; Farber et al., 1963; Lombardi and Recknagel, 1962; Windmueller, 1964; Smuckler and Benditt, 1965; Smuckler et al., 1962).

According to Lombardi the common and characteristic feature of fatty liver belonging to this group is the deposition of triglycerides and decreased concentration of plasma lipids. The available evidence points toward a deficient secretion of lipoprotein into the ER and release from the cell. A model system for decreased lipid binding, and deficient transport is orotic acid toxicity ("e and f"). This is shown in the upper right-hand corner of the diagram (Novikoff et al., 1966).

b. INCREASED RATE OF SYNTHESIS, NORMAL UTILIZATION. Increased rates in synthesis of hepatic triglycerides occur in situations where either decreased oxidation or increased synthesis of fatty acids takes place or where increased uptake of plasma fatty acids or nonesterification of fatty acids occurs. This situation could be precipitated by hormonal action such as growth hormones and epinephrine which are known to stimulate the release of free fatty acids by the adipose tissue and cause fatty liver.

c. DECREASED RATE IN HEPATIC TRIGLYCERIDE SYNTHESIS, DECREASED UTILIZATION. In alcohol toxicity the increased pressure of glycerol 3-phosphate in combination with decreased metabolism of free fatty acids has been thought to be the cause of triglycerate accumulation. In such cases fatty liver could be accompanied by either normal or higher levels of plasma triglycerides.

d. LOCALIZATION IN VARIOUS COMPARTMENTS. Synthesis of triglycerides in the cellular compartments other than ER has been invoked as an explanation of fatty liver, and, indeed, the accumulation of lipid droplets occurs in the cytoplasm of cells and not in the lumen of the ER. Recent studies, however, have postulated that this accumulation of lipids in the cytoplasm is a normal reaction of cells and does not indicate abnormality *per se*, however, the amount of stored lipids in the liver indicates the metabolic defect. In this scheme the fatty liver appears as an imbalance of two variables at the basis of any pathogenic mechanism, the rate at which hepatic triglycerides are synthesized and the rate at which they are utilized or a combination of these. In lipodystrophies, for example, synthesis is increased beyond the maximal rate at which hepatic triglycerides can be utilized.

e. MISCELLANEOUS CHANGES IN LIPID METABOLISM.   Bailey *et al.* (1972) proposed that cultured cells provide a promising system for studying the regulation of lipid metabolism because the homogeneous character of the cells allows examination of events separated from complex physiological interactions encountered *in vivo*. Moreover, nutritional environmental conditions can be more easily manipulated. In these studies the authors found that cells cultured in lipid-free media synthesized lipids from simple metabolic precursors, a process which is inhibited by the addition of serum. When serum lipid was present, cells preferentially utilized fatty acids as a source of energy. These are subsequently esterified intracellularly to make glycerides and phospholipids. When triglycerides are used as a source of cell lipids it is first hydrolyzed before being taken up.

In a recent report by Spitzer and Spitzer (1972) an interesting change in myocardial metabolism in dogs during hemolytic shock was reported. Both the myocardial uptake and oxidation of free fatty acids decreased markedly while lactate in cells and blood also changed significantly. During the control period, free fatty acid was the major and lactate was the second most important substrate utilized by the myocardium and fatty acids. After hemorrhage, free fatty acid supplied only a minor portion of metabolized substrates. A greater portion came from glycogen. The authors conclude that following severe hemorrhage and the manifestation of myocardial hypoxia the major change in myocardial metabolism is a decreased uptake and oxidation of free fatty acids and an increased metabolism of glycogen and of other carbohydrates.

Studies by Hagopian *et al.* (1972) suggested directed action of reserpine on the heart, and among the changes the author suggested the reduced metabolic rate is related to the lipid accumulation. As in other types of cardiac fatty change, the lipid droplets are in proximity to mitochondria, often indenting them into cup-shaped profiles.

In the study of experimental vitamin B6 deficiency in the rat, it was noted that collecting duct epithelial cells developed irregular homogeneous osmiophilic lipid bodies by 28 days, which became more numerous after 42 days, and that large, round intracytoplasmic lipid bodies developed prominency after 10 days, the earliest detection of oxalate crystals. Some extremely large myelin forms, possibly lysosomal, occurred in the interstitial cells.

Gordon and Lough (1972) studied liver during the regression of fatty liver in alcoholism. During regression the rough ER regained its lamellar appearance and showed disappearance of the vesiculation of the smooth reticulum by the third day. Abnormal mitochondria were still present on the fifth day even though the magnesium-stimulated ATPase had returned to normal. The accumulated lipid was slowly moved from the liver, as observed in the electron micrographs and confirmed by biochemical analysis. Evidence of glycogen and the concentration of this reached normal levels in 24 hours after the removal of ethanol from the diet. By the third day to the seventh day, ultrastructure of the liver parenchyma cells of the ethanol-induced fatty liver was similar to that of the liquid controls.

Little agreement exists in the literature regarding the etiology of the changes produced in parenchymal cells of the liver by chronic consumption of ethanol. While metabolic imbalance is invoked by one group of investigators (Ruebner *et al.*, 1972), direct toxic effects of ethanol on the liver cell is postulated by other investigators. In chronic ethanol intake the smooth ER has become very prominent (Gordon and Lough, 1972). This proliferation of smooth ER has been observed in fatty liver owing to a number of hepatotoxic agents such as ethionine and *orotic* acid. The idea of increased enzyme activity and proliferation of the ER has been supported by Rubin and Lieber (1968) and Rubin *et al.* (1970). Di Luzio and Hartmann (1969) and other investigators postulated a depression of hepatic triglyceride oxidation as a factor in ethanol induced fatty liver. Furthermore, the development of lipoperoxidases and hydroperoxidases or polymers have been invoked.

Some of the common cell reactions to injury are summarized in Fig. 58.

Acknowledgments

The authors would like to acknowledge the following who contributed pictures and assisted in the preparation of this manuscript. Mrs. Gloria Taylor, Dr. Greta Tyson, Mrs. Jane Dees, Dr. Elizabeth M. McDowell, Dr. Jon Valigorsky, Robert Pendergrass, Dr. Kook Kim, Dr. Zdenek Hruban, Ray Jones, and Dr. Lucy Barrett.

References

Afifi, A. K., Ibrahim, Z. M., Bergman, R. A., Haydar, N. A., Mire, J., Bahuth, N., and Kaylani, F. (1972). *J. Neurol. Sci.* **15**, 271.
Aiyar, A. S., Fatterpaker, P., and Sreenivasan, A. (1964). *Biochem. J.* **90**, 558.
Albahary, C. (1972). *Amer. J. Med.* **52**, 367.
Alexander, C. (1972). *Amer. J. Med.* **53**, 395.
Allison, A. C. (1968). *Advan. Chemother.* **3**, 253.

Allison, A. C., and Mallucci, L. (1965). *J. Exp. Med.* **121**, 463.

Allison, A. C., and Sandelin, K. (1963). *J. Exp. Med.* **117**, 879.

Allison, A. C., and Young, M. R. (1961). *Life Sci.* **3**, 1407.

Allison, A. C., Harington, J. S., and Birbeck, M. (1966a). *J. Exp. Med.* **124**, 141.

Allison, A. C., Magnus, I. A., and Young, M. R. (1966b). *Nature (London)* **209**, 874.

Amick, C. J., and Stenger, R. J. (1964). *Lab. Invest.* **13**, 128.

Arakawa, M., and Tokunaga, J. (1972). *Lab. Invest.* **27**, 366.

Armstrong, J. A., and Hart, P. d'Arcy. (1971). *J. Exp. Med.* **134**, 713.

Arstila, A. U., and Trump, B. F. (1968). *Amer. J. Pathol.* **53**, 687.

Arstila, A. U., and Trump, B. F. (1969). *Virchows Arch., B.* **2**, 85.

Arstila, A. U., and Trump, B. F. (1972). *Virchows Arch. B* **10**, 344.

Arstila, A. U., Bradford, W. D., Kinney, T. D., and Trump, B. F. (1970). *Amer. J. Pathol.* **58**, 419.

Arstila, A. U., Jauregui, H. O., Chang, J., and Trump, B. F. (1971). *Lab. Invest.* **24**, 162.

Arstila, A. U., Shelburne, J. D., and Trump, B. F. (1972a). *Lab. Invest.* **27**, 317.

Arstila, A. U., Smith, M. A., and Trump, B. F. (1972b). *Science* **175**, 530.

Ashford, T. P., and Porter, K. R. (1962). *J. Cell Biol.* **12**, 198.

Baba, N., and Ruppert, R. D. (1972). *Amer. J. Clin. Pathol.* **57**, 306

Bachi, T., and Howe, C. (1972). *J. Cell Biol.* **55**, 10a.

Bahr, G. F., and Zeitler, E. (1962). *J. Cell Biol.* **15**, 489.

Bailey, E., Taylor, C. B., and Bartley, W. (1967). *Biochem. J.* **104**, 1026.

Bailey, J. M., Howard, B. V., Dunbar, L. M., and Tillman, S. F. (1972). *Lipids* **7**, 125.

Baker, H. (1956). *J. Pathol. Bacteriol.* **71**, 135.

Barankay, T., Horpacsy, G., Nagy, S., and Petri, G. (1969). *Med. Exp.* **19**, 267.

Barber, A. A., and Bernheim, F. (1967). *Advan. Gerontol. Res.* **2**, 355–403.

Baringer, J. R., and Swoveland, P. (1972). *Proc. Electron Microsc. Soc. Amer.* **30**, 320.

Baserga, R., and Wiebel, F. (1969). *Int. Rev. Exp. Pathol.* **7**, 1–30.

Bassi, M., and Bernelli-Zazzera, A. (1964). *Exp. Mol. Pathol.* **3**, 332.

Beaver, D. L. (1961). *Amer. J. Pathol.* **39**, 195.

Beaver, D. L., and Burr, R. E. (1963). *Amer. J. Pathol.* **42**, 609.

Beck, F., Lloyd. J. B., and Griffiths, A. (1967). *Science* **157**, 1180.

Behnke, O. (1963). *J. Cell Biol.* **18**, 251.

Bennet, M. V. L. (1973). *Fed. Proc., Fed. Amer. Soc. Exp. Biol.* **32**, 65.

Bennett, H. S. (1963). *J. Histochem. Cytochem.* **11**, 14.

Berenbom, M. C., Chang, P. I., Betz, H. E., and Stowell, R. E. (1955a). *Cancer Res.* **15**, 1.

Berenbom, M. C., Chang, P. I., and Stowell, R. E. (1955b). *Lab. Invest.* **4**, 315.

Bernelli-Zazzera, A., Caradonna, D., and Cassi, E. (1960). *Exp. Cell Res.* **20**, 592.

Bernhard, W., and Granboulan, N. (1968). *In* "The Nucleus" (A. J. Dalton and F. Haguenau, eds.). Acad. Press, New York, London, pp. 81–149.

Bessis, M. C., and Breton-Gorius, J. (1959). *Blood* **14**, 423.

Biava, C. (1964). *Lab. Invest.* **13**, 301.

Bitensky, L. (1963). *In* "Lysosomes Ciba Foundation Symposium" (A. V. S. de Revck and P. M. Cameron, eds.), pp. 362–375. Little Brown, Boston.

Bitensky, L., Chayen, J., Cunningham, G. J., and Fine, J. (1963). *Nature (London)* **199**, 493.

Björksten, J. (1971). *Suom. Kemistisenran. Tiedonantoja* **80**, 23.

Black, L., and Berenbom, M. C. (1964). *Exp. Cell Res.* **35**, 9.

Boime, I., Smith, E. E., and Hunter, F. E. (1968). *Arch. Biochem.* **128**, 704.

Braasch, W., Gudbjarnason, S., Pui, P. S., Ravens, K. G., and Bing, R. J. (1968). *Circ. Res.* **23**, 429.

Bracker, C. E., and Grove, S. N. (1971). *Protoplasma* **73**, 15.

Bradford, W. D., Elchlepp, J. G., Arstila, A. U., Trump, B. F., and Kinney, T. D. (1969). *Amer.*

J. Pathol. **56**, 201.

Bradley, D. F. (1961). *Trans. N.Y. Acad. Sci.* [2] **24**, 64.

Brady, R. O., Fishman, P. H., and Mora, P. T. (1973). *Fed. Proc., Fed. Amer. Soc. Exp. Biol.* **32**, 102.

Brandes, D., Gyorkey, F., and Groth, D. P. (1962). *Lab. Invest.* **11**, 339.

Brinkley, B. R., and Rao, P. N. (1972). *J. Cell Biol.* **55**, 28a.

Brodie, B. B., Axelrod, J., Copper, J. R., Gaudette, L., La Du, B. N., Mitoma, C., and Udenfriend, S. (1955). *Science* **121**, 603.

Brodie, B. B., Gillette, J. R., and La Du, B. N. (1958). *Ann. Rev. Biochem.* **27**, 427.

Bruni, C. (1960). *Lab. Invest.* **9**, 209.

Brunk, U., and Brun, A. (1972). *Histochemie* **29**, 140.

Brunk, U., and Ericsson, J. L. E. (1972). *J. Ultrastruct. Res.* **38**, 1.

Bucher, N. L. R., and Berkley, P. (1972). *J. Cell Biol.* **55**, 31a.

Bulger, R. E., and Trump, B. F. (1968). *Exp. Cell Res.* **51**, 587.

Bulger, R. E., and Trump, B. F. (1969a). *J. Morphol.* **127**, 205.

Bulger, R. E., and Trump, B. F. (1969b). *J. Ultrastruct. Res.* **28**, 301.

Bulger, R. E., Griffith, I. D., and Trump, B. F. (1966). *Science* **151**, 83.

Bulos, B., Shukla, S., and Sacktor, B. (1972). *Arch. Biochem. Biophys.* **149**, 461.

Burger, M. M. (1973). *Fed. Proc. Fed. Amer. Soc. Exp. Biol.* **32**, 91.

Burger, P. C., and Herdson, P. B. (1966). *Amer. J. Pathol.* **48**, 793.

Caesar, R. (1961). *Verh. Deut. Ges. Pathol.* **45**, 278.

Cameron, G. R. (1951). *In* "Pathology of the Cell," pp. 262–274 and 381–405. Thomas, Springfield, Illinois.

Canonico, P. G., and Bird, J. W. C. (1969). *J. Cell Biol.* **43**, 367.

Carafoli, E., Tiozzo, R., Pasquali-Ronchetti, I., and Laschi, R. (1971). *Lab. Invest.* **25**, 516.

Caulfield, J., and Klionsky, B. (1959). *Amer. J. Pathol.* **35**, 489.

Charvat, I., Ross, I., and Cronshaw, J. (1972). *J. Cell Biol.* **55**, 38a.

Christensen, H. N. (1968). *Proc. Nat. Acad. Sci. U.S.* **63**, 948.

Christensen, H. N. (1973). *Fed. Proc., Fed. Amer. Soc. Exp. Biol.* **32**, 19.

Claude, A. (1970). *J. Cell. Biol.* **47**, 745.

Cohn, Z. H. (1971). *In* "Cell Membranes: Biological and Pathological Aspects" (G. W. Richter and D. G. Scarpelli, eds.), pp. 129–135. Williams & Wilkins, Baltimore, Maryland.

Conney, A. H. (1967). *Pharm. Rev.* **19**, 317.

Coward, J. E., Harter, D. H., and Morgan, C. (1970). *Virology* **40**, 1030.

Cresti, M., Pacini, E., and Sarfatti, G. (1972). *J. Submierosc. Cytol.* **4**, 33.

Criddle, R. S., and Schatz, G. (1969). *Biochemistry* **8**, 322.

Croker, B. P., Saladino, A. J., and Trump, B. F. (1970). *Amer. J. Pathol.* **59**, 247.

Dales, S., and Mosbach, E. H. (1968). *Virology* **35**, 564.

Dallman, P. R., and Goodman, J. R. (1970). *Blood* **35**, 496.

Danielli, J. F. (1967). *J. Theor. Bio.* **15**, 179.

Daniels, C. A., Bradford, W. D., and Trump, B. F. (1973). In preparation.

Davis, W. L., Schuster, R. J., Goodman, D. B. P., and Allen, J. E. (1972). *J. Cell Biol.* **55**, 56a.

de Duve, C. (1959). *Exp. Cell Res. Suppl.* **7**, 169.

de Duve, C. (1964). *In* "Injury, Inflammation and Immunity" (L. Thomas, J. W. Uhr, and L. Grant, eds.), pp. 283–311. Williams & Wilkins, Baltimore, Maryland.

de Duve, C. (1969). *Ann. N.Y. Acad. Sci.* **168**, 369.

de Duve, C., and Baudhuin, P. (1966). *Physiol. Rev.* **46**, 323.

de Duve, C., and Beaufay, H. (1959). *Biochem. J.* **73**, 610.

de Duve, C., and Wattiaux, R. (1966). *Annu. Rev. Physiol.* **28**, 435.

De La Iglesia, F. A., and Lumb, G. (1972). *Lab. Invest.* **27**, 17.

DiLuzio, R., and Hartmann, A. D. (1969). *Exp. Mol. Pathol.* **11**, 38.

De Reuck, A. V. S., and Knight, J., eds. (1964). "Cellular Injury," Ciba Found. Little, Brown, Boston, Massachusetts.

Deter, R. L., and de Duve, C. (1967). *J. Cell Biol.* **33**, 437.

Dingle, J. T. (1963). *In* "Lysosomes" (A. V. S. De Reuck and M. P. Cameron, eds.), p. 384. Ciba Foundation Symposium. Little, Brown, Boston, Mass.

Dingle, J. T., and Fell, H. B., eds. (1969). "Lysosomes in Biology and Pathology," Vol. , Part I, pp. 3–508. North-Holland Publ., Amsterdam.

Donnelly, W. H., and Yunis, E. J. (1971). *Amer. J. Pathol.* **62**, 87.

Douglas, S. D., and Fudenberg, H. H. (1969). *Hosp. Pract.* **4**, 29.

Douglas, S. D., Davis, W. C., and Fudenberg, H. H. (1969a). *Amer. J. Med.* **46**, 901.

Douglas, S. D., Davis, W. C., and Fudenberg, H. H. (1969b). *New Engl. J. Med.* **281**, 329.

Dourmashkin, R. R., and Rosse, W. F. (1966). *Amer. J. Med.* **41**, 699.

Ekholm, R., and Edlund, Y. (1960). *Proc. Int. Conf. Electron Microsc., 4th, 1958* Vol. 2, p. 273.

Emmelot, P., and Beneditti, E. L. (1967). *In* "Carcinogenesis: A Broad Critique," p. 771. Williams & Wilkins, Baltimore, Maryland.

Enwonwu, C. O. (1972). *Lab. Invest.* **26**, 626.

Ericsson, J. L. E. (1965). *Lab. Invest.* **14**, 16.

Ericsson, J. L. E., and Trump, B. F. (1964). *Lab. Invest.* **13**, 1427.

Ericsson, J. L. E., Biberfeld, P., and Seljelid, R. (1967). *Acta Pathol. Microbiol. Scand.* **70**, 215.

Ernster, L., and Luft, R. (1963). *Exp. Cell Res.* **32**, 26.

Ernster, L., Ikkos, D., and Luft, R. (1959). *Nature (London)* **184**, 1851.

Ernster, L., Nordenbrand, K., Orrenius, S., and Dus, M. L. (1968). *Hoppe Seyler's Z. Physiol. Chem.* **349**, 1604.

Estable-Puig, R. F. de, and Estable-Puig, J. F. de (1971). *Acta Neuropathol.* **17**, 287.

Estable-Puig, R. F. de, Estable-Puig, J. F. de, and Romero, C. (1971). *Virchows Arch. B* **8**, 267.

Farber, E., and Magee, P. N., eds. (1965). "Biochemical Pathology," pp. 1–242. Williams & Wilkins, Baltimore, Maryland.

Farber, E., Lombardi, B., and Castillo, A. E. (1963). *Lab. Invest.* **12**, 873.

Farber, E., Liang, H., and Shinozuka, H. (1971). *Amer. J. Pathol.* **64**, 601.

Farrell, E. C., Baba, N., Brierley, G. P., and Grimer, H. D. (1972). *Lab. Invest.* **27**, 209.

Fell, H. B., and Thomas, L. C. (1960). *J. Exp. Med.* **111**, 719.

Fisher, E. R., and Fisher, B. (1963). *Lab. Invest.* **12**, 929.

Flax, M., and Tisdale, W. A. (1964). *Amer. J. Pathol.* **44**, 441.

Fletcher, M. J., and Sanadi, D. R. (1961). *Biochim. Biophys. Acta* **51**, 356.

Flickinger, C. J. (1971). *Exp. Cell Res.* **68**, 381.

Fonnesu, A., and Severi, C. (1956). *J. Biophys. Biochem. Cytol.* **2**, 293.

Fouts, J. R. (1962). *Fed. Proc., Fed. Amer. Soc. Exp. Biol.* **21**, 1107.

Frei, J. V., and Sheldon, H. (1961). *J. Biophys. Biochem. Cytol.* **11**, 724.

Gear, A. R., and Bednarek, J. M. (1972). *J. Cell. Biol.* **54**, 325.

Gelfant, S., and Smith, J. Jr. (1972). *Science* **178**, 357.

Gertz, E. W., Hess, M. L., Lanin, R. F., and Briggs, F. N. (1967). *Circ. Res.* **20**, 477.

Ginn, F. L., Shelburne, J. D., and Trump, B. F. (1968). *Amer. J. Pathol.* **53**, 1041.

Ginn, F. L., Hochstein, P. E., and Trump, B. F. (1969). *Science* **164**, 843.

Glas, U., and Bahr, G. F. (1966). *J. Cell Biol.* **29**, 507.

Glaumann, H. (1970). *Biochim. Biophys. Acta* **224**, 206.

Glaumann, H. (1971a). *Chem. Biol. Interactions* **3**, 268.

Glaumann, H. (1971b). "Structural and Functional Heterogeneity of the Endoplasmic Reticulum in the Liver Cell," pp. 5–24. Department of Pathology at Sabbatsberg Hospital, Karolinska Institutet, Stockholm.

Glaumann, H., and Dallner, G. (1970). *J. Cell Biol.* **47**, 34.

Glaumann, H., and Jakobsson, S. (1969). *Proc. Intern. Congr. Pharmacol. 4th* **4**, 79.
Glende, E. A. Jr., and Recknagel, R. O. (1969). *Exp. Mol. Pathol.* **11**, 172.
Gold, P., and Freedman, S. O. (1965). *J. Exp. Med.* **121**, 439.
Goldblatt, P. J. (1969). *In* "Handbook of Molecular Cytology" (A. Lima-de Faria, ed.), p. 1101–1129. North-Holland Publ., Amsterdam.
Goldblatt, P. J., and Williams, G. M. (1969). *Amer. J. Pathol.* **57**, 253.
Goldblatt, P. J., Sullivan, R. J., and Farber, E. (1969). *Lab. Invest.* **20**, 283.
Goldblatt, P. J., Trump, B. F., and Stowell, R. E. (1965). *Amer. J. Pathol.* **47**, 183.
Goldfeder, A., and Mukerjee, H. (1972). *J. Cell Biol.* **55**, 87a.
Goldfischer, S. (1963). *Amer. J. Pathol.* **43**, 511.
Goldman, R. D. (1972). *J. Cell Biol.* **52**, 246.
Goldstone, A., and Koenig, H. (1972). *J. Cell Biol.* **55**, 89a.
Gonzalez-Licea, A. (1972). *Lab. Invest.* **26**, 403.
Goode, D., and Maugel, T. K. (1972). *J. Cell Biol.* **55**, 90a.
Gordon, E. R., and Lough, J. (1972). *Lab. Invest.* **26**, 154.
Gordon, G. B. (1972). *J. Cell Biol.* **55**, 91a.
Goyer, R. A. (1968). *Lab. Invest.* **19**, 71.
Goyer, R. A., and Krall, R. (1969). *J. Cell Biol.* **41**, 393.
Goyer, R. A., Krall, A., and Kimball, J. P. (1968). *Lab. Invest.* **19**, 78.
Green, H., Fleischer, R. A., Barrow, P., and Goldberg, B. (1959). *J. Exp. Med.* **109**, 511.
Griffin, C. C., Waravdekar, V. S., Goldblatt, P. J., Trump, B. F., and Stowell, R. E. (1965a). *Arch. Pathol.* **79**, 595.
Griffin, C. C., Waravdekar, V. S., Trump, B. F., Goldblatt, P. J., and Stowell, R. E. (1965b). *Amer. J. Pathol.* **47**, 833.
Griffin, J. L., Stein, M. N., and Stowell, R. E. (1969). *J. Cell. Biol.* **40**, 108.
Grinstein, M., Bannerman, R. M., and Moore, C. V. (1959). *Blood* **14**, 476.
Gritzka, T. L., and Trump, B. F. (1968). *Amer. J. Pathol.* **52**, 1225.
Hagopian, M., Gershon, M. D., and Nunez, E. A. (1972). *Lab. Invest.* **27**, 99.
Hamilton, R. C. (1972). *Proc. Electron Microsc. Soc. Amer.* **30**, 40.
Handel, M. A. (1971). *J. Exp. Zool.* **178**, 523.
Haust, M. D., Orizaga, M., Bryans, A. M., and Frank, H. F. (1969). *Exp. Mol. Pathol.* **10**, 141.
Havel, R. J. (1972). *N. Engl. J. Med.* **287**, 1186.
Hawiger, J., Hawiger, A., and Koenig, M. G. (1972). *J. Yale Biol. Med.* **45**, 42.
Hawkins, H. K., Ericsson, J. L. E., Biberfeld, P., and Trump, B. F. (1972). *Amer. J. Pathol.* **68**, 225.
Hay, E. D., and Revel, J. P. (1963). *J. Cell. Biol.* **16**, 29.
Hayflick, L. (1966). *In* "Perspectives in Experimental Gerontology" (N. W. Shock *et al.*, eds.), p. 195–211. Thomas, Springfield, Illinois.
Hayflick, L. (1968). *Sci. Amer.* **218**, 32.
Hayflick, L., and Moorhead, P. S. (1961). *Exp. Cell Res.* **25**, 585.
Helminen, H. J., and Ericsson, J. L. E. (1970). Exp. Cell Res. **60**, 419.
Helminen, H. J., and Ericsson, J. L. E. (1971a). *Exp. Cell Res.* **68**, 411.
Helminen, H. J., and Ericsson, J. L. E. (1971b) *J. Ultrastruct. Res.* **33**, 528.
Helminen, H. J., and Ericsson, J. L. E. (1972). *J. Ultrastruct. Res.* **39**, 443.
Henderson, N. S. (1972). *J. Cell Biol.* **55**, 111a.
Henson, P. M. (1972). *Amer. J. Pathol.* **68**, 593.
Herdson, P. B., Garvin, P. J., and Jennings, R. B. (1964). *Amer. J. Pathol.* **45**, 157.
Herdson, P. B., Sommers, H. M., and Jennings, R. B. (1965). *Amer. J. Pathol.* **46**, 367.
Hers, H. G. (1965). *Gastroenterology* **48**, 625.
Higgins, J. A., and Barrnett, R. J. (1972). *J. Cell Biol.* **55**, 282.

Higgins, J. A., Levine, A. M., and Barrnett, R. J. (1972). *J. Cell Biol.* **55**, 113a.

Hinkley, R. E., and Samson, F. E. (1972). *J. Cell Biol.* **53**, 258.

Hirsch, J. G., and Cohn, Z. A. (1960). *J. Exp. Med.* **112**, 1005.

Hochstein, P., and Ernster, L. (1964). *Cell. Injury, Ciba Found. Symp., 1963* pp. 123–135.

Hoffstein, S., Zurier, R. B., and Weissmann, G. (1972). *J. Cell Biol.* **55**, 115a.

Horie, A., Takino, T., Herman, L., and Fitzgerald, P. J. (1971). *Amer. J. Pathol.* **63**, 299.

Howes, E. L., Price, H. M., and Blumberg, J. M. (1964). *Amer. J. Pathol.* **45**, 599.

Hruban, Z., and Rechcigl, M., Jr. (1969). *Int. Rev. Cytol. Suppl.* **1**, 1–251.

Hruban, Z., Swift, H., and Wissler, R. W. (1962). *J. Ultrastruct. Res.* **7**, 273.

Hruban, Z., Spargo, B., Swift, H., Wissler, R. W., and Kleinfeld, R. G. (1963). *Amer. J. Pathol.* **42**, 657.

Hruban, Z., Slesers, A., and Hopkins, E. (1972). *Lab. Invest.* **27**, 62.

Huebner, G., and Bernhard, W. (1961). *Beitr. Pathol. Anat.* **125**, 1.

Hugon, J. S., Maestracci, D., and Menard, D. (1972). *Histochemie* **29**, 189.

Ikeda, M., and Otsuji, H. (1971). *Toxicol. Appl. Pharmacol.* **20**, 30.

Inbar, M., Ben-Bassat, H., and Sachs, L. (1972). *Nature (London), New Biol.* **236**, 3.

Iturriaga, H., Posalaki, I., and Rubin, E. (1969). *Exp. Mol. Pathol.* **10**, 231.

Jacob, H. S. (1970). *Semin. Hematol.* **7**, 341.

Jago, M. V. (1969). *Amer. J. Pathol.* **56**, 405.

James, R., Keith, A., and Branton, D. (1972). *J. Cell Biol.* **55**, 123a.

Janigan, D. T., Santamaria, A., and Trump, B. F. (1960). *J. Histochem. Cytochem.* **8**, 385.

Janoff, A. (1964). *In* "Shock" (S. G. Hershey, ed.), pp. 93–111. Little, Brown, Boston, Massachusetts.

Jasper, D. K., and Bronk, J. R. (1972). *J. Cell Biol.* **55**, 124a.

Jennings, R. B., Baum, J. H., and Herdson, P. B. (1965). *AMA Arch. Pathol.* **79**, 135.

Jennings, R. B., Herdson, P. B., and Sommers, H. M. (1969). *Lab. Invest.* **20**, 548.

Jöbsis, F. F. (1964). *In* "Handbook of Physiology" (Amer. Physiol. Soc., J. Field, ed.), Sect. 3, Vol. I, pp. 63–124. Williams & Wilkins, Baltimore, Maryland.

Jockusch, B. M., and Blessing, J. (1971). *Exp. Cell Res.* **69**, 465.

Johnson, H. A., and Amendola, F. (1969). *Amer. J. Pathol.* **54**, 35.

Johnson, H. A., and Pavelec, M. (1972). *Amer. J. Pathol.* **66**, 557.

Jonek, J., Konecki, J., Grzybek, H., and Olkowski, Z. (1971). *Histochemie* **26**, 28.

Jordan, S. W. (1964). *Exp. Mol. Pathol.* **3**, 183.

Judah, J. D., and Rees, K. B. (1959). *Biochem. Soc. Symp.* **16**, 94.

Katchalsky, A., and Curran, P. F. (1965). "Nonequilibrium Thermodynamics in Biophysics." Harvard Univ. Press, Cambridge, Massachusetts.

Kessler, D. (1972). *J. Cell Biol.* **55**, 134a.

King, M. E., and King, D. W. (1971). *Lab. Invest.* **25**, 374.

King, M. E., Godman, G. C., and King, D. W. (1972). *J. Cell Biol.* **53**, 127.

Kleinfeld, R. G., Greider, M. H., and Frajola, W. J. (1956). *J. Biophys. Biochem. Cytol.* **2**, Suppl 7, 435.

Klion, F. M., and Schaffner, F. (1968). *Digestion* **1**, 2.

Kovacs, J. (1971). *Acta Biol. Acad. Sci. Hung.* **22**, 287.

Krishan, A., and Whitlock, S. (1972). *J. Cell Biol.* **55**, 142a.

Krohn, P. L. (1966). "Topics in the Biology of Aging." Interscience, New York.

Kübler, W., and Spieckermann, P. G. (1970). *J. Mol. Cell. Cardiol.* **1**, 351.

Laguens, R. P., and Gomez-Dumm, C. L. (1967). *Circ. Res.* **21**, 271.

Laiho, K. U., Shelburne, J. D., and Trump, B. F. (1971). *Amer. J. Pathol.* **65**, 203.

Laiho, K. U., and Trump, B. F. (1973). Unpublished observation.

Lampert, P. W. (1969). *Lab. Invest.* **20**, 127.

Lampert, P. W., and Schochet, S. S. (1968). *J. Neuropathol. Exp. Neurol.* **27**, 527.

Leaf, A. (1959). *Ann. N.Y. Acad. Sci.* **72**, 396.

Leaf, A. (1970). *Amer. J. Med.* **49**, 291.

Leduc, E. H., and Wilson, W. J. (1959). *J. Biophys. Biochem. Cytol.* **6**, 427.

Lehninger, A. L. (1964). "The Mitochondrion." W. Benjamin, New York.

Lehninger, A. L. (1970). "Biochemistry." Worth Publ., New York.

Lessin, L. S., Jensen, W. N., and Klug, P. (1972). *Arch. Intern. Med.* **129**, 306.

Lewis, M. R. (1923). *Bull. Johns Hopkins Hosp.* **34**, 373.

Ling, G. N., Miller, C., and Ochsenfeld, P. (1973). *In* "Physico State of Ions and Water in Living Tissue and Model Systems" (C. Hazelwood, ed.). *Annals New York Acad. Sci.* **204**, 6–49.

Littau, V. C., Alfrey, V. G., Frenster, J. H., and Mirsky, A. E. (1964). *Proc. Nat. Acad. Sci. U. S.* **52**, 93.

Lloyd, J. B., Beck, F., Griffiths, A., and Parry, L. M. (1968). *In* "The Interaction of Drugs and Subcellular Components in Animal Cells" (P. N. Campbell, ed.), pp. 171–200. Little, Brown, Boston, Massachusetts.

Loewenstein, W. R. (1973). *Fed. Proc., Fed. Amer. Soc. Exp. Biol.* **32**, 60.

Lombardi, B. (1965). *In* "Biochemical Pathology" (E. Farber and P. N. Magee, eds.), pp. 1–15. Williams & Wilkins, Baltimore, Maryland.

Lombardi, B., and Recknagel, R. O. (1962). *Amer. J. Pathol.* **40**, 571.

Longnecker, D. S. (1972). *Lab. Invest.* **26**, 459.

Lubin, M. (1967). *Nature (London)* **213**, 451.

Lucy, J. A., Dingle, J. T., and Fell, H. B. (1961). *Biochem. J.* **79**, 500.

Luft, R., Ikkos, D., Palmieri, G., Ernster, L., and Afzelius, B. (1962). *J. Clin. Invest.* **41**, 1776.

Lundquist, P., Igarashi, M., Wersall, J., Guilford, F. R., and Wright, W. K. (1971). *Acta Otolaryngol.* **72**, 68.

Luse, S. A., Burch, H. B., and Hunter, F. E. (1962). *Electron Microsc., Proc. Int. Cong. (Stockholm), 5th, 1962* Vol. 2, VV–5.

Lutzner, M. A., Tierney, J. H., and Benditt, E. P. (1965). *Lab. Invest.* **14**, 2063.

McCallister, B. D., and Brown, A. L. (1965). *Lab. Invest.* **14**, 692.

McKay, D. G., Whitaker, A. N., and Cruse, V. (1969). *Amer. J. Pathol.* **56**, 177.

Mahley, R. W., Bennett, B. D., and Morre, D. J. (1971). *Lab. Invest.* **25**, 435.

Majno, G., La Gattuta, M., and Thompson, T. E. (1960). *Virchows Arch. Path. Anat.* **333**, 421.

Majno, G. (1964). *In* "The Liver: Morphology, Biochemistry, Physiology" (Ch. Rouiller, ed.), Vol. II, p. 267. Academic Press, New York.

Mallory, F. B. (1914). "The Principles of Pathologic Histology." Saunders, Philadelphia, Pennsylvania.

Marchesi, V. T. (1971). *In* "Cell Membranes: Biological and Pathological Aspects" (G. W. Richter and D. G. Scarpelli, eds.), pp. 145–150. Williams & Wilkins, Baltimore, Maryland.

Massover, W. H. (1971). *Ultrastruct. Res.* **36**, 603.

Max, S. R. (1972). *Biochem. Biophys. Res. Commun.* **46**, 1394.

May, J. F., and Paule, W. J. (1972). *J. Cell Biol.* **55**, 168a.

Mergner, W. J., and Trump, B. F. (1970). *Lab. Invest.* **22**, 505.

Mergner, W. J., Garbus, J., Valigorsky, J. M., and Trump, B. F. (1972a). *Amer. J. Pathol.* **66**, 36a.

Mergner, W. J., Smith, M. A., and Trump, B. F. (1972b). *Lab. Invest.* **27**, 372.

Merkow, L. P., Epstein, S. M., Sidransky, H., Verney, E., and Pardo, M. (1971). *Amer. J. Pathol.* **62**, 57.

Miller, R., and Garbus, J. (1971). *Science* **175**, 1010.

Miller, J. H., Gilliam, R. H., and Villarejos, V. M. (1972). *Proc. EMSA* **30**, 152.

Miranda, A., and Godman, G. C. (1972). *J. Cell Biol.* **55**, 178a.

Mirsky, A. E., and Osawa, S. (1961). *In* "The Cell" (J. Brachet and A. E. Mirsky, eds.), Vol. 2, p. 677. Academic Press, New York.

Monserrat, A. J., Ghoshal, A. K., Hartroft, W. S., and Porta, E. A. (1969). *Amer. J. Pathol.* **55**, 163.

Moser, H. W. (1970). *N. Engl. J. Med.* **282**, 337.

Mueller, C. C. (1969). *Fed. Proc., Fed. Amer. Soc. Exp. Biol.* **28**, 1780.

Mueller, P., and Rudin, D. O. (1969). *Curr. Top. Bioenerg.* **3**, 157.

Murayama, M. (1966). *Science* **153**, 145.

Nadler, H. L., and Egan, T. J. (1970). *N. Engl. J. Med.* **282**, 302.

Napolitano, L. (1963). *J. Cell Biol.* **18**, 478.

Nayyar, R., and Koenig, H. (1972). *J. Cell. Biol.* **55**, 187a.

Netter, H. (1970). *In* "Theoretical Biochemistry" (J. H. Ohawan, and F. M. Irvine, transl.), pp. 1–855. Wiley (Interscience). New York.

Nordlander, R. H., and Singer, M. (1972). *Z. Zellforsch. Mikrosk. Anat.* **126**, 157.

Normann, S. J., and Stone, C. M. (1972). *Lab. Invest.* **27**, 236.

Norseth, T., and Brendeford, M. (1971). *Biochem. Pharmacol.* **20**, 1101.

Novikoff, A. B. (1959). *J. Biophys, Biochem. Cytol.* **6**, 136.

Novikoff, A. B., and Essner, E. (1962). *J. Cell Biol.* **15**, 140.

Novikoff, A. B., Roheim, P. S., and Quintana, N. (1966). *Lab. Invest.* **15**, 27.

Oliver, J., MacDowell, M., and Lee, Y. C. (1954). *J. Exp. Med.* **99**, 589.

Opie, L. H. (1972). *Circulation* **45**, 483.

Orci, L., and Stauffacher, W. (1971). *J. Ultrastruct. Res.* **36**, 499.

Orrenius, S. (1968). *In* "The Interaction of Drugs and Subcellular Components in Animal Cells" (P. N. Campbell, ed.), p. 97. Little, Brown, Boston, Massachusetts.

Orrenius, S., and Ernster, L. (1971). *In* "Cell Membranes: Biological and Pathological Aspects" (G. W. Richter and D. G. Scarpelli, eds.), pp. 38–53. Williams & Wilkins, Baltimore, Maryland.

Orrenius, S., Ericsson, J. L. E., and Ernster, J. (1965). *J. Cell Biol.* **25**, 627.

Oudea, P. R. (1963). *Lab. Invest.* **12**, 386.

Pacer, J. C., and Welt, L. G. (1972). *Arch. Intern. Med.* **129**, 320.

Paterson, R. A., Layberry, R. A., and Nadkarni, B. B. (1972). *Lab. Invest.* **26**, 755.

Pauling, L., Itano, H. A., Singer, S. J., and Wells, I. C. (1949). *Science* **110**. 543.

Peracchia, C. (1972). *J. Cell. Biol.* **55**, 202a.

Perutz, M. F., Kendrew, J. C., and Watson, H. C. (1965). *J. Molec. Biol.* **13**, 669.

Peters, T. J., Muller, M., and De Duve, C. (1972). *J. Exp. Med.* **136**, 1117.

Petrovic, A. G. (1972). *J. Cell Biol.* **55**, 202a.

Pinto da Silva, P. (1972). *J. Cell Biol.* **53**, 777.

Policard, A., Collet, A., Daniel-Moussard, H., and Pregerman, S. (1961). *J. Biophys. Biochem. Cytol.* **9**, 236.

Poole, B., and Wibo, M. (1972). *J. Cell Biol.* **55**, 205a.

Porter, K. R., and Bruni, C. (1959). *Cancer Res.* **19**, 997.

Prescott, D. M. (1972). *Ca.* **22**, 262.

Price, H. M., Pease, D. C., and Pearson, C. M. (1962). *Lab. Invest.* **11**, 549.

Prieur, D. J., Davis, W. C., and Padgett, G. A. (1972). *Amer. J. Pathol.* **67**, 227.

Pycock, C. J., and Nahorski, S. R. (1971). *J. Mol. Cell. Cardiol.* **3**, 229.

Rafferty, R. E. (1973). *Sci. Amer.* **229**, 26.

Raine, C. S., Wisniewski, H., and Prineas, J. (1969). *Lab. Invest.* **21**, 316.
Rand, R. P. (1964). *Biophys. J.* **4**, 303.
Rand, R. P., and Burton, A. C. (1964). *Biophys. J.* **4**, 115.
Rather, L. J. (1966). *AMA Arch. Pathol.* **82**, 197.
Recknagel, R. O. (1967). *Pharmacol. Rev.* **19**, 145.
Reddy, J., Bunyaratvej, S., and Svoboda, D. J. (1969). *Amer. J. Pathol.* **56**, 351.
Remington, C. C. R. (1937). *C. R. Trav. Lab. Carlsberg* **22**, 454.
Remmer, H., Schenkman, J., Estabrook, R. W., Sesame, H., Gilette, J., Navashimburhn, S., Cooper, D. Y., and Rosenthal, I. (1966). *Mol. Pharmacol.* **2**, 187.
Reynolds, E. S. (1963). *J. Cell Biol.* **19**, 139.
Reynolds, E. S. (1965). *J. Cell Biol. Suppl.* **25**, 53.
Reynolds, E. S., and Ree, H. J. (1971). *Lab. Invest.* **25**, 269.
Rhodes, R. S., and Karnovsky, M. J. (1971). *Lab. Invest.* **25**, 220.
Riede, U. N., and Rohr, H. P. (1971). *Virchows Arch., B* **8**, 350.
Riley, R. K., and Schraer, H. (1972). *J. Cell Biol.* **55**, 216a.
Robbins, E., and Marcus, P. I. (1963). *J. Cell Biol.* **18**, 237.
Robbins, S. L. (1967). "Pathology," 3rd ed Saunders, Philadelphia, Pennsylvania.
Robinson, J. D. (1968). *J. Theor. Biol.* **19**, 90.
Rohlich, P., Anderson, P., and Uvnas, B. (1971). *J. Cell Biol.* **51**, 465.
Romen, W., and Bannasch, P. (1972). *Virchows Arch., B* **10**, 51.
Rosenbluth, J. (1972). *J. Cell Biol.* **55**, 220a.
Rubin, E., and Lieber, C. S. (1968). *Science* **162**, 690.
Rubin, E., Beattie, D. S., and Lieber, C. S. (1970). *Lab. Invest.* **23**, 620,
Rubin, E., Beattie, D. S., Toth, A., and Lieber, C. S. (1972a). *Fred. Proc.,* **31**, 131.
Rubin, R. W., Everhart, L. P., Porter, K. R., Prescott, D. M., and Frye, J. (1972b). *J. Cell Biol.* **55**, 222a.
Ruebner, B. H., Brayton, M. A., Freedland, R. A., Kanayama, R., and Tsao, M. (1972). *Lab. Invest.* **27**, 71.
Sahaphong, S., and Trump, B. F. (1971). *Amer. J. Pathol.* **63**, 277.
Sakiyama, H., and Robbins, P. W. (1973). *Fed. Proc.* **32**, 86.
Saladino, A. J., and Trump, B. F. (1968). *Amer. J. Pathol.* **52**, 737.
Saladino, A. J., Bentley, P. J., and Trump, B. F. (1969). *Amer. J. Pathol.* **54**, 421.
Saladino, A. J., Hawkins, H. K., and Trump, B. F. (1971). *Amer. J. Pathol.* **64**, 271.
Sarma, D. S. R., Reid, I. M., Verney, E., and Sidransky, H. (1972). *Lab. Invest.* **27**, 39.
Savage, N., and Hackett, A. (1972). *Proc. Electron Microsc. Soc. Amer.* **30**, 286.
Scarpelli, D. G. (1971). *In* "Cell Membranes: Biological and Pathological Aspects" (G. W. Richter and D. G. Scarpelli, eds.), p. 151–174. Williams & Wilkins, Baltimore, Maryland.
Scarpelli, D. G., and Trump, B. F. (1971). "Cell Injury." Upjohn Company, Kalamazoo, Michigan.
Schafer, D. (1972). *Cytobiologie* **5**, 463.
Schaffner, F., Loebel, A., Weiner, H. A., and Barka, T. (1963). *J. Amer. Med. Ass.* **183**, 343.
Schatz, G. (1970). *In* "Membranes of Mitochondria and Chloroplasts" (E. Racker, ed.), p. 251–314. Van Nostrand-Reinhold, Princeton, New Jersey.
Schofield, B. H., and Grossman, I. W. (1968). *Arch. Pathol.* **86**, 208.
Schumacher, H. R., and Phelps, P. (1971). *Arthritis Rheum.* **14**, 513.
Sciver, C. R. (1970). *Hosp. Prac.* **5**, 92.
Scott, C. R., Lagunoff, D., and Trump, B. F. (1967). *J. Pediat.* **71**, 357.
Seil, F. J., Lampert, P. W., and Klatzo, I. (1969). *J. Neuropathol. Exp. Neurol.* **28**, 74.
Sekhri, K. K., Alexander, C. S., Nagasawa, H. T., and Derr, R. F. (1972). *Proc. Electron Microsc. Soc. Amer.* **30**, 28.
Shelburne, J. D., and Trump, B. F. (1968). *Fed. Proc. Fed. Amer. Soc. Exp. Biol.* **27**, 410.

Shelburne, J. D., Arstila, A. U., and Trump, B. F. (1973). *Amer. J. Pathol.* **72**, 521.
Sheldon, H., and Zetterqvist, H. (1956). *Exp. Cell Res.* **10**, 225.
Shinozuka, H. (1971). *Exp. Cell Res.* **64**, 380.
Shinozuka, H., Goldblatt, P. J., and Farber, E. (1968). *J. Cell Biol.* **36**, 313.
Shofe, G. I. (1964). *J. Ultrastruct. Res.* **10**, 224.
Sidransky, H., Epstein, S. M., Verney, E., and Horovitz, C. (1972). *Amer. J. Pathol.* **69**, 55.
Siekevitz, P. (1972). *Annu. Rev. Physiol.* **34**, 117.
Silver, B. B., and Lawwill, T. (1972). *Proc. Electron Microsc. Soc. Amer.* **30**, 54.
Sjodin, R. A. (1971). *In* "Biophysics and Physiology of Excitable Membranes" (W. J. Adelman, ed.). Van Nostrand Reinhold, New York.
Sjöstrand, F. S., Cedesgren, E. A., and Karlsson, U. (1964). *Nature (London)* **202**, 1075.
Smith, U., and Ryan, J. W. (1972). *J. Cell Biol.* **55**, 244a.
Smuckler, E. A., and Arcasoy, M. (1969). *Int. Rev. Exp. Pathol.* **7**, 305–418.
Smuckler, E. A., and Benditt, E. P. (1965). *Biochemistry* **4**, 671.
Smuckler, E. A., and Trump, B. F. (1968). *Amer. J. Pathol.* **53**, 315.
Smuckler, E. A., Iseri, O. A., and Benditt, E. P. (1962). *Exp. Med.* **116**, 55.
Sobel, B. E. (1972). *Hosp. Pract.* **7**, 59–71.
Sohal, R. S., McCarthy, J. L., and Allison, V. F. (1972). *J. Ultrastruct. Res.* **39**, 484.
Sommers, H. M., and Jennings, R. B. (1964). *Lab. Invest.* **13**, 1491.
Soslau, G., and Nass, M. M. (1971). *J. Cell Biol.* **51**, 514
Spencer, P. S., Raine, C. S., and Peterson, E. R. (1972). *J. Cell Biol.* **55**, 247a.
Spitzer, J. J., and Spitzer, J. A. (1972). *Amer. J. Physiol.* **222**, 101.
Springer, A., and Perdue, J. F. (1972). *J. Cell Biol.* **55**, 247a.
Stäubli, W., Hess, R., and Weibel, E. R. (1969). *J. Cell Biol.* **42**, 92.
Steiner, J. W., and Baglio, C. M. (1963). *Lab. Invest.* **12**, 765.
Steiner, J. W., and Carruthers, J. S. (1962). *Amer. J. Pathol.* **40**, 253.
Steiner, J. W., Miyai, K., and Phillips, M. J. (1964). *Amer. J. Pathol.* **44**, 169.
Steinman, R. M., and Silver, J. M. (1972). *J. Cell Biol.* **55**, 249a.
Stenger, R. J. (1963). *Amer. J. Pathol.* **43**, 14a.
Stevens, B. J. (1964). *J. Ultrastruct. Res.* **11**, 329.
Stowell, R. E., and Lee, C. S. (1950). *AMA Arch. Pathol.* **50**, 519.
Sugioka, G., Posta, E. A., and Hartroft, W. S. (1969). *Amer. J. Pathol.* **57**, 431.
Suko, J., Vogel, J. H. K., and Chidsey, C. A. (1970). *Circ. Res.* **27**, 235.
Sun, C. N., White, H. J., and Flanigan, S. (1972). *Proc. Electron Microsc. Soc. Amer.* **30**, 96.
Svoboda, D. J., (1962). *Cancer Res.* **22**, 1197.
Swartzendruber, D. C., and Mateer, H. (1972). *J. Cell Biol.* **55**, 255a.
Szubinska, B. (1971). *J. Cell Biol.* **49**, 747.
Szubinski, B. (1972). *J. Cell Biol.* **55**, 256a.
Tandler, B., Erlandson, R. A., Smith, A. L., and Wynder, E. L. (1969). *J. Cell Biol.* **41**, 477.
Tauchi, H., and Sato, T. (1968). *J. Gerontal.* **23**, 454.
Tolnai, S., and Beznak, M. (1971). *J. Mol. Cell. Cardiol.* **3**, 193.
Tosteson, D. C. (1963). *In* "The Cellular Functions of Membrane Transport" (J. F. Hoffman, ed.), 3–22. Prentice-Hall, Englewood Cliffs, New Jersey.
Travis, D. F., and Travis, A. (1972). *J. Ultrastruct. Res.* **39**, 124.
Tribe, M. A., and Ashhurst, D. E. (1972). *J. Cell Sci.* **10**, 443.
Trump, B. F. (1961). *J. Ultrastruct. Res.* **5**, 291.
Trump, B. F. (1970). *Proc. Int. Cong. Nephrol., 4th, 1969* Vol. p. 88
Trump, B. F. (1972). *Encycl. Sci. Technol.* **1**, 32–35.
Trump, B. F. (1973). *Amer. J. Pathol.* **70**, 295.
Trump, B. F., and Arstila, A. U. (1971). *In* "Principles of Pathobiology" (M. F. La Via M. F. and R. B., Hill, eds.), pp. 9–95. Oxford Univ. Press, London and New York.

Trump, B. F., and Benditt, E. P. (1962). *Lab. Invest.* **11**, 753.

Trump, B. F., and Bulger, R. E. (1968a). *Lab. Invest.* **18**, 721.

Trump, B. F., and Bulger, R. E. (1968b). *Lab. Invest.* **18**, 731.

Trump, B. F., and Bulger, R. E. (1971). *Fed. Proc., Fed. Amer. Soc. Exp. Biol.* **30**, 22.

Trump, B. F., and Ericsson, J. L. E. (1965). *In* "The Inflammatory Process" (B. W. Zweifach, L. Grant, and R. T. McCluskey, eds.), 1st ed., pp. 35–120. Academic Press, New York.

Trump, B. F., and Ginn, F. L. (1969). *In* "Methods and Achievements in Experimental Pathology" (K. Bajusz, and G. Yasmin, eds.), Vol. IV, p. 1–29. Yearbook Publ., Chicago, Illinois.

Trump, B. F., and Janigan, D. T. (1962). *Lab. Invest.* **11**, 395.

Trump, B. F., Goldblatt, P. J., and Stowell, R. E. (1962). *Lab. Invest.* **11**, 986.

Trump, B. F., Goldblatt, P. J., Griffin, C. C., Waravdekar, V. S., and Stowell, R. E. (1964). *Lab. Invest.* **13**, 967.

Trump, B. F., Goldblatt, P. J., and Stowell, R. E. (1965a). *Lab. Invest.* **14**, 343.

Trump, B. F., Goldblatt, P. F., and Stowell, R. E. (1965b). *Lab. Invest.* **14**, 1946.

Trump, B. F., Goldblatt, P. J., and Stowell, R. E. (1965c). *Lab. Invest.* **14**, 1969.

Trump, B. F., Goldblatt, P. J., and Stowell, R. E. (1965d). *Lab. Invest.* **14**, 2000.

Trump, B. F., Tisher, C. C., and Saladino, A. J. (1969). *Biol. Basis Med.* **6**, 387–394.

Trump, B. F., Duttera, S. M., Byrne, W. L., and Arstila, A. U. (1970). *Proc. Nat. Acad. Sci. U. S.* **66**, 433.

Trump, B. F., Croker, B. P., and Mergner, W. J. (1971). *In* "Cell Membranes: Biological and Pathological Aspects" (G. W. Richter, and D. G. Scarpelli, eds.), pp. 84–128. Williams & Wilkins, Baltimore, Maryland.

Trump, B. F., Dees, J. H., Kim, K. M., and Sahaphong, S. (1972). *In* "Urolithiasis: Physical Aspects" (B. Finlayson, L. L. Hench, and L. H. Smith, eds.), pp. 1–42. Nat. Acad. Sci., Washington, D. C..

Trump, B. F., Dees, J. H., and Shelburne, J. D. (1973a). *In* "The Liver" (E. A. Gall and F. K. Mistofi, ed.), pp. 80–121. Williams & Wilkins, Baltimore, Maryland.

Trump, B. F., Valigorsky, J. M., Dees, J. H., Mergner, W. J., Kim, K. M., Garbus, J., Jones, R. T., Pendergrass, R., and Cowley, R. A. (1973b). *Hum. Path.* **4**, 89.

Trump, B. F., Valigorsky, J. M., Arstila, A. V., Mergner, W. J., and Kinney, T. D. (1973c). *Amer. J. Pathol.* **72**, 295.

Tyson, G. E., and Bulger, R. E. (1972). *Anat. Rec.* **172**, 669.

Tzagoloff, A, (1971). *Curr. Top. Membranes Trans.* **2**, 157.

Vanderkooi, G. (1972). *Ann. N.Y. Acad. Sci.* **195**, 6.

Van Lancker, J. L., and Holtzer, R. L. (1959). *Amer. J. Pathol.* **35**, 563.

Verbin, R. S., Longnecker, D. S., Liang, H., and Farber, E. (1971). *Amer. J. Pathol.* **62**, 111.

Vickerman, K. (1960). *Nature (London)* **188**, 248.

Virchow, R. (1858). *In* "Cellular Pathology, As Based upon Physiological and Pathological Histology, 1858" (transl. from 2nd German edition by Chabce, F., 1860; Introduction by L. J. Rather, Dover, New York, 1971).

Vogt, M. T., and Farber, E. (1968). *Amer. J. Pathol.* **53**, 1.

Warren, L., Fuhrer, J. P., and Buck, C. A. (1973). *Fed. Proc.* **32**, 80.

Webb, J. L. (1962). *Biochim. Biophys. Acta* **65**, 47.

Weber, R. (1964). *J. Cell Biol.* **22**, 481.

Weed, R. I., and LaCelle, P. L. (1969). *In* "Red Cell Membrane Structure and Function" (G. A. Jamieson, and T., Greenwalt, eds.), pp. 318–338. Lippincott, Philadelphia, Pennsylvania.

Weed, R. I., LaCelle, P. L., and Merrill, E. W. (1969). *J. Clin. Invest.* **48**, 795.

Weibel, E. R., Staubli, W., Gnagi, H. R., and Hess, F. A. (1969). *J. Cell Biol.* **42**, 68.

Weinstein, R. S. (1969). *In* "Red Cell Membrane Structure and Function" (G. A. Jamieson and T. Greenwalt, eds.), pp. 36–82. Lippincott, Philadelphia, Pennsylvania.

Weiss, M., and Meyer, J. (1972). *J. Ultrastruct. Res.* **38**, 411.

Weissmann, G. (1971). *Hospital Practice* **6**, 43.

Weissmann, G., Zurier, R. B., and Hoffstein, S. (1972). *Amer. J. Pathol.* **68**, 539.

Welt, L. G. (1967). *Trans. Ass. Amer. Physicians* **80**, 217.

Wengler, G., and Wengler, G. (1972). *Eur. J. Biochem.* **27**, 162.

Werb, Z., and Cohn, L. A. (1972). *J. Biol. Chem.* **247**, 2439.

Westerman, M. P., Balcerzak, S. P., and Heinle, E. W. Jr. (1968). *J. Lab. Clin. Med.* **72**, 663.

White, J. G., and Estensen, R. D. (1972). *Amer. J. Pathol.* **68**, 289.

Williams, J. P., and Wacker, W. E. C. (1967). *J. Amer. Med. Ass.* **201**, 96.

Williamson, D. H., Krebs, H. A., Stubbs, M., Page, M. A., Morris, H. P., and Weber, G. (1970). *Cancer Res.* **30**, 2049.

Wills, E. J. (1965). *J. Cell Biol.* **24**, 511.

Windmueller, H. G. (1964). *J. Biol. Chem.* **239**, 530.

Wohlrab, H., and Jacobs, E. (1967). *Biochem. Biophys. Res. Commun.* **28**, 998.

Wu, B. C., Valle, R. T., White, L. A. E., Sohal, R. S., and Arcos, J. C. (1971). *Virchows Arch., B.* **9**, 97.

Yee, A. G. (1972). *J. Cell Biol.* **55**, 294a.

Yunis, E. J., and Samaha, F. J. (1971). *Lab. Invest.* **25**, 240.

Zimmerman, A. N. E., Daems, W., Hulsmann, W. C., Snijder, J., Wisse, E., and Durrer, D. (1967). *Cardiovasc. Res.* **1**, 201.

Zollinger, H. U. (1948). *Amer. J. Pathol.* **24**, 545.

Zucker-Franklin, D., and Hirsch, J. G. (1964). *J. Exp. Med.* **120**, 569.

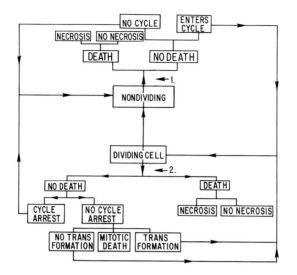

Fig. 1. This is a diagram showing the possible effects of injury on dividing and nondividing cells; (1) indicates injury to a nondividing cell and (2) injury to a dividing cell. For further explanation see text.

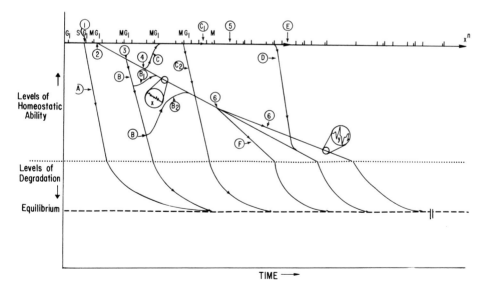

Fig. 2. Conceptualization of the effects of injury and ageing on cells. For explanation see text.

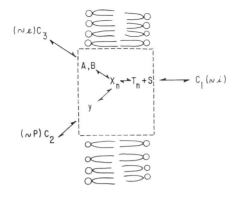

Fig. 3. Relationship between biological energy states and cell membrane. Modified from Mueller and Rudin (1969). ($\sim e$) Electron transfer energy is released by passing down the respiratory chain components (A, B). Phosphate group transfer energy ($\sim P$) is released by passing to water via Y. Ion electrochemical transfer energy ($\sim i$) is released by passing down a concentration gradient across the membrane by translocation-selector system (T + S). X, hypothetical intermediate through which energy is transmitted. C_1–C_3 indicates conformational states.

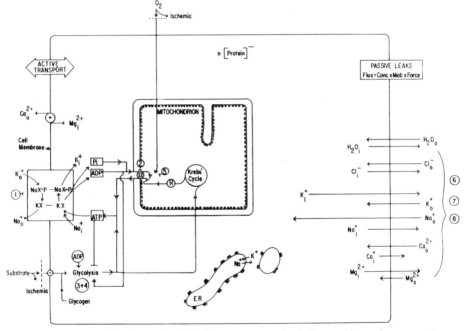

Fig. 4. Diagram showing relationships between energy metabolism and ion and water regulation in a typical cell. Along the left side of the cell, mechanisms involved with active transport are shown; along the right side, conditions affecting passive leaks. A hypothetical mechanism for a typical ion pump, the sodium–potassium pump, is shown in relation to utilization of ATP. Modified from Sjodin (1971). The symbol ⊣ indicates inhibition; the symbol → indicates stimulation. 1. Inhibition of plasma membrane Na + K-stimulated pump by ouabain. 2. Atractyloside inhibition of ATP/ADP exchange. 3. Inhibition of enzymes of anaerobic glycolysis by rising hydrogen ion concentration. 4. Inhibition of glyceraldehyde-3-phosphate dehydrogenase by iodoacetate and inhibition of glucose metabolism by 2-deoxyglucose. 5. Membrane damage and phosphorylation inhibitors. 6. Membrane activation by alteration of SH groups via mercurials and PCMB(S). 7. Inophorous antibiotics causing selective leaks of ions, valinomycin, gramicidin, and amphotericin. 8. Membrane damage with complement.

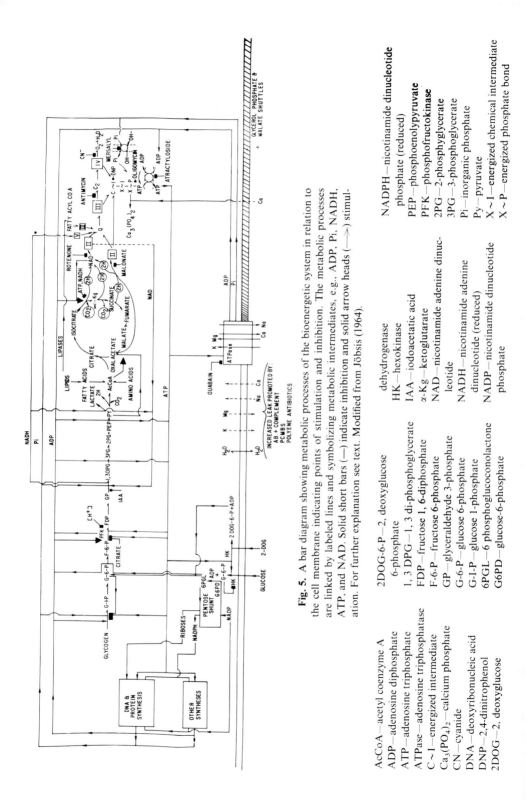

Fig. 5. A bar diagram showing metabolic processes of the bioenergetic system in relation to the cell membrane indicating points of stimulation and inhibition. The metabolic processes are linked by labeled lines and symbolizing metabolic intermediates, e.g., ADP, Pi, NADH, ATP, and NAD. Solid short bars (—) indicate inhibition and solid arrow heads (→) stimulation. For further explanation see text. Modified from Jöbsis (1964).

AcCoA—acetyl coenzyme A
ADP—adenosine diphosphate
ATP—adenosine triphosphate
ATPase—adenosine triphosphatase
C∼I—energized intermediate
Ca$_3$(PO$_4$)$_2$—calcium phosphate
CN—cyanide
DNA—deoxyribonucleic acid
DNP—2,4-dinitrophenol
2DOG—2, deoxyglucose

2DOG-6-P—2, deoxyglucose 6-phosphate
1, 3 DPG—1, 3 di-phosphoglycerate
FDP—fructose 1, 6-diphosphate
F-6-P—fructose 6-phosphate
GP—glyceraldehyde 3-phosphate
G-6-P—glucose 6-phosphate
G-1-P—glucose 1-phosphate
6PGL—6 phosphoglucoconolactone
G6PD—glucose-6-phosphate

dehydrogenase
HK—hexokinase
IAA—iodoacetic acid
α-Kg—ketoglutarate
NAD—nicotinamide adenine dinucleotide
NADH—nicotinamide adenine dinucleotide (reduced)
NADP—nicotinamide dinucleotide phosphate

NADPH—nicotinamide dinucleotide phosphate (reduced)
PEP—phosphoenolpyruvate
PFK—phosphofructokinase
2PG—2-phosphyglycerate
3PG—3-phosphoglycerate
Pi—inorganic phosphate
Py—pyruvate
X∼I—energized chemical intermediate
X∼P—energized phosphate bond

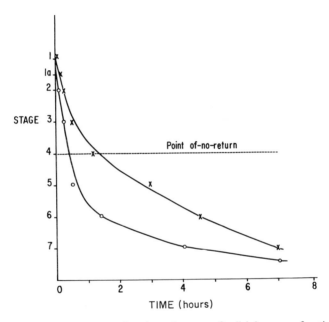

Fig. 6. Diagram showing progression through stages of cell injury as a function of time, comparing inhibition of ATP synthesis with antimycin plus IAA to primary damage to the cell membrane produced by PCMBS. X—X, antimycin + IAA; O — O, PCMBS.

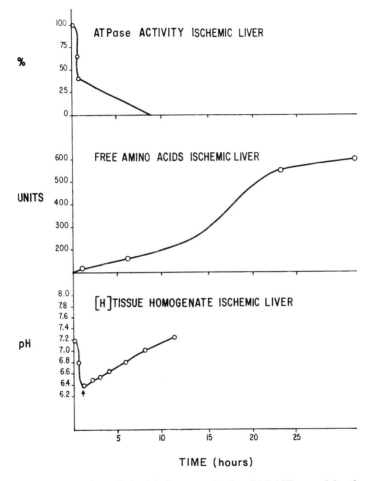

Fig. 7. Diagram showing relationship between mitochondrial ATPase activity, free amino acids, and cell pH. Note that there is a very rapid decline in ATPase activity following ischemia which roughly parallels the decline in tissue homogenate pH. Later, as equilibration occurs with the extracellular space, the pH tends to rise; still later, presumably as lysosomes become leaky, digestion of intracellular components with release of soluble components such as free amino acids occurs. Data: Mergner *et al.* (1972a), Mergner and Trump, (1970) (ATPase), Majno (1964) (amino acids, pH).

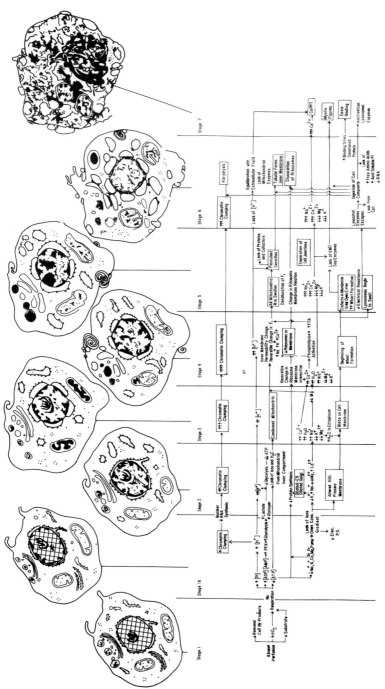

Fig. 8. Diagram showing relationship of earlier stages to the course of reaction to cell injury. Plotted along the abscissa is time and along the ordinate is the range of homeostatic ability.

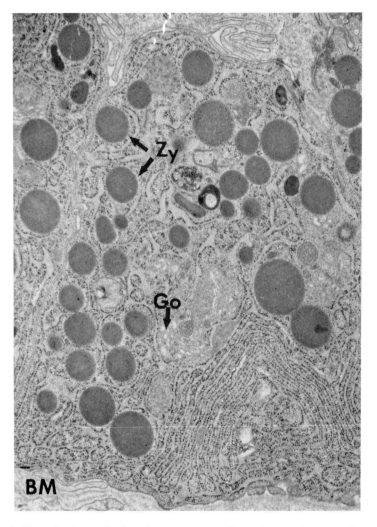

Fig. 9. Normal acinar cells from human pancreas illustrating relationships of zymogen granules (Zy), Golgi apparatus (Go), rough endoplasmic reticulum, and basement membrane (BM). Magnification 15,000 × . Courtesy of Raymond T. Jones.

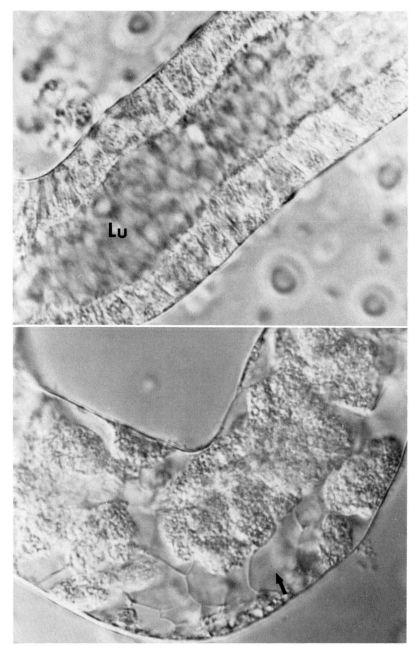

Fig. 10. (top) Light micrograph, using Nomarski optics, of isolated flounder kidney tubule showing normal appearance of the columnar cells. Note the widely patent tubular lumen (Lu). Magnification 903 ×.

Fig. 11. (bottom) Same technique as Fig. 11. Flounder tubule a few minutes after adding 10^{-3} M PCMBS showing marked cell swelling with appearance of large watery vacuoles (arrow). In these clear regions the viscosity of the cytoplasm was lowered as evidenced by markedly intensified Brownian motion. Magnification 903 ×.

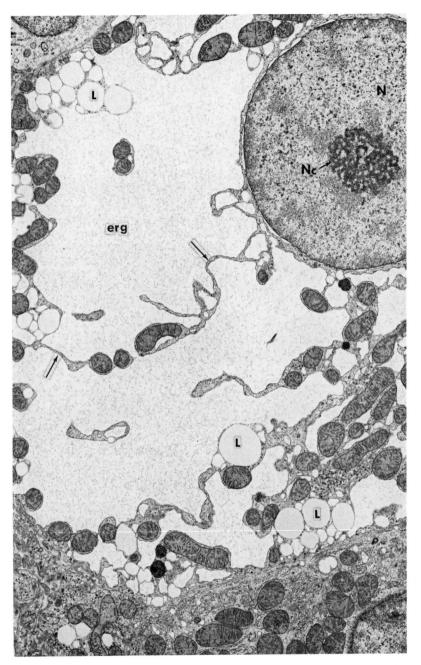

Fig. 12. Rat hepatic parenchymal cell 3 hours after oral administration of chloroform showing marked dilatation of cisternae of rough-surfaced endoplasmic reticulum (erg). This is stage 2 reaction following cell injury. The dilated cisternae contain a flocculent-appearing material of low density which is presumably high in water content. L indicates lipid droplets, nucleolus, and N, nucleus. Magnification 13,300 × .

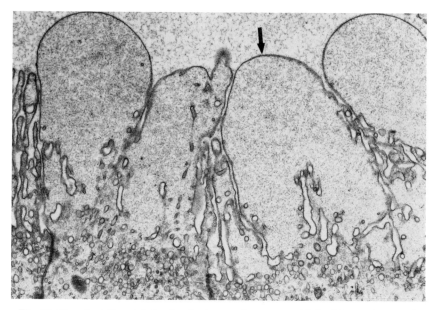

Fig. 13. Flounder kidney tubule after 5 minutes of treatment with 3 mM potassium cyanide showing marked apical blebbing (arrow). Note that the blebs have an electron lucent interior, indicating a low cytoplasmic viscosity. Compare with light micrograph in Fig. 12. Magnification 12,50 ×.

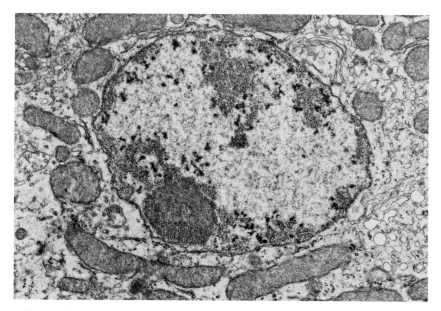

Fig. 14. Flounder kidney tubule 15 minutes after application of 3 mM potassium cyanide showing marked clumping of nuclear chromatin. Magnification 10,500 ×.

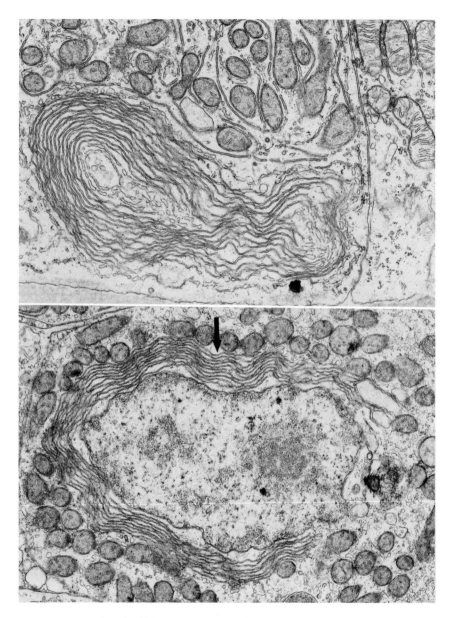

Fig. 15. (top) Flounder kidney tubule immersed 15 minutes in medium containing 3 m*M* potassium cyanide and then restored for 30 minutes to oxygenated media. Note the whorl formed by disordered cytoplasmic membranes. Magnification 15,000 ×.

Fig. 16. (bottom) Same treatment as Fig. 16, showing partial reversibility of chromatin clumping but marked irregularity of cytoplasmic membrane systems (arrow). Magnification 15,000 ×.

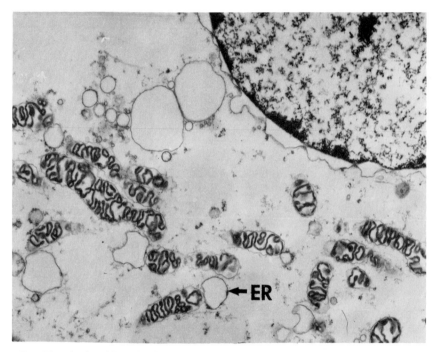

Fig. 17. Mitochondria-rich cell of toad bladder 5 minutes after adding amphotericin B showing stage 3 changes with marked condensation of mitochondria, dilatation of endoplasmic reticulum (ER), and swollen cell sap. Magnification 15,000 ×.

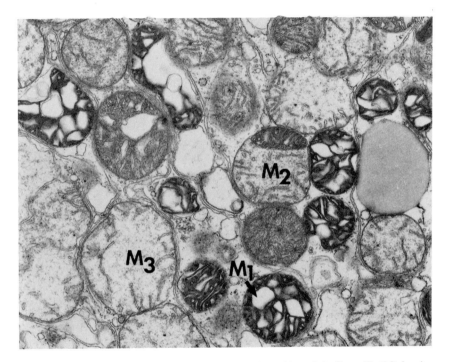

Fig. 18. Rat kidney cortex slice, immersed 24 hours in Robinson's buffer at $0°$–$4°C$ showing typical stage 4 findings. Some mitochondria (M_1) are condensed, others (M_3) are swollen; still others (M_2) show one inner compartment swollen and one inner compartment condensed. Magnification 18,000 × .

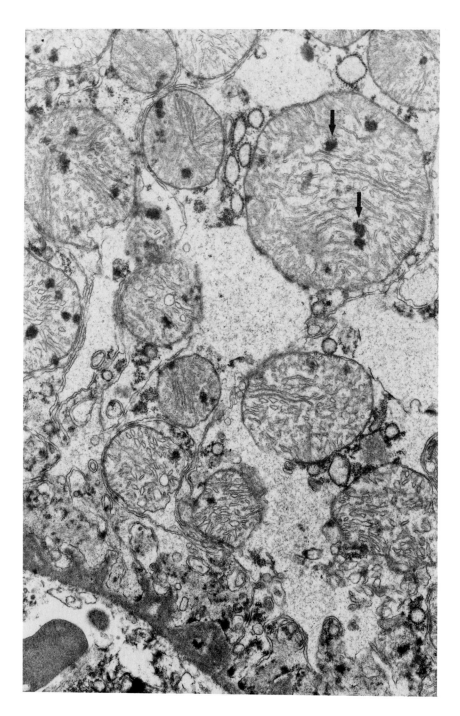

Fig. 19. Rat kidney cortex showing effects of ischemia for 2 hours. Note the marked swelling of mitochondria with typical flocculent densities (free arrows). Magnification 18,500 ×.

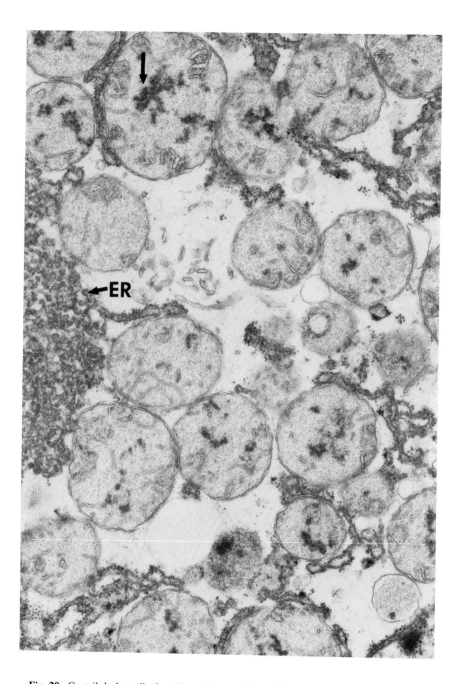

Fig. 20. Centrilobular cell of rat liver 12 hours after administration of carbon tetrachloride showing typical findings of a necrotic cell with swollen mitochondria. Note the flocculent densities (free arrow). Clumps of endoplasmic reticulum (ER) with absence of ribosomes and appearance of dense material between cisternae can be seen. These resemble effects of membrane peroxidation *in vitro*. Magnification 30,000 ×.

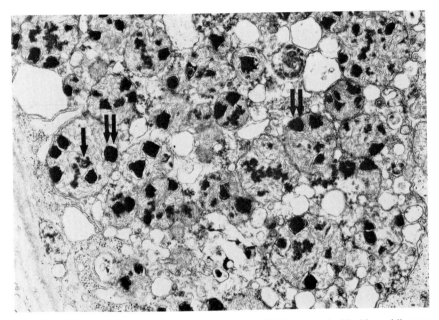

Fig. 21. Rat pars recta 48 hours after administration of 16 mg mercuric chloride per kilogram body weight showing necrotic cells with calcification. Note the swollen mitochondria contain two types of density. The flocculent densities are indicated by the free arrow; the calcifications by the double arrow. Magnification 20,000 × .

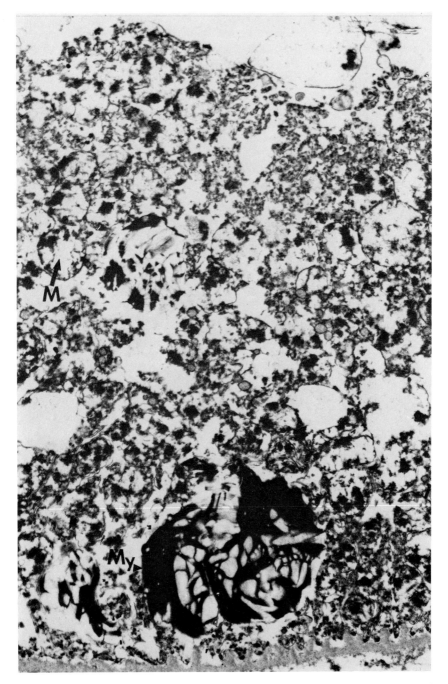

Fig. 22. Rat kidney tubule exposed to ischemia for 12 hours displaying typical changes of stage 7 reaction following cell injury. M, altered mitochondrion. Magnification 15,000

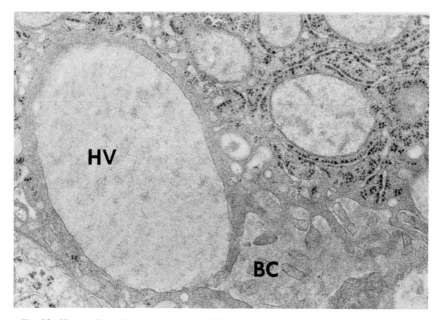

Fig. 23. Human liver. Hypoxic vacuoles (HV) are seen adjacent to a bile canaliculus (BC); in a human liver cell following hemorrhagic shock. Magnification 12,000.

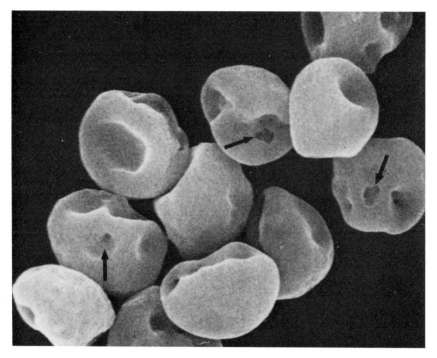

Fig. 24. Scanning electron micrograph of human red blood cells exposed to primaquine. Note the typical invagination of plasma membrane (arrows), causing a marked deformity of the normally doughnut-shaped human red blood cell. Magnification × 3,500.

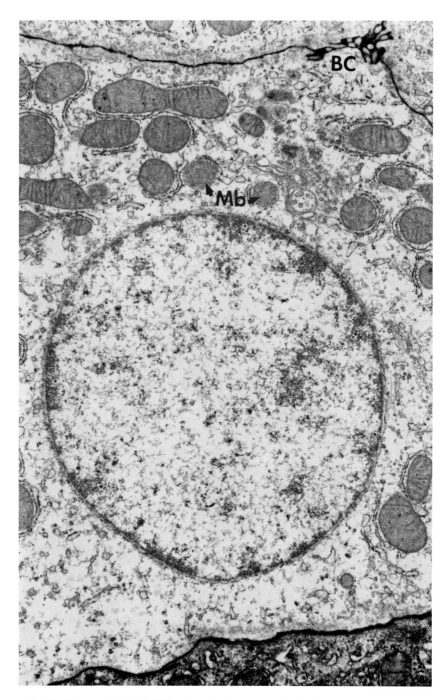

Fig. 25. Micrograph of well-differentiated rat hepatoma showing features resembling normal rat hepatocyte. Colloidal lanthanum was present in the fixative and shows staining of surface and rather uniform penetration of intercellular spaces. mb, microbody; BC, bile canaliculus. Magnification 15,000 ×.

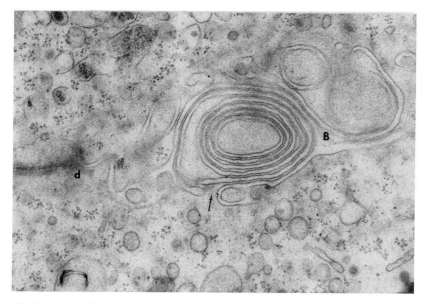

Fig. 26. Area of bile canaliculus (B) in mouse liver during necrosis *in vitro* produced by incubation for 1 hour at 37°C. Instead of the normal microvilli, canaliculus is occupied by a series of attenuated cell processes forming membrane-limited cytoplasmic segments resulting in a myelinlike structure. Continuity of one of these with adjacent cytoplasm is indicated by the arrow. Cell attachment complex including intermediate and tight junctions is indicated by d. Magnification 16,160 × From Trump *et al,* (1962).

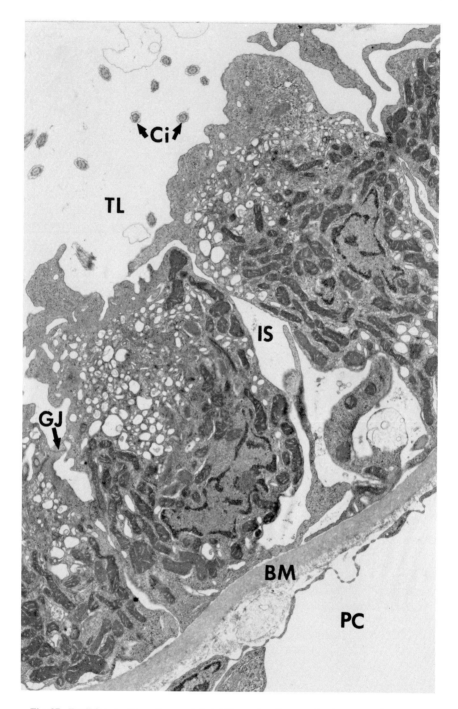

Fig. 27. English sole (Parophrys vetulus) kidney showing proximal segment incubated in calcium-deficient medium. Note the change in the overall shape of the cells with changes in the orientation of apical processes. Numerous cilia (Ci) can be seen in the lumen. Note dilatation of intercellular spaces (IS). In some regions the cells are still attached by gap junctions (GJ). BM, basement membrane; PC, peritubular capillary; TL tubular lumen; Ci, cilia. × 10,000 From Trump and Bulger (1971).

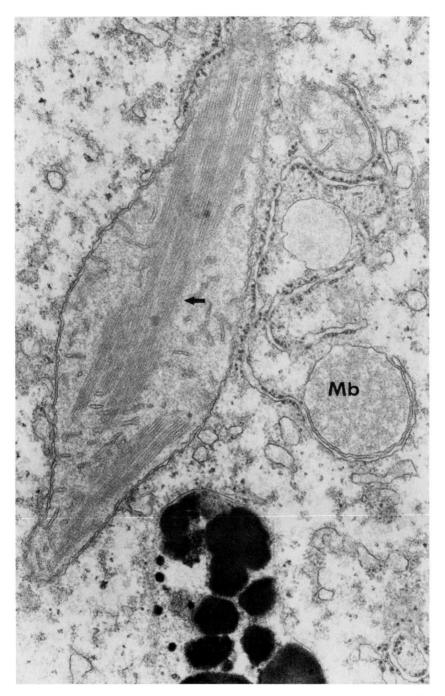

Fig. 28. Megamitochondrion with paracrystalline inclusions seen in human liver cells. (Mb) microbody showing relationship to ER. Arrow points to paracrystalline array. Magnification 38,000 ×.

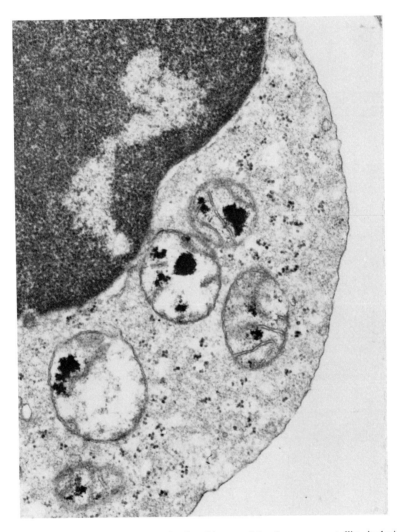

Fig. 29. Human erythroblast with mitochondria containing iron paracrystalline inclusions in the mitochondrial matrix from a patient with sideroblastic anemia. Magnification 17,000 ×. From Trump *et al*, 1973c.

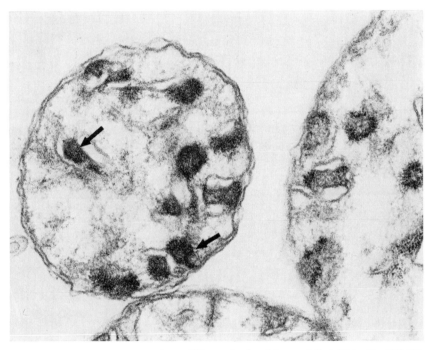

Fig. 30. Calcium accumulation in rat kidney mitochondria, partially inhibited by PCMBS. Magnification 26,200 × .

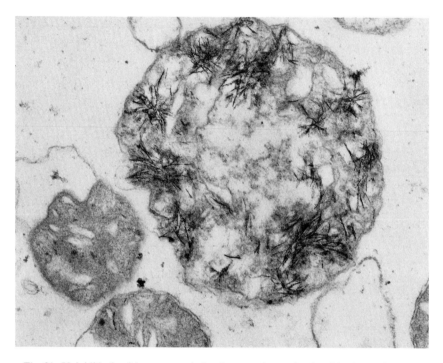

Fig. 31. Uninhibited calcium accumulation in normal rat mitochondria. Note the marked needlelike development of crystalline calcium apatite within the matrix space. Magnification 17,000 ×.

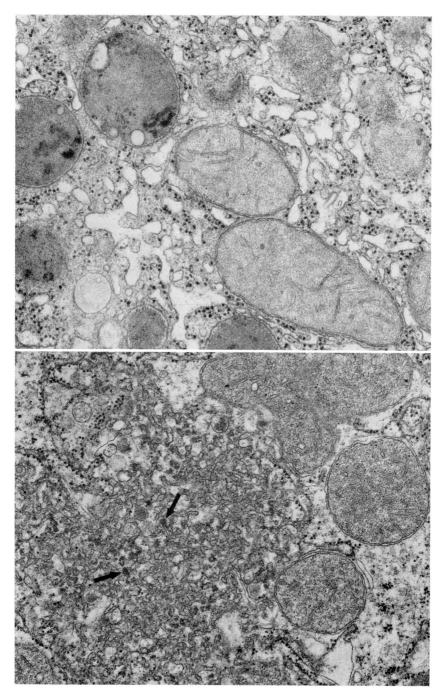

Figs. 33 (top) and 34 (bottom).

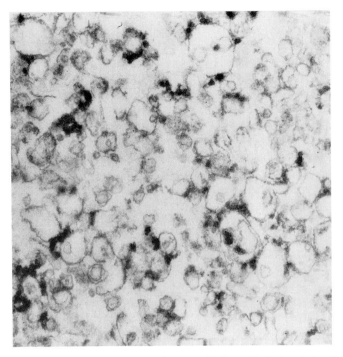

Fig. 35. Hepatic microsomes from a rat after peroxidation with the iron-induced NADPH-dependent system first described by Hochstein and Ernster; note the aggregation of vesicles and the densities between microsome profiles. Magnification 23,000 ×.

Fig. 33. Section of rat liver parenchymal cell 1 hour after administration of carbon tetrachloride showing early dilatation of endoplasmic reticulum and beginning detachment and dissociation of polysomes. Magnification 18,500 ×.

Fig. 34. Hepatic parenchymal cell 24 hours after administration of carbon tetrachloride showing typical cluster of collapsed ER cisternae with dense smudges, probably representing membrane peroxidation. Magnification 17,000 ×.

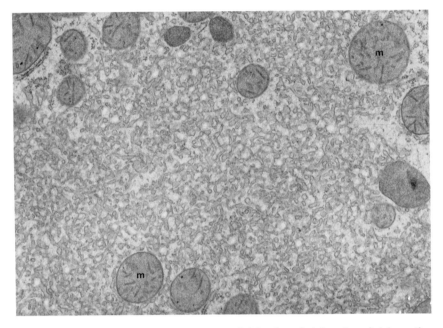

Fig. 36. Portion of rat hepatic parenchymal cell following administration of alphanapthye isothiocyanate showing prominent proliferation of smooth endoplasmic reticulum. Such alterations have been reported following a variety of chemical compounds which have been shown to induce synthesis of rough and smooth endoplasmic reticulum. m, mitochondrion. Magnification 14,320 × . From Steiner and Baglio (1963).

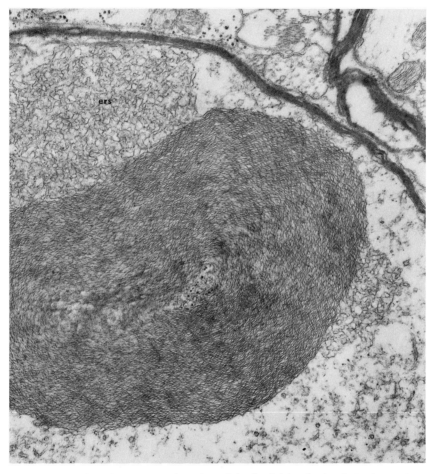

Fig. 37. Axon from the cuneate nucleus of a rat fed a diet deficient in vitamin E. The axoplasm appears toward the lower left, the myelin toward the upper right. Observe the large lamellated body composed of concentrically disposed membranes some of which are continuous with the adjacent proliferations of smooth endoplasmic reticulum (ERS). Magnification 25,350 ×. Courtesy of Dr. Peter W. Lampert.

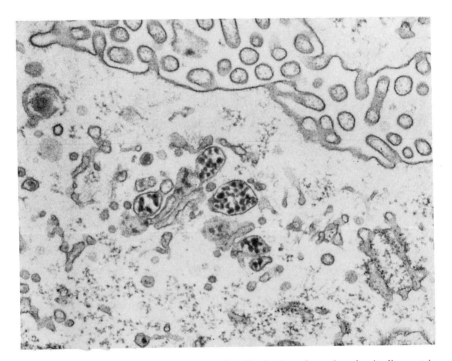

Fig. 38. Rat hepatic parenchymal cell showing distribution of very low density lipoprotein granules (VLDL) in control rat using the osmium impregnation method described by Claude (1970). Note that the granules are confined to Golgi saccules and membrane-bound bodies adjacent to them. Magnification 16,000 ×.

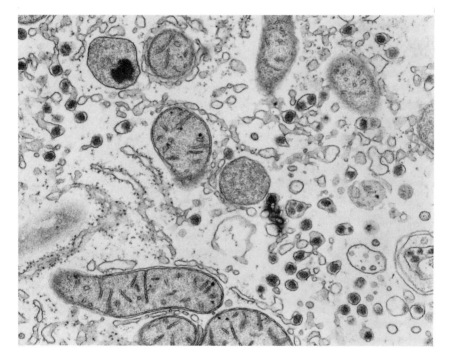

Fig. 39. Rat hepatic parenchymal cell 2 hours after ethionine administration showing change in the distribution of the VLDL: The profiles now appear within elements of the smooth- and rough-surfaced endoplasmic reticulum. Magnification 18,200 ×.

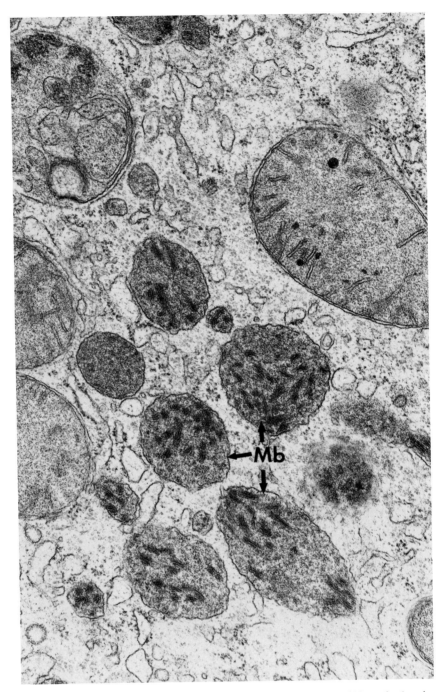

Fig. 40. Hepatic parenchymal cell of a rat fed 0.5 % aspirin in chow diet *ad libitum* for 6 weeks, showing proliferation of abnormal microbodies (Mb) with numerous contained paracrystalline corelike material. Magnification 34,000 ×. Unpublished micrograph courtesy of Dr. Zdenek Hruban.

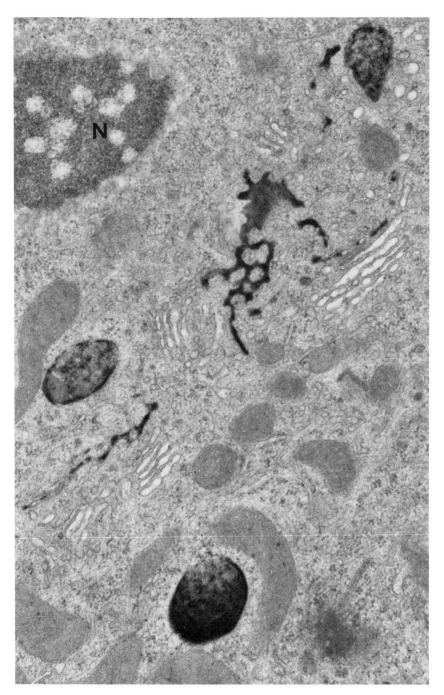

Fig. 41. Mid-cell area of pars recta of rat kidney incubated to show acid phosphatase activity. Activity is localized to lysosomes and within cisternae located at the basal aspects of the Golgi stacks. One cisterna is cut en-face and its fenestrated extremity is evident N, nucleus. Magnification 38,000 ×. Unpublished micrograph courtesy of Dr. E. M. McDowell.

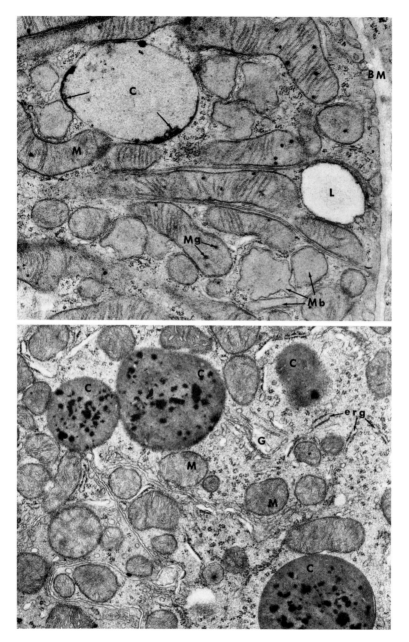

Fig. 42. (top) Portion of a proximal tubular cell from a normal rat kidney showing the appearance of cytosomes (C) and microbodies (Mb), basement membrane (BM), mitochondrion (M), mitochondrial matrix granules (Mg), and lipid droplet (L). Stained with lead hydroxide. Magnification 17,010 × .

Fig. 43. (bottom) Cell similar to that shown in Fig. 43, showing localization of acid phosphatase activity in the cytosomes (C). The black granular deposits in the cytosomes represent precipitates of lead phosphate. M, mitochondria; G, Golgi apparatus; erg, rough endoplasmic reticulum. Specimen fixed in buffered glutaraldehyde; acid phosphatase, demonstrated by modified Gomori technique on frozen section; sections postfixed in s-collidine-buffered osmium tetroxide; specimen stained with lead hydroxide. Magnification 19,440 × .

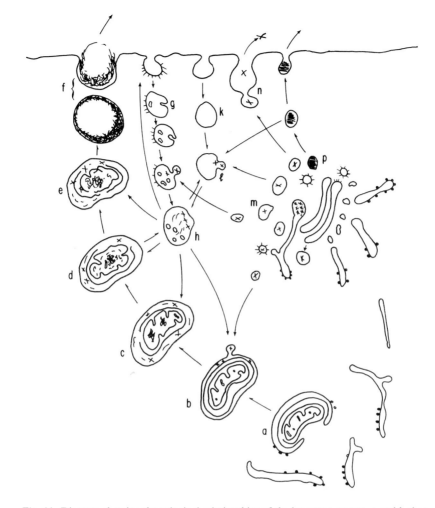

Fig. 44. Diagram showing the principal relationships of the lysosome system. a and b show formation of autophagic vacuoles with addition of hydrolytic enzymes to the outer compartment from elements such as primary or secondary lysosomes. The enzyme is indicated by the small x. c is an ambilysosome containing materials taken in by both heterophagy and autophagy. Note the gradual disintegration of the enclosed mitochondrion in d, conversion to residual body in e and f. g shows pinocytic or phagocytic uptake with exotropic budding forming multivesicular bodies. Note addition of enzyme by fusion with the primary lysosome; enzyme indicated by "X," giving finally a typical ambiphagic secondary lysosomes (H) with both vesicles and enzymes; k illustrates a phagosome without budding forming simpler secondary lysosome (1). Note that fusions in both directions between h and l and h and d are postulated. The Golgi apparatus is shown with a convex forming face with transitional vesicles bearing materials from the rough ER, a concave maturing face with coated and uncoated vesicles leaving the Golgi saccules; m indicates hydrolase-containing vesicles or tubules in the vicinity of the Golgi apparatus representing so-called primary lysosomes; also shown along the forming face is a saccule in continuity with the rough endoplasmic reticulum representing the so-called GERL of Novikoff; p illustrates an exocrine or endocrine secretory granule with secretion to the outside under normal conditions or fusing with (L) in the process known as crinophagy; n indicates typical exocrine or endocrine secretion with fusion to the extracellular space only.

Fig. 45. Survey picture of proximal convoluted tubule from a rat which received 300 mg lyophilized homologous hemoglobin per 100 3m of body weight 4 hours prior to sacrifice. The hemoglobin absorption droplets ($Hb_{1\ 6}$) present in the cytoplasm are illustrative of different stages observed during this process. Immediately after their formation through pinocytosis, the content is rather pale ($Hb_{1\ 2}$); later, a condensation appears to occur with formation of focal, very dense areas usually near the periphery (Hb_2). At this stage some droplets are very dark (Hb_4), though they still contain recognizable irregular, even darker areas.

They then appear to move toward the base of the cell, usually forming a polarized stream toward the Golgi–cytosome region and again attain a rather pale background matrix ($Hb_{5\ 6}$). It appears that at least some of the droplets fuse with, or deliver their content into, cytosomes (C,C), which appear to contain only the irregularly clumped, very dense material. The cytosomes can be identified by their content of vesicular, dense, and filamentous material (arrows in the cytosomes). TL, tubular lumen; BM, basement membrane; Mb, microbody; G, Golgi apparatus; BB, brush border. Specimen fixed by dripping 2% osmium tetroxide buffered with *s*-collidine on the surface of the kidney for 15 minutes (fixation *in vivo*); section stained with lead hydroxide. Magnification 10,500 ×. From Ericsson (1965).

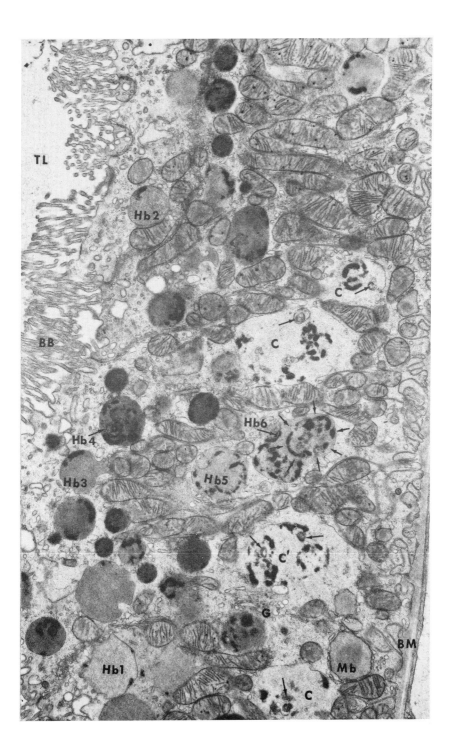

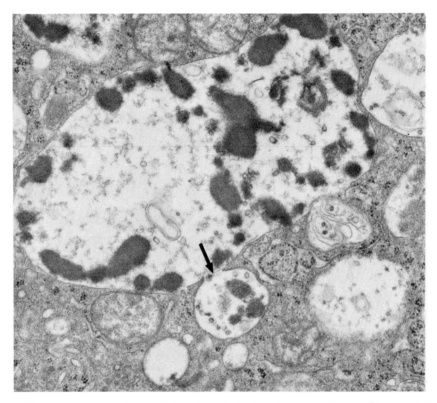

Fig. 46. Micrograph showing fusions (arrow) of enlarged secondary lysosomes in mannitol nephrosis. Magnification 29,000 × .

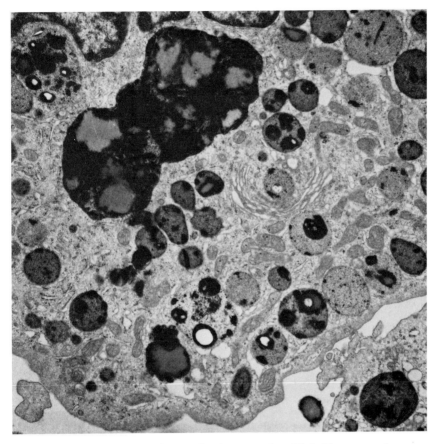

Fig. 47. "Heart failure" cell in the lung showing macrophage filled with numerous lysosomes containing iron pigment. Magnification 10,500 × . Unpublished micrograph courtesy of Jane H. Dees.

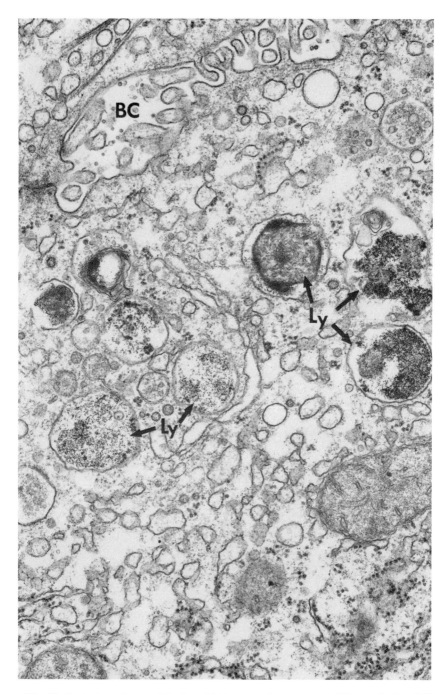

Fig. 48. Single iron dextran injection. 14 Days, rat hepatocyte. A bile canaliculus (BC) between two cells. The Golgi apparatus is present at this site and on either side of it are several lysosomes (Ly) containing aggregates of hemosiderin and ferritin. Magnification 37,500 ×. From Trump *et al.* (1973c).

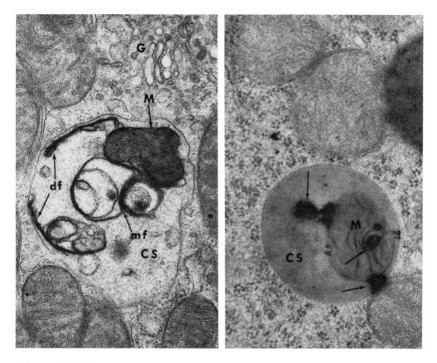

Fig. 49. (left) Cytosegresome (CS) from normal rat proximal tubular epithelium containing a recognizable mitochondrion (M). In addition to the mitochondrion, this cytosegresome contains many dense filamentous (df) and granular aggregates and a myelinlike figure (mf). These aggregates are found in fully formed cytosomes and may be derived from organelle breakdown (see text). G, Golgi apparatus. Fixation and staining as in Fig. 43. Magnification 32,000 ×.

Fig. 50. (right) Electron micrograph showing localization of acid phosphatase activity in a cytosegresome (CS) from a normal rat proximal tubular cell. The black precipitates (arrows) represent lead phosphate reaction product. Technique same as Fig. 43. Magnification 40,000 ×.

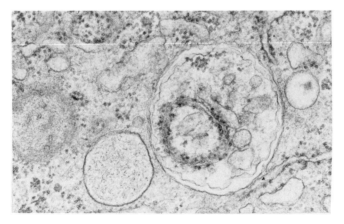

Fig. 51. Early double-walled autophagic vacuole from an immediate autopsy specimen of human liver. Note contained profiles of endoplasmic reticulum and cell sap.

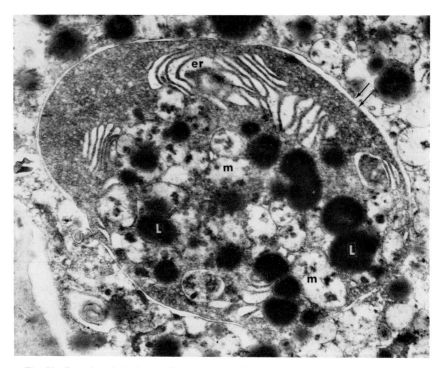

Fig. 52. Cytoplasmic inclusion from a mouse hepatic parenchymal cell in experimental murine hepatitis. The inclusion is surrounded by two membranes (arrows) and contains structures which probably represent degenerating mitochondria (m), lipid droplets (L), and endoplasmic reticulum (er). Such inclusions are thought to correspond to the "Councilman bodies" demonstrable by light microscopy and to represent increased cytosegresome formation following cell injury (see text). Magnification 10,710 ×. From Svoboda (1962).

Fig. 53. Pulmonary capillary from "immediate autopsy" specimen of individual suffering acute hemorrhagic shock showing adherent polymorph with disintegration and release of granules (arrows) into capillary lumen. Magnification 16,200 ×. Micrograph by Jane H. Dees.

Fig. 54. Hepatic parenchymal cell from "immediate autopsy" of patient suffering several episodes of shock over a 30-day period, illustrating large residual bodies filled with myelin. Magnification 12,500 ×. From Trump et al. (1973c).

Fig. 55. Glomerular epithelial cell from child with neurovisceral lipidosis showing characteristic clear lysosomes containing mucopolysaccharide and small amounts of phospholipid as evidenced by the myelin forms. Magnification 15,000 ×.

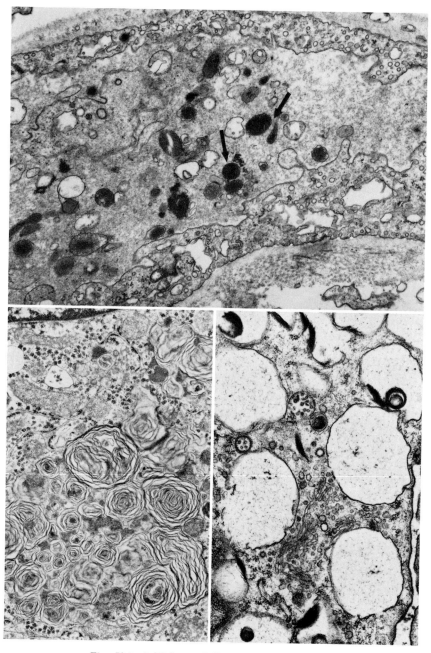

Figs. 53 (top), 54 (bottom left), and 55 (bottom right).

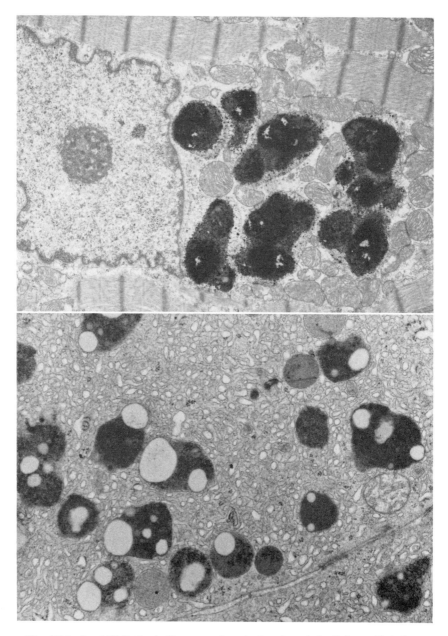

Figs. 56 (top) and 57 (bottom). Heart muscle and adrenal cortical cell from elderly human patient obtained at "immediate autopsy" showing abundant lipofuscin pigment. Magnification 11,800 ×.

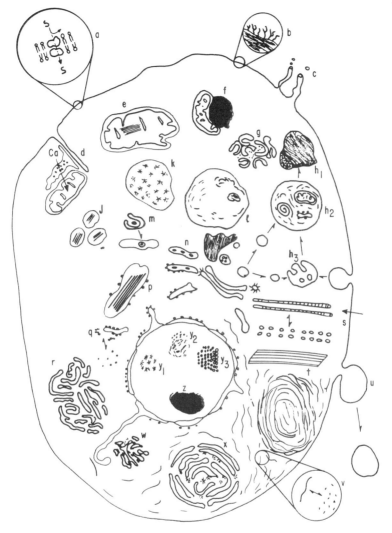

Fig. 58. Diagram showing chronic reactions to cell injury. The letters in sequence are as follows: a, alteration of transmembrane transport processes; b, alteration of cell surface coat, e.g., neoplastic transformation; c, alterations of cell surface activity, e.g., tubular forms; d, calcium shift from sarcoplasmic reticulum to mitochondria in heart failure; e, megamito-chondria; f, lipid droplet; g, exotropy, induced by polio virus; h, lipofuscin; h_2, autophagic vacuole; h_3, multivesicular body; i, alcoholic hyaline; j, formation of new peroxisomes; k and l, lysosomal storage; m, virus budding into ER; n, lipoprotein in ER; o, storage in dilated ER cisterna; p, protein crystals in ER, e.g., Russell bodies; q, separation of polyribosomes from membrane; r, proliferation of SER; s, microtubule—disassembly; t, microtubules—crystal formation; u, exotropy at surface; v, microfilament—disassembly; w, peroxidation lesions of ER; x, glycogen body; y_1, virus production; y_2, stratification of elements in nucleolus; y_3, crystalline virus inclusion; z, protein inclusion in nucleus, e.g., Pb poisoning.

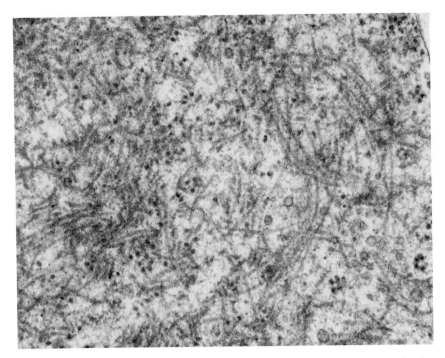

Fig. 59. Hepatic parenchymal cell from an individual with alcoholic hepatitis showing typical alcoholic hyaline. Magnification 15,000 ×. Unpublished picture courtesy of Dr. Kook M. Kim

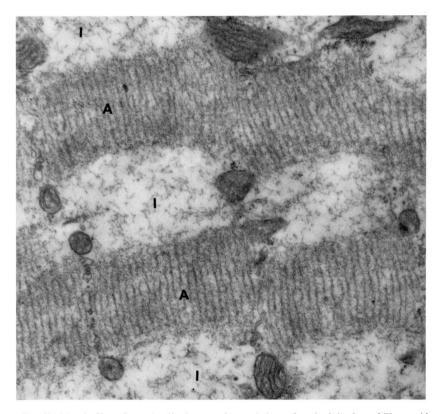

Fig. 60. Muscle fibers from the diaphragm of a rat 3 days after the injection of Plasmocid showing complete dissolution of I-band components, including actin filaments, and absence of Z lines. Although the A bands retain normal orientation, the actin filaments cannot be identified. At this time the sarcoplasmic reticulum appeared normal. Note the normal appearing mitochondria. Magnification, 35,000 × . Courtesy of Dr. Harold M. Price.

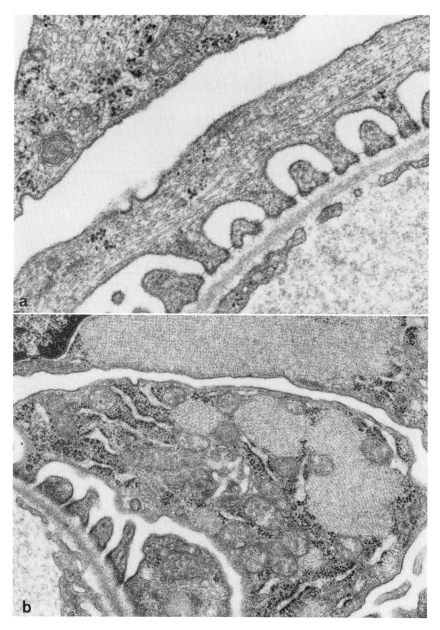

Fig. 61. (a) Rat kidney. Normal untreated podocytes with numerous microtubules. Magnification 36,000 ×. Courtesy of Dr. G. Tyson. (b) Rat kidney. Visceral epithelium from animal given IV injections of vinblastine—showing paracrystals of microtubular protein in cytoplasm. Magnification 26,000 ×. Courtesy of Dr. G. Tyson.

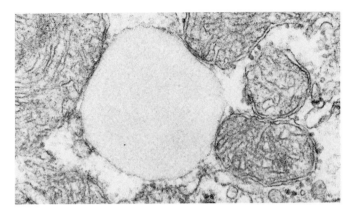

Fig. 62. Triglyceride droplet in a hepatic parenchymal cell from a patient with shock obtained at "immediate autopsy."

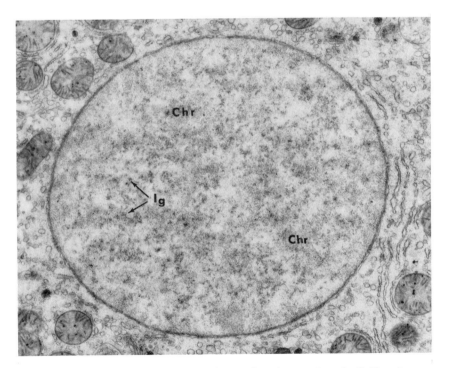

Fig. 63. Interphase nucleus from a normal mouse hepatic parenchymal cell. Note the even, diffuse dispersion of the chromatin (Chr) and interchromatinic granules (Ig). Magnification 8500 ×.

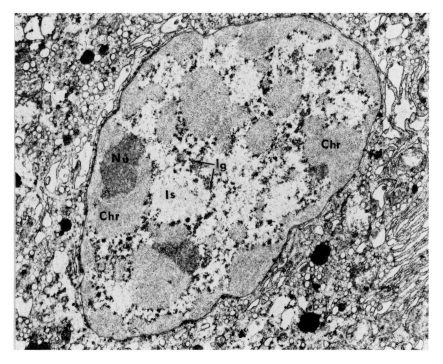

Fig. 64. Interphase nucleus from a mouse liver slice undergoing necrosis *in vitro* (4 hours incubation at 37°C). The chromatin fibrils (Chr) are aggregated together and form clumps along the nuclear membrane and around the nucleolus (Nu). The interchromatinic granules (Ig) are aggregated along the interface between the chromatin and the interchromatin substance (Is) which is extremely prominent. Magnification 8500 × .

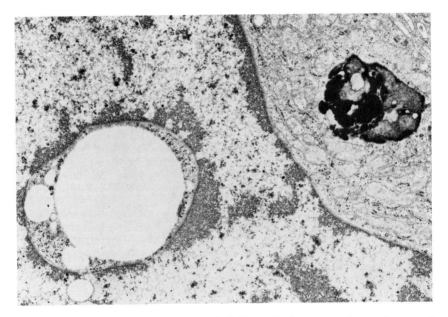

Fig. 65. Hepatic parenchymal cell from an individual suffering several episodes of shock and showing evidence of hepatic regenerative activity showing nuclear pseudo-inclusions. Magnification 30,000 ×

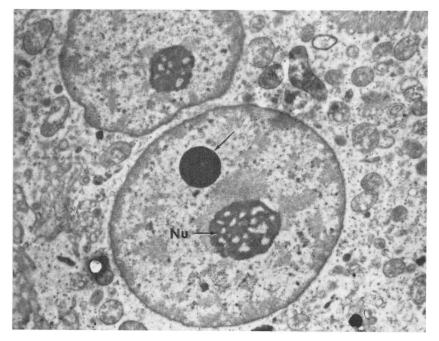

Fig. 66. Interphase nucleus in proximal tubular epithelial cell from a rat which had received large amounts of bismuth. Note the round, dense homogeneous inclusion (arrow) above the nucleolus (Nu). Tissue was embedded in methacrylate. Magnification 9000 ×. From Beaver and Burr (1963).

Fig. 67. Regenerating pars recta cell in the rat kidney 2 days after administration of mercuric chloride showing early regenerating cells with abundant free polysomes, small mitochondria, and randomly oriented rough endoplasmic reticulum. Note necrotic cells in the lumen. Magnification 7500 ×.

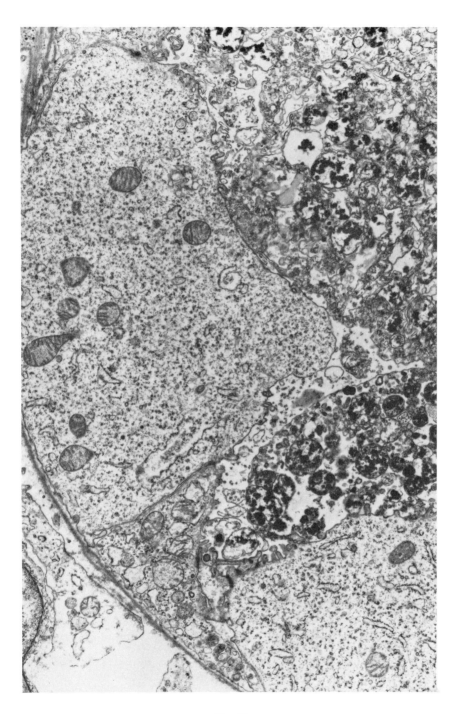

Fig. 67.

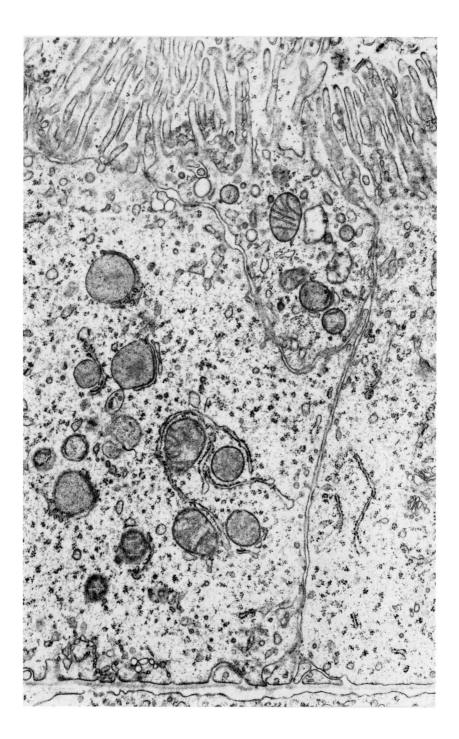

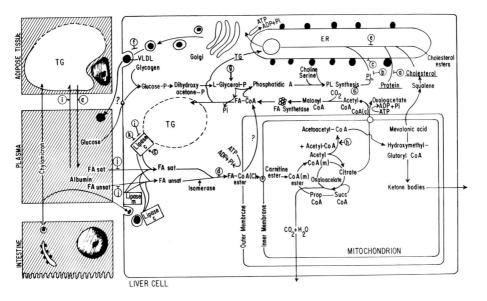

LIVER CELL

Fig. 69. Shows four compartments or tissues which consist of the blood space of the intestine, the adipose tissue, and the liver tissue. Lipid metabolism depends on the interplay between cells of these tissues. Fat and lipids enter the body by absorption by intestinal cells and are released as chylomicrons or very low density lipoproteins into the plasma from where they reach the adipose tissue and are stored as triglycerides and lipid substances in the adipose cells. Secondary to hormonal action triglycerides are released from the adipose tissue into the plasma from where they reach the liver cells. The liver is a major checking point in metabolism of lipids. The following conditions lead to accumulation of lipid substances in the liver: increased release from adipose tissue; defective metabolism of FA; defective production of proteins and phospholipids; defective coupling of protein and lipids; and defective release of lipoproteins. The letters indicate the inhibitions and stimulations possible in this metabolic process: a, inhibition of protein synthesis by CCl_4, puromycin, ethionine, phosphorus, and alcohol; b, choline deficiency associated with deficient biosynthesis of phospholipids; c, release of FA + L-glycerol-P from adipose tissue by epinephrine and growth hormones; d, deficient esterification of free fatty acids and decreased oxidation induced by alcohol; e, effect of orotic acid which may prevent coupling of proteins with lipids; f, effect of orotic acid which may prevent release of lipoproteins into plasma; g, increased production of L-glycerol-P in starvation; h, effect of diabetic acidosis; i, effect of insulin; j, effect of detergents; and k, effect of prostaglandins.

Fig. 68. Same conditions as Fig. 68, but 1 week after administration of mercuric chloride showing late state in regeneration with formation of microvilli and beginning formation of basalar cell processes. Note abundant free polysomes and curving profiles of rough ER with newly formed peroxisomes. Magnification 8500 × .

Chapter 4

LYSOSOMAL MECHANISMS IN THE INFLAMMATORY PROCESS

ROCHELLE HIRSCHHORN

I. Introduction

Of all the components of the cell, the lysosome is an obvious candidate for a role in the inflammatory process. After the initial delineation of this class of subcellular organelles, the nature of their contents, capable of lysing or degrading a variety of biological substrates, suggested that they might represent the source of the "cytases" described by Eli Metchnikoff (1905) during his classic studies of the role of the phagocyte in inflammation. However, in order to better define what this role may be, it is necessary to examine more closely what is encompassed by the word lysosome, for unlike other subcellular organelles, such as nuclei or mitochondria, lysosomes may vary widely.

Specific components which may be peculiar to the lysosomes of phagocytic cells will be discussed in greater detail in the chapter dealing specifically with the macrophage and the polymorphonuclear leukocytes.

A. Biochemical

The manner in which lysosomes were discovered has greatly influenced and modified some of the subsequent investigations and ideas concerning this subcellular organelle. Although lysosomes are visible under the light, as well as the electron microscope, their existence as a separate class of organelles was not appreciated by morphologists. Rather, this class of subcellular organelles was discovered through the application of deductive reasoning to a mass of complex biochemical data in order to predict the existence of these previously undescribed morphological entities. Thus, de Duve and his co-workers initially (Berthet and de Duve, 1951) observed that the activity of the enzyme acid phosphatase appeared to be relatively low in freshly prepared homogenates of liver, but was greatly increased when these homogenates were "aged" or left in storage. Utilizing the then newly developed methods of differential centrifugation to fractionate cells, they also separated the contents of disrupted liver cells into different subcellular components or "fractions" rich in nuclei, mitochondria, or "microsomes." They observed that this increase in activity of acid phosphatase on aging was most pronounced in what was called the "mitochondrial-rich" fraction. They also made the crucial observation that, parallel with the increase in activity of acid phosphatase in "aged" homogenate, the enzyme activity could no longer be sedimented with this mitochondrial fraction. Of all the possible explanations for these phenomena, they chose to consider the possibility that acid phosphatase normally existed within a subcellular structure consisting of a surrounding membrane which separated the enzyme from its substrate, serving both to render it latent and to cause the enzyme complex to sediment between the mitochondria and the microsomes. During "aging," they postulated this membrane was disrupted, allowing the enzyme free access to substrate, as well as allowing the enzyme to become nonsedimentable. Starting with this hypothesis, they performed a series of experiments which demonstrated that there were several enzymes which behaved in a similar fashion, in that they sedimented together between the mitochondrial and microsomal elements when osmotically buffered homogenates of cells were subjected to different centrifugal forces. These enzymes, which shared similar acid pH optima and were predominantly hydrolytic in nature, all appeared to be relatively inactive until they were aged or left in storage. The effect of storage could also be mimicked by a variety of treatments such as diminished osmotic pressure, exposure to surface active agents, vigorous homogenization or freezing, and thawing, all of which would presumably rupture biomembranes. Based essentially on these observations (Appelmans *et al.*, 1955; de Duve *et al.*, 1955; de Duve, 1959; de Duve and Wattiaux, 1966), together with the insight to disregard for the moment some apparently nonconfirmatory data (Conchie and Levvy, 1963), they predicted the existence of an intracellular organelle which was membrane bounded, between 0.2 and 0.8 μm in size and which contained at least five hydrolytic enzymes [acid phosphatase, acid ribonuclease, acid deoxyribonuclease, cathepsin (D), and β-glucuronidase]. Because of the lytic nature of these enzymes, the name lysosome was proposed.

B. Morphological

A purposeful search soon revealed the morphological equivalent of the biochemical construct. Novikoff (who had been conducting experiments along similar lines) (Novikoff, 1961; Novikoff *et al.*, 1956) collaborating with de Duve examined with the electron microscope fractions from rat liver presumably rich in these lysosomes. He observed clusters of what had previously been called the pericanalicular dense bodies of the liver. These ranged in size from 0.2 to 0.8 μm in size, and he suggested that they were the containers of hydrolytic enzymes or lysosomes. Histochemical staining for acid phosphatase activity revealed that these structures did indeed exhibit such enzyme activity both in subcellular fractions and in the whole tissue, and thus the lysosome had been identified both biochemically and morphologically. Parallel with these investigations in liver, Strauss (1954, 1967) had collected similar data utilizing kidney tissue.

It was soon apparent that the lysosome, as seen microscopically, was not as morphologically uniform as mitochondria or nuclei. It was perhaps because of this pleomorphic nature of the organelle that its identification had to await enzymic definition. However, in the process of drawing a meaningful generalization from complex biochemical data, it was realized early that an idealized subcellular structure had been described. Histochemical evidence suggested that the generalized lysosome included a wide range of structures with slightly different constituents and functions in different cell types (cf. Ericsson, 1964; Mausbach, 1966; Bainton and Farquhar, 1966). These structures could be called lysosomes in that they shared the common property of containing acid hydrolases within a semipermeable membrane. Lysosomes have since then not only been described in many if not all vertebrate tissues, but have been found in such widely divergent sources as fungi (Matile, 1966), unicellular organisms (Muller, 1967), and insects (Locke and Collins, 1968).

II. Formation, Classification, and Fate of Lysosomes

In order to understand the structure, function, and content of lysosomes as they might relate to the pathogenesis of inflammation, their natural history must be considered. Lysosomes appear to be dynamic structures interacting and merging with other portions of the membranous systems of cells. As will become apparent, their content and form depend on the cell in which they are found, their prior history, as well as the prior history of the cell in which they are found. The major events in the formation of lysosomes have been outlined from observations in several different types of cells, most notably including macrophages (Cohn, 1968; Nichols et al., 1971), polymorphonuclear leukocytes (Bainton and Farquhar, 1968), kidney cells (Strauss, 1967), and nervous tissue (Holtzman and Novikoff, 1965). Although the details may be slightly different from tissue to tissue, several generalizations can be made. In the initial search for the origin of the primordial lysosome, the granules of the polymorphonuclear leukocyte and of the macrophage were examined, since it had been demonstrated that these numerous, clearly visible granules (Cohn and Hirsch, 1960; Cohn and Weiner, 1963) fulfilled the criteria for lysosomes. Investigation of the manner of formation of these granules has demonstrated that the synthesis and packaging of lysosomal enzymes appears to follow, in general, lines previously delineated by Palade (Caro and Palade, 1964; Palade, 1966) for the synthesis and packaging of pancreatic secretory proteins and for many other proteins (Peters et al., 1971). Enzyme protein is apparently synthesized on ribosomes, transferred to the endoplasmic reticulum and concentrated within the Golgi apparatus. For example, the lysosomal enzymes of the azurophilic granules of the polymorphonuclear leukocyte (as opposed to the specific granules) are found (using histochemical techniques) in the endoplasmic reticulum and the proximal face of the Golgi complex during the progranulocyte stage of development. It is during this phase of granulocyte maturation that the azurophilic granule is formed (Bainton and Farquhar, 1968). Similar studies have demonstrated that the "granule" of the bone marrow and blood macrophage and the eosinophile are formed in a similar fashion (Nichols et al., 1971; Bainton and Farquhar, 1970). These granules have been considered to represent the primordial, primary, or virgin lysosome, but they may well represent a specialized form of this granule, one meant for storage.

Beginning with the work of Novikoff in 1964 (Novikoff et al., 1964), it has been clear that there are other pathways for formation of primary lysosomes, or lysosomes which have not yet met with substances for digestion. Lysomal enzymes may be sequestered directly from the endoplasmic reticulum or Golgi into small vesicles in macrophages (Cohn et al., 1966; Nichols et al., 1971) or directly into larger vacuoles, such as the dense bodies of neurons. However, it is possible that the latter form of dense body is a secondary lysosome with intracellular digestion having occurred within the endoplasmic reticulum (Novikoff, 1967). It now appears that this pathway is also utilized in the pancreas, where, on continued stimulation, enzyme is sequestered within vacuoles directly from the endoplasmic reticulum (Jamieson and Palade, 1971). In most cells, the primary or virgin lysosome, which can be defined as a packaging of lysosomal enzymes which have not previously met substrate, may occur most often as a small vesicle. They have been so elusive to define in most cell types other than circulating white blood cells both because they appear to be morphologically indistinguishable from other small vesicles and because they are relatively short lived.

The fate of these primary lysosomes is clear in the white blood cell. After phagocytosis, the ingested particulate matter is present within a vacuole formed by the invagination of the outer cell membrane. The membranes of the PMN granules (both lysosomal and specific) fuse with this vacuole, thus adding their enzymes and other constituents to its content (Hirsch and Cohn, 1960). This combined vacuole is now one of the several forms of secondary lysosomes, variously called phagolysosomes or heterophagic vacuoles. However, such fusion is not limited to phagocytosing cells in which it is firmly established that uptake of particulate matter occurs by this process of engulfment. It is now obvious that in most cell types, in addition to transport across the plasma membrane by what may be loosely called "permeation," bulk transport of smaller soluble substances occurs by a similar process of vesicular transport (Chapman-Andresen, 1963, 1964; Ryser, 1967). After a suitable stimulus (Cohn and Parks, 1967), a portion of the surrounding fluid environment is incorporated within a vacuole formed by invagination of the plasma membrane, with subsequent joining and internalization of the newly formed vesicle. This has been referred to as pinocytosis, and together with phagocytosis the ingestion of foreign matter is called endocytosis.

Both in isolated cells, such as the macrophage, and in nonphagocytic tissues, such as the kidney, the primary lysosome also fuses with pinocytic vesicles. Numerous elegant studies have utilized substances (Daems et al., 1969; Strauss, 1964), such as horseradish peroxidase, ferritin, thorotrast, dextran, carbon, and DNA coacervates, to mark the uptake of bulk material (both soluble and particulate) through this process of endocytosis into pinocytic or endocytic vesicles. These substances may all be visualized under the electron microscope. These studies have demonstrated the combination of these vesicles with preexisting lysosomes, identified histochemically as vacuoles staining for acid phosphatase.

The fate of the secondary lysosome is then variable. It may fuse with additional primary lysosomes, as during phagocytosis, where several granules will discharge into a single phagocytic vacuole (Hirsch and Cohn,

1960). Secondary lysosomes, after having expended their enzymes in a digestive effort, may become a third form of lysosome known as a residual body, or bodies containing indigestible material, such as lipofuscin granules or myelin figures (Koenig, 1964; Novikoff, 1963). The most obvious form of this type of granule is seen in the inherited lysosomal diseases (Brady et al., 1971; Resibois et al., 1970) where, because of the absence of specific normal degradative enzymes, the substrate accumulates in multiple residual bodies. This may be a specialized form of residual lysosomes in that there is an increase in activity of the other lysosomal enzymes in the cell, whereas residual bodies of the class of lipofuscin granules presumably are relatively deficient in enzyme.

In addition, a fourth type of membrane-bounded vesicle which stains for hydrolytic enzymes has also been identified. This type of granule is distinguished by its contents, recognizable as parts of the cell itself, such as partially digested mitochondria and ribosomes (Ericsson, 1964; 1969; Novikoff and Essner, 1962). These vacuoles are classed together as autophagic vacuoles, or vacuoles in which the cell literally eats part of itself. The initial vacuole appears to consist of a segregated portion of the cell, which then fuses with primary or secondary lysosomes and by a mechanism which is not yet defined, often may have double membrane. They are seen most often after several different forms of sublethal injury or during periods of starvation. However, autophagy is seen in many normal cells and is most probably a normally occurring physiological process for dealing with aging of components of the cell (Ericsson and Trump, 1964).

The eventual fate of the secondary lysosome, the residual body, and the autophagic vacuole may vary in different cells. The most widely held view is that all these vacuoles, through a process of continued fusion, intralysosomal digestion, and dehydration, eventually become compact residual bodies. Thus, no "defecation" or exocytosis of indigestible substances sequestered in lysosomes of macrophages or of lysosomal proteins could be detected (Cohn and Benson, 1965). Such exocytosis from lysosomes would be an important mechanism for the participation of the contents of lysosomes in the inflammatory response. Exocytosis of either intact granules or of their contents may perhaps be limited to specialized cell types. Thus, it is now evident that contents of lysosomes can be released during phagocytosis without prior cell death (Weissmann et al., 1971b; Henson, 1971). Additionally, extracellular secretion of lysosomal enzymes from cartilaginous limb bone rudiments has been reported on addition of complement-sufficient antibody prepared against lysosomes, but apparently acting via an effect on the plasma membrane (Dingle et al., 1967; Dingle, 1969). Similar effects have also been found in HeLa cells (Güttler, 1971). Secretion of lysosomal enzymes without concomitant release of cytoplasmic enzymes has also been reported in the adrenal medulla after stimulation by carbamycholine (Schneider, 1968). Electron micrographs of apparently intact residual and autophagic granules in extracellular spaces have been published both in normal kidney tissue (Mausbach, 1966) and in liver after toxin (Kerr, 1970).

In all the above transformations, lysosomes are essentially acting as a primitive digestive system similar to that found in amoebae. As such, they are the means by which a cell deals with foreign material present in the external environment, sequestering it and altering or presumably degrading such matter completely to small molecules capable of diffusing out of the organelle, through the lysosomal membrane into the cytoplasm. It has even been suggested that such uptake serves as a major pathway for providing normal metabolites necessary for cellular maintenance (Chapman-Andresen and Holter, 1964).

Just as the digestive system of higher organisms is interrelated with more highly specialized organs, so the lysosomal system is related to other granules of the cell. The most obvious example of this interrelationship is provided by the predominant cell type of acute inflammation, the polymorphonuclear leukocyte (PMN). It was believed for some time that all the visible granules of the PMN were lysosomes. It is now clear that there are at least two different types of granules, the azurophilic granule containing classic lysosomal proteins, as well as peroxidase and cationic proteins, and the other, or specific granule, containing alkaline phosphatase. Although they are formed at different times during differentiation of the cell and from different faces of the Golgi apparatus, the two granule populations both appear to share one protein, lysozyme. Additionally, the acid hydrolase containing azurophilic granule contains an enzyme activity (peroxidase) normally sequestered, in other tissues, in a separate form of granule, the peroxisome. Both forms of granule empty into the phagocytic vacuole, and thus their contents become combined in a single vesicle (Bainton and Farquhar, 1966; Wetzel et al., 1967; Baggiolini et al., 1969; Zeya and Spitznagel, 1969). These events, as well as the interrelationships of other granules such as the eosinophiles, will be dealt with in greater detail in later chapters. In addition, classic lysosomal granules fuse with secretory vacuoles in many endocrine glands and play a role in the processing and secretion of specific hormones. It has been proposed that lysosomes comprise one portion of a vacuolar system which is common to all cell types (de Duve and Wattiaux, 1966). The vacuolar system also includes such specialized organelles as secretory vacuoles of the exocrine and endocrine glands, certain granules of the eosinophiles, as well as the classic hydrolase-containing digestive lysosomes. It is, therefore, not surprising that functions in addition to simple intracellular digestion of unwanted materials have been proposed for the lysosome, nor that lysosomes should contain substances other than hydrolytic enzymes.

III. Structure and Contents of Lysosomes

A. Membrane

The factors which control fusion of the membranes of the vacuolar system during these transitions from one form of lysosome to another are poorly understood. Knowledge of the properties and structure of the limiting membrane should explain the manner in which, and the mechanism for, the fusion of lysosomal membranes. Currently membranes are conceived of as being composed of 40% lipids (primarily phospholipid and cholesterol) arranged in a lamellar bilayer with the polar groups of the lipids oriented to the water surfaces (Danielli and Davson; 1934–1937, Singer and Nicolson, 1972; Bretscher, 1973). There is some evidence that the phospholipids are not randomly arranged in the bilayer but that they differ in composition in the inner cytoplasmic layer as compared with the outer layer. The protein components can be thought of as in solution within this lipid bilayer. Some protein molecules extend across the bilayer with portions protruding both extra- and intracellularly. Other proteins, such as many glycoproteins, extend primarily into the extracellular space. In addition, proteins may be limited to the intramembranous or extend only into the intracellular portion of the bilayer. The proteins appear to be freely movable laterally within this bilayer. It can be visualized that interaction between two proteins on neighboring membranes could lead to their clustering together, as is seen during the phenomenon of lymphocyte "capping." This local alteration in lipid protein interactions could possibly play a role in the multiple membrane fusions of lysosomes.

1. Lipid

It may be suspected that analysis of the lipid content of lysosomes as compared with that of other organelles should reflect differences in membrane structure, since it has been found that almost all the lipid of lysosomes (Sawant et al., 1964) and mitochondria is associated with the membranes. However, in preliminary studies, analysis of these lipids has until now not consistently demonstrated any major qualitative differences. Comparison of the lipids of mitochondria, microsomes, and lysosomes revealed that the major components were qualitatively similar in all (Tappel, 1969), consisting of sphingomyelin, lecithin, cephalin, neutral triglycerides, and cholesterol. The phospholipids have been further investigated and no qualitative differences between lysosomal and plasma membranes have been found in those phospholipids (Thines-Sempoux, 1967; Dingle, 1968), which are known to affect the properties of artificial lipid membranes (Sessa and Weissmann, 1968). Also, no major differences have been found in the fatty acid composition (Wynn *et al.*, 1967). However, the difficulties inherent in obtaining a very pure lysosomal membrane fraction suggest that a quantitative difference or differences in a minor but crucial constituent might easily be overlooked. Data would suggest that lysosomal membranes might contain considerably more sterol than do mitochondrial membranes. It is clear that plasma membranes differ significantly in lipid composition from mitochondrial membranes and from "smooth internal membranes," having a greatly increased cholesterol to phospholipid ration and containing more sphingomyelin and less cardiolipin than does the mitochondrial membrane (Weinstein *et al.*, 1969; Coleman and Finean, 1966; Bosmann *et al.*, 1968; Dodd and Gray, 1968; Korn, 1966). Addition of several agents have demonstrated a different response (Weissmann, 1969) of mitochondrial, lysosomal, and plasma membranes, presumably dependent on a difference in lipid composition (Iqbal *et al.*, 1969). Differential responses of portions of the vacuolar system might well be important for determining differential responses to exogenous material.

2. PROTEIN

The antigenic properties of the extrinsic proteins of the membrane and their attached carbohydrate and lipid side chains, as well as any immunogenic carbohydrate and lipid, have been examined by Trouet (1964, 1968). He has determined the antigenic properties of the lysosomal membrane and has shown that they share common antigens with the plasma membrane and the microsomal membrane. Additionally, lysosomal membranes contain antigens not present on microsomal membrane but do not contain some antigens present on plasma membranes. This could be interpreted either as addition of immunogenic groups to a basic structure or to actual differences in structural macromolecules. It is well established that enzymes capable of adding carbohydrate groups to molecules are present in the Golgi apparatus (Wagner and Cymkin, 1971), thus providing a means for addition of groups known to be capable of conferring antigenic specificity. In addition, some of these antigens may well represent enzyme protein with specific membrane localization, such as ATPase (Emmelot *et al.*, 1964) or adenyl cyclase (Robison *et al.*, 1968). Naturally occurring antibodies to specific organelles have been described in disease states, as well as in experimental situations, again suggesting that there are indeed compositional differences of a type capable of eliciting specific antibodies. Although it is interesting to speculate as to the possible pathogenetic importance of these antibodies in various diseases, they may well represent a secondary response to the existence of partially destroyed cellular components in the circulation (McKay, 1966; Waksman, 1966).

Under normal circumstances, the immune system is tolerant to self, and the existence of these autoantibodies (Dameshek, 1965) has been considered to represent an aberration of the immune response. However, injection of subcellular fractions into genetically homologous experimental animals is known to result in production of antibodies. In this case presumably, alteration of the organelles has occurred, so that new antigenic specificities have developed. These experiments suggest that lysosomal enzymes acting on membranes within autophagic vacuoles or in the fluid of an inflammatory exudate can result in partial digestion of macromolecules, thus altering their antigenic properties, either exposing previously hidden embryonic antigens or giving rise to new antigens (Weissmann, 1966). In support of this concept, lymphocytes from patients with lupus erythematosis respond more vigorously to denatured DNA than to native DNA (Patrucco et al., 1967).

B. Enzymatic Contents

Enzymes capable of degrading all the classes of macromolecules which are found in mammalian tissues have been described within lysosomes. These include over 60 enzyme activities, as well as several biologically active, nonenzymatic substances. However, the evidence for the coexistence of even more than two enzymes in the same vesicle is not extensive, and it is very likely that not all the enzymes are present in every lysosome in every cell. Additionally, the contents of secondary lysosomes, as well as auto-phagic vacuoles and residual bodies, may be different from those of newly formed lysosomes. Therefore, all enzyme localizations discussed apply to the generalized, idealized lysosome.

Classicly, the list of contents of lysosomes has been developed by first isolating a lysosome-rich subcellular fraction (variously referred to as "light mitochondrial" or "large granule") and then determining if a specific enzyme activity is concentrated in that fraction and exhibits the property of latency. Similar criteria have been applied to localize other molecules to lysosomes. Some enzyme activities, as well as metals, can also be identified histochemically and electron microscopically and thus by localized to single membrane-bounded bodies, preferably to those containing a previously identified lysosomal enzyme (Goldfischer et al., 1970b; Schnitka and Seligman, 1971). Although this has been an extremely productive approach, it is not without its pitfalls. For example, most enzyme activities exist as multiple molecular forms or isozymes (Harris, 1969). These isozymes may have similar or different subcellular localizations, e.g., aryl sulfatase A and B, which are lysosomal, as opposed to aryl sulfatase C (Roy, 1960). It is now clear that many enzyme activities optimally active at acid pH and found in the lysosome are also present in other areas of the cell (Fishman et al., 1969;

Ide and Fishman, 1969). In some cases it would appear probable that macromolecules displaying the same enzyme activity are very different in structure (Patel and Tappel, 1969, 1970), while in some cases, as for α-glucosidase, the same molecule may have two or more apparently different activities (Jeffrey et al., 1970; Bruni, 1970). Since proteins are synthesized primarily in the endoplasmic reticulum, it is not surprising to detect the presence of many "lysosomal" enzyme activities in this fraction. Additionally, isozymes may be generated by the attachment of carbohydrate side groups such as N-acetyl neuraminic acid to a core protein molecule. Data suggest that as enzymes progress through the endoplasmic reticulum and Golgi to vacuoles, they acquire such carbohydrate groups (Peters et al., 1971; Heath, 1971). By this mechanism, enzymes with the same amino acid sequence could exist in two apparently different molecular forms with two different subcellular localizations. There is some evidence to suggest that this occurs with lysosomal enzymes (Goldstone and Koenig, 1971). Another group of difficulties in assigning subcellular localizations is essentially due to artifact. For example, during separative procedures, proteins may be differentially adsorbed onto subcellular components other than those in which they are normally found in the intact cell (Tartakoff et al., 1971). In addition, substances present within lysosomes may have entered via the route of endocytosis and represent materials either present in the external milieu or in their breakdown products. All these considerations apply as well to molecules other than enzymes and must be taken into account before attributing an effect to enzymes of lysosomes.

An exhaustive survey of the contents of lysosomes is beyond the scope of this chapter. The enzymic contents have been reviewed by Barrett (1969) and Tappel (1969), and the biologically active substances will be considered in detail in chapters dealing with white cells and mediators of inflammation. Table I lists some of the enzyme activities and contents which have been described. However, in order to develop some idea as to the nature and functioning of the enzyme content of lysosomes, it would be informative to examine one of these classes of enzymes in some detail. The group of enzymes which might well play a role in the inflammatory process are those capable of degrading structural proteins or enzymatically activating protein mediators of inflammation.

1. PROTEIN DEGRADATION

Information concerning this group of proteolytic enzymes has been developed in several ways. As discussed previously, the capacity of lysosome-rich subcellular fractions to hydrolyse denatured proteins, such as hemoglobin (Anson, 1939), and artificial substrates has been examined, and the presence of enzymes inferred by correlating their properties with those of

TABLE I[a]

DEGRADATIVE ENZYME ACTIVITIES FOUND IN LYSOSOMES

A. Enzymes acting on proteins and peptides

Cathepsin D
- Cathepsin E
Histonase
Neutral proteinase
Cathepsin A
Cathepsin B and B[1]
Cathepsin C
Arylamidase
Dipeptidase (tyrosyl glycine)
Collagenase
Elastase
Kininogen activator
Plasminogen activator
Renin
Chemotactic factor generating protease
β-Asparytl glucosylamine amido hydrolase
O-Seryl-N acetyl galactosaminide glycosidase

B. Enzymes acting on lipids

Acid lipase
Phospholipase A_1
Phospholipase A_2
Cholesterol esterase
Organophosphate resistant esterase
Spingomyelinase
Glucocerebrosidase
Galactocerebrosidase

C. Enzymes acting on carbohydrates

Lysozyme
Neuraminidase
α-Glucosidase
β-Glucosidase
α-Galactosidase
β-Galactosidase
α-Mannosidase
α-Acetyl glucosaminidase
α-Acetyl galactosaminidase
β-Acetyl galactosaminidase
β-Glucuronidase
β-Xylosidase
α-L-Fucosidase
β-D-Fucosidase
Sucrase
Hyaluronidase

TABLE I*a* (continued)

DEGRODATIVE ENZYME ACTIVITIES FOUND IN LYSOSOMES

D. Enzymes acting on nucleic acids

Acid ribonuclease
Acid deoxyribonuclease

E. Miscellaneous enzymes

Aryl sulfatase
Acid phosphatase(s)
Phosphodiesterase(s)
Phosphoprotein phosphatase

---

*a*Adapted from Barrett (1969) and Tappel (1969).

previously purified enzymes. In relatively few cases, enzymes have actually been purified from lysosomal fractions (Barrett, 1969). Secondly, the effect of lysosomal contents, either as isolated from tissues (Coffey and de Duve, 1968) or as partially reconstituted from purified components (Goettlich-Riemann et al., 1971) on substrates, has been determined. Lastly, the fate of proteins including some identifiable by electron microscopy has been observed either after injection into the whole animal (Strauss, 1964) or *in vitro* (Ehrenreich and Cohn, 1967, 1968). Until now, no proteolytic enzyme activity has been localized to lysosomes by the finding of an inherited storage disease, as has been the case for some of the other classes of enzymes (O'Brien, 1972).

It has been found that proteins are hydrolyzed to dipeptides and amino acids by the contents of lysosomes (Coffey and de Duve, 1968). Ingestion of labeled protein by intact cells with segregation in lysosomes has been followed by the rapid degradation of almost 90 % of the protein and the appearance of labeled amino acids in the surrounding fluid (Ehrenreich and Cohn, 1967). Several enzymes capable of bringing this about have been described including one of the first enzymes localized to lysosomes, Cathepsin D. Cathepsin D appears to be capable of hydrolysing many different peptide bonds in the β chain of insulin (Woessner and Shamberger, 1971), as well as in its classic substrate, hemoglobin (Anson, 1939). However, it does not have a generalized nonspecific affinity for all proteins, as indicated by its slow rate of attack on albumin (Barrett, 1970). Another major endopeptidase, Cathepsin E (Lapresle and Webb, 1962), has been localized to lysosomes and is capable of digesting albumin relatively rapidly. Other acid proteases or cathepsins, labeled A, B, and C, which attack either the ends of proteins or peptides, have also been localized to lysosomes. Cathepsin A (Iodice et al., 1966; Coffey and de Duve, 1968) appears to act as a carboxypeptidase and has been shown to be capable of degrading glucagon sequentially from the carboxyl terminus of the chain (Iodice, 1967). Cathepsin B (Keliova *et al.*, 1968; Bouma and Gruber, 1966) appears to consist of two thiol-dependent endopeptidases capable of hydrolyzing gelatin, but has classicly been determined by the hydrolysis of a synthetic substrate, benzoyl L arginine amide, which is also attacked by trypsin. The last of the classic acid proteases is Cathepsin C, also a thiol-dependent enzyme, which apparently has little or no effect on the usual proteins used in similar assays, but appears to be capable of transferring terminal dipeptides, as well as hydrolyzing glycyl-L-phenylalanine amide (Metrione *et al.*, 1966).

Enzymes capable of splitting off the carboxyl terminal group from a di- or tripeptide (Jablonski and McQuillan, 1967), as well as a dipeptidase, (Tappel *et al.*, 1967), have also been described in lysosomes. However, most of the dipeptidase activity of liver cell homogenates was localized to the soluble cytoplasm (Coffey and de Duve, 1968).

In addition, a class of enzymes known as arylamidases, or enzymes causing hydrolysis of amino acids from napthylamide, have been reported to be lysosomal (Mahadevan and Tappel, 1967a) and may utilize protein or peptides as natural substrates.

Proteases active at neutral as well as acid pH have also been reported to exist in lysosomes. For example, a neutral protease active on hemoglobin (Janoff and Zeligs, 1968) as well as one active on histone (Davies *et al.*, 1971) have also been found in lysosomes of white blood cells.

In addition, enzymes capable of degrading other specific protein components of connective tissues have been described. An apparently true collagenase active on undenatured collagen was found in rat bone lysosomes (Woods and Nichols, 1965). Lysosomal collagenase has been further identified in other tissues (Wynn *et al.*, 1967) and in granules of the white blood cell (Lazarus *et al.*, 1968a,b). This collagenase does not completely degrade native collagen but breaks it down into two large fragments as seen on acrylamide gel electrophoresis.

An enzyme capable of degrading elastin both in its native form and as an artificial substrate has been described in PMN's and will be discussed more extensively (Janoff and Scherer, 1968). Although the enzyme or combination of enzymes have not been isolated, electron micrographs suggest that macrophage lysosomes can degrade ingested amyloid (Shirahama and Cohen, 1971).

Some of these enzymes have been shown to act synergistically in the hydrolysis of proteins (Goettlich-Riemann *et al.*, 1971). The concerted action of the several enzymes described above could in theory account for the complete degradation of proteins within lysosomes, and apparently massive amounts of hemoglobin can be completely cleared and degraded by liver lysosomes in the intact animal (Goldfischer *et al.*, 1970a). When denatured γ-globulin was incubated for prolonged periods of time *in vitro* with extracts of lysosomes, the degradation of 70% of the protein occurred, as compared with that brought about by acid hydrolysis. Approximately one-half of the available amino acids were released plus small peptides, primarily as dipeptides. However, proteins not previously denatured showed differential susceptibilities to *in vitro* hydrolysis by lysosomal enzymes. It was suggested that this was dependent on whether the protein was susceptible to acid denaturation (Coffey and de Duve, 1968). Similar experiments with shorter periods of incubation have also shown a differential susceptibility of various proteins to *in vitro* hydrolysis by lysosomal enzymes. Ryan and Lee (1970) have shown that the rate of hydrolysis of proteins by lysosomal enzymes appears to correlate with the antigenicity of the protein used. Thus, tetanus toxin and keyhole limpet hemocyanin, two good immunogens, were almost totally undegraded under conditions where hemoglobin and insulin, both poor immunogens, were almost totally hydrolyzed. Bovine serum albumin and γ-globulin were intermediate in susceptibility to attack. Further investigation of the substrate specificities of lysosomal enzymes individually and in concert utilizing natural molecules is needed.

Evidence for limited proteolysis by lysosomal enzymes is provided by the finding of enzymes with very specific actions on specific proteins. Thus lysosomal localization has been found for an enzyme with an alkaline pH optima which is capable of converting serum plasminogen to plasmin, that is, a plasminogen activator (Ali and Evans, 1968). Lysosomal localization has also been reported for a tissue kininogen activator (Carvalho and Diniz, 1966) or of an enzyme, again with an alkaline pH optimum, capable of liberating free bradykinin from precursors. The alkaline pH optima of these last two enzymes suggests that separation by the more discriminatory technique of zonal ultracentrifugation might reveal that they are localized in a specialized granule similar to the specific granules of polymorphonuclear leukocytes. A lysosomal kininogen activator active at neutral or acid pH has been described in human PMN's (Melmon and Cline, 1967) and rabbit PMN's (Greenbaum and Kim, 1967).

A neutral protease has also been localized to rabbit PMN lysosomes which can split the fifth component of human complement (C5) into fragments which are active in inducing chemotaxis (Ward and Hill, 1970). Release of such a protease either following phagocytosis or with cell death would lead to the self-perpetuation of the inflammatory exudate. (See Volume II, Chapter 7.) A neutral protease has also been found in tissue extracts which cleaves C3 into chemotactically active products (Hill and Ward, 1969). This might well be lysosomal and would provide a means for triggering the emigration of PMN's into an area of acute tissue injury such as that brought about any mechanical or thermal means.

2. Lipid Degradation

Other degradative activities potentially important for tissue injury and inflammation are those by which the lipid components of biomembranes might presumably be damaged. Isolated lysosomes can hydrolyse lipids extensively under different conditions. For example, various classes of neutral lipids and phospholipids were degraded on incubation with lysosome-rich subcellular fractions from liver (Fowler and de Duve, 1969). Lysosomes of kidney, liver, and PMN's have been found to contain specific lipolytic activities classified as acid and neutral lipases, as well as phospholipases A1 and A2 (Elsbach and Rizack, 1963; Mellors and Tappel, 1967; Mahadevan and Tappel, 1968; Stoffel and Greten, 1967; Hayase and Tappel, 1970; Elsbach and Kayden, 1965). The action of a phospholipase on lecithin (phosphatidyl choline) either by removing the first acyl fatty acid chain (phospholipase A1) or the second (phospholipase A2) results in the generation of lysolecithin. Lysolecithin has the capacity to rapidly disrupt biomembranes, as well as to cause cell fusion with formation of multinuclear cells (Lucy, 1970). It has been reported that significant amounts of lysolecithin are generated during intralysosomal digestion of lipids (Fowler and de Duve, 1969). However, other studies could not detect generation of any appreciable amounts of lysolecithin from lecithin by highly purified fractions of lysosomes, and it was felt that only a single phospholipase which removed both chains simultaneously was present (Mellors and Tappel, 1967). However, a phospholipase A2, active at neutral pH, has been reported to be associated with the membrane of the lysosome (Rahman and Verhagen, 1970). Attachment of this enzyme to phospholipids present on the plasma membrane or to other phospholipid-rich internal membranes could result in hydrolysis with subsequent membrane fusions and/or extracellular lysosomal enzyme release. The same mechanism could account for damage to target cell membranes by lysosomal enzymes released into an exudate.

3. Carbohydrate Degradation

The cell membrane also contains many glycoproteins, alteration in which can cause changes in permeability, electrostatic charge, and antigenic characteristics (Cook, 1968). Additionally, glycosaminoglycans form an essential component of connective tissue. When glycoproteins were incubated *in vitro* with purified lysosomal extracts, the protein moiety was rapidly degraded and sialic acid removed, but there was a relatively slow rate of attack on the other carbohydrate linkages (Aronson and de Duve, 1968). However, in addition to neuraminidase (Horvat and Touster, 1968; Tulsiani and Carubelli, 1970), specific enzyme activities capable of attacking numerous sugar linkages have been demonstrated within lysosomes (Barrett,

1969). These are apparently biologically significant, since the genetic absence of any or several of these enzymes is associated with specific storage diseases (O'Brien, 1972; Hirschhorn and Weissmann, 1967). In addition to enzymes for various carbohydrate linkages, enzyme activities have been reported in lysosomes which hydrolyse two of the most common linkages between carbohydrate and polypeptides in glycoproteins. Thus an aspartyl glucosylamine amidase (Mahadevan and Tappel, 1967b) and an enzyme hydrolyzing the link between serine and N-acetyl galactosamine (Tappel, 1969) have been found in lysosomes. Enzymes for the degradation of various glycosaminoglycans have also been described in lysosomes (Hutterer, 1966; Aronson and Davidson, 1967). Lysozyme, which hydrolyzes a polysaccharide component of the cell wall of certain bacteria, has also been localized to lysosomes, including those of the monocyte and PMN.

Lysosomal extracts can also degrade nucleic acids from various sources (Arsenis et al., 1970) and have been demonstrated to contain several specific enzymes capable of this activity, such as acid RNase and acid DNase (Hunter and Korner, 1968; Van Dyck and Wattiaux, 1968). Interestingly, the double-stranded RNA of the reovirus appears to be resistant to hydrolysis within lysosomes (Silverstein and Dales, 1968) and again suggests substrate-dependent specificity of lysosomal enzymes.

Other enzyme activities in lysosomes are capable of hydrolyzing phosphate and sulfate bonds. These include various acid phosphatases (Barrett, 1969) and aryl sulfatase A and B (Roy, 1960).

C. Nonenzymatic Contents

Several nonenzymatic substances have been localized to polymorphonuclear leukocytes or to their granules and are therefore presumably lysosomal. Some of these substances, which have obvious potential significance for the inflammatory process, will be considered in detail in a later chapter. In brief, PMN granules contain cationic proteins which can cause degranulation of mast cells, increase vascular permeability, and are capable of killing bacteria (Janoff and Zweifach, 1964; Janoff et al., 1965; Zeya and Spitznagel, 1963, 1966; Movat et al., 1964, 1971; Ranadive and Cochrane, 1967; Cochrane, 1968). Additionally, endogenous pyrogen has also been localized to PMN's (Atkins and Bodel, 1971). A chemotactic factor is also present within PMN's but may well be extralysosomal (Borel et al., 1969).

Lysosomes also appear to contain acid mucopolysaccharides (Olsson and Gardell, 1969). It has also been postulated that lysosomes contain a relatively solid, highly anionic matrix in which the cationic enzymes are maintained in an inactive form by electrostatic bonds (Koenig, 1969).

This presumably would account for the fact that lysosomal proteases do not appear to degrade other lysosomal proteins *in situ*.

Metallic ions, including iron (Kent *et al.*, 1965) and copper (Goldfischer and Moskal, 1966) have also been found to be concentrated within lysosomes.

V. Morphology

From the previous discussion, it is clear the lysosomes are a morphologically heterogeneous population. Although all are organelles sharing the property of being limited by a single membrane, they cannot definitively be identified on the basis of fine structure alone. Even this broad definition does not always hold true, since autophagic vacuoles are often bounded by double membranes. By light microscopy, lysosomes are perhaps best identified by utilizing histochemical markers. However, they can be tentatively identified under phase microscopy as phase dense granules (Cohn, 1968), as well as by vital staining (Allison and Young, 1969). Thus, several dyes, including acridine orange, trypan blue, and neutral red appear to be selectively concentrated within lysosomes. Of these, trypan blue can also be visualized with the electron microscope (Trump, 1961).

Lysosomal enzymes which can be demonstrated histochemically include acid phosphatase (Novikoff, 1963), aryl sulfatase (Goldfischer, 1965), β-glucuronidase (Hayashi *et al.*, 1968), acid lipase (Lake, 1971), and *N*-acetyl β-glucosaminidase (Hayashi, 1967). As with biochemical procedures, the existence of isozymes with different localizations must be considered.

Lysosomes have also been identified morphologically following the fusion of endocytic vacuole-containing specific substances with primary lysosomes. Horseradish peroxidase (Strauss, 1967), fluorescein conjugated proteins (Cohn and Benson, 1965), radioactively labeled proteins, ferritin, latex particles, as well as various colloidal particles such as gold, have been used (Daems *et al.*, 1969). In phagocytic cells, bacteria, zymosan, virus, etc., also have served to mark the vacuolar system.

IV. Functions of Lysosomes

A. General

The lysosomal system functions in several ways. First and most clearly, lysosomes provide a means whereby cells digest compounds ingested from their external environment. The role this plays in the economy of the whole organism depends on the cell type and ranges from the ingestion and destruction of potentially harmful bacteria by phagocytes to the sequestration of other potentially harmful molecules to a mechanism for providing simple molecules for energy metabolism and/or synthesis of new types of macromolecules. Secondly, the lysosomal system provides one means for regulating the turnover and destruction of intracellular components without total cell destruction. This ranges from the sequestration and destruction or autophagy of apparently damaged intracellular components following sublethal injury to the physiological sequestration within vacuoles and subsequent breakdown of glycogen in liver following administration of glucagon or the intracellular destruction of secretory hormones in response to various stimuli (Ericsson, 1969; Farquhar, 1969). Lysosomes have been postulated to function in several other physiological and pathological processes, and evidence has been provided for some of these. These include the capacitation of sperm (Dott and Dingle, 1968), bone resorption response to parathyroid hormone (Vaes, 1968), metamorphosis (Weber, 1969), teratogenesis (Lloyd and Beck, 1969), and carcinogenesis, as well as the inflammatory process.

B. As a Mediator of Inflammation

Lysosomes have been shown to contain enzyme activities theoretically capable of completely destroying all the components of cells and their organelles, as well as the intercellular matrix. Incubation of various parts of cells and tissue such as mitochondria, nuclei, or basement membrane with lysosomes results in their degradation. In addition, lysosomes of at least some tissues contain either compounds capable of propagating an inflammatory response or enzymes capable of activating precursors of such compounds. Therefore, it seems clear that lysosomes and their contents obviously might play a role in the inflammatory response, whether it be as an initiating agent or only to propagate it.

There are essentially three major ways in which lysosomal enzymes and contents have been observed to escape from their normal sequestration within the vacuolar system of the cell and thus be capable of causing tissue injury and propagating inflammation.

First, primary lysis of cells may occur with subsequent liberation of enzymes. Thus, agents, which disrupt the integrity of the cell membrane such as lysolecithin, interfere with major metabolic pathways for energy or for the synthesis of essential components of the cell and will lead to cell disruption with eventual release of lysosomal enzymes.

Second, agents may act directly on lysosomal membranes, resulting in leakage of enzymes and contents into the cytoplasm with subsequent cell death and leakage of enzymes into the intercellular space. Allison *et al.* (1966b) has provided evidence that selective intracellular rupture of lysosomes can lead to cellular death. Thus activation, by light, of the dye neutral red after it had been concentrated within lysosomes was followed by apparent rupture of lysosomal membranes with leakage of enzyme into the cytoplasm and cell death. Phagocytosis of isolated heterologous lysosomes by rabbit PMN's was followed by rapid degranulation and apparent cell death, whereas ingestion of latex particles did not cause damage over the same length of time (Hirschhorn and Weissmann, 1967). Phagocytosis of silica has also been shown to result in dissolution of the lysosomal membrane with the same consequences of enzyme leakage into the cytoplasm followed by cell death (Allison *et al.*, 1966a). These findings have also been confirmed by Nadler and Goldfischer (1970) utilizing horseradish peroxidase to tag the lysosome and its contents. Evidence for a similar series of events following the uptake of monosodium urate crystals has been provided (Phelps and McCarty, 1966; Wallingford and McCarty, 1971; Weissmann *et al.*, 1971b). In both of these situations, phagocytosis of other compounds did not result in such damage.

Additionally, correlative evidence has also suggested that lysosomes are important in the inflammatory process. Thus, several compounds have been found to have differential effects on the stability of lysosomal membranes, acting either as "stabilizing" or "labilizing" agents. Agents such as glucocorticoid which stabilizes the membrane are also antiinflammatory. Conversely, many agents, such as streptolysin S, which disrupt lysosomes *in vitro*, also can produce an acute or chronic inflammatory reaction after injection (Weissmann, 1969).

Third, enzymes could be released without concomitant cell death. Thus there is extensive evidence for the release of lysosomal enzymes from macrophages during phagocytosis of particulate matter such as immune complexes, bacteria, or zymosan. In some of these studies, the absence of cell death has been determined by monitoring the absence of release of a suitable enzyme of the cell sap (Movat *et al.*, 1964; Tew *et al.*, 1969; Parish, 1969; Henson, 1971; Weissmann *et al.*, 1971b).

Extrusion or secretion of lysosomal enzymes, without preceding cell damage, can also occur as part of a phenomena termed "frustrated phagocytosis" (Henson, 1971). When PMN's are incubated with immune complexes coated onto millipore membranes, the cells attempt to phagocytose such complexes, as they normally would do. Although the white blood cells can no longer engulf these attached complexes, the cells still secrete lysosomal hydrolases as if they had actually ingested the immune complex. Secretion of lysosomal enzymes is not limited to the wandering phagocyte, since it has been reported to occur in bone (Vaes, 1968), adrenal medulla (Schneider, 1968), and cartilage (Dingle, 1969).

The inflammation of joints, or arthritis, has been investigated most extensively as a possible prototype for the involvement of lysosomes in the inflammatory response. The initial data which led to these investigations, as well as the experimental evidence which has been collected to support such a role, has been reviewed in great detail by several authors (Weissmann, 1966, 1967; Lack, 1969). In brief, several of the mechanisms for lysosomal enzyme release discussed previously have been described in the different forms of arthritis. Thus, in gout, after ingestion of crystalline monosodium urate by phagocytes, the crystal interacts with the membrane of the phagosomes, releasing lysosomal enzymes into the cytoplasm and eventually into the joint (Phelps and McCarty, 1966; Wallingford and McCarty, 1971; Weissmann *et al.*, 1971a). Although there is extensive evidence that this series of events does indeed occur, the observation that high levels of uric acid seen in secondary hyperuricemia are often unaccompanied by gouty arthritis indicates that other factors, such as genetic and endocrine, must also be operative.

Additionally, release of lysosomal enzymes might well occur at sites of the membrane-associated antigen–antibody complexes seen in such conditions as vasculitis, nephritis, and systemic lupus erythematosis. This release would represent the *in vivo* equivalent of the *in vitro* "frustrated phagocytosis" phenomenon.

Many of these release phenomena, involving active bulk translocation of enzymes out of the cell, can be modified *in vitro* by the addition of several classes of compounds. These include cyclic nucleotides and specifically cyclic AMP and cyclic GMP; compounds which alter intracellular levels of cyclic AMP; such as some of the prostaglandins (e.g., PGE_1); as well as compounds such as cytochalasin and colchicine, which affect the musculoskeletal system of the cell or, respectively, the microfilaments and microtubules (Weissmann *et al.*, 1971b,c, 1972; Bensch and Malawista, 1969).

It is not clear if these several agents all work along the same pathway. However, one can postulate that attachment of a particle at the cell membrane results in alteration in the intracellular level of cyclic nucleotides, which would result in activation of several protein kinases. Such a series of events has been documented in several tissues where cyclic AMP acts as a "second messenger" following attachment of polypeptide hormones to receptor sites (Robison *et al.*, 1968). Phosphorylation of microfilaments and microtubular proteins by such protein kinases would then alter the contractility of these proteins, thus affecting phagocytosis-associated hydrolytic enzyme release. Many of these agents demonstrate a biphasic effect, whereby they stimulate the phenomena being observed at one concentration and inhibit the same phenomena at other concentrations. Thus the enzyme-release phenomena while initially propogating and locally amplifying an inflammatory response could be terminated by the same mechanism which initially started it. This may well be the explanation for some of the data demonstrating both an antiinflammatory and inflammatory effect of prostaglandin E_1 or the protective effect upon lysosomes of serum from rats with adjuvant arthritis (Zurier and Quagliata, 1971; Persellin, 1972; Kaley and Weiner, 1971). Indeed, as suggested by Ramsey and Grant (Chapter 5) and as will be discussed further in Chapter 5, this would provide a very economical control mechanism whereby the generation of an inflammatory response could carry within itself the means for self-limitation.

In other forms of arthritis, such as rheumatoid arthritis, there is evidence for the involvement of lysosomes of lymphocytes and of the synovial cell itself, as well as those of PMN's. In brief, there is a marked increase in lysosomal contents of synovial cells (Barland et al., 1964). Second, phagocytosis of complexes of rheumatoid factors and IgG with release of lysosomal enzymes has been reported (Astorga and Bollet, 1965). Third, several lysosomal enzymes are present in increased concentration in synovial fluid of inflamed joints. Last, injection of compounds which disrupt lysosomes in vitro, as well as of PMN granules themselves, can initiate chronic arthritis (Weissmann, 1967; Weissmann et al., 1965, 1967; Weissmann and Spilberg, 1968).

Although the PMN leukocyte with its pominent granules containing "cytases" is an obvious candidate for bringing about destruction of tissue, another cell type, the lymphocyte, has also been shown to be a "killer" cell. Thus the small lymphocyte is an effector cell in graft-versus-host reactions in vivo. Lymphocytes on stimulation in vitro by a variety of agents can bring about the destruction of a variety of target cells. During the process of lymphocyte stimulation, there is elaboration and secretion into the surrounding media of cytotoxic factors together with a number of other "mediators." These include a factor which inhibits the migration of macrophages, as well as two chemotactic factors and factors causing increased cell division (Bloom and Glade, 1971). Although these have been considered to be mediators of cellular immunity because their appearance is often dependent on immunological reactions, they may equally well be considered mediators of inflammation.

During the process of lymphocyte stimulation, when these products appear, labilization of lysosomal enzymes as well as a marked increase in lysosomes and their contents has been demonstrated (Hirschhorn et al., 1968, 1967, 1965). It is therefore quite possible that the factors synthesized and released by the activated lymphocytes are originally contained within their lysosomes. The observation that, following the stimulus of phagocytosis, the polymorphonuclear leukocyte secretes enzymes contained within vacuoles (Henson, 1971) and synthesizes additional ones (Axline and Cohn, 1970) may be due to similar mechanisms.

It is quite clear from what has been said in this chapter that the lysosome and its multipotential contents are a prime candidate for the physiological mediator of the inflammatory process and its pathological results.

References

Ali, S. Y., and Evans, L. (1968). *Biochem. J.* **107**, 293.

Allison, A. C., and Young, M. R. (1969). *In* "Lysosomes in Biology and Pathology" (J. T. Dingle and H. B. Fell, eds.), Vol. 2, pp. 600–628. North-Holland Publ., Amsterdam.

Allison, A. C., Harrington, J. S., and Birbeck, M. (1966a). *J. Exp. Med.* **124**, 141.

Allison, A. C., Magnus, I. A., and Young, M. R. (1966b). *Nature (London)* **209**, 874.

Anson, M. L. (1939). *J. Gen. Physiol.* **23**, 695.

Appelmans, F., Wattiaux, R., and de Duve, C. (1955). *Biochem. J.* **59**, 438.

Aronson, N. N., and Davidson, E. A. (1967). *J. Biol. Chem.* **242**, 437.

Aronson, N. N., Jr., and de Duve, C. (1968). *J. Biol. Chem.* **243**, 4564.

Arsenis, C., Gordon, J. S., and Touster, O. (1970). *J. Biol. Chem.* **245**, 205.

Astorga, G., and Bollet, A. J. (1965). *Arthritis Rheum.* **8**, 511.

Atkins, E., and Bodel, P. (1971). *Pyrogens Fever, Ciba Found. Syrup.* p. 81.

Axline, S. G., and Cohn, Z. A. (1970). *J. Exp. Med.* **131**, 1239.

Baggiolini, M., Hirsch, J. G., and de Duve, C. (1969). *J. Cell Biol.* **40**, 529.

Bainton, D. F., and Farquhar, M. G. (1966). *J. Cell Biol.* **28**, 277.

Bainton, D. F., and Farquhar, M. G. (1968). *J. Cell Biol.* **39**, 299.

Bainton, D. F., and Farquhar, M. G. (1970). *J. Cell Biol.* **45**, 54.

Barland, P., Novikoff, A. B., and Hamerman, D. (1964). *Amer. J. Pathol.* **44**, 853.

Barrett, A. J. (1969). *In* "Lysosomes in Biology and Pathology" (J. T. Dingle and H. B. Fell, eds.), Vol. 2, pp. 245–312. North-Holland Publ., Amsterdam.

Barrett, A. J. (1970). *Biochem. J.* **117**, 601.

Bensch, K. G., and Malawista, S. E. (1969). *J. Cell Biol.* **40**, 95.

Berthet, J., and de Duve, C. (1951). *Biochem. J.* **50**, 174.

Bloom, B. R., and Glade, P. R., eds. (1971). "*In Vitro* Methods in Cell-Mediated Immunity". Academic Press, New York.

Borel, J. F., Keller, H. U., and Sorkin, E. (1969). *Int. Arch. Allergy Appl. Immunol.* **35**, 194.

Bosmann, H. B., Hagopian, A., and Eylar, E. H. (1968). *Arch. Biochem. Biophys.* **128**, 51.

Bouma, J. M. W., and Gruber, M. (1966). *J. Biol. Chem.* **243**, 3757.

Brady, R. O., Johnson, B., and Uhlendorf, W. (1971). *Amer. J. Med.* **51**, 423.

Bretscher, M. S. (1973). *Science* **181**, 622.

Bruni, C. B. (1970). *Biochim. Biophys. Acta* **212**, 470.

Caro, L. G., and Palade, G. E. (1964). *J. Cell Biol.* **20**, 473.

Carvalho, I. F., and Diniz, C. R. (1966). *Biochim. Biophys. Acta* **128**, 136.

Chapman-Andresen, C. (1963). *C. R. Trav. Lab. Carlsberg* **33**, 73.

Chapman-Andresen, C. (1964). *Methods Cell Physiol.* **1**, 277.

Chapman-Andresen, C., and Holter, H. (1964). *C. R. Trav. Lab. Carlsberg* **34**, 211.

Cochrane, C. G. (1968). *Advan. Immunol.* **9**, 97.

Coffey, J. W., and de Duve, C. (1968). *J. Biol. Chem.* **243**, 3255.

Cohn, Z. A. (1968). *Advan. Immunol.* **9**, 163.

Cohn, Z. A., and Benson, B. (1965). *J. Exp. Med.* **122**, 455.

Cohn, Z. A., and Hirsch, J. G. (1960). *J. Exp. Med.* **112**, 983.

Cohn, Z. A., and Parks, E. (1967). *J. Exp. Med.* **125**, 213.

Cohn, Z. A., and Weiner, E. (1963). *J. Exp. Med.* **118**, 991.

Cohn, Z. A., Fedorko, M. E., and Hirsch, J. G. (1966). *J. Exp. Med.* **123**, 757.

Coleman, R., and Finean, J. B. (1966). *Biochim. Biophys. Acta* **125**, 197.

Conchie, J., and Levvy, G. A. (1963). *Biochem. Soc. Symp.* **23**, 86.

Cook, G. M. W. (1968). *Brit. Med. Bull.* **24**, 119–123.

Daems, W. T., Wisse, E., and Brederoo, P. (1969). *In* "Lysosomes in Biology and Pathology" (J. T. Dingle and H. B. Fell, eds.), Vol. 1, p. 65. North-Holland Publ., Amsterdam.

Dameshek, W. (1965). *Ann. N. Y. Acad. Sci.* **124**, 6.

Danielli, J. F., and Davson, H. (1934–1935). *J. Cell. Comp. Physiol.* **5**, 495.

Davies, P., Rita, G. A., Krakaver, K., and Weissmann, G. (1971). *Biochem. J.* **123**, 559.

de Duve, C. (1959). *In* "Subcellular Particles" (T. Hayashi, ed.), pp 128–159. Ronald Press, New York.

de Duve, C., and Wattiaux, R. (1966). *Physiol. Rev.* **28**, 35.

de Duve, C., Pressman, B. C., Gianetto, R., Wattiaux, R., and Appelmans, F. (1955). *Biochem. J.* **60**, 604.

Dingle, J. T. (1968). *Brit. Med. Bull.* **24**, 141.

Dingle, J. T. (1969). *In* "Lysosomes in Biology and Pathology" (J. T. Dingle and H. B. Fell, eds.), Vol. 2, pp. 421–436. North-Holland Publ., Amsterdam.

Dingle, J. T., Fell, H. B., and Coombs, R. R. A. (1967). *Int. Arch. Allergy Appl. Immunol.* **31**, 283.

Dodd, B. J., and Gray, G. M. (1968). *Biochim. Biophys. Acta* **150**, 397.

Dott, H. M., and Dingle, J. T. (1968). *Exp. Cell Res.* **58**, 523.

Ehrenreich, B. A., and Cohn, Z. A. (1967). *J. Exp. Med.* **126**, 941.

Ehrenreich, B. A., and Cohn, Z. A. (1968). *J. Cell Biol.* **38**, 244.

Elsbach, P., and Kayden, H. J. (1965). *Amer. J. Physiol.* **209**, 765.

Elsbach, P., and Rizack, M. A. (1963). *Amer. J. Physiol.* **205**, 1154.

Emmelot, P., Bos, C. J., Benedetti, E. L., and Rumke, P. H. (1964). *Biochim. Biophys. Acta* **90**, 126.

Ericsson, J. L. E. (1964). *Acta Pathol. Microbiol. Scand., Suppl.* **168**. 1.

Ericsson, J. L. E. (1969). *In* "Lysosomes in Biology and Pathology" (J. T. Dingle and H. B. Fell, eds.), Vol. 2, pp. 345–394. North-Holland Publ., Amsterdam.

Ericsson, J. L. E., and Trump, B. F. (1964). *Lab. Invest.* **13**, 1427.

Farquhar, M. G. (1969). *In* "Lysosomes in Biology and Pathology" (J. T. Dingle and H. B. Fell, eds.), Vol. 2, pp. 462–482. North-Holland Publ., Amsterdam.

Fishman, W., Ide, H., and Rufo, R. (1969). *Histochemie* **20**, 287.

Fowler, S., and de Duve, C. (1969). *J. Biol. Chem.* **244**, 471.

Goettlich-Riemann, W., Young, J. O., and Tappel, A. L. (1971). *Biochim. Biophys. Acta* **243**, 137.

Goldfischer, S. (1965). *J. Histochem. Cytochem.* **13**, 520.

Goldfischer, S., and Moskal, J. (1966). *Amer. J. Pathol.* **48**, 305.

Goldfischer, S., Novikoff, A. B., Albala, A., and Biempica, L. (1970a). *J. Cell Biol.* **44**, 512.

Goldfischer, S., Schiller, B., and Sternlieb, I. (1970b). *Nature* (*London*) **228**, 172.

Goldstone, A., and Koenig, H. (1971). *Proc. Amer. Soc. Cell Biol.* Abstr. No. 203, p. 106.

Green, D. E. (1971). *Science* **174**, 867.

Greenbaum, L. M., and Kim, K. M. (1967). *Brit. J. Pharmacol. Chemotner.* **29**, 238.

Güttler, F. (1971). *Biochim. Biophys. Acta* **237**, 43.

Harris, H. (1969). *Proc. Roy. Soc., Ser. B* **174**, 1.

Hayase, K., and Tappel, A. L. (1970). *J. Biol. Chem.* **245**, 169.

Hayashi, M. (1967). *J. Histochem. Cytochem.* **15**, 83.

Hayashi, M., Shirahama, T., and Cohen, A. S. (1968). *J. Cell Biol.* **36**, 289.

Heath, E. S. (1971). *Annu. Rev. Biochem.* **40**, 29.

Henson, P. M. (1971). *J. Exp. Med.* **134**, 1145.

Hers, G., and van Hoof, F. (1969). *In* "Lysosomes in Biology and Pathology" (J. T. Dingle and H. B. Fell, eds.), Vol. 2, pp. 19–40. North-Holland Publ., Amsterdam.

Hill, J. H., and Ward, P. A. (1969). *J. Exp. Med.* **130**, 505.

Hirsch, J. G., and Cohn, Z. A. (1960). *J. Exp. Med.* **112**, 1005.

Hirschhorn, R., and Weissmann, G. (1967). *Nature (London)* **214**, 892.

Hirschhorn, R., Kaplan, M. J., Hirschhorn, K., and Weissmann, G. (1965). *Science* **147**, 55.

Hirschhorn, R., Hirschhorn, K., and Weissmann, G. (1967). *Blood* **30**, 84.

Hirschhorn, R., Brittinger, G., Hirschhorn, K., and Weissmann, G. (1968). *J. Cell Biol.* **37**, 412.

Hirschhorn, R., Grossman, J., and Weissmann, G. (1970). *Proc. Soc. Exp. Biol. Med.* **133**, 1361.

Holtzman, E., and Novikoff, A. B. (1965). *J. Cell Biol.* **27**, 651.

Horvat, A., and Touster, O. (1968). *J. Biol. Chem.* **243**, 4380.

Hunter, A. R., and Korner, A. (1968). *Biochim. Biophys. Acta* **169**, 488.

Hutterer, F. (1966). *Biochim. Biophys. Acta* **115**, 312.

Ide, H., and Fishman, W. H. (1969). *Histochemie* **20**, 300.

Iodice, A. A. (1967). *Arch. Biochem. Biophys.* **121**, 241.

Iodice, A. A., Leong, V., and Weinstock, I. M. (1966). *Arch. Biochem. Biophys.* **117**, 477.

Iqbal, M., Dingle, J. T., Moore, M., and Sharman, I. M. (1969). *Brit. J. Nutr.* **23**, 31.

Jablonski, P., and McQuillan, M. T. (1967). *Biochim. Biophys. Acta* **132**, 454.

Jamieson, J. J., and Palade, G. E. (1971). *J. Cell Biol.* **50**, 135.

Janoff, A., and Scherer, J. (1968). *J. Exp. Med.* **128**, 1137.

Janoff, A., and Zeligs, J. D. (1968). *Science* **161**, 702.

Janoff, A., and Zweifach, B. W. (1964). *J. Exp. Med.* **120**, 747.

Janoff, A., Schaeffer, S., Scherer, J., and Bean, M. A. (1965). *J. Exp. Med.* **122**, 841.

Jeffrey, P. L., Brown, D. H., and Brown, B. I. (1970). *Biochemistry* **9**, 1403.

Kaley, G., and Weiner, R. (1971). *Nature (London), New Biol.* **234**, 1114.

Keilova, H., Blaha, K., and Keil, B. (1968). *Eur. J. Biochem.* **4**, 422.

Kent, G., Minick, O. T., Orfei, E., Volini, F. I., and Madera-Orsini, F. (1965). *Amer. J. Pathol.* **48**, 803.

Kerr, J. F. R. (1970). *J. Pathol.* **100**, 99.

Koenig, H. (1964). *Trans. Amer. Neurol. Ass.* **89**, 212.

Koenig, H. (1969). *In* "Lysosomes in Biology and Pathology" (J. T. Dingle and H. B. Fell, eds.), Vol. 2, p. 136. North-Holland Publ., Amsterdam.

Korn, E. D. (1966). *Science* **153**, 1491.

Lack, C. H. (1969). *In* "Lysosomes in Biology and Pathology" (J. T. Dingle and H. B. Fell, eds.), Vol. 1, pp. 493–508. North-Holland Publ., Amsterdam.

Lake, B. D. (1971). *J. Clin. Pathol.* **24**, 617.

Lapresle, C., and Webb, T. (1962). *Biochem. J.* **84**, 455.

Lazarus, G. S., Daniels, J. R., Brown, R. S., Bladen, H. A., and Fullmer, H. M. (1968a). *J. Clin. Invest.* **47**, 2622.

Lazarus, G. S., Brown, R. S., Daniels, J. R., and Fullmer, H. M. (1968b). *Science* **159**, 1483.

Lindahl-Magnusson, P., Leary, P., and Gresser, I. (1972). *Nature (London), New Biol.* **237**, 120.

Lloyd, J. B., and Beck, F. (1969). *In* "Lysosomes in Biology and Pathology" (J. T. Dingle and H. B. Fell, eds.), Vol. 1, pp. 433–449. North-Holland Publ., Amsterdam.

Locke, M., and Collins, J. V. (1968). *J. Cell Biol.* **36**, 453.

Lucy, J. A. (1970). *Nature (London)* **227**, 815.

McKay, R. (1966). *In* "Controversy in Internal Medicine" (F. J. Ingelfinger, A. S. Relman, and M. Finland, eds.), p. 517. Saunders, Philadelphia, Pennsylvania.

Mahadevan, S., and Tappel, A. L. (1967a). *J. Biol. Chem.* **242**, 2369.

Mahadevan, S., and Tappel, A. L. (1967b). *J. Biol. Chem.* **242**, 4568.

Mahadevan, S., and Tappel, A. L. (1968). *J. Biol. Chem.* **243**, 2849.

Matile, P. (1966). *Science* **151**, 86.

Mausbach, A. B. (1966). *J. Ultrastruct. Res.* **16**, 197.

Mellors, A., and Tappel, A. L. (1967). *J. Lipid Res.* **8**, 479.

Melmon, K. L., and Cline, M. J. (1967). *Nature (London)* **213**, 90.

Metchnikoff, E. (1905). "Immunity in Infective Diseases" (reprint) Johnson Reprint Corp., New York, 1968.

Metrione, R. M., Neves, A. G., and Fruton, J. S. (1966). *Biochemistry* **5**, 1597.

Movat, H. Z., Urihara, T., Macmorine, D. R. L., and Burke, J. S. (1964). *Life Sci.* **3**, 1025.

Movat, H. Z., Urihara, T., Takeuchi, Y., and Macmorine, D. R. L. (1971). *Int. Arch. Allergy Appl. Immunol.* **40**, 197.

Muller, M. (1967) *Chem. Zool.* **1**, 351–380.

Nadler, S., and Goldfischer, S. (1970). *J. Histochem. Cytochem.* **18**, 368.

Nichols, B. A., Bainton, D. F., and Farquhar, M. G. (1971). *J. Cell Biol.* **50**, 498.

Novikoff, A. B. (1961). *In* "The Cell" (J. Brachet and A. E. Mirsky, eds.), Vol. 2, pp. 423–488. Academic Press, New York.

Novikoff, A. B. (1963). *Lysosomes Ciba Found. Symp.,* 1963.

Novikoff, A. B. (1967). *Proc. Amer. Soc. Cell Biol. Abstr.* 708, p. 208.

Novikoff, A. B., and Essner, E. (1962). *J. Cell Biol.* **15**, 140.

Novikoff, A. B., Beaufay, H., and de Duve, C. (1956). *J. Biophys. Biochem. Cytol.* **2**, Suppl., 179.

Novikoff, A. B., Essner, E., and Quintana, N. (1964). *Fed. Amer. Soc. Exp. Biol.* **23**, 1010.

O'Brien, J. S. (1972). *Advan. Hum. Genet.* **3** (in press).

Olsson, I., and Gardell, S. (1969). *Exp. Cell Res.* **54**, 318.

Palade, G. E. (1966). *J. Amer. Med. Ass.* **198**, 815.

Parish, W. E. (1969). *Brit. J. Dermatol.* **81**, 28.

Patel, V., and Tappel, A. (1969). *Biochim. Biophys. Acta* **191**, 653.

Patel, V., and Tappel, A. L. (1970). *Biochim. Biophys. Acta* **220**, 622.

Patrucco, A., Rothfield, N. F., and Hirschhorn, K. (1967). *Arthritis Rheum.* **10**, 32.

Persellin, R. H. (1972). *Arthritis Rheum.* **15**, 144.

Peters, T., Jr., Fleischer, B., and Fleischer, S. F. (1971). *J. Biol. Chem.* **246**, 240.

Phelps, P., and McCarty, D. J. (1966). *J. Exp. Med.* **124**, 115.

Rahman, Y. E., and Verhagen, J. (1970). *Biochem. Biophys. Res. Commun.,* **38**, 670.

Ranadive, N. S., and Cochrane, C. G. (1967). *Fed. Amer. Soc. Exp. Biol.* **26**, 574.

Resibois, A., Tondeur, M., Mockel, S., and Dustin, S. (1970). *Int. Rev. Exp. Pathol.* **9**, 93.

Robison, G. A., Butcher, R. W., and Sutherland, E. W. (1968). *Annu. Rev. Biochem.* **37**, 149.

Roy, A. B. (1960) *Advan. Enzymol.* **22**, 205.

Ryan, W. L., and Lee, J. W. (1970). *Immunochemistry* **7**, 251.

Ryser, H. J. P. (1967). *Nature (London)* **215**, 934.

Sawant, P. L., Shibko, S., Kumta, U. S., and Tappel, A. L. (1964). *Biochim. Biophys. Acta* **85**, 82.

Schneider, F. H. (1968). *Biochem. Pharmacol.* **17**, 848.

Schnikta, T. K., and Seligman, A. M. (1971). *Annu. Rev. Biochem.* **40**, 375.

Sessa, G., and Weissmann, G. (1968). *J. Lipid Res.* **9**, 310.

Shirahama, T., and Cohen, A. S. (1971). *Amer. J. Pathol.* **63**, 463.

Silverstein, S. C., and Dales, S. (1968). *J. Cell Biol.* **36**, 197.

Singer, S. J., and Nicolson, G. L. (1972). *Science* **175**, 720.

Stoffel, W., and Greten, H. (1967). *Hoppe-Seyler's Z. Physiol. Chem.* **348**, 1145.

Strauss, W. (1954). *J. Biol. Chem.* **207**, 745.

Strauss, W. (1964). *J. Cell Biol.* **20**, 497.

Strauss, W. (1967). *In "Enzyme Cytology"* (D. B. Roodyn, ed.), pp. 239–319. Academic Press, New York.

Tappel, A. L. (1969). *In* "Lysosomes in Biology and Pathology" (J. T. Dingle and H. B. Fell, eds.), Vol. 2, pp. 207–244. North-Holland Publ., Amsterdam.

Tappel, A. L., Beck, C., Mahadevan, R., Brightwell, R., Mellors, A., Navaguba, J., and Dillard, C. (1967). *Fed. Amer. Soc. Exp. Biol.* **26**, 797.

Tartakoff, A. M., Greene, L. J., Jamieson, J. D., and Palade, G. E. (1971). *Proc. Amer. Soc. Cell Biol.* Abstr. No. 591, p. 300.

Tew, J. G., Hess, W. M., and Donaldson, D. M. (1969). *J. Immunol.* **102**, 743.

Thines-Sempoux, D. (1967). *Biochem. J.* 20P.

Trouet, A. (1964). *Arch. Int. Physiol. Biochim.* **72**, 698.

Trouet, A. (1968). *J. Cell Biol.* **39**, 137a.

Trump, B. F. (1961). *J. Ultrastruct. Res.* **5**, 291.

Tulsiani, D. R. P., and Carubelli, R. (1970). *J. Biol. Chem.* **245**, 1821.

Vaes, G. (1968). *J. Cell Biol.* **39**, 676.

Van Dyck, J. M., and Wattiaux, R. (1968). *Eur. J. Biochem.* **7**, 15.

Wagner, R. R., and Cymkin, M. A. (1971). *J. Biol. Chem.* **246**, 143.

Waksman, B. (1966). *In* "Controversy in Internal Medicine" (F. J. Ingelfinger, A. S. Relman, and M. Finland, eds.), p. 530. Saunders, Philadelphia, Pennsylvania.

Wallingford, W. R., and McCarty, D. J., Jr. (1971). *J. Exp. Med.* **133**, 100.

Ward, P. A., and Hill, J. H. (1970). *J. Immunol.* **104**, 535.

Weber, R. (1969). *In* "Lysosomes in Biology and Pathology" (J. T. Dingle and H. B. Fell, eds.), Vol. 2, pp. 437–461. North-Holland Publ., Amsterdam.

Weinstein, O. B., Marsh, J. B., Glick, M. C., and Warren, L. (1969). *J. Biol. Chem.* **244**, 4103.

Weissmann, G. (1966). *Arthritis Rheum.* **9**, 834.

Weissmann, G. (1967). *Annu. Rev. Med.* **18**, 97.

Weissmann, G. (1969). *In* "Lysosomes in Biology and Pathology" (J. T. Dingle and H. B. Fell, eds.), Vol. 1, pp. 276–298. North-Holland Publ., Amsterdam.

Weissmann, G., and Spilberg, I. (1968). *Arthritis Rheum.* **11**, 162.

Weissmann, G., Becher, B., Wiederman, G., and Bernheimer, A. W. (1965). *Amer. J. Pathol.* **46**, 129.

Weissmann, G., Pras, M., and Rosenberg, L. (1967). *Arthritis. Rheum.* **10**, 325.

Weissmann, G., Rita, G. A., Zurier, R. B., and Mortara, M. (1971a). *J. Clin. Invest.* **50**, 97a.

Weissmann, G., Zurier, R. B., Spieler, P. J., and Goldstein, I. M. (1971b). *J. Exp. Med.* **134**, 149s.

Weissmann, G., Dukor, P., and Zurier, R. B. (1971c). *Nature (London)*, New Biol. **231**, 131.

Weissmann, G., Zurier, R. B., and Hoffstein, S. (1972). *Amer. J. Pathol.* **68**, 539.

Wetzel, B. K., Spicer, S. S., and Horn, R. G. (1967). *J. Histochem. Cytochem.* **15**, 311.

Woessner, J. F., and Shamberger, R. J. (1971). *J. Biol. Chem.* **246**, 1951.

Woods, J. F., and Nichols, G. (1965). *Nature (London)* **208**, 1325.

Wynn, C. H., Iqbal, M., and Davies, I. (1967). *Biochem. J.* **105**, 19P.

Zeya, H. I., and Spitznagel, J. K. (1963). *Science* **142**, 1085.

Zeya, H. I., and Spitznagel, J. K. (1966). *J. Bacteriol.* **91**, 750.

Zeya, H. I., and Spitznagel, J. K. (1969). *Science* **163**, 1069.

Zurier, R. B., and Quagliata, F. F. (1971). *Nature (London)* **234**, 305.

Chapter 5

CHEMOTAXIS

W. SCOTT RAMSEY AND LESTER GRANT

I. Introduction

A. General Statement of the Problem

Chemotaxis can be defined as that property of certain biologically active substances which enables them to attract cells and microorganisms. So named by the early botanists (Pfeffer, 1884) and applied to white cells by Leber in 1888, chemotaxis has been confirmed many times by many techniques *in vitro* (Commandon, 1917, 1919; McCutcheon *et al.*, 1934; Harris, 1953a; Boyden, 1962; Bessis and Burté, 1964; Ramsey, 1972a), but it has never been demonstrated, beyond a doubt, by direct observation *in vivo*, even though the technology now seems available to achieve this, and *in vivo* correlations with *in vitro* results are hard to come by. Indeed, chemotaxis remains after many years of study a little understood phenomenon.

An illustration of this lack of correlation can be found in the case of experiments performed with antigen–antibody complexes. In *in vitro* experiments, using fresh serum, there seems no doubt that these complexes are chemotactic (Boyden, 1962). In *in vivo* experiments, the effect is ambiguous. Cliff found, for example, that more white blood cells actually moved away from injection sites (in a ratio of 4:1) than moved toward the injection sites (Cliff, 1965, 1966a,b). Cliff wondered, therefore, if results could be explained on the basis of negative chemotaxis, an awkward formulation for the white blood cell, or if in fact the slow centrifugal expansion of the population of emigrated leucocytes might make it unnecessary to invoke negative chemotaxis to rationalize his results. Yet the circumstantial evidence that chemotaxis is a true biological event is impressive. The assumption has been made, for almost a century, that chemotaxis is a primordial reaction of living cells that explains, in large part, one of the elementary defense sequences in biology, and there is hardly a biologist who does not believe in it.

Metchnikoff, in fact, saw chemotaxis as a quite basic activity of living cells, on a level with phagocytosis and excretion (1892). More recent evidence suggests that the complement system is present in lower vertebrates, such as the frog, and in several lines of phylogenetically divergent invertebrates (Day *et al.*, 1970a,b), where adaptive immunity seems not to have yet emerged in the evolutionary scheme. Since chemotactic reactions proceed quite vigorously in the absence of complement, there is some question about the importance of complement in this phenomenon. However, assuming a significant role for complement, there is evidence that the appearance of complement antedates immune reactions and therefore it may play a role in the initiation of primitve inflammatory responses (Gewurz *et al.*, 1967; Page *et al.*, 1968; Cochrane, 1969; Ward and Hill, 1970; see also discussion of this point in Chapter 1 by Ebert and Grant). If there is any validity to this kind of thinking, then the continuing preoccupation of the biomedical community with chemotaxis represents a research thrust that strikes deep into the roots of biology and conceivably may lay open, at a molecular level, one of the most significant of cellular mechanisms.

Failure to demonstrate, control, and manipulate the phenomenon *in vivo*, however, is not only disconcerting but it also raises questions about the relevancy, in living systems, of many of the factors that seem to influence chemotactic reactions *in vitro*. Whatever the triggering molecule, if there be one, that sets off the chemotactic response, the response itself has been demonstrated in bacterial systems, in plants, and in a variety of animal species ranging from amoebae to mammals. Recent evidence even suggests that tumor tissues contain substances specifically chemotactic for cancer cells (Yoshida *et al.*, 1970; Ozaki *et al.*, 1971).

There may be a rather wide distribution of chemotactic defects in the human population that can be correlated with the genesis or aggravation of disease states. These come about as the result of factors lacking in the serum, of the existence of inhibitors in the serum, or of apparent deficiencies in white blood cells. Defects of this type are said to be characterized by recurrent and sometimes uncontrollable infections and, in a growing series of notations in the literature, have been stated to include such conditions as diabetes mellitus (Mowat and Baum, 1971a); congenital agammaglobulinemia (Steerman *et al.*, 1971); the Chediak-Higashi syndrome (Clark and Kimball, 1971); cirrhosis of the liver associated with alcoholism (De Meo and Anderson, 1972); and rheumatoid arthritis (Mowat and Baum, 1971b) for which there may be experimental correlates (Zvaifler, 1969; Ward and Zvaifler, 1971; De Shazo *et al.*, 1971, 1972; Persellin, 1972). It should also be noted that chemotactic function in the human neonate is less vigorous than in the human adult, according to Miller (1971). That chemotaxis may subserve a useful defense mechanism in human disease can be inferred from the report that infection of primary rabbit kidney cells with herpes simplex virus leads to the release of a cell factor or factors that on incubation with serum results in the cleavage of the fifth component, C5, of complement (Brier *et al.*, 1970). The product of the cleavage, C5a, is chemotactic for neutrophils and could be responsible for the accumulation of these cells at the site of herpetic lesions.

A related study by Snyderman and co-workers, in which rabbit kidney cells were infected with herpes simplex virus, demonstrated additionally that the interaction of antiviral antibody and complement with viral antigens absorbed to the surface of cells (before penetration) also resulted in the generation of chemotactic activity but did not cause injury to the cells (Snyderman *et al.*, 1972). The most recent addition to the analysis of clinical inflammatory syndromes comes from Berenberg and his colleagues in a study of tick-bite injury, which they characterized by the interesting expression that such injury is mediated by a complement-derived chemotictic chemotactic factor (Berenberg *et al.*, 1972). They found that tick salivary gland extracts have no intrinsic chemotactic activity but they can generate this activity from human or dog serum. Activity can also be generated from human C5 complement component but not from C3. Antibodies to C5 eliminate chemotactic activity produced in human serum. The chemotactic factor appeared to be a C5 cleavage product with a low sedimentation velocity in sucrose density grandients. The investigators noted that the action of tick salivary gland extract on C5 is not a unique story: Other proteolytic enzymes such as trypsin (Ward and Newman, 1969) and a bacterial protesase derived from the β-hemolytic streptococcus (Ward et al., 1971a) can interact with C5 to generate a neutrophil chemoattractant. A similar cleavage product of C5 may result from the activation of the complement system by bacterial endotoxin (Synderman et al., 1968). It is suggested that the tick bite study may represent a nonimmunological model of tissue injury analogous to the immune models of the Arthus reaction (Ward and Cochrane, 1965) and of acute nephrotoxic nephritis (Unanue and Dixon, 1964).

The neutrophil (polymorphonuclear leukocyte) has been the most assiduously studied of the white cells that participate in chemotactic responses, but the eosinophil (Rosegger, 1932; Ingraham and Wartman, 1939; Harris, 1954) and mononuclear phagocyte (Chambers and Fell, 1932; Lasfargues, 1946; Harris, 1954; Ward, 1968; Sorkin et al., 1970) also react chemotactically. Harris could not demonstrate chemotaxis for lymphocytes (1953b) and noted (1954) that in vitro or in vivo there was no evidence up to that time that lymphocytes participated in chemotactic responses, a viewpoint that was consistent with evidence from Clark (Clark et al., 1936) and others (Ebert et al., 1940; Bessis and Burté, 1964). This led Harris to conclude that either the right stimulus had not been found for the lymphocyte or the cell does not in fact exhibit chemotaxis. The first of these possibilities seems to have been the correct one, for Ward and his colleagues have shown recently that the products of antigen-stimulated lymphoid cells cause emigration of other lymphocytes through membrane filters (Ward et al., 1971b). A remarkable, if not bewildering, fact from these experiments is that a trypsin fragment of C5, rabbit serum, treated with heterologous immune complexes, and a bacterial factor, are each chemotactically active for rabbit neutrophils and mononuclear cells but they are inactive for rat lymphoid cells (Ward, 1968; Ward et al., 1965, 1969; see also discussion by Ward, 1971c). Ward pointed out that these differences in leukotactic responses of each of the three cell types cannot be caused by some functional peculiarity of the rat lymphocyte, since the latter cell can respond to the culture fluids from antigen-stimulated lymphoid cells. Thus far, the factor in culture fluids from antigen-stimulated lymphoid cells is the only chemotactic factor found to induce migration of lymphocytes, and this conceivably could represent one of the more important mediators generated in reactions of delayed hypersensitivity of the tuberculin type. (For further comments on the pathophysiology of these cells, see appropriate chapters in Volumes I and III by Steinman and Cohn, Hirsch, McGregor and Mackaness, Dumont, and Spector.)

Until recently, Harris' dictum that only starch granules and bacteria are chemotactic for white blood cells was a generally accepted principle, largely because of the uniqueness and elegance of the *in vitro* system introduced by Harris in 1953 (Harris, 1953a) and the sharply critical view he took of many experimental procedures up to that time. In recent years, however, Boyden has introduced a chamber technique, using a membrane filter, that has produced results indicating, among other things, that antigen–antibody complexes are chemotactic for white blood cells, the reaction often, if not exclusively, mediated by various components of the complement system (Boyden, 1962). Correlates for this hypothesis, *in vivo*, though meager, are emerging, an example being the observation of Snyderman and his colleagues (Snyderman *et al.*, 1971a) who demonstrated that intraperitoneal injections into guinea pigs of glycogen or endotoxin yielded a fluid that was chemotactic for neutrophils and contained in it a complement fraction, C5a. Similar injections into C5-sufficient mice gave similar results, but injections into C5-deficient mice produce a peritoneal fluid that gave no chemotactic activity *in vitro*, and the subsequent harvest of neutrophils from the mouse peritoneum was depressed. Hill and Ward (1971), moreover, have extracted from infarcted rat myocardium an enzyme that cleaves the third component of complement into leukotactic fragments, as judged by the ability of the substance to elicit chemotaxis in white cells in a Boyden chamber. The studies suggest a nonimmunological role for C3 in the mediation of the inflammatory response in nonspecific tissue injury. Yet substantial evidence has accumulated that chemotaxis can proceed in the absence of complement; indeed, Lotz and Harris (1956) demonstrated that chemotaxis exerted by *Staphylococcus albus* on neutrophils occurred in the absence of serum, complement, or glucose and in solutions containing chelating agents to remove as much calcium and magnesium as possible. Harris also produced impressive evidence from his own experiments that dead granulocytes and tissues autolyzed, damaged, or digested by various enzymes do not induce chemotaxis, a principle that tends to make difficult the construction of a unitary hypothesis for the role of chemotaxis in biology. A decade of evidence from others (Allison *et al.*, 1955; Weimar, 1957; Hurley and Spector, 1961a,b; Buckley, 1963; Bessis and Burté, 1964; Grant, 1974; Grant *et al.*, 1967) seems to contradict, but may not refute, Harris' view on this point.

It is of interest to note that Policard *et al.* (1961) also stated that neutrophils pay no attention to dead cells. However, Bessis and Burté emphasized, in experiments in which they killed cells with laser beams, that the granulocytes failed to react to cells that have been "dead for a long time," although they did not specify the time in question. When the cells did pick up the signal—whatever the signal is—from a dead neutrophil, lymphocyte, or red cell, they moved to the kill rapidly. Approximately 1 second after the destruction of one of these cells there was a pronounced movement of certain leukocytes toward the damaged cell, the neutrophils approaching the target in a manner that varied from a straight line to a highly tortuous path. Thereafter, Bessis describes a series of events fraught with enough violence to constitute the basis of a children's television show, as "these cells literally tear the corpse apart." Phagocytosis usually takes place by morsels, each phagocyte carrying off part of the prey (Policard and Bessis, 1953). In a few minutes, no traces of the dead cell remain. From the films it appeared that it is not until after the cell had plasmolysed and the cellular contents had escaped that neighboring cells moved toward it, sometimes as far as 500 μm. The newly arrived neutrophils could be seen to push aside vigorously the phagocytes which already had surrounded the dead cell in order to capture their prey. In a literary flight not commonly found in short scientific communications, Bessis and Burté stated that on a cellular level the phenomenon suggested "the violent feeding orgy of sharks, in which blood escaping from a wound causes one attacker to fasten on another of its kind." They also reported observing that on occasion a leukocyte would abandon a piece of a previously ingested corpse; even though other cells were close to the egested material, they were not attracted to it. It is conceivable that in this situation, as perhaps in Harris' experiments, there comes a time when attractant material in a cell has become exhausted or inactivated and therefore no longer has chemotactic properties.

On balance, 85 years after Leber's early studies (Leber, 1888, 1891), the phenomenon of chemotaxis seems at one and the same time to be more secure and yet more confounding than ever in a sprawling literature that is growing with some rapidity and might even be considered as exhibiting some chemotactic properties of its own. This review covers a wider spectrum of the subject than is normally attempted, including the expression of chemotaxis in microorganisms and plants, in lower and higher forms of animal life, and a review of direct observations *in vivo* where the suggestion is permissible that recent work with thin tissue preparations may have overcome some early obstacles and where evidence seems to be emerging that the ground rules may be different from the more precise, more quantitative, more reproducible, but more artificial *in vitro* systems (Allison *et al.*, 1955; Buckley, 1963; Grant, 1974). It is our hope that by drawing together in one chapter materials and experimental data from a wide variety of investigations of chemotaxis, particularly the simpler and more direct studies of the microbiologists, it may be possible to accelerate a certain amount of cross-fertilization in the research enterprise. It is also hoped that a treatment such as this may yield generalizations about the process which might be less obvious with a narrower focus.

Reviews of special aspects of the problem have been published in recent years, among them Harris (1954, 1960), Weibull (1960), Boyden *et al.* (1965), Doetsch and Hageage (1968), Keller and Sorkin (1968b), Adler (1969), Becker (1969), Müller-Eberhard (reviews of serum complement, 1968, 1969, and in 1971) and Sorkin *et al.* (1970). Chemotaxis in plants is reviewed by Rosen (1962), Ziegler (1962), Shaffer (1962), and Machlis and Rawits-cher-Kunkel (1963). A review of chemotaxis in lower plants can be found in Rothschild's work (1956). Harris' astringent monograph of 1954 was the best single summation of the phenomenon of chemotaxis in the literature up to that time and he followed this 6 years later with a more up to date review. No attempt has been made in this chapter to reanalyze in detail the material that Harris covered with such provocative excellence, nor do we take into account the phenomenon of phagocytosis which may be so closely related to chemotaxis that the two terms, chemotaxis and phagocytosis, may be simply aspects of one broad pattern of cell ativity. (For a full discussion of phagocytosis, please see Chapter 6 by Elsbach, in which chemotaxis is viewed as the first of four phases in the process of phagocytosis). Please also make reference to chemotaxis in Volumes I–III, Chapters by Hirsch, Steinman and Cohn, Grant, Cochrane and Janoff, Austin and Stechschulte, and Nelson.

B. *Historical Review*

Early investigators of the inflammatory process knew, before the word chemotaxis came into general use, that leukocytes were attracted by certain chemical substances or by factors produced by the injury created by chemicals and other agents. They were impressed that injury—mechanical, chemical, or thermal—caused the formed elements of the blood, notably white cells, to adhere to the vessel wall. Von Haller, (1757) may have been the first person to call attention to the margination and emigration of white blood cells, but it is not clear whether the globules he described coating the mesenteric veins, and the extravascular appearance of spherical and yellow cells, were in fact red cells or white cells. Dutrochet (1824) and Wagner (1833, 1839) may have had priorities here. Addison (1843), Waller (1846), Wharton-Jones (1851), and Cohnheim (1882) all inflamed amphibian and mammalian vascular beds in a variety of ways, Addison noting that the application of a crystal of salt to the web of a frog's foot led to adherence of "lymph globules" to the vessel wall and that later such globules could be seen to be extravascular. Metchnikoff (1887, 1893) saw that bacteria could attract leukocytes which then ingested the organisms.

By the 1880's, the botanists had described many examples of chemotaxis in the plant kingdom (Engelmann, 1881, 1883; Pfeffer, 1884), but Leber first used the term with reference to leukocytes. Leber injected bacterial molds, putrified tissue, and extracts of *Staphylococcus aureus* into the cornea or anterior chamber of the eyes of frogs and rabbits and noted an accumulation of leukocytes in the injured and infected areas. Early in the reaction he excised the affected area and examined it under the microscope, observing leukocytes moving toward the injection site. His conclusion was that the extracts offered proof of the chemotactic attraction of microbial metabolic products for leukocytes.

Except for Leber's direct observations of leukocyte movement on isolated fragments of guinea pig cornea, early experiments on chemotaxis were performed either with some variation of a capillary tube technique or by injecting the test substance into the tissues of an animal and then examining the injection site. Harris (1954) has underscored the serious criticism of both methods: In one case, the objects being studied may enter the capillary tubes passively, and in the second case, the fact that the capacity of a substance to cause emigration of leukocytes from blood vessels is no indication of its chemotactic power, thus negating a fair amount of poorly controlled histological analyses of these preparations. As Harris noted, almost all substances, including physiological saline, will produce some degree of leukocyte emigration when injected into tissues.

In the present century, Commandon (1917), Clark and Clark (1920, 1922), McCutcheon *et al.* (1934), McCutcheon and Dixon (1936), and Harris (1953a) all made original contributions to the study of chemotaxis. Commandon spread a thin film of blood between a slide and cover slip and recorded the movements of leukocytes in the film with time-lapse cinematography. He showed that avian red cells, parasitized with *Haemamoeba danilewski*, were chemotactic for avian leukocytes and that various bacteria, including *Streptococci*, *Corynebacterium diphtheriae*, and *Bacillus anthracis* could attract human leukocytes. Clark and Clark made their observations on the transparent tail of the tadpole with the amphibian larva anesthetized in a special microaquarium that made possible for long periods of time the continuous microscopic examination of the tail vasculature. Clark and Clark injected test substances into the tail as droplets or they introduced various substances through small capillary tubes. They found that leukocytes accumulated focally in response to a wide variety of materials, including powdered carbon, carmine, olive oil, cream, egg yolk, croton oil, bacteria, starch, agar, gelatin, and gum arabic. They were most impressed with the leukocytic response to various preparations of starch.

Using Commandon's slide–coverslip technique, McCutcheon and his colleagues (1934; McCutcheon and Dixon, 1936) demonstrated that a clump of dried *Staphylococcus albus* caused nearby leukocytes to move toward it but there was no such clear-cut effect if a clump of dead leukocytes was the test object. However, they did offer evidence that the living cells were attracted to the dead ones "weakly and from no great distance." Some measure of attraction was also shown for paraffin wax and for fragments of glass. Other studies with many bacterial species showed that all leukocytes within a certain range of the bacterial clump moved directly toward it.

Harris (1953a) made a striking contribution to the study of chemotaxis by devising a slide chamber constructed by placing a drop of blood on a coverslip and incubating this in a moist chamber. During incubation, many leukocytes in the blood clot adhered to the coverslip. After washing away clot, serum, and red cells, he was left with a pure population of leukotytes which were then incorporated into a film of plasma about 20 μm deep, laid down between the coverslip and a slide. The plasma was allowed to clot, and when a solid or semisolid object was to be tested, it was placed on the surface of the slide so that it was incorporated in the plasma film also. A drill-hole opening on a perspex slide permitted the study of test substances in fluid. Movements of the white cells were recorded photomicrographically by dark ground illumination. Harris demonstrated, as many others before him, the chemotactic effect on leukocytes of various microorganisms but he found that dead leukocytes, injured and autolyzed tissues, peptic and tryptic tissue digests, and inflammatory exudates were not chemotactic for the white cells, contrary to other evidence that various digests of protein act as attractants for such cells (Menkin, 1938a,b,c; Duthie and Chain, 1939; Cullumbine and Rydon, 1946).

On the other hand, Hurley (1963) entered a disclaimer to Harris' conclusion that the products of disintegrating tissues were not chemotactic to granulocytes. He incubated minced liver or granulocytes with serum and tested the serum for chemotactic activity in Boyden chambers and for activity in causing *in vivo* migration of rat leukocytes. There was a parallelism in results. Hurley speculated that Harris' negative results with dead tissue fragments, autolyzing tissue, or peptic or tryptic digests may have been caused by the absence of serum in the preparations tested and suggested that the Harris system was unable to demonstrate chemotaxis by substances in solution—nothing in this state tested by Harris gave a positive response. Harris also studied inflammatory exudates induced both by intraperitoneal injection of turpentine into the pleural cavity of rabbits, a technique used by Menkin, and by intraperitoneal injection of isotonic saline (de Haan, 1917). The pleural fluid evoked by the turpentine killed white cells. A cell-free exudate extracted by Menkin's method, for the preparation of leukotaxine, a substance Menkin thought to be chemotactic, was taken up in saline and was highly toxic to leukocytes. The peritoneal exudates, on the other hand, contained living leukocytes; the cell-free fluid was not toxic to living cells, nor was it chemotactic in the drill-hole preparations.

The introduction of the Boyden membrane filter chamber in 1962 facilitated the *in vitro* analysis of materials that could be tested for chemotactic properties by placing the white blood cells on one side of the filter and the test material on the other side. Approximately 20% of the cells migrate through the filter under optimal chemotactic conditions, and this does not increase with time. There is no clear explanation of why the majority of cells do not respond to chemotactic stimuli in the same way. In other test systems, such as those devised by Harris and by Ramsey, all cells exposed to chemotactic stimuli move toward the attractant. Among these various systems, the heaviest concentrations of cells is in the membrane technique, and it is possible that such a concentration causes some sort of mechanical block to cell movement. In any event, although reproducibility sometimes may be a problem, in expert hands experimental results seem internally consistent and the technique has led to such prodigious efforts that *in vitro* experimental work in chemotaxis in the decade of the 1960's has been virtually dominated by variations on the Boyden method. A large part of these studies has to do with the precise elaboration of those components of complement which are and are not chemotactic for white blood cells. An analysis of such results is given in some detail below and in Volume III, Chapter 3, Cochrane and Janoff discuss further those experiments believed to demonstrate the primacy of complement in chemotactic reactions.

II. Chemotaxis in Bacteria

The term chemotaxis has been used historically with varying degrees of rigidity. Early workers devised an elaborate terminology for various types of animal responses, codified by Fraenkel and Gunn (1940). The term "taxis" was reserved for those types of responses in which the organism oriented its axis of movement so as to become nearer to or farther from the effector chemical. "Kineses" were responses which took the form of alterations in the speed of movement or in the frequency of turning. This included the avoiding reaction in which an organism altered its direction of movement in response to changes in concentration of effector, as well as trapping, in which organisms collected at a site because of the reduction in speed. It has proved very difficult, however, to apply these definitions to actual cases of cell and microorganism behavior. In many cases, the observed response falls into more than one class, and often it is not clear that the behavior resulting in the changes in cell distribution in fact has been observed. As research proceeded, conclusions concerning the mechanism of response have been found to be incomplete. For example, Pfeffer (1888) used the term chemotaxis with reference to bacteria, because of the belief that such cells did orient toward an effector, an observation which has proved incorrect. Since so little is known about the mechanisms that result in chemotactic responses, there would appear to be little advantage in adhering to a classification system which is not known to reflect realities at the cellular level. MacInnis (1966) has suggested that "chemical attraction," a term which does not imply a mechanism, be used. In this chapter, we will use "chemotaxis" to refer to instances in which functional organisms or cells, using their own motility, alter their distribution in response to what almost certainly is, or seems to be, a chemical signal. Specifically excluded are cases in which immobile cells are passively carried by currents and those in which otherwise motile cells collect because of the toxic effect of a chemical.

Weibull's (1960) carefully documented monograph on bacterial motility includes the best review of early work on bacterial chemotaxis. A number of other reviews (Rosen, 1962; Ziegler, 1962; Jahn and Bovee, 1965; Holwill, 1966; Doetsch and Hageage, 1968) also touch on this subject. Bacterial chemotaxis was discovered and extensively studied in the late 1800's by Engelmann (1881), Pfeffer (1884, 1888), Rothert (1901), Jennings (1904, 1906), and Beyerinck (1893), whose ingenious and careful experiments form the basis of our present knowledge. A rather quaint nomenclature has grown up around the study of chemotaxis in microorganisms. Types of cellular behavior are referred to, variously, as the avoiding reaction, tumbling, swarming, and milling. In the case of myxococcus, one can speak of aggregation. In the case of amoeba, one can use the expression scavenging. It is important to recognize that these terms refer only to reasonably precise descriptions of cell behavior and of course they carry no quantitative implications.

A. Cell Behavior

1. AVOIDING REACTION

It is clear that photosynthetic bacteria are able to collect in areas of optimum light intensity by means of an avoiding reaction (Manten, 1948; Clayton, 1964). A cell which swims into a region of lower light intensity stops, changes direction, and resumes swimming, generally in a new direction. If the new direction leads to lowered light intensity, the process is repeated, thus causing cells to accumulate in regions of relatively high light intensity. There are few data on the behavior of individual bacteria during chemotaxis, probably because of the difficulty of making accurate observations on such small objects. Jennings and Crosby (1901) reported that *Spirillum*, as well as several unidentified species, made avoiding reactions during chemotaxis to oxygen.

2. TUMBLING

Baracchini and Sherris (1959) reported that *Pseudomonas* cells either reversed their directions of movement or made a series of uncoordinated movements during chemotaxis. Adler and Dahl (1967) while studying chemotaxis in *Escherichia coli* found that cells during chemotaxis often made "tumbling" motions which were only rarely seen in the absence of chemotaxis. A cell was said to tumble when it halted movement, appeared to quiver or tremble, and then resumed movement, usually in a new direction, a procedure which would resemble an avoiding reaction.

MacNab and Koshland (1972) have examined *Salmonella* during chemotaxis and they conclude that the rate of tumbling increases when the cell experiences a decrease in concentration of attractant and, conversely, the rate of tumbling decreases as the cell senses an increase in attractant concentration. Berg and Brown (1972) have followed individual *Escherichia coli* cells during chemotaxis using a tracking microscope which records the movement of cells in three dimensions. Computer analysis of these tracks indicates that these cells respond to increasing concentrations of attractant by decreasing their rate of directional changes; movement in uniform concentration of attractant was similar to that in decreasing concentration. These results are consistent with Nossal and Chen's report (1973) that there is no change in the speed of individual cells during chemotaxis.

Keller and Segel (1971a) have presented a theoretical mathematical analysis of chemotaxis in which they view the process as analogous to Brownian movement. They suggest that local evaluations of chemical concentrations give fluctuations in cellular paths which, over a period of time, cause a macroscopic flux of organisms. Application of this theory to movement of bands of *E. coli* during chemotaxis has resulted in reasonable agreement with predicted rates of movement (Keller and Segel, 1971b).

B. *Myxococcus: Aggregation*

Many myxobacteria have life cycles similar to that of cellular slime molds (see below) in which individual cells migrate over a surface, collect, and form fruiting bodies (Dworkin, 1966). The involvement of chemotaxis in this process was shown by McVittie and Zahler (1962), who demonstrated the response of vegetative cells to a substance produced by fruiting bodies which could pass through a cellophane membrane. Experiments suggesting chemotaxis in liquid media were reported by Fluegel (1963).

C. *Proteus: Swarming*

Proteus cells inoculated in the center of an agar plate exhibit a curious behavior pattern called swarming. Cells migrate out of the inoculum for up to 1 cm and then stop, forming a band of growth. As this process is repeated, additional concentric rings of growth appear on the plate. Lominski and Lendrum (1947) reported experiments which indicated that *Proteus* swarmed as a negative chemotactic response to metabolites produced by heavy growth. This could explain the formation of successive rings. Kopp and Muller (1965; also Kopp *et al.*, 1966) examined the effects of a number of inhibitors on swarming and found that *p*-nitrophenyl glycerol selectively inhibited swarming while not affecting flagella structure and function. It was concluded that this compound has a specific effect on negative chemotaxis; by inhibition of the production of the active metabolites or by inhibition of the response of the cells to those products.

D. Pseudomonas: Oxygen as an Attractant

Smith and Doetsch (1968) studied negative chemotaxis in *Pseudomonas fluorescens*. Suspensions of cells in capillary tubes formed sharp bands which moved away from plugs at the ends of the tubes which contained highly acidic or basic agar. It was suggested that the cells did avoiding reactions on entering the acidic or basic regions, although that would not account for the sharpness of the bands on the side toward the middle of the tubes. In addition, cells which entered the acidic region were observed to be immobilized, which complicated the analysis. Attempts to inhibit the negative chemotaxis without affecting motility were not successful. These authors also have studied the survival advantage of motility (Smith and Doetsch, 1969). Equal numbers of flagellated and nonflagellated *P. fluorescens* were mixed and incubated 24 hours in aerated and nonaerated cultures. In aerated cultures the ratio of flagellated to nonflagellated cells remained constant while it became 10:1 in the nonaerated cultures. It was suggested that this fascinating observation reflects the ability of flagellated cells to remain near the surface by means of positive chemotaxis to oxygen.

The earliest observation of bacterial chemotaxis was Engelmann's discovery that motile bacteria collected around illuminated algal cells. These observations have been extended in studies on the chemotactic response of *Pseudomonas* to oxygen (Sherris *et al.*, 1957; Baracchini and Sherris, 1959). Suspensions of cells in capillary tubes developed a band of cells 3–4 mm below the meniscus when exposed to air; if nitrogen were substituted for air the band moved up and dispersed; if oxygen were substituted, the band moved down the tube. It was concluded that the band formed as a chemotactic response to oxygen with positive chemotaxis to optimum concentrations and negative chemotaxis to excessive concentrations. In the absence of oxygen, motility was lost, unless the amino acid arginine were present. It was suggested that anaerobic metabolism of this amino acid provided energy for motility, a situation similar to that described by Adler (1966a). When a number of different types of bacteria were examined, a correlation was found between positive chemotaxis to oxygen and ability of bacteria to grow aerobically. It may be noted parenthetically that although many organisms exhibit positive chemotaxis to oxygen, this element is generally not a good attractant for study, since motility is often lost in its absence.

E. *Escherichia: Evidence for Receptors*

Adler and his group have used three methods to study chemotaxis in *E. coli* (Adler, 1966b, 1969). (1) In the capillary tube method, motile cells were introduced into one end of a melting-point capillary tube containing aerated amino acid or sugar solution. Under certain conditions, discrete bands of cells formed and migrated down the tube. These bands were not caused by heterogeneity of the bacteria. Band movements could easily be measured with a densitometer or ruler. Cells in the bands often tumbled and, in general, moved in a jerky manner; movement of the bands could be characterized as an enhanced diffusion constant for the bacteria (Adler and Dahl, 1967). (2) In the soft agar method, bacteria were inoculated in the center of a plate containing soft agar. Concentric rings were observed to form after incubation. (3) In the Pfeffer assay, a modification of the method devised by Pfeffer in the 1880's, a 1-λ micropipette containing a solution of the chemical to be tested was inserted into a drop of bacterial suspension. After incubation of 1 hour, the micropipette was washed off and the bacteria inside the micropipette diluted and plated for viable counts. Figure 1 indicated the results of testing various concentrations of glucose.

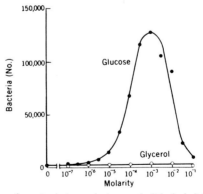

Fig. 1. Graph showing chemotaxis toward glucose (solid circles) but not toward glycerol (open circles). Wild-type (strain W3110) bacteria, grown on glycerol, were used, and the experiment lasted 1 hour. From Adler (1969).

The threshold concentration where accumulation began was about 10^{-6} M glucose. It was clear that this figure did not indicate the actual threshold concentration for individual cells, as attractant diffused into the drop and also was metabolized; nevertheless, a figure useful for comparative purposes was obtained. Inactivity of attractant at high concentrations was presumably caused by saturation of the bacterium's response mechanism; that is, the concentration was so high that the chemical gradient was obscured. Note also that there was a linear relationship over a certain range between the number of responding bacteria and the log of attractant concentration.

The following picture of chemotactic behavior in *E. coli* has emerged from use of the capillary tube and soft agar methods (Adler, 1966a,b; Adler and Templeton, 1967). Bands or rings of bacteria formed after the bacteria exhausted the nutrient or oxygen and moved toward higher concentrations. For example, when bacteria were put into capillary tubes in the presence of galactose, an anaerobically usable energy source, the first band was shown to utilize all the oxygen and part of the galactose, whereas the second band used all the remaining galactose anaerobically. When no energy sources were present, only one band was formed, which used all the oxygen, presumably by means of an endogenous energy source. No oxygen ring appeared with the soft agar method because the oxygen over the plate could not be exhausted. If a number of attractants were present, the bacteria preferentially used all of one and then another. Chemotaxis was demonstrated toward oxygen, galactose, glucose, aspartic acid, threonine, and serine. Serine, the only amino acid which could be utilized both aerobically and anaerobically, was also the only amino acid to support the formation of two bands in the capillary tube method. An increase in the serine concentration was without effect on the movement of the first (oxygen) band although it caused the second (serine) band to move slower. When oxygen was excluded there was no oxygen band, but the serine band moved normally. Theoretical treatment of the rate of movement of these rings has been given by Nossal (1972a,b).

Fleming *et al.* (1967; also Fleming and Williams, 1968) studied the effect of *p*-fluorophenylalanine and chloramphenicol on *E. coli* chemotaxis toward galactose using a soft agar technique. The former inhibitor nonspecifically reduced motility, growth, and chemotaxis. Chloramphenicol, on the other hand, was without great effect on the percentage of motile cells or on the rate of motility, although it delayed formation of the galactose ring. It was concluded that the chemotactic system for galactose was induced by incubation in the presence of this sugar. Chloramphenicol was thought to inhibit chemotaxis by preventing this induction.

The ease of obtaining and analyzing mutants has contributed to the popularity of *E. coli* in many field of research, and chemotaxis is no exception.

Armstrong *et al.* (1967) described isolation of 40 nonchemotactic mutants, all which had normal flagella, were fully motile when examined microscopically, and were sensitive to *chi* phage, a phage which attacks only motile bacteria. One mutant studied in detail was found to be completely nonchemotactic to oxygen, glucose, serine, threonine, and aspartic acid, although its ability to utilize all these compounds, as well as its growth characteristics, were identical with the wild type.

Armstrong and Adler (1969a,b) used the abortive transduction method to divide the nonchemotactic mutants into three complementation groups, *cheA*, *cheB*, and *cheC*. These complementation groups were distinct from nonflagellated (*fla*) or nonfunctional flagellated (*mot*) mutants. When the chemotactic genes were mapped, it was found that they were located near the *fla* and the structural gene for flagellin (*H*), although the occurrance of other genes in this area made it unlikely that those controlling chemotaxis and flagella synthesis and function were all part of the same operon. It is intriguing, however, to speculate that the chemotactic mechanism may be located on or near the flagella.

Hazelbauer *et al.* (1969) have studied in detail two mutants, one deficient in chemotaxis to L-serine and, to a lesser degree, to glycine, alanine, and cysteine (serine-blind); the other deficient in chemotaxis to D-galactose and related sugars including fucose, L-arabinose, xylose, and L-sorbose (galactose-blind). The serine-blind mutant did not have defects in uptake or oxidative metabolism of L-serine. The galactose-blind mutant, however, suffered a defect in the galactose uptake system, suggesting the existence of a common component between galactose uptake and chemotaxis. This was confirmed by the demonstration that chemotaxis to galactose is dependent on a galactose binding protein which is a common element in both chemotaxis and galactose uptake (Hazelbauer and Adler, 1971). Further work (Adler *et al.*, 1973) demonstrated the existence of 9 different sugar chemoreceptors in *E. coli*.

Mesibov and Adler (1972) pursued the effects of amino acids on chemotaxis in a wide-ranging study with *E. coli*. They found that the organism was attracted to the L-amino acids alanine, asparagine, aspartate, cysteine, glutamate, glycine, methiodine, serine, and threonine, but not to arginine, cystine, glutamine, histidine, isoleucine, leucine, lysine, phenylalanine, trypophan, tyrosine, or valine. Bacteria grown in a proline-containing medium were, in addition, attracted to proline. They found that chemotaxis toward amino acids is shown to be mediated by at least two detection systems, the aspartate and serine chemoreceptors. The aspartate chemoreceptor was nonfunctional in the aspartate taxis mutant, which showed virtually no chemotaxis toward aspartate, glutamate, or methionine and reduced taxis toward alanine, asparagine, cysteine, glycine, and serine. The serine chemo-receptor was nonfunctional in the serine taxis mutant, which was defective in taxis toward alanine, asparagine, cysteine, glycine, and serine and which showed no chemotaxis toward threonine.

The thrust of Adler's work (1969) has led to the conclusion that *E. coli* possesses specific receptors for specific chemicals and responds to external gradients of these chemicals rather than to products of their metabolism. It has been suggested (Clayton, 1964) that photosynthetic bacteria respond phototactically not to light per se but to the decrease in internal ATP which characterized the entering of a dark zone. The evidence that a similar mechanism does not work in *E. coli* chemotaxis may be summarized as follows. Some compounds which were extensively metabolized (glycerol) do not attract bacteria. Some compounds which are not metabolized do attract. (D-Fucose, a nonmetabolizable analogue of galactose, was found to be an attractant; mutants unable to utilize galactose did respond to it.) Bacteria are able to make a chemotactic response to one compound in the presence of a large excess of another which was extensively utilized for energy production. Structurally related compounds blocked chemotaxis to each other (if galactose were present in both the drop and micropipette in the Pfeffer assay, no chemotaxis to D-fucose in the micropipette would occur). Finally, certain mutants, such as the serine-blind mutant, were unable to respond to serine even though they were normal in ability to take up and metabolize this compound.

These experiments suggested the formal existence of discrete specific receptors for chemotactic response. In blocking experiments, a high concentration of one chemical was put in both the drop of bacterial suspension and the micropipette used in the Pfeffer assay. If the bacteria responded to a second chemical found only in the micropipette, it was said that the bacteria did not use the same receptor for both chemicals. Such experiments indicated existence of at least five receptors—galactose, glucose, ribose, aspartate, and serine—each receptor except glucose and ribose could also detect certain related compounds. The physical nature of the receptors remains unknown, although the possibility exists that they may be permeases.

An intriguing aspect of bacterial chemotaxis is the fact, reported by Pfeffer (1884) and abundantly confirmed since, that chemotaxis follows the Weber rule. This states that an organism will respond to a proportional change in concentration of effector rather than to an absolute concentration. One might find, for example, that cells suspended in 10^{-6} M attractant would respond to 10^{-5} M, whereas cells suspended in 10^{-5} M would respond to 10^{-4} M. It is clear that the concentration gradient over the length of a bacterium would be very small. As Adler (1969) has pointed out, however, it would not be necessary for a motile cell to detect a concentration gradient over its length if it could continually sample the medium as it moved and could detect changes in concentration with time.

F. Salmonella: Effects of Gradients

Dahlquist *et al.* (1972) studied chemotaxis in *Salmonella typhimurium* by imposing various gradients of serine on a uniform cell suspension in a tube. Concentrations of cells were quantitated by light scattering caused by projection of a laser beam through the length of the tube. It was concluded that the cells followed the Weber rule through a wide range of concentrations, although there was an element of dependence on absolute concentration. The cells tumbled less frequently while descending gradients of repellents or ascending gradients of attractants (Tsang *et al.*, 1973).

III. Chemotaxis in Plants

A number of reviews deal with chemotaxis in plants (Rosen, 1962; Ziegler, 1962; Shaffer, 1962; Machlis and Rawitscher-Kunkel, 1963).

A. Algae: Influence of Pheromones

Chemotaxis is involved in fertilization in some algae, apparently caused by the presence of pheromones. Cook *et al.* (1948) found that sperm of the marine alga *Fucus* were attracted to the eggs. The chemotactic principle surprisingly could be extracted from egg suspension by bubbling an inert gas through the suspensions. A number of hydrocarbons, particularly *n*-hexane, as well as some ethers and alcohols, mimicked the chemotactic factor (Cook and Elvidge, 1951). Attempts to determine the structure of the natural chemotactic factor using mass spectroscopy were not successful. Rawitscher–Kunkel and Machlis (1962) found that sperm in the green alga *Oedogonium* were attracted to a protoplasmic papilla which briefly protruded from the oogonial pore leading to the eggs. This would appear to be an example where chemotaxis aids movement of male gametes to a relatively hidden female gamete. Müller has described chemotaxis of male gametes of the brown alga *Ectocarpus siliculosus* toward an attractant produced by the female gamete (1967, 1968). The attractant was found to be highly volatile and was collected by passing an air stream through a suspension of female gametes followed with passage through a cold trap. Gas chromatography indicated that the attractant was a homogeneous substance. Male gametes in suspension reacted to the attractant by collecting at the meniscus. This process appeared to have elements of orientation of movement toward attractant as well as elements of trapping through movements in tight circles. (The attractant was found to have the odor of gin, the general significance of which is not clear). Its structure has been determined recently (Müller et al., 1971). Again, a number of organic compounds simulated the attractant. A possible chemotactic involvement in another brown alga *Giffordia* has been reported (Müller, 1969). Cultures of these organisms had a distinct sweet odor, although the odor was found in asexual as well as sexual cultures.

B. Cellular Slime Molds: Influence of Acrasin

Aggregation in the cellular slime mold *Dictyostelium discoideum* has long been a subject of study (for extensive review, see Shaffer, 1962), and it is appropriate that this provides one of the most exciting chapters in the field of chemotaxis today. The life cycle of this asexual organism may be said to begin as individual amoebae move about on a surface, eat bacteria, and multiply. When the bacteria are gone, individual cells aggregate into a pseudoplasmodium which moves about and, when in an appropriate place, stops and differentiates into a fruiting body, a structure with stalk cells supporting spores. These spores fall to the surface, germinate, and resume the individual amoeboid cell phase. Runyon (1942) reported that motile cells, separated by cellophane from aggregation centers, formed aggregates directly over the original aggregation centers. Bonner (1947) extended these observations and demonstrated in a rigidly controlled system the involvement of a soluble, diffusible chemotactic factor which he named acrasin. Despite extensive work, it is not known what initiates the formation of an aggregation center, although the territory or area of cells incorporated into one aggregate was found to be constant for each species and independent of the density of cells on the agar (Bonner and Dodd, 1962; Konijn, 1968). It has been suggested (Keller and Segel, 1970) that aggregation resulted from certain inhomogeneities invariably present in a uniform distribution of cells and did not reflect heterogeneity of the population. Shaffer (1956, 1957) presented theoretical considerations supporting the idea that an attractant would be most efficient if it were unstable and emitted in pulses. He also showed that acrasin was indeed unstable, apparently because of the production of an enzyme which caused its destruction. There also is some evidence that acrasin is emitted in pulses from the attracting center (Gerisch et al., 1966). This is based on the rhythmic movements of aggregating cells. A theoretical treatment of chemotaxis in response to pulses of acrasin has been presented by Cohen and Robertson (1971a,b). The first direct evidence for a role of acrasin pulses was offered by Robertson *et al.* (1972). They presented cells with periodic pulses of cAMP from an electrically controlled micropipette. These pulses seemed to entrain the cell movement and resulted in aggregate formation at the tip of the micropipette.

Konijn *et al.* (1967) reported that culture filtrates of *E. coli* had acrasin activity for preaggregation amoebae of *D. discoideum*, and an active compound could be isolated which had physical characteristics consistent with cAMP. Pure cAMP was found to have acrasin activity at low concentrations, and it was suggested that this compound might be the naturally occurring acrasin, particularly since the cells exhibited greatest sensitivity to it just before aggregation. It was later reported (Konijn, 1969) that a variety of bacteria would, under certain conditions, produce material that attracted preaggregative cells, and that the bacterial attractant at high concentrations caused dispersal of aggregates while even higher concentrations caused amoebae to stop moving. Further work (Konijn *et al.*, 1968) indicated that cAMP could be isolated from cultures of another cellular slime mold, *Polysphondylium pallidum*. It was suggested that difficulties in isolating this compound from *D. discoidium* was caused by the naturally occurring acrasinase which destroyed the cAMP as it was produced. Chang (1968) found that *D. discoidium* cultures contained a phosphodiesterase which catalyzed conversion of cAMP to 5-adenosine monophosphate. This enzyme seems to be primarily extracellular, since the amoebae contained only 4 % of the activity in the culture. A membrane-associated phosphodiesterase with a much lower Michaelis constant (15 μmoles *vs.* 2 mmoles) was reported by Pannbacker and Bravard (1972). Dithiothreitol inhibited this enzyme and thus enhanced cellular response to cAMP. Concurrent with this finding was the observation of Chassy (1972), who reported isolation of an extracellular phosphodiesterase of low Michaelis constant that was converted spontaneously to one of high constant. This conversion could be prevented in the presence of dithiothreitol.

Gerisch and associates (Riedel and Gerisch, 1971; Gerisch *et al.*, 1972) studied a specific phosphodiesterase inhibitor found in liquid cultures of *D. discoidium*. This inhibitor was shown to be an extracellular heat-stable protein of 40,000 daltons, the production of which is responsible for the observed decrease in phosphodiesterase activity in starving cells. A number of aggregation mutants had defects in the phosphodiesterase-inhibitor system. It was suggested that the function of the inhibitor is to control development in *D. discoidium*.

Other effects of cAMP included an increase in rate of cellular motility, increase in adhesion of cells to each other, inhibition of new aggregation center formation, and, in high concentrations, the formation of centers of reduced territory size. This work was made possible by a new technique for assay of acrasin activity (Konijn, 1970). In this assay, a drop containing sensitive amoebae was placed on specially washed hydrophobic agar and a drop containing the material to be tested placed adjacent to it. After incubation for 30–45 minutes, cells migrated outside the boundary of the original drop if acrasin were present in the test drop (Fig. 2). Low concentrations of acrasin caused the cells to collect at the margin of the drop, and very high concentrations caused the cells to migrate out of the drop in all directions, probably because high concentrations saturated the agar everywhere around the amoebae until a gradient was created by action of the acrasinase. The assay was made quantitative by diluting solutions to be tested until only a certain percentage of cells responded.

The success of this technique depended on careful pretreatment of the cells to obtain uniform populations at the most sensitive stage. A modification of this technique (Konijn *et al.*, 1968) involved incorporation of substances to be tested into an agar block which was placed on an agar plate among amoebae; cells streamed toward the block if acrasin were present. Ordinary agar could be used in this technique, although, again, sensitive cells were required.

A membrane filter method similar to that devised by Boyden (1962) may also be used to study *Dictyostelium* chemotaxis (Bonner *et al.*, 1971). Acrasin could be isolated from cultures of *D. dictystelium* (Barkley, 1969) by growing the amoebae on a dialysis membrane and collecting the cAMP which diffused through the membrane, thus excluding the diesterase. It was also shown that cAMP could be isolated from such cultures by absorption on ion-exchange resins. In each case, the acrasin was identified as cAMP by paper chromatography. A large number of compounds were tested for acrasin activity (Konijn *et al.*, 1969). The cyclic 3'–5'-monophosphates of guanosine, uridine, cytidine, inosine, and theymidine as well as tubercidin-3'–5'-cyclic monophosphate, N^6-2-O-dibutyl cAMP, and 5'-methyl cAMP had some

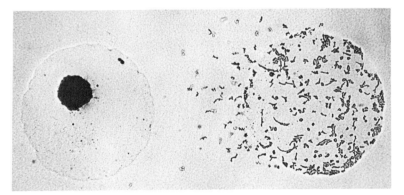

Fig. 2. Chemotaxis in *Dictyostelium discoideum*. The aggregation in the drop on the left attracts myxameobae outside the boundary of the drop on the right. From Konijn (1970).

activity but all were less active than cAMP. It was suggested that cAMP was first used to detect food bacteria, and then through evolution became involved in the mechanism of aggregation.

The acrasin work was summed up in a paper (Bonner *et al.*, 1969) which considered relationships between acrasin production, acrasin sensitivity, and acrasinase production during the life cycle of *D. discoidium*. At the onset of aggregation there is an increase of 100 times in both the production and sensitivity to acrasin. Acrasinase activity does not appear to vary over the life cycle however, although quantitative assay is difficult. The importance of acrasinase is indicated by the demonstration that antibody prepared against *D. discoidium* cAMP diesterase inhibited enzyme activity *in vitro* and inhibited amoeboid aggregation *in vivo* (Goidl *et al.*, 1972). Aggregationless mutants were found to be perpetually similar to vegetative amoebae in acrasin production and sensitivity. It was suggested that initiation of aggregation occurs when a few cells prematurely begin to produce acrasin in large amounts or when other cells become more sensitive to the attractant.

Bonner (1970) reported isolated unaggregated cells were stimulated to become differentiated stalk cells by high concentrations of cAMP (10^{-3} M). Acrasin production in the pseudoplasmodium was found only at the anterior end, the part which eventually becomes the stalk. It was suggested that cAMP may nonspecifically stimulate catabolism and thus lead to differentiation. Evidence for a second attractant in *E. coli* filtrates, which specifically attracts vegetative amoebae, has been presented (Bonner *et al.*, 1970). This new attractant is heat-stable, nondialyzable, negatively charged, and inactivated by an enzyme produced by the amoebae. This attractant, identified recently as folic acid (Pan *et al.*, 1972), was thought to be involved in food gathering, whereas cAMP serves as acrasin. Murray *et al.* (1971) examined the phosphodiesterases of the acellular slime mold *Physarum polycephalum* and found two distinct enzymes, one associated with particles in the mycelium and another soluble and excreted into the medium. These enzymes exhibited different patterns of kinetics and inhibition. The biological role of the soluble enzyme was believed to be to destroy cAMP, which might be found in the environment, and thus prevent this compound from interfering with normal differentiation. Production of this "acrasinase" in a nonchemotactic acellular slime mold suggests a possible second role for acrasinase in the cellular slime molds. A survey of 7 slime molds (Bonner *et al.*, 1972) supports this view (see also Konijn and Koevenig, 1971).

C. *Phycomycetes: Milling; Influence of Plant Roots and Sirenin*

There has been a good deal of recent work on chemotaxis of plant pathogen *Phycomycete* zoospores toward the roots of host plants (Dukes and Apple,

1961; Turner, 1963; Zentmyer, 1966; Ho and Hickman, 1967; Schmidt, 1963; Rai and Strobel, 1966; Spencer and Cooper, 1967; Bimpong and Clerk, 1970). In general, zoospores were found to respond to roots of the natural hosts (as well as to nonhosts), to exudates and extracts from roots, and to sugars and amino acids found in root exudates. Royle and Hickman (1964a,b) have analyzed in detail chemotaxis of *Pythium aphanidermatum* to pea roots. Zoospores which reached the roots attached to the root hairs, encysted, and then germinated with the germ tube directed toward the source of attractant. In the absence of attractant, zoospores swam about at random. When attractant was present, they apparently oriented their paths toward the source; as cells approached they began to move in a jerky, disjointed, and looping fashion called milling. The behavior of individual cells under influence of attractant was very complex, although elements of directed motility and trapping appeared to be involved. Of the substances tested, only glutamic acid and casein hydrolysate, plus some sugars, caused milling, although dilution experiments made it clear that the activity of root exudate could not be accounted for by its glutamic acid content alone.

Study of chemotaxis in the water mold *Allomyces* has led to a fascinating story of attraction on two levels. In the life cycle of this organism there are five motile forms. The diploid plant produces motile diploid mitospores as well as motile haploid meiospores. Meiospores form haploid plants which produce both motile male and female zoospores. Formation of a motile zygote leads to the diploid plant. Female zoospores produce an attractant for male zoospores called sirenin (Machlis, 1958). In a monumental accomplishment, 2.5 g of sirenin were isolated (Machlis *et al.*, 1966) and its structure determined by mass spectroscopy and nuclear magnetic resonance (NMR) (Machlis *et al.*, 1968). Male zoospores responded to sirenin at concentrations from 10^{-10}–$10^{-5} M$, apparently by orientation toward the source, although there is a suggestion of an avoiding reaction. Sirenin is inactivated by male gametes (Carlile and Machlis, 1965a). Further work on these organisms (Machlis, 1969a; Carlile and Machlis, 1965b) indicates that all motile forms except gametes respond chemotactically to casein hydrolysate, owing to L-leucine and L-lysine in the hydrolysate. Within 5 minutes after formation, zygotes also responded to amino acids (Machlis, 1969b), Thus, two gametes (one responding to sirenin but neither sensitive to amino acids) form a zygote which within 5 minutes responds to amino acids.

D. Ferns: Influence of Malic Acid

Rothschild (1956) has reviewed the role of chemotaxis in fertilization in lower plants. Bracken fern sperm responded to malic acid, but not to fumarate and succinate, and Rothschild suggested that the *cis* form is necessary for activity. Brokaw (1958a,b) examined cheomtaxis of bracken sperm to malic acid in a pH gradient and found that chemotaxis occured only in the pH range in which the *cis* bimalate ion predominated, rather than the *trans* malic acid or malate ion. He also derived formula for determining the concentration of material diffusing from a capillary tube and suggested the mechanism of chemotaxis might involve electrochemical orientation of the cells toward the high concentration end of a chemical gradient.

IV. Chemotaxis in Lower Animal Forms

Some reviews of interest include Allen (1961), Dryl and Grebecki (1966), Sandon (1963), and Jahn and Bovee (1964, 1967, 1969). These articles, however, are in the main about cell motility, treating chemotaxis only in passing. The pioneering papers of Jennings (1904) and a later somewhat broader treatment by the same author (Jennings, 1906) are highly recommended.

A. Amoeba: Scavenging

In a series of impressive papers, Jeon and Bell have presented the first picture of positive chemotaxis in an amoeba, *Amoeba proteus*. This organism was shown to respond to portions of *Hydra* or *Tetrahymena* (Jeon and Bell, 1962) or to heparin solution (Bell and Jeon, 1962), although later work suggested that the response to heparin was caused by contamination (Jeon and Bell, 1965). The response took the form of local production of pseudo-pods in the region nearest attractant when pieces or extracts of *Hydra* were presented with a micromanipulator (Fig. 3). Such pseudopods formed on the rear as well as the front of the cell, on forming or retreating pseudopods, in all cases without affecting cytoplasmic flow in old pseudopods. Such behavior led Bell (1961) to suggest that the key feature in ameobid movement is the production of a new membrane on the pseudopod. Bingley *et al.* (1962) found that the relative electrical potential inside *A. proteus* was negative with respect to the medium. This potential was reduced when cells were bathed with chemotactic solutions, and it was suggested that chemotaxis might be correlated with local depolarization of the cell owing to chemotactic stimuli. This idea was supported by discovery (Bingley and Thompson, 1962) of a potential gradient within the cell, with the pseudopod top positive with respect to the rest of the cell. A negative potential applied at the rear of the cell caused movement away from the electrode whereas a positive potential had the opposite effect. When large portions of hydra were placed on a slide among an

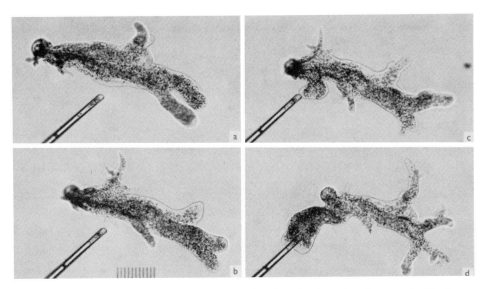

Fig. 3. Serial photographs to show an amoeba forming a local pseudopod toward the tip of a hydra-containing fine glass pipette. Note the initial thin hyaline pseudopods in picture b. Scale interval, 10 μm. From Jeon and Bell (1965).

even suspension of *A. proteus*, the cells were observed to move toward the hydra fragments and to form food cups around them (Jeon and Bell, 1965). Water extracts of fresh or dried hydra induced pseudopod formation; amoebae immersed in such extracts lost motility and irregularily projected and retracted blunt pseudopods. Attempts to enhance the release of attractant from hydra using proteolytic enzymes led to the discovery that a substance in crude papain induced pseudopod formation. A high molecular weight, water-soluble active fraction was isolated. It contained protein, was without proteolytic action, reacted with heparin (suggesting a basic protein), migrated as one band on electrophoresis, and contained a high percentage of basic amino acids. The papain extract was labeled with fluorescein dye and demonstrated to attach only to the cell surface. It was also shown (Jeon and Bell, 1964) that this material could be removed from the cell surface by treatment with neuraminidase and trypsin and by forcing pseudopods into capillary tubes, supporting the idea that the papain extract absorbed to the mucous coat rather than the cell membrane. Brewer and Bell (1969) determined the effect on *Amoeba* of long-chain charged compounds, on the supposition that these molecules might affect the lipid portion of the cell membrane. Cationic quaternary ammonium compounds and succinyl dicholine in agar at 10^{-3} M induced pseudopod formation. All active compounds were positively charged, although many positively charged molecules were not active. Because the effect was reversible and did not seem to depend solely on chain length, it was suggested that the compounds absorbed on the mucous coat.

McIntyre and Jenkin (1969) have studied chemotaxis in the free-living amoeba *Hartmannella rhysodes* using a modification of the Boyden method for determining chemotaxis. This amoeba was attracted to intact bacteria or cell walls of *Pseudomonas fluorescens*. Incubation of bacteria with intact amoebae or amoeba extracts gave enhanced chemotactic activity, suggesting that the amoebae excreted material, presumably enzymatic, that increased the ability of bacteria to be an attractant.

B. *Paramecium: Avoiding Reaction*

In a series of classic papers (1904), Jennings developed the idea of the avoiding reaction to account for chemotactic behavior of a number of micro-organisms, including *Paramecium*. These animals were observed to swim about at random in gently curving lines; after moving into an unfavorable region they were found to stop, back up (and in the process turn to the aboral side), and resume forward movement in a new direction. Thus the animals were said to accumulate in favorable areas by avoiding unfavorable ones. One would have positive chemotaxis if the unfavorable region were down the gradient of the attractant and negative chemotaxis if the unfavorable region were up the gradient of the repellent. Jennings suggested this avoiding reaction might allow animals to collect in regions where food organisms had caused the water to become slightly acidic. He was unable, however, to relate chemotaxis to avoidance of toxic regions. Dryl (1952) found that paramecia exhibited avoiding reactions at pH outside the range 5.2–6.2. The pH extremes causing 50 % deaths were 4.6 and 9.1. The chemotactic effect of a number of salts was shown to be due to their effect on pH. When a series of homologous alcohols was tested (Dryl, 1959a), it was found, with one exception, that the most toxic caused the greatest avoiding reactions. Thus within closely related compounds there was a relationship between avoiding reactions and toxicity. Of greater interest was the discovery (Dryl, 1959b) that incubation of animals for 24 hours in solutions of $MgCl_2$, NaCl, or with greatest effect KCl prevented subsequent chemotaxis. These ions, as it turned out, affected motility in a quite unexpected manner (Dryl, 1961). Chemotaxis was determined by suspending the animals in water on a glass plate inscribed with a grid. Side-lighting provided a dark-field effect which was recorded by long exposure photography. Solutions to be tested were added to the suspension of animals over various grids which, after allowing time for the animals to react, we rephotographed. When KCl was tested in this manner, high counts suggested positive chemotaxis, but it became apparent that animals entering the high KCl region were becoming trapped owing to reduced motility. It was found (Dryl, 1963) that animals in KCl not only exhibited the normal range of behavior of swimming in long gentle curves and avoiding reactions, but in addition often made a motor response which lasted 4–5 seconds at a time and consisted of rotations around the transverse axis of the body. In an extensive review (Dryl and Grebecki, 1966), a number of new types of movements (partial, periodic, and continuous ciliary reversal) caused by various ionic concentrations are described and the relationships among the ionic environment, resting potential within the animals, and ciliary movement are discussed.

In the same manner, Naitoh and Kaneko (1972) treated paramecia with a detergent and determined the relationship between ciliary behavior and concentration of Ca^{2+} ions. They reported normal beating of cilia at less than $10^{-6}\ M\ Ca^{2+}$, but reversal of the beat above this concentration. Eckert (1972) correlated these results with studies on the membrane potential. Mechanical, electrical, or chemical stimulation of the cells caused depolarization of the membrane and a simultaneous increase in intracellular Ca^{2+} ions. This, in turn, caused a shift in the direction and an increase in the frequency of ciliary beat, resulting in an avoiding reaction. Hyperpolarization of the membrane caused an increase in beat frequency in the normal direction. Each step of the response was graded so that the degree of response reflected the intensity of stimulation.

C. Euglena: Avoiding Reaction

Bessis and Burté (1964) noted that laser irradiation of a suspension of *Euglena* caused animals to move away from a killed cell. The mechanism for this negative chemotaxis appeared to be an avoiding reaction similar to that found in paramecia.

D. Hydroids: Specificity of Pheromones

Miller and Nelson (1962; Miller, 1966a) have described the role of chemotaxis in fertilization in the hydroids *Campanularia* and *Tubularia* and have produced evidence to show a more precise role for pheromones. In these organisms, eggs are contained in a funnel-shaped gonangium which has only a few openings through which sperm could pass; it would not be surprising, therefore, to find chemotaxis involved. In the case of the hydroid *Gonothyrea* (Miller 1970), the eggs are located at the base of the tentacles. Sperm were attracted to the female, stuck to the tentacles, and began to migrate along them. Those sperm migrating toward the tentacle tip continued up one side and down the other. Occasionally, sperm were observed to change direction without apparent reason. Chemotactic reactions between sperm and extracts from female animals were specific between species of the same genus; there was some cross reaction between the three genera. Alcoholic extracts of the female animals were prepared and analyzed by gel filtration (Miller, 1966b). *Campanularia* and *Tubularia* yielded distinct single peaks of molecular weight 600 and 240, respectively. Two peaks of activity were found from *Gonothyrea*.

In further studies of chemotaxis in *Campanularia* (Miller, 1966c), movies were made of sperm as they approached a source of attractant. Sperm were found to swim normally in gentle curves or, when in contact with a surface, in circles. In the presence of attractant the sperm began to increase speed and to describe tight circles (Fig. 4). There was no consistent behavior on the part of every sperm; many swam away from the attractant. Nevertheless, many

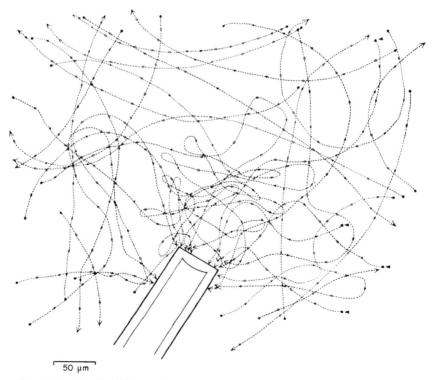

50 µm

Fig. 4. Plotted trails of *Campanularia* sperm and pipette injecting an active extract of female gonangia. Solid circles represent start of each trail and open circles are ten frames (0.45 second) apart. From Miller (1966c).

sperm made turns which resulted in contact with the gonangium. Miller and Brokaw (1970) examined chemotaxis in individual *Tubularia* sperm using stroboscopic illumination and time-exposure photography. These cells were in contact with a glass slide, and the behavior observed may not have corresponded with that of cells suspended in water. It was concluded that chemotactic behavior under these conditions could be explained by assuming that a sperm decreased the radius of curvature of its path on entering a region of decreasing concentration of attractant. Sometimes the sperm also reacted on approaching the source of attractant; the explanation offered that such turns might cause an even more rapid approach to the sources seems unlikely, as such turns would also cause the sperm to move away from the attractant.

V. Tissue Culture Studies: Chemotactic Factors in Tumors

Chemotaxis has been suggested as a factor in the movement of some cells in tissue culture. Twitty and Niu (Twitty, 1944; Twitty and Niu, 1948, 1954) found that newt melanophores in tissue culture moved faster when confined under a glass coverslip. (See discussion of locomotion in Section VI, A, 1.) Further experiments with individual cells in capillary tubes indicated that cells moved away from each other, but the experiment may be subject to the hazards of the capillary tube technique (Pfoehl, 1898; see discussion in Harris, 1954). Twitty and Niu interpreted the result as a reflection of negative chemotaxis to metabolic products. However, they found that chick heart fibroblasts and neural crest cells, not thought to be chemotactic, exhibited the same behavior as the melanophores. (See discussion of negative chemotaxis in Section VI,4.) Somewhat similar observations on cultures of leukocytes were reported by Oldfield (1963). Outgrowth of chick leukocytes from adjacent explants of clots appeared to avoid a "no man's land" between the explants, and negative chemotaxis was postulated as the mechanism to explain this. There were, however, no direct observations to chart the movements of the cells. [For additional comment on experiments of this type, see Trinkaus (1969).]

Recent work from Hayashi's laboratory has led to the isolation of a pseudoglobulin fraction, 70,000 MW from some tumor tissues which is said to be chemotactic for cancer cells (Hayashi *et al.*, 1970; Yoshida *et al.*, 1970; Ozaki *et al.*, 1971). The material was said to be similarly active for rat ascites hepatoma AH109A cells, mouse ascites hepatoma MH134 cells, and mouse myeloid leukemia C-1498 cells, which suggested to the investigators a common chemotactic action. It was not chemotactic for neutrophils, as judged by Boyden chamber studies. Intracutaneous injection of the protein into rats and mice caused local accumulation of circulating tumor cells. It was hypothesized that the cancer cell chemotactic factor might be associated with malignant invasion. The work merits critical evaluation and confirmation in other assay systems.

VI. Chemotaxis in White Blood Cells

A. *In Vitro Studies*

1. LOCOMOTION AND CHEMOTAXIS

Dixon and McCutcheon (1936) analyzed the chemotactic movements of neutrophils in clotted blood and concluded that chemotaxis was a function only of directional movement and was without effect on cell speed. This generalization was supported by Ramsey, who analyzed movements of large numbers of isolated neutrophils (1972a), showing that individual cells could respond quickly and repeatedly to shifts in the location of the attractant source. Cells moved by extending a flat empty membrane (lamellipodium) along the substratum into which the cell contents flowed, in agreement with earlier studies by Robineaux (1964). No differences in the mechanism of locomotion in the presence and absence of chemotactic materials were revealed by high magnification cinemicrographs (Ramsey, 1972b). The lamellipodia seemed to be extended at random on all sides of the cells. Chemotaxis was characterized by preferential flow into lamellipodia on the side of the attractant.

The rate of movement of white cells toward an attractant is difficult to calculate. The cells do not approach the attractant by continuous uninterrupted movement, but make their way toward chemotactic materials in a more or less apparently haphazard start and go fashion. From an extended or spread position on the glass surface, the cell first protrudes up into the medium, creating a hump as it prepares to take a step. During this phase, there is no movement forward. From the protruded or humped up position, the cell extends a fold of membrane into which cytoplasmic contents flow, reducing the height of the protrusion. Finally, with most of the cell material in what started out as the new membrane fold, the cell, having advanced one step, then flattens out to its original spread position. This cycle is then repeated. Some students of locomotion exclude the immobile cells in calculating rates of movement. Also, speed of movement is controlled in part by environmental conditions, certain media, such as serum, tending to promote movement, in contrast to other media, such as Gey's solution, with albumin, in which movement is slower. Dixon and McCutcheon found that neutrophils moved at an average speed of $33 + 8$ μm/minute in clotted whole blood, in agreement with von Phillipsborn (1925, 1928, 1930, 1957, cited by Dittrich, 1962), who used siliconized glass slides and found a rate of migration for neutrophils of 34–37 μm/minute or about 3mm/hour. Ramsey, however, in a study of white cell movement on a glass slide with a cover slip some distance above the cells themselves, so as to avoid compression, found neutrophils moving a serum at a rate of $10 \pm 1\mu$m/minute and in Gey's solution with 2% bovine serum albumin at 6.5 ± 1 μm/minute. Cliff (1966b) observed the rate of movement of white blood cells in rabbit ear chambers and found the average speed to be 7.4 ± 0.9 μm/minute. In studies of the upward movement of white blood cells, taken from a buffy coat, in capillary tubes, Ketchel *et al.* (1958) reported a wide variation in the average motility of leukocytes from various individual donors. It is not clear, however, whether the technique permitted statements about individual variations in movement or simply noted the end result of movement, that is, a mass migration proceeding more or less in one direction but without taking into account possible free myriad movements within the mass.

Bryant and his colleagues (1966) pursued this question with a modification of the microhematocrit method described originally by Ketchel and Favour (1955) to permit an evaluation of the separate effects of leukocyte adhesiveness, intrinsic cell motility, and leukocyte clumping. Among other things, they found that leukocyte motility is unimpaired by wide variations in glucose, electrolyte, and hydrogen ion concentrations, in accord with the observations of Lotz and Harris (1956) that migration increased with increasing temperatures over a range of 25° to 40°C, that adhesion to glass required the presence of magnesium ion, was totally independent of calcium ion, and was partially dependent on heat-labile plasma factors. They noted that serum or plasma factors necessary for leukocyte migration in glass capillary tubes were heat sensitive and hydrazine sensitive but differed from complement as classically defined. They suggested that such factors appeared to resemble the heat-labile noncomplement opsonic substances which facilitate ingestion of microbes by leukocytes (Hirsch and Church, 1960; Cohn and Morse, 1960). They added that the function of serum factor or factors may be related more to cellular adherence to glass than to intrinsic cell motility; leukocyte adhesion to the sides of capillary tubes was reduced in heated serum, whereas individual cell motility observed on horizontal surfaces was only slightly impaired. They made the interesting observation that leukocyte migration was significantly reduced after phagocytosis of viable coagulase-positive, heat-killed, and coagulase-negative staphylococci, as well as after ingestion by the white blood cells of latex particles. It was noted that the literature contains few references to reduced leukocyte migration following phagocytosis, among them Allgower and Block (1949) and Martin *et al.* (1950) who showed that the ingestion of tubercle bacilli resulted in decrease leukocyte motility and cell aggregation.

Martin and Chaudhuri (1952) reported that leukocyte migration was inhibited by purified products obtained from gram-negative bacteria but intact staphylococci or pneumococci were without effect. It was felt that the system employed by these investigators would not favor phagocytosis, and effects noted were not attributed to phagocytosis. In Bryant's experiments, inhibition of leukocyte migration in capillary tubes following phagocytosis was mediated both by cellular aggregation and by decreased intrinsic cellular motility. Individual nonaggregated cells were observed to move at reduced rates following phagocytosis. Decrease in individual cell motility was directly proportional to the number of bacteria ingested. Cohn and Morse (1960) demonstrated increase leukocyte oxygen consumption, glucose utilization, and phagocytic activity after ingestion of staphylococci, and similar effects were described following ingestion of polystyrene, latex, and starch particles (Sbarra and Karnovsky, 1959; Strauss and Stetson, 1960). As Bryant pointed out, since cell motility is decreased as gross indices of cellular metabolism are increased, phagocytosis may divert cellular energy stores from motility to the more important functions of particle ingestion and destruction. Increasing cellular metabolism, decreasing motility, and cellular aggregation, following phagocytosis, may favor localization and concentration of neutrophils in areas of bacterial invasion.

2. ATTRACTANTS OF WHITE BLOOD CELLS

a. BACTERIAL ATTRACTANTS, Keller and Sorkin (1967c) analyzed the chemotactic relationships among bacterial culture supernatents, washed bacterial walls, endotoxin, and complement. Culture supernatents of *Staphylococcus albus* and *Escherichia coli* were dialyzable attractants which did not require the presence of serum and therefore were presumably complement free. These results were confirmed by Ramsey (1972a). Washed *S. albus* and *E. coli* cells, as well as various endotoxin preparations, required fresh serum for activity. Ward *et al.* (1968) extended the work on culture supernatent fluids by showing that chemotactic activity was a function of the density of bacterial growth and resided in a compound of less than 3600 MW. Konijn's evidence, noted above, that culture filtrates of *E. coli* produced a compound that had the characteristics of cAMP led Leahy *et al.* (1970) to study cAMP as an attractant for rabbit neutrophils. They found cAMP in a concentration of 10^{-5} M to be chemotactic for the white cells in the absence of serum. The Boyden technique was used and the optimum cAMP concentration gave positive results in only 14 of 24 trials, the number of cells responding to the specific attractant being less than those responding to casein. Gamow *et al.* (1971) and Ramsey (1972a) found cAMP to be chemotactic for horse and human neutrophils, respectively. In Gamow's slide culture technique, which included the use of a capillary tube, buffy coat cells in serum were used, leaving open the possibility that complement could be activated in this system. Ramsey's technique was complement-free. It should be noted that Wissler *et al.* (1972c) were unable to find any chemotactic activity for cAMP per se *in vitro*.

b. ROLE OF COMPLEMENT IN CHEMOTAXIS. 1. *The Boyden chamber.* Virtually all recent work on complement and chemotaxis stems from Boyden's seminal paper in which the membrane filter technique for determining chemotaxis was introduced (Boyden, 1962; see also a review, Boyden *et al.*, 1965). In the Boyden technique, leukocytes are allowed to settle on a membrane filter separating them from a chamber containing material to be tested as attractant. Chambers are incubated for 1 to 3 hours and the filters fixed, stained, cleared, and the cells which migrated through (or sometimes into) the filter counted. It is perhaps prophetic that in the original paper the filter pore size was omitted, apparently through an oversight. One group of workers feels that 0.65 μm filters should be used for PMN experiments and 3 μm filters for other leukocytes. They found high control counts when larger pore sizes were used with PMN's. In various experiments, these workers have counted only the PMN which migrated all the way through to the opposite side of the filter (Ward *et al.*, 1965) or those cells which migrated into the filter (Ward and Becker, 1970a). Another group believes better results were obtained when 3 μm filters were used with PMN and only those cells which migrated all the way through the filter counted (Stecher and Sorkin, 1969; Keller and Sorkin, 1967b). In either case, the results were expressed as cells per microscopic field or as a ratio between cells per field in control and experimental chambers rather than as absolute numbers. Little consideration has been given to the possibility that cells might migrate through the filter and drop off the other side or that cells might lyse and thereby be lost to the experiment.

Keller, indeed, addressed himself to this question recently after noting in conventional Boyden chambers that cells that had migrated through the filter do not in fact stick firmly to the lower side as had been assumed (Keller *et al.*, 1972; Keller, 1972). He claims to have gotten around this bit of awkwardness, with some ease, by placing under the cell-permeable filter a second filter with a pore size of 0.45 mμ, which is too small to permit cell passage. This enables him to count all the neutrophils which have migrated through the filter by adding the number of cells found on the lower surface of the upper filter to the cells which have accumulated on top of the lower filter. He found that this caused a striking shift in cell counts gained by the conventional technique because the average loss of cells in such a system, during a 3-hour incubation period, amounted to 50% of the neutrophils that had actually passed through the filter.

The most fundamental question that can be raised about the Boyden technique concerns the proportion of cells placed on the filter that actually respond to attractant. Observation of chemotaxis in PMN on glass microscope slides indicates that essentially every cell responds (Harris, 1953a; Ramsey, 1972a). Photographs of filters after chemotaxis however, show that only about 20 % of the cells placed on the filter migrated to the other side (Ward et al., 1965; Ward, 1968). Indeed, slices of membrane filters after chemotaxis (Fig. 5) show that while many cells were distributed throughout the filter, large numbers remained on the upper surface (Synderman et al., 1968). The failure of most cells to migrate into the filter did not appear to be a function of length of incubation, as migration leveled off with time (Ward, 1968).

It has been suggested that chemotaxis by the Boyden technique really reflected increased random migratory activity (Spector and Willoughby, 1963). This seems unlikely since experiments in which attractant was placed on both sides of the filter resulted in low counts (Boyden, 1962). In most experiments, leukocytes have been collected from the rabbit peritoneal cavity after injection of a glycogen or casein solution. Thus the cells may be thought of as having already made a chemotactic response, and it has been suggested that most of these cells may have exhausted a component necessary for further response (Becker and Ward, 1969). Other experiments suggest that this is not the whole answer, since PMN collected from peripheral blood without intervention of a chemotactic stimulus still did not all respond in Boyden chambers (Carruthers, 1966; Ward and Becker, 1970b). It is to be noted, however, that in the study by Ward and Becker, comparing chemotactic responsiveness of exudate neutrophils and blood neutrophils, there was a slightly greater responsiveness of the cells taken from peripheral blood. In addition, experiments demonstrating the reversal of direction of chemotaxis indicate individual cells are able to undergo repeated chemotactic responses (Cornely, 1966; Ramsey, 1972a).

Zigmond and Hirsch (1973) have made an extensive study of the Boyden technique in comparison with slide culture methods. They feel that the most reliable results are obtained if one measures the advancing front of cells into the filter, rather than counting cells which emerge from the filter. Their discovery that some substances stimulate locomotion in low concentrations and inhibit it in high concentrations is of particular interest, as it suggests that the lack of migration in Boyden chambers observed when attractant is on both sides of the filter may in some cases be due to locomotion effects. On the other hand, Gallin et al. (1973) claimed the greatest accuracy for a technique that involved 51 CR-labeling of granulocytes and the counting of radioactivity in a double membrane filter system.

2. *Evidence for a role for complement in chemotaxis.* Müller-Eberhard (1968, 1969, 1971) has reviewed the subject of serum complement. This system consists of 11 serum globulins which are normally inactive enzymes

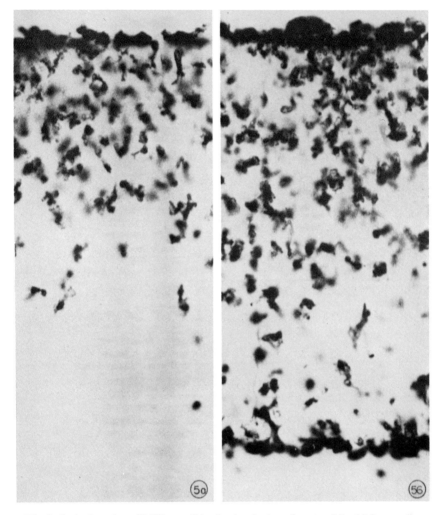

Fig. 5. Sagittal section of Millipore disk after incubation of neutrophils. (a) Serum alone. (b) Chemotactic factor generated by LPS and serum. Top of figure represents surface on which neutrophils were applied while bottom of figure represents counting surface. × 655. From Snyderman *et al.* (1968).

(with the exception of the first component which is normally active). In the presence of an antigen–antibody reaction, the first component, C1, reacts to cause the sequential activation of the remaining components, which results in lysis of a susceptible cell. In addition, there is a second system ("alternate") which activates C3 without the involvement of C1, C2 and C4 (Sandberg *et al.*, 1970; Frank *et al.*, 1971). Active components are indicated by a bar, as C3̄. Fragments of components are designated with small letters, as C5a. Several components may form complexes, as C5,6,7. Individuals of various animals have been found with genetic complement deficiencies, e.g., human C2 (Polley and Müller-Eberhard, 1967), guinea pig C4 (Frank et al., 1971), mouse C5 (Cinader et al., 1964; Nilsson and Müller-Eberhard, 1965), man C5 (Miller and Nillson, 1970), and rabbit C6 (Rother et al., 1966). Heating serum at 56°C for 30 minutes destroys substantial complement activity, but this is nonspecific inasmuch as heating may also affect other components of the serum.

Delaunay et al. (1951) reported that complement may play a role in chemotaxis. They observed movement of leukocytes on a slide toward starch granules in the presence of serum and found that chemotaxis was prevented by heating the serum at 56°C for 30 minutes. Lotz and Harris (1956), however, challenged these findings, as discussed below. Boyden (1962) reported that rabbit PMN were attracted to a number of proteins and other nondialyzable molecules with these materials phylogenetically most distant from the rabbit the most active. The response was greatly increased if the material was in the presence of corresponding antibody, and this activity was not found if the serum in both parts of the Boyden chamber had been heated at 56°C for 30 minutes. Heating the serum after the antibody–antigen reaction had taken place was without effect on chemotactic activity. Virtually all subsequent workers have used some modification of Boyden's technique.

Hurley (1963, 1964) incubated minced liver or granulocytes with serum and tested the serum for chemotactic activity in Boyden chambers and for activity in causing in vivo migration of rat leukocytes. There was a parallelism between these activities. Serum incubated in the absence of tissues or granulocytes was without either activity. Hill and Ward (1969) confirmed these findings and showed the chemotactic factor to be a fragment of C3, cleaved by the action of a neutral tissue protease present in most normal tissues.

Chemotaxis toward serum which had been incubated with antigen–antibody complexes or aggregated human γ globulin was reported by Keller and Sorkin (1965a). Again this activity could be prevented by heating serum before but not after incubation, although complement activity, in the sense of complement fixation, was not necessary for chemotaxis. Complement fixation alone did not induce chemotaxis; treatment of serum so as to prevent subsequent complement fixation did not inhibit induction of chemotactic activity. Further work (Keller and Sorkin, 1965b) indicated that a variety of fresh normal sera were chemotactic after incubation with complexes of human serum albumin and rabbit antibody. Activity also resulted from incubation of fresh normal rabbit serum with heat-aggregated γ globulin, PPD, glycogen, Proteus endotoxin, or heat-killed S. albus (inactive in heated serum or the absence of serum), although a peptone was chemotactic in the absence of serum. It was concluded that serum components were required for chemotaxis in all cases except that of peptone.

Miles (1969) found that interaction of sera from precolostal germ-free piglets with rough strains of *E. coli* resulted in complement fixation and generation of chemotactic activity. Such activity was complement dependent and, since antibodies do not pass the pig placenta, independent of antibodies. Harvey *et al*. (1970) found that protein A, a wall protein from staphylococci, generated a complement-dependent chemotactic activity for PMN. A complement-dependent activity for macrophages was generated by heat-killed *Mycobacterium tuberculosis* (Symon *et al*., 1972). This factor was more attractive for macrophages than for neutrophils. Walker *et al*. (1969) isolated a protein from *S. aureus* supernatent which is nondialyzable and heat labile, depends on serum for its activity, and which is an attractant for rabbit neutrophils.

Keller and Sorkin (1967c) introduced the term cytotaxin for substances chemotactic for leukocytes and cyotaxigen for substances which induced the formation of cytotaxins (see also review, Keller and Sorkin, 1968b). It is helpful to keep this distinction in mind, although these terms are not in general usage.

3. *C567*. Ward *et al*. (1965) were the first to examine the various components of complement for chemotactic activity. Intact antibody was required for generation of antigen–antibody induced activity. Chemotactic factor was not generated in mouse and rabbit sera genetically deficient in C5 and C6, respectively; complement-deficient rabbit serum became active, however, if human C6 were added. The first four complement components were chemotactically inactive whereas C5 and C6 became active after incubation with the first four components and an antigen–antibody complex. The C5,6 behaved as a complex and could be isolated. Further work (Ward *et al*., 1966) indicated a parallel between ability of *N*-CBZ-glycyl-L-phenylalanine and *N*-CBZ-α-glutamyl-L-tyrosine to inhibit formation of chemotactic activity in serum, cause loss of preformed activity, and cause dissociation of C5,6. Evidence for involvement of C7 in this complex was also presented.

Keller and Sorkin (1967a) activated serum by incubation with aggregated bovine γ globulin and fractionated the serum by gel filtration. Activity was found in fractions other than that expected for C567 complex. Activity for PMN was found in two fractions, both different from the one fraction active for monocytes. In addition, later work (Stecher and Sorkin, 1969) using C6-deficient individual or pooled rabbit sera indicated there were no differences between these sera and normal sera in ability to generate chemotactic activity. Inclusion of rabbit anti-C6 antibody into normal serum did not reduce the amount of activity. It is not clear why these results should be so diametrically opposed to those of Ward *et al*. (1965). Yet the studies of

Ward and his colleagues (1965, 1966) would seem to indicate that chemo-tactic activity generated in serum by immune complexes is C5-C6-C7-de-pendent. The work of Stecher and Sorkin (1969) indicates that activity can be generated in sera lacking C6. These discrepancies are hardly surprising in view of the new knowledge of the complement system. There are two sequential pathways for activation: one requiring, the other independent of, $C\overline{142}$. Additionally, a heterogeneity of complement-derived chemotactic factors exists and all are derivatives either of C3 or C5, with or without C6 and C7. Thus it is now known that C5 cleavage products with chemotactic activity can be produced in C4-deficient guinea pig serum. Perhaps in the case of C5 or C6 deficiency, C3 will substitute in the formation of chemotactic activity. The realization of the complexities of the complement system and the various ways by which factors can be generated suggest that what on the surface appear to be irreconcilable differences may all eventually fall into an understandable perspective. It is by no means clear, of course, that when this perspective unfolds there will stand a case for complement as the dominant, or possibly even significant, controlling mechanism in chemotaxis. Yet no matter how the complement story is pieced together ultimately, whether as a relevant mechanism in chemotaxis or not, there is no doubt that the elegant biochemistry that this system has stimulated in the last decade has opened up a productive and important area of biomedical research. The cell–cell inter-relationships in the complement story surely have added new dimensions to the exploration of molecular biology.

4. *C3 fragments.* Taylor and Ward (1967) reported a new chemotactic activity by the action of plasminogen and streptokinase on rabbit serum. Plasminogen is a trypsinlike enzyme active in blood clotting and strepto-kinase is a proteolytic enzyme from streptococci. These enzymes were active only in a certain concentration ratio and also destroyed the chemotactic activity of $C\overline{567}$ complex. This was thought to be an example of a nonimmune reaction in which a foreign protein may change the normal function of blood proteins. Additional work indicated that streptokinase plus purified human plasminogen could release a chemotactic factor from C3 (Ward, 1967). The active fragment was shown to consist of about 4% of the intact C3 molecule and differed from the $C\overline{567}$ complex in several respects. The molecular weight of C3a was about 6000, passed dialysis membranes, was heat labile, and had a higher electrophoretic mobility than $C\overline{567}$. It is interesting to note in this regard that Borel and Sorkin (1969; see also Wilkinson *et al.*, 1969) found differences between plasma and serum in chemotactic activity for neutrophils and macrophages. Plasma alone was not active for either cell type, although serum alone had some activity for each; immune complexes increased activity for neutrophils but decreased activity for macrophages. It was suggested that plasminogen reacted with serum components to produce the chemotactic activity.

On the other hand, Hausman and his colleagues found that heparinized guinea pig plasma was equal in chemotactic activity to guinea pig serum in experiments using mononuclear leukocytes (Hausman *et al.*, 1972), which is at variance with the results reported by Borel and Sorkin and by Wilkinson cited above. Hausman pointed out that the discrepancy possibly can be explained on the basis of the use of high concentrations of heparin in plasma without equivalent heparined serum controls. In low doses of the anticoagulant, Hausman found no significant differences in the chemotactic activity for mononuclear cells in serum and plasma.

Hill and Ward (1969), in agreement with Ryan and Hurley (Hurley, 1963; Ryan and Hurley, 1966; see also Hurley and Spector, 1961a,b), found incubation of various rat tissues in homologous serum resulted in generation of a factor chemotactic for neutrophils. Purified C3 could replace the serum, and trypsin inhibitors or anti-C3 antibody prevented generation or expression of the factor. Gel filtration indicated the principal activity was in a fragment of about 14,000 MW, although activity was found in several fractions. It was suggested that this attractant may be active in cases of acute inflammation.

Ward (1968) examined activated serum for chemotactic activity for mononuclear cells. Such cells responded to a factor induced by antigen–antibody complexes similar but not identical to C$\overline{567}$ and to a plasmin-split factor (as well as to soluble bacterial factors and lysates from neutrophils).

5. C5 fragments. Snyderman *et al.* (1968) reported that incubation of guinea-pig serum with endotoxic lipopolysaccharide from *Serratia marcescens* resulted in generation of a new heat-stable chemotactic attractant. This was shown to have about 15,000–30,000 MW and was not generated under conditions which prevented complement fixation. Further studies (Shin *et al.*, 1968) using ^{125}I-labeled C5 indicated that treatment of C5 with sheep red blood cells plus the first four complement components resulted in splitting the C5 into two fragments with sedimentation constants of 1.5s and 7.4s. The smaller fragment, about 15,000 MW, was chemotactic for rabbit PMN. In order to establish identity of this fragment with the previously observed lipopolysaccharide-induced factor, ^{125}I-labeled C3 and C5 were incubated separately with guinea pig serum and lipopolysaccharide (Snyderman *et al.*, 1969). Both complement components were cleaved, but chemotactic activity was found only in the C5 cleavage products. Most of the activity was found in the fraction containing the 15,000 MW fragment. Rabbit antibody against C5 inhibited generation of this activity, but antibody against C3 did not. The C5a fragment was found to be the major attractant in activated rabbit and guinea pig sera (Snyderman *et al.*, 1970). It was suggested that other chemotactic activities were associated with binding of C5a with antigen–antibody complexes.

Ward and Newman (1969) reported generation of a chemotactic factor of about 8500 MW by the action of trypsin on human C5. This could also be produced by incubation of C5 with sensitized sheep red blood cells plus the first four components of complement and was probably the same fragment found by Snyderman *et al.* (1969). It was suggested that this fragment might be identical with F(a)C5, a fragment with anaphylactic activity (Cochrane and Müller-Eberhard, 1968). The C5 fragment could also be produced by action of a trypsinlike enzyme isolated from lysosomal granules of rabbit neutrophils on C5 (Ward and Hill, 1970). (See discussion below of lysosome-complement interactions.) It was suggested that this fragment may be responsible for reports of the chemotactic activity of neutrophil extracts in experiments in which serum was used to suspend the cells.

As already noted, Snyderman *et al.* (1971a) demonstrated the apparent participation of C5a as a chemotactic attractant for neutrophils, and the Snyderman group followed this with a second study (Snyderman *et al.*, 1971b) showing mononuclear chemotaxis to C5a (also found independently by Ward. 1971b). They suggested that this may be of importance in *in vivo* immune responses. Other more recent attempts to correlate pathological states and the presence of complement fragments derive from a crucial basic study by Zvaifler (1969), who demonstrated a correlation between breakdown products of C3 in the synovial fluid and the incidence of rheumatoid arthritis. Ward and Zvaifler (1971; also Ward, 1971a) followed this with an extended study along the same lines that showed, for the first time, the presence of complement-derived chemotactic factors in pathological human fluids. They were able to relate, in rheumatoid synovial fluids, chemotactic activity and the fifth (C5) and sixth (C6) components of human complement. They suggested that the activity was attributable to $C\overline{567}$ and C5a, a cleavage product of $C\overline{5}$. Inflammatory nonrheumatoid synovial fluids contained chemotactic activity related to C3a, and they also found a C3-cleaving enzyme, capable of producing C3a. Of other synovial fluids examined, those taken from patients with systemic lupus erythematosis arthritis were remarkable for their total lack of chemotactic activity. Two parallel studies from Cochrane's laboratory (De Shazo *et al.*, 1971, 1972) of experimental arthritis in the rabbit knee joint demonstrated a requirement for complement in the development of the lesion. They reported that rabbits genetically deficient in C6 showed delay in the hallmarks of the inflammatory reaction: vascular permeability, appearance of neutrophils, and the character of histological lesions. Rabbits with a C6 deficiency had synovial vascular permeability averaging approximately one-third less than that in animals without a deficiency of C6. Use of cobra venom factor to deplete C3 in normal or C3-deficient rabbits also hindered development of vascular permeability. Evidence was also adduced for a chemotactic attraction of neutrophils *in vivo*. Antigen–antibody-complement complexes in the walls of blood vessels attracted neutrophils placed in the joint space of neutrophil-depleted rabbits. They reported that omission of either antigen or antibody from this replacement system prevented the migration of neutrophils.

Many studies, of which those cited above are examples, attempt to delineate the role of complement in the inflammatory process in systems where animals are depleted of complement by such agents as cobra venom (Cochrane *et al.*, 1970; see also Nelson, 1966, and Chapter 3 by Cochrane and Janoff and Chapter 2 by Nelson in Volume III) or in situations such as glomerulonephritis, where complement deficiencies have been demonstrated (Gewurz *et al.*, 1966) or in lower and higher animals genetically deficient in certain components of complement (Cinader *et al.*, 1964; Klemperer *et al.*, 1966; Rother *et al.*, 1966). In some of these studies, differences in inflammatory responses in normal and complement-deficient animals cannot be demonstrated (Frank *et al.*, 1971) or differences show up only with variations in the timing of immunological challenge (Cinader *et al.*, 1971). Thus, while there appear to be rather clear-cut experimental differences between normal and complement-deficient animals in some cases (De Shazo *et al.*, 1971, 1972), other results remain somewhat ambiguous. (For a more detailed discussion of these points and a discussion of an alternate pathway of complement activation, see Chapter 3 by Cochrane and Janoff in Volume III.)

6. *Lysosome-complement interactions.*   Cornely showed (1966) that there is some chemotactic factor associated with the lysosomal fraction of rabbit leukocytes which is active in the presence of fresh serum, suggesting a mechanism mediated by complement. However, she also demonstrated that some such factor is present which does not require fresh serum for its activity and this one, therefore, is complement free. Borel *et al.* (1969) found, however, that lysosomes can generate chemotactic factors from fresh serum, and Hurley and Spector injected intradermally into rats leukocyte extracts which appeared to be chemotactic on the basis of careful histologic studies. Similar results were obtained with injected leukocytes suspended in serum and in physiological saline and other tissues and tissue extracts treated in the same way. Incubation with serum favored chemotaxis.

Other evidence (Ward and Hill, 1970; Taubman *et al.*, 1970; Taubman and Lepow, 1971) clearly links the chemotactic activity of white cell lysosomes with a complement effect. Such evidence suggests that lysosomal enzymes— in the absence of immune reactions—can induce alterations usually associated with sequential, immunological activation of the complement system. Weissmann and Dukor (1970) speculated, on the basis of the foregoing, that it is likely that when leukocytes in plasma endocytose inert particles or immune precipitates they may also take up components of the complement system in various stages of activation. This extends the lysosomal–complement interaction away from total dependence on immune mechanisms, invests it with greater generality, and creates a broader view of intravascular events. Whether such a mechanism can be extended to cover processes operative outside of vessels—that is, after the white cells have emigrated—is not yet clear. However, since Cornely demonstrated that fresh serum is not required for this type of activity, such an extension, real or not, may not be necessary. Most of the studies actually indicate that, in the absence of serum, extracts of lysosomal granules from neutrophils have very limited chemotactic activity. Yet possibly the significant point from these interesting experiments, in terms of chemotaxis, is that degranulating leukocytes may have chemotactic propensities, suggesting that inflammatory foci, where massive degranulation can occur, may possess the same capacity. It is interesting that Ward and Zvaifler (1973a,b) have shown the release of a lysosomal-bound C5-cleaving enzyme from neutrophils during the process of phagocytosis, suggesting that the release of the enzyme may exacerbate the inflammatory response in tissue where phagocytosis is occurring.

7. *Chemotactic factors in antigen-stimulated lymphocytes.* When lymph node lymphocytes obtained from guinea pigs exhibiting delayed hypersensitivity are stimulated *in vitro* by specific antigen, a soluble factor is produced that is chemotactic *in vitro* for mononuclear macrophages (Ward *et al.*, 1969). The material is nondialyzable, relatively heat stable, and elutes from Sephadex G-100 in the fraction containing molecules smaller than immunoglobulins. When the Sephadex fractions containing chemotactic factor are further fractionated by disk electrophoresis, mononuclear chemotactic activity is consistently found in the gel fraction which also contains albumin, but in contrast migration inhibitory factor (MIF) is found in a gel fraction anodal to albumin (Ward *et al.*, 1970), Ward and his colleagues also demonstrated a chemotactic factor for neutrophils produced by sensitized lymphocytes that was clearly distinguishable by disk electrophoresis from the other two factors. It was surmised that the neutrophil chemotactic factor produced by antigen-stimulated lymph node cells might have relevance to the "product of antigenic recognition" (PAR) reported by Ramseier (1969), who was able to induce accumulations of neutrophils following injection of the material into the skin of normal hamster hosts. The finding that MIF, chemotactic factor for mononuclear cells, and chemotactic factor for neutrophils can each be differentiated by their electrophoretic behavior implies that these three factors are separate and distinct molecular entities.

The work of Ward and his colleagues could open up an extremely productive line of investigation in chemotaxis, laying out the ground rules to account for differences in focal accumulation of cells at different times during the inflammatory response as well as pin-pointing special characteristics of delayed hypersensitivity reactions (see Volume III, Chapter 7).

c. NONCOMPLEMENT-MEDIATED REACTIONS. Whatever the significance of complement in mediating chemotactic reaction, it is clear that chemotaxis can proceed vigorously in the absence of complement. As noted above, in the section on bacterial-produced attractants and cAMP, Keller and Sorkin,

Ward *et al.*, and Ramsey all used complement-free systems in their studies of factors attractant for neutrophils. Lotz and Harris (1956) took note of the report by Delaunay *et al.* (1951) that calcium, serum, and complement were necessary for chemotaxis to occur in leukocytes and that other substances, such as citrate, azide, and fluoride, could abolish the chemotactic response without impairing the motility of the cell. Using Harris' photographic trace technique, with *S. albus* as the test object, Lotz and Harris demonstrated that chemotaxis can occur in the absence of complement, serum, or glucose and in solutions relatively free of ionized calcium or magnesium. The neutrophils were able to withstand large increases or decreases in the tonicity of the ambient medium, the degree of hypertonicity they can tolerate varing with the substance added. It appeared that much greater increases in tonicity could be withstood when these were produced by substances which enter the cell freely, such as urea, than by substances which do not, such as sucrose and mannitol.

Lotz and Harris pointed out that the ability of neutrophils to survive and remain motile for considerable periods in solutions devoid of any known source of energy suggests that these cells may have an intrinsic energy store. The fact that the cells remained for many hours in solutions containing 0.001 and even 0.011 M sodium cyanide or 0.005 M sodium azide suggested that their survival is not acutely dependent on a supply of oxygen. Lotz and Harris also failed to find evidence for the assertion that chemotaxis can be inhibited without impairing the motility of the cell. They found that chemotaxis was suppressed only when motility was suppressed, that is, under conditions toxic for the cell. Lotz and Harris suggested that discrepancies between their results and those of Delaunay might be due, in part, to differences in technique. In Harris' photomicrographic trace technique, chemotaxis was said to have occurred when clear-cut directional response of the white cell toward the test object was recorded. In Delaunay's experiments, the adherence of leukocytes to grains of starch was considered evidence of chemotaxis. This adherence might under certain circumstances indicate that chemotaxis had occurred, it was conceded, but the phenomenon may involve more than chemotaxis as noted by Nelson and Lebrun (1956), who offered evidence that starch is not immunologically inert and demonstrated that there are at least two components of serum which are specifically required for phagocytosis of starch: a heat-labile component identified as complement and a heat-stable component identified as specific antibody. Keller and Sorkin (1965b) used Boyden chambers to study the chemotactic effect of *S. albus* on rabbit neutrophils and found that chemotaxis could not be demonstrated in the absence of serum.

It was suggested that the use by Lotz and Harris of human white cells, instead of rabbit cells, might explain the difference in results, but Keller and Sorkin offered an alternative explanation that the bacteria in the Lotz and Harris experiment were contaminated by a chemotaxis-producing factor present in the bacteriological culture medium. Keller and Sorkin pointed out that Witte's peptone and Bacto-Casitone, widely used in bacteriological media, were found to be chemotactic in their serum-free test system. Aside from peptone and Bacto-Casitone as attractants in serum-free systems, Keller and Sorkin also showed that casein has chemotactic properties, in the absence of complement, inducing migration of both neutrophils and mononuclear cells through Boyden chamber filters (1967c).

As noted, Keller, Sorkin, and Cornely showed that chemotaxis could be induced in rabbit neutrophils in the complete absence of serum, Keller (1966) suspending the cells in Gey's solution plus 2% human serum albumin and Cornely suspending them in Hanks' solution with heat-treated normal rabbit serum. Keller also demonstrated a low level of chemotactic activity in normal, untreated serum. In Keller's experiments, the Boyden (1962) method was found to correlate well with Harris' slide chamber technique (1953a). It was observed that activated serum (and normal serum to a lesser degree) seemed to enhance the random motility of white blood cells in the absence of a gradient of attractant but caused direction movement with such a gradient (Keller and Sorkin, 1966). Comparison of rabbit exudate cells indicated that culture filtrates of *E. coli*, *S. albus*, Witte's peptone, casitone, or casein, as well as various serum related factors, attracted neutrophils, whereas only casein attracted mononuclear cells (Keller and Sorkin, 1967d).

Recently, several new noncomplement-related factors have been found. Stecher *et al.* (1971) noted that normal blood clotting released attractant factors from rabbit blood. If clotting was prevented or allowed to take place in the absence of buffy coat cells, no attractant was produced. Kay *et al.* (1971) reported that incubation of sensitized guinea pig lung tissue with the specific antigen produced a substance specifically chemotactic for eosinophils. A substance attractant for eosinophils (as well as for neutrophils) was found by Cohen and Ward (1971). They reported that when lymphocytes from guinea pigs stimulated to produce delayed hypersensitivity reactions were incubated with the specific antigen, an active supernatant was obtained, which generated attractant for the white blood cells when subsequently incubated with the specific antigen–antibody complex. They noted the uniqueness of this reaction in that other systems require either immune complexes or substances released in lymphocyte culture but not both. It was conceded that the lymphoid cells could conceivably have synthesized a complement fragment, but the evidence to support this view was not impressive.

The kallikrein fragment of the clotting mechanism also yielded a noncomplement-mediated attractant in the hands of Kaplan *et al.* (1972). In the process of blood clotting, prekallikrein is converted to kallikrein, which, in turn, leads to the production of bradykinin. The conversion of prekallikrein to kallikrein produces a chemotactically active material, according to Kaplan.

It is of interest that Wissler and his colleagues (1972a) studied a leukotactic binary serum peptide system related to anaphylatoxin, noting that the two low molecular weight peptides studied—cocytotaxin and anaphylatoxin—displayed no significant chemotactic activity when used singly, but on recombination and depending on their molar ratio and the absolute concentration of each of the peptides they exhibited cell-specific chemotactic activity for neutrophil and eosinophil leukocytes. In an extensive parallel series of studies, Wissler and his colleagues characterized chemically the two peptides (Wissler, 1972a, b; Wissler et al., 1972b). Wissler's group suggested that cocytotaxin, a basic peptide, acts as a Bronstedt or Lewis acid and accounts for the activation of cells by the binary peptide system (Wissler et al., 1972c). Although the signal for chemotaxis may turn on the level of entropy which the peptide transmits, it seems necessary to postulate the existence of a specific chemical conformation on the cell surface for chemotaxis.

Yoshida et al. (1968) reported the isolation of a chemotactic attractant "leucogresin" from the skin of rabbits subjected to Arthus reactions. Purification of this material showed it to be a protein of about 140,000 MW with a sedimentation coefficient of 6.585. The material had no effect on vascular permeability and was proposed as the natural mediator of the Arthus reaction (Yoshinaga et al., 1971b). A possible relationship of this material to antibody IgG was indicated by the demonstration, using agar immunoelectrophoresis and immunodiffusion, that leucogresin and IgG shared common antigens. Treatment of leucogresin with anti-IgG antibody caused loss of soluble attractant activities (Yamamoto et al., 1971). Furthermore, treatment of normal rabbit IgG with a purified protease derived from Arthus-inflamed skin resulted in a generation of chemotactic activity (Yoshinaga et al., 1971a), as did treatment of mouse, rabbit, and human IgG with papain (Yoshinaga et al., 1972).

d. STUDIES OF EXTRAVASCULAR INJURY THAT LEAVE OPEN THE QUESTION OF COMPLEMENT INVOLVEMENT.   Two studies, one by Weimar (1957) involving rat cornea and the second based on direct observations of Arthus reactions by Grant and his colleagues (Grant et al., 1967), elicited chemotactic responses in extravascular tissue but the role of complement was not studied in either case. Weimar caused sterile injuries in the corneas of rats and studied the accumulation of leukocytes at the injury site in the first 6 hours. The origin of the white blood cells is not clear, but it is unlikely that the acute injury itself created changes in distal limbal vessels, and it seems probable that materials released at the injury site, assuming sterility of the system, elicited the leukocyte invasion. Weimar noted that the reaction was inhibited by sodium salicylate and soy bean trypsin inhibitor, which suggested to her that the activation of a proteolytic system liberated chemotactic substances (she guessed that they might be polypeptides) that had chemotactic properties.

In in vivo study which was combined with electron micrographic studies of inflammatory sites, Grant and his colleagues immunized rabbits with ferritin and then placed antigen on the subcutaneous areolar connective tissue of the rabbit ear chamber and on the immune mesentery. The procedure bypassed the conventional difficulties in the study of the Arthus reaction where materials are forced intracutaneously, under high pressure, into all compartments of the skin. A brisk inflammatory reaction ensued, characterized by white cell sticking and, after a delay of 5 or 10 minutes, emigration of cells into the extravascular spaces. Electron micrographs of tissue taken from sites of injury revealed aggregates of material that was considered to be antigen–antibody complex in the extravascular tissue, often perivascularly, inside and outside of white blood cells, but the clumps were never found intraluminally. The results were interpreted as evidence that such reactions have their genesis in the extravascular deposition of immune complexes, not in the vessel wall as is claimed with intradermal injections. (See discussion in Volume III, Chapter 3, by Cochrane and Janoff of vessel wall injury.)

In a flow sheet of postulated events to explain such reactions, Grant and his colleagues suggested that injury products, produced in the extravascular tissue, generated chemotactic materials which eventually impinged on blood vessels, causing them to become adhesive, which, in turn, caused white blood cells to stick to the vessel walls. With a gradient of attractants outside of the vessels, the white blood cells emigrated, setting up inflammatory foci which drew more and more phagocytic cells into the arena.

Whether such a mechanism requires complement as a mediator is an open question at this point. The fact that there appears to be an extravascular pool of complement (Alper and Rosen, 1967) makes the possibility of complement mediation not unreasonable. On the other hand, the disparity in experimental chemotaxis studies, many of which demonstrate that complement is not required for chemotaxis, leaves open the possibility that other injury products, operating through other mechanisms, may be critical determinants in the evoking of emigrating white blood cells and in controlling their directional movements in tissues. It is perhaps worth noting that if one injures a blood vessel in such a way as to confine the injury to the intravascular space, there is no emigration of white blood cells in the wake of the reaction (Grant and Becker, 1965, 1966; Grant, 1974). On the contrary, one gets thrombus formation unless the injury is so extensive that the vessel is sheared and its contents spilled into the extravascular space. Depending on the extent of such an injury, and in all likelihood whether extravascular tissue is involved, there may or may not be white blood cell emigration. This would make it appear that in classically produced Arthus reactions, which are believed to be generated by complement, the injury stimulus is a widespread one, both intra- and extravascular, and that the chemotactic effects, whether mediated by complement or not, come from outside the blood vessel, not from vessel wall alteration.

In a differently designed experiment, where extravascular injuries were achieved with a laser beam (Grant, 1973), a microburn of collagen also induced a chemotactic response in rabbit subcutaneous tissue. The experiment raises questions similar to those raised by the Arthus reaction and is discussed below in the section dealing with chemotaxis *in vivo*.

3. INHIBITION OF CHEMOTAXIS

Chemotaxis may be inhibited at several levels; by destruction, alteration, or preventing the generation of attractant; by inhibition of the ability of the cell to detect or respond specifically to the attractant; or by a general inhibition of the motility of the cell. Unfortunately, many studies on inhibition of chemotaxis do not adequately distinguish between treatments which affect chemotaxis specifically and those which inhibit motility in general.

a. INHIBITION BY PHOSPHONATES.   An impressive body of work has been produced by Ward and Becker concerning the effects of some phosphonates on chemotaxis (for review, see Becker, 1969).

Ward and Becker (1967) studied the effect of a number of phosphonates on chemotaxis of rabbit PMN using the $C\overline{567}$ attractant. Phosphonates were known to inhibit irreversibly a large number of esterases which have serine residues in their active sites, such as trypsin, chymotrypsin, and acetyl cholinesterase. It was found that treatment of PMN with certain phosphonates would inhibit subsequent chemotaxis, called *cell-dependent inhibition*. Treatment of cells in the presence of chemotactic attractant resulted in *chemotactic factor-dependent inhibition*. Differences in the effect of various phosphonates, the time courses of inhibition, dose-response curves, and structure–activity relationships supported the idea that these two inhibitions reflected action of the phosphonates on two different cell bound esterases. One esterase (activated) was active in the cell before exposure to attractant; the other became active (and therefore susceptible to inhibition) only after exposure to attractant (activatable esterase). There were no effects of phosphonates on attractant. Treatment of cells with trypan blue indicated that substantial inhibition of chemotaxis could occur without allowing dye uptake, suggesting that inhibition was not caused by a general cell damage. No determinations of the effect of phosphonates on motility were made.

Cell-dependent inhibition was studied further in an attempt to learn more of the nature of the esterases (Becker and Ward, 1967). Treatment of an esterase with certain esters, presumably those related to the natural substrate of the enzyme, will block subsequent irreversible inactivation of the esterase by phosphonates. Leukocytes were therefore treated with a variety of esters followed by phosphonates, and chemotaxis was determined. Protection against inhibition was found to be very specific and occurred only with acetate esters. These esters were also the only ones which prevented chemotaxis when present in Boyden chambers, presumably by saturating the esterase. It was concluded that the cell-dependent esterase was an enzyme capable of specifically reacting with acetates.

Incubation of rabbit PMN in the presence of attractant rendered the cells incapable of subsequent chemotactic response in a gradient of the attractant (Ward and Becker, 1968). Phosphonates would prevent this deactivation of the cells. This implied involvement of the activatable esterase, otherwise phosphonates would have prevented all subsequent chemotaxis. Acetate esters did not prevent deactivation of the leukocyte, although aromatic amino acid esters did, suggesting that aromatic amino acid residues were involved in the activity of the activatable esterase.

Becker and Ward (1969) extended this work by examining rabbit PMN for esterases capable of hydrolyzing aromatic amino acid esters. Three activities were found, esterase 1, 2, and 3. Esterase 1 was most inhibited by phosphonates, esterase 2 less so, and esterase 3 not at all. It was not possible to show an increase in esterase 1 activity during chemotaxis nor could this enzyme be found in an inactive form. It was suggested that esterase 1 may have been activated while the PMN made a (postulated) chemotactic response to glycogen while migrating to the peritoneal cavity before collection. Evidence supporting this view has been presented by Ward and Becker (1970b). Comparisons of neutrophils from rabbit peripheral blood and peritoneal exudates indicated that the blood cells were distinctly more active chemotactically and had slightly more esterase 1 activity. The difference in esterase activity was statistically significant. Likewise, a small amount of esterase activity could be activated by incubation of the blood leukocytes with chemotactic factor. It was suggested that the activatable esterase may be a proteolytic enzyme.

Becker (1972) raised a question about the generality of proesterase 1 in chemotaxis. Phosphonate-inhibition profiles were found to be similar in cells responsing to C3a, C5a, C$\overline{567}$, and bacterial factor. He showed increases in esterase activity in cells responding to C3a and C5a but not in those responding to bacterial factor. It was concluded that activation of proesterase 1 is a general step in leukocyte chemotaxis, although such activation was not as great in response to bacterial factor as to complement factors.

Woodin and Wiencke (1969, 1970) have studied the effects of phosphonates on the action of leukocidin on leukocytes. Leukocidin was found to be a complex of two proteins produced by *Staphylococcus* which kills leukocytes by damaging the cellular potassium ion pump. Phosphonates in the presence of suboptimal concentrations of leukocidin caused enhance leakage of enzymes, which suggested that the effect of phosphonates on chemotaxis might be caused by disruption of permeability mechanism rather than an effect on esterases. The relatively high concentrations required for phosphonate inhibition of chemotaxis supports this contention, although experiments with esters do not. Further studies (Becker, 1971) suggest that the phosphonate effect on chemotaxis is caused by a phosphorylation reaction and not by a detergent effect. Woodin and Harris (1973) disagreed sharply with this view in experiments that showed an inhibitory effect of phosponates on locomotion per se, suggesting that this, not enzyme inhibition, may account for the effect on chemotaxis.

b. NONPHOSPHONATE INHIBITORS OF CHEMOTAXIS. Lotz and Harris (1956) studied chemotaxis in PMN moving on glass slides and found that treatments which killed the cells, in the sense of stopping motility, were the only treatments which inhibited chemotaxis. From this they concluded that chemotaxis could not be suppressed without affecting motility. Ketchel et al. (1958) found hydrocortisone greatly inhibited random motility of leukocytes although there was no effect caused by tetrahydrocortisone and desoxycorticosterone. Ward (1966) reported that hydrocortisone, methyl prednisolone, and chloroquine inhibited the response of rabbit PMN to the $C\overline{567}$ complex attractant. He suggested that hydrocortisone and chloroquine prevented inflammation by preventing response of leukocytes to attractants.

Glovsky et al. (1968) found that maleopimaric acid inhibited complement-mediated chemotaxis if it were present when serum was activated. Maleopimaric acid was dialyzed out of the preparation before being tested for chemotaxis; its effect therefore was to prevent production of attractant. It was also shown (Glovsky et al., 1969) that a less toxic analog, fumaropimaric acid, suppressed Forssman, reversed passive Arthus and noncomplement-dependent passive cutaneous anaphylaxis reactions, and also caused the dissociation of the $C\overline{567}$ complex.

Keller and Sorkin (1968a) found that chemotaxis was inhibited if cells were incubated with washed immune complexes. Incubation in filtered chemotactically active serum did not prevent chemotaxis, leading to the suggestion that the unresponsive form was a result of phagocytosis of attractant.

Malawista (1965) reported that 10^{-3} M colchicine would inhibit random motility of human PMN on glass slides. Caner (1965) found chemotaxis of human leukocytes in Boyden chambers was inhibited by 1.5×10^{-7} M colchicine, suggesting a specific role for this compound in inhibiting chemotaxis. Ward and Becker (1970a) discovered 10^{-4}–10^{-6} M oubain caused an approximate 50 % inhibition of chemotaxis. This effect was partially reversed by potassium ions, which suggested the existence of a sodium–potassium-stimulated ATPase. Recent observations (Ramsey and Harris, 1973) indicate that 10^{-4} M oubain reduced by about 50% the average speed of human neutrophils moving on glass slides. The effect of such speed reduction on chemotaxis is not known, however, other experiments suggested that although inhibitors of microtubule function inhibited motility, they did so only at relatively high concentrations, while cytochalasin B, an inhibitor of microfilament function (Wessells et al., 1971), inhibited motility at concentrations to be expected if microfilaments were involved in motility.

Becker *et al.* (1972) found cytochalasin B, in concentrations of 2–4 $\mu g/ml$, inhibited motility and chemotaxis. Paradoxically, chemotaxis was stimulated by 0.1–1.0 $\mu g/ml$, while motility was inhibited by as little as 0.2 $\mu g/ml$ cytochalasin B.

Carruthers (1966, 1967) studied the chemotactic movement of human leukocytes through membrane filters using starch particles as attractant. Puromycin at 10^{-3} M and actinomycin D at 10 $\mu g/ml$ were said to have a greater effect on chemotactic response than on motility. Phelps and Stanislaw (1969) found that chemotaxis to *E. coli* cells in Boyden chambers was inhibited by ethyl alcohol and caffein, as well as by small variations in pH. It was also found (Phelps, 1969a,b) that the process of phagocytosis of urate crystals in the absence of plasma produced a chemotactic factor which would induce chemotaxis in other PMN. Production of this factor could be inhibited by the presence of colchicine. Interestingly, there was some inhibition of phagocytosis as well (Phelps, 1970a). Colchicine also prevented formation of chemotactic activity in synovial fluid of dogs after injection of monosodium urate crystals (Phelps, 1970b). A model for quantitating extravascular leukocyte accumulation has been described in which labeled neutrophils and mononuclear cells (non-lymphocytes) are adoptively transferred to isologous recipients (Perper *et al.*, 1974a). Agents that alter microtubular function, such as colchicine, inhibit neutrophil but not mononuclear accumulation, whereas nonsteroidal antiinflammatory agents and other membrane-active agents selectively inhibit mononuclear chemotaxis (Perper *et al.*, 1974b).

Anderson and Van Epps (1972) reported that Streptolysin O inhibited chemotaxis in human neutrophils at concentrations below those causing lysis or morphological changes in the cells. Since their experiments also demonstrated that the agent inhibited random migration, the effect that they found may have had less to do with chemotaxis than with a nonspecific effect on motility.

4. NEGATIVE CHEMOTAXIS

There are scattered reports in the literature describing a phenomenon known as negative chemotaxis (Gabritchewsky, 1890; Wells, 1918; McCutcheon *et al.*, 1939), a difficult concept to understand if one accepts the viewpoint that the function of chemotaxis is to help the organism or the cell to attain a position in order to isolate, by engulfment, noxious materials. Negative chemotaxis might be of some use to a white blood cell or to free-living organisms (see earlier discussion of chemotaxis in bacteria and lower animal forms: *re* avoiding reaction). However, a white blood cell fleeing an area of injury would be absolutely useless to the tissue it is guarding. Yet this view tends to have teleological overtones, however rational it may appear when looked at from the viewpoint of tissue under assault. Metchnikoff himself recognized the trap one could fall into by imputing motivation to cell activities and he dismissed this kind of thinking by substituting concepts that grow out of evolutionary theory (see discussion of this point in Chapter 1 by Ebert and Grant). In our present state of understanding of what is happening at the molecular level, therefore, it is perhaps best not to dismiss negative chemotaxis on the grounds that it would be bad for the species and consequently does not exist, but to reserve a conclusion on this point until cell–cell interactions are more clearly defined. Although negative chemotaxis could be bad for the species, perhaps it happens anyway. Gabritchewsky classified various chemical substances as positively chemotactic, negatively chemotactic, and indifferent in their effect on leukocytes. He used a capillary tube method, a questionable assay because of the interference of convection currents [see Pfoehl (1898) and Harris' discussion of this point (1954)]. Gabritchewsky's criteria for determining chemotaxis, moreover, were arbitrary; if few leukocytes accumulated in the capillary tubes, the test substance was said to be negatively chemotactic, and if a large number accumulated, positively chemotactic. Actually he did not demonstrate, nor could the technique be expected to demonstrate, the avoidance of white cells for test materials.

Wells tested many drugs *in vitro* and added a long list to these three classes. What might be mistaken for negative chemotaxis is the effect, noted by Clark and Clark (1922), of various chemotactic substances, some of which are stronger in their attraction for white blood cells than others. Thus paraffin oil is virtually indifferent as a chemotactic agent, whereas gelatinized starch is strongly chemotactic on a spectrum that includes such intermediate materials as carbon, carmine granules, uncooked starch, olive oil, emulsions of cream, and yolk of egg. All are positively chemotactic to one degree or another, and the Clarks found no instance of a white cell fleeing from a foreign material. It would be possible, on the other hand, to find material so toxic to the white cells that it would kill them, in all liklihood killing the tissue around them, too, but this situation would have nothing to do with chemotaxis in any form [see comments by Harris (1954) on turpentine as an inflammatory agent].

McCutcheon reported that rabbit neutrophils exhibited negative chemotaxis to kaolin particles, that is, the white cells moved away from the particles. There was a suggestion of negative chemotaxis to β-hemolytic streptococcus, although a number of other bacteria did not appear to elicit such a response. Lotz and Harris (1956), on the other hand, found no negative chemotaxis to kaolin but rather normal phagocytosis of particles after chance encounters. Cliff's observations (Cliff, 1965, 1966a,b), referred to earlier, should also be noted. He suggested that perhaps what seem to be ambiguous results in the study of chemotaxis *in vivo* might be explained by analysis of centrifugal expansion in a population of emigrated white blood cells, one that might tend to create an impression of negative chemotaxis but would not, in fact, be a true explanation of the movements of cells in relation to an inflammatory focus.

As noted earlier, Bessis and Burté found that *Euglena* exhibited negative chemotaxis to *Euglena* cells that had been killed by ultraviolet radiation or laser microbeams. They chose to describe such a phenomenon as "necrophobia." Paramecium (see earlier discussion) also seem to have the capacity for negative chemotaxis. Thus, it is conceivable that even the most primitive forms of animal life, such as one-celled organisms, may be equipped with some faculty for avoiding, as a positive step, certain noxious material in the environment. However, when Bessis and Burté killed individual leukocytes and red blood cells by UV and laser stimuli, positive chemotaxis toward these dead cells was shown by neutrophils and, to a lesser degree, by eosinophils and monocytes.

In summary, the concept of negative chemotaxis for white blood cells can be said to be an awkward one, biologically; the evidence for it is weak, and the evidence against it seems substantial.

B. *Chemotaxis in vivo: Direct Observations*

In observations on the transparent tail of the tadpole, Clark and Clark reported in 1920 that white blood cells move toward a globule of injected croton oil, and in this study and a subsequent one in 1922 they reported that the accumulation of leukocytes and of "wandering cells" from the tissue was observed to occur with a large number of test substances, including powdered carbon, carmine, olive oil, cream, and yolk of egg. They stated that carbon and carmine were the least effective of the substances they used, that olive oil, cream, and egg yolk were more effective; that croton oil produced a dense zone of leukocytic infiltration at some distance from the injected droplet; and that starch and agar were the most effective chemotactic substances.

Subsequently, the Clarks produced evidence, also from their microaquarium studies, that macrophages of amphibian larvae seem chemotactically attracted to products of aseptically injured cells and to erythrocytes (Clark and Clark, 1930). They made the statement that when a cell begins to die the macrophages of the neighborhood make a "bee-line" for it. "If a single macrophage reaches the dead cell, or its remnants, it proceeds to ingest them," the Clarks reported. "Frequently two or three macrophages reach the dead cell simultaneously, whereupon a struggle occurs over it or its remains."

In a later study along the same lines (Clark and Clark, 1935), they studied the adhesion of white blood cells to vessel walls, using the inflammatory substances noted above, and came to the conclusion that if sticking precedes the emigration of white cells from the vessel, as it does, then some other event must occur to cause the white blood cell to emigrate into the extravascular spaces. They reasoned that a change in the endothelium itself is a necessary precursor to sticking and "a further change in the wall, beyond that of stickiness alone, appears to be necessary before such cells can penetrate the endo-thelium, as was shown by the observation that a reversal from this latter phase may occur so abruptly as to trap leucocytes in the act of emigrating, in addition to preventing further diapedesis of the leucocytes adherent to the inner wall."

Metchnikoff (1893) had suggested that white cell sticking could be attributed to chemotactic attraction of the cells from outside the blood vessel, but the Clarks took the position that chemotaxis alone was an inadequate explanation for leukocyte emigration, asserting that emigration occurred in the absence of any localized focus of attraction in the outside tissue. Although minimally plausible, this is a weak point in the Clarks' argument, for a chemotactic stimulus would not have to be narrowly restrictively focal, in juxtaposition to the vessel wall, for example, to be chemotactically active provided the presumed chemical signal could reach the vessel from near or far. On balance, then, the Clarks may have been correct but possibly for the wrong reason. The Clarks also cited examples in which emigration of leukocytes from nearby vessels failed to take place in the presence of a foreign substance in the tissue which exerted a positive chemotactic influence on the same types of leukocytes just outside the vessels, the attractants in this case being cream and yolk of egg emulsions. This is a stronger point and does suggest, as Florey (1962) implied, that the factors that control the sticking of white cells to endothelium may not necessarily be the same as those control-ling the movement of white cells in the extravascular tissues.

The Clarks concluded their lengthy studies of chemotaxis *in vivo* in rabbit ear chamber studies and, by and large, confirmed their earlier amphibian studies, but they did not injure the ear chamber tissue to follow the sequence of sticking and emigration. They noted, in a reference to earlier studies in larvae, that neutrophils present in the tissue may move directly toward an injected foreign substance in the absence of any emigration of neutrophils from the bloodstream, and they added that neutrophils may be attracted positively toward an area of injury or toward a foreign substance and yet fail to take part in its phagocytosis.

Sandison's introduction of the ear chamber (1924, 1931) technique opened the possibility that chemotaxis could be demonstrated *in vivo*. The thin (30–40 μm) connective tissue preparations permit careful viewing for long periods without upsetting the physiological balance of the chamber system, but experimental pathologists are, in a sense, trapped in their own definition of chemotaxis. The definition demands that the phenomenon be demonstrated by some method which shows a direct convergence of white blood cells on an inflammatory focus, a relatively simple achievement on a glass slide or in similar preparations. In a thin transparent tissue, such as mesentery, cheek pouch, or ear chamber, the path of the white cell in its progress toward an inflammatory focus is likely to be indirect or at least not on a course as straight as an arrow. In tissues, white cells crawl across and through various structures in their path, requiring footing such as connective tissue fibers (Sandison, 1931) and the highways are not laid out like a modern turnpike.

As Zweifach has noted (see Volume II, Chapter 1), the alterations in tissue from gel to sol states in inflammatory reactions may pose the problem for the white cell whether to walk or swim, and it is by no means clear that the white cell does both with equal facility or, for that matter, swims at all. With changes in extravascular pressure, it is conceivable that the white cell, once it has escaped the endothelial barrier, is buffeted by forces that may direct it away from, as well as toward, injury sites, accounting for randomness of movement. Although the Clarks reported volumes of evidence that white blood cells seemed to accumulate around inflammatory foci, their experiments lacked precision and are open to the criticism that too many events intervened in the course of the inflammatory reactions they observed to enable one to narrow the interpretation to chemotaxis solely. Sanders reported through Harris (1954) that leukocytes behave indifferently toward tissue breakdown products *in vivo*, a point that Florey subscribed to (Florey and Jennings, 1970). Sanders' observation was based on the study of a thermal injury in the rabbit ear chamber where polymorphonuclear leukocytes were seen to emigrate from the vessels in the vicinity of the injury, moving about in a haphazard way and showing no tendency to move toward the injured tissue or to collect around it.

In more precise studies of thermal injury, Allison *et al.* (1955) reported that white cells emigrated from blood vessels and then moved at random extravascularly, although frequently they seemed to follow the route of least resistance between fibrous bands in the connective tissue. In this way, the cells were directed by chance toward, away from, or parallel to the injured area. Their motion was not influenced by the movement of edema fluid or by the tissue pulsations produced by vasodilatation. In spite of their random movement, however, they eventually became concentrated about the site of injury. Within 6 hours, a considerable number of leukocytes had congregated in the area of stasis, after 12 hours the cells had moved into the central ischemic area, and 24 hours after injury the tissue of the ischemic area was densely packed with motile leukocytes. One could not make out a case for chemotaxis on this evidence—Allison did not do so—but the results are suggestive of it, although it is possible that cells reached the injured area in a wholly fortuitous way and then became trapped there. If this were the case, it is an interesting and unexplained point that the cells accumulating at the injury site remained motile, possibly, but not necessarily, suggesting that they were not really "trapped."

Buckley (1963) came a bit closer. He injured a minute area of tissue in rabbit ear chambers with a radiofrequency generator under conditions where it seems quite unlikely that the tissue was contaminated. The injury was followed within hours by damage to surrounding small blood vessels over a wider area, and large numbers of granulocytes migrated into the region of damage. In one experiment, focal aseptic heat injury of a small group of isolated macrophages was followed by migration of granulocytes into the region of injury, where they continued to move about. He concluded that the damage appearing around a focus of heat injury was most simply interpreted as indicating injury to vascular endothelium by diffusible toxic products of heat-injured tissue.

Buckley drew a parallel between the delayed increased capillary permeability reported by Sevitt (1957, 1958) and Wilhelm and Mason (1960) and the delayed vascular damage noted in his experiments. He suggested that both may have a common antecedent cause in the form of diffusible chemical mediators liberated from the initially burned tissue. The accumulation of leukocytes around the area of injury was believed to support the view that the products of aseptically injured cells are chemotactic for leukocytes, a conclusion that ran counter to one drawn by Harris, who stated that dead tissue fragments, autolyzing tissue, and peptic and tryptic digests had no attractive power for leukocytes under circumstances where bacteria were chemotactic (Harris, 1953a). Harris (1954) pointed out that Leber is sometimes said to have demonstrated that products of the breakdown of tissue are chemotactic for leukocytes (Leber, 1891). Leber used extracts of tissues which had been allowed to putrify, evidence of the attractive power of microbial metabolic products for leukocytes rather than tissue breakdown products.

However, Weimar (1957) caused sterile injuries in the corneas of rats and studied the accumulation of leukocytes at the injury site in the first 6 hours. The reaction was inhibited by sodium salicylate and soy bean trypsin inhibitor, suggesting to Weimar that the activation of a proteolytic enzyme system was an essential step leading to the leukocyte invasion. The working hypothesis for the experiment was that the proteolytic system liberated chemotactic substances (probably polypeptides) leading to leukocyte invasion.

Whether the experiment is evidence for chemotaxis under these conditions of corneal injury might be debated—it seems to favor it—but it does fit Buckley's conclusions *in vivo*, and it seems clear that there was no reported evidence of contamination of the specimens.

Because of the preciseness of the microburn imparted by a laser beam (Grant and Becker, 1965, 1966), Grant recently investigated the problem of chemotaxis *in vivo* anew (1974). Rabbits were injected via the central artery of the ear with 1% solutions of Alphazurine A, a highly diffusible dye. The dye imparted a blue-green color to the subcutaneous areolar connective tissue of the ear chamber under physiological circumstances that created no inflammatory artefacts in the test tissue. The color thereby invested the tissue with

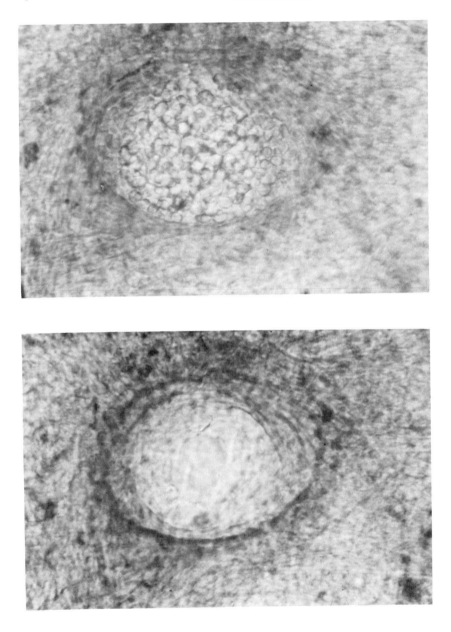

the capacity to absorb laser energy, making it possible to inflict a microburn on areas outside of the blood vessels. A single microburn was created (Fig. 6a), producing what appeared to be a more or less clear crater, rimmed by blue tissue which had somewhat the character of a whorl. Intermittent observations over a 3-hour period revealed little or no change in the injury, the crater remaining free of cells. On examination of the lesion at 4 hours, however, it was obvious that the crater had filled up with cells. The cells seemed to have a regular orientation around the rim of the injury (Fig. 6b) and they were randomly massed in the center of the lesion. The injury at this point looked something similar to a basket of eggs, with discrete cell margins showing in a heterogeneous pattern and creating the appearance that the cells were more than one layer thick.

The lesion was made in an area at least 1mm from a venule or arteriole, and there was no obvious reaction, from any blood vessels, to suggest that there had been direct stimulation of the vessels to cause white cell adherence to vessel walls and emigration of white cells through the vessel walls. Thus one could not account for the focal accumulation of cells on the basis of a chemotactic response that elicited intravascular neutrophils; nor was it apparent that the cells came from nearby capillaries, although this is a somewhat more difficult point to be sure of because the smallest vessels, owing to their unpredictability in carrying blood, are less easily visualized.

The movement of cells into the microburn occurred, apparently, with some rapidity, actually probably in a 40-minute period, between the third and fourth hour of the reaction. Yet the focal accumulation could hardly be considered fortuitous because there were no other such accumulations in the tissue, which was normal in every way except for the single microburn approximately $15–20$ μm in diameter.

It is of possible interest to note that Houck and his colleagues have reported that enzymatic digestion of collagen yielded a number of peptides that, when placed in a chamber embedded in an epidermal-free area of the skin of rats, elicited a focal accumulation of neutrophils (Houck and Chang, 1971; see also extensive earlier studies of this group: Houck and Jacob, 1959, 1961; Jacob and Houck, 1959; Houck *et al.*, 1967; Chang

---

Fig. 6. (a) Photomicrograph of a laser lesion in the subcutaneous tissue of the rabbit ear. Note the clear, cell-free central area rimmed by tissue which represents the stain imparted by the infusion of dye. There is one spot (arrow) in the lower center of the microburn, which serves as orientation for (b). × 500. (b) Photomicrograph of the same laser lesion as in (a). The laser crater has filled with cells, which have a rather regular orientation around the rim of the injury and which centrally give the impression of a basket of eggs more than one layer deep, and randomly massed. This was the only area of focal injury in the tissue. It is not clear whether the cells are neutrophils or macrophages, or both, and their origin is obscure. × 500. From Grant (1974).

and Houck, 1970). They asserted that their leukotactic collagenolysis products were made up of at least eight polypeptides with MW's of 30,000 and 1,000. Seven of these peptides were leukotactic *in vivo* at concentrations of 10^{-10} M. Although there is no direct evidence at this time to support a correlation of the observations of Houck and Chang and those of Grant, it is not unreasonable to speculate that the laser burn may have released degradation products of collagen with chemotactic properties.

That such an injury represents an example of chemotaxis *in vivo* seems to be beyond question, but one can only speculate at this point about the biological mechanisms that created it. Whether complement need be invoked as a necessary intermediary in the reaction cannot be stated for certain. This would seem unlikely unless one assumes that extravascular depots of complement or complement fragments have leaked from the blood vessel and reside in the extravascular space and that these react with degraded proteins produced by thermal injury. There are several pieces of evidence indeed that might make such a viewpoint plausible. Since most normal tissues contain a neutral protease capable of cleaving C3 into chemotactic fragments (Hill and Ward, 1969) and since a reserve of C3 exists in the extravascular fluid, it is possible to reconstruct a complement-mediated reaction to account for chemotactically directed accumulation of neutrophils in response to thermal injury induced by a laser beam.

In a study of the *in vivo* behavior of human C3 in normal subjects and in patients with diseases in which complement is thought to play a pathophysiological role, Alper and Rosen (1967) demonstrated the existence of an extravascular pool of complement, in equilibrium with the plasma.

Rosen notes that in this study one can extrapolate turnover curves back to the origin to achieve a plasma fraction of 0.7, indicating that 0.3 or 30%, of the total complement pool is extravascular. In studies using fluorescent antibody as an endpoint, Cochrane, moreover, found C3a in the extravascular space and concluded that this is evidence that C3a may be formed in the union of antigen and antibody, regardless of the area where immunological reactants unite (C. G. Cochrane, personal communication, 1973). Support for the view that these observations may have some bearing on the involvement of the complement system in burn pathology can be found in a series of studies by Ishizaka (Ishizaka and Ishizaka, 1959, 1960; Ishizaka *et al.*, 1961), where it was demonstrated that aggregated human and rabbit globulin, obtained by heating, gave immediate skin reactions in normal guinea pigs and inactivated complement, the aggregation fixing C1,4, followed by inactivation of C2, the inactivation of C3 by the aggregate being inhibited in the presence of EDTA. Putting this together into a somewhat speculative construction, it can be imagined that an innocuous complement pool bathes all small vascular beds and that this physiological state is altered by many types of insult—infection, burns, antigen–antibody complexes, and indeed even such agents as starch (Nelson and Lebrun, 1956)—causing complement to be cleaved and to release chemotactic fragments into the affected zone of injury. Indirect support for such a view comes from Stecher (see summary by Stecher, 1970) who has shown that macrophages and fibroblasts from a variety of species, including human, can synthesize complement components.

VII. Possible Modifying Mechanisms in Chemotaxis

A review of the literature of chemotaxis can create the impression that this remarkable phenomenon is arranged to work in only one direction: toward the continual accumulation of white blood cells at inflammatory foci where bacteria and proteolytic debris are sought out, ingested, and degraded. On this basis, even trivial injuries conceivably could be never ending sources of a continuing inflammatory process as white cells cannibalize each other to bring new white blood cells into the field to ingest and create new fodder for the same process.

To accept such a construction one would have to believe that proteolytic end products of tissue destruction are in themselves chemotactic for white cells, an attractive idea that recurs repeatedly in the literature but for which there is little direct proof that can stand up under critical examination and against which Harris produced striking evidence. Yet, clearly, even given the assumption that injured cells beget more injured cells . . . ad infinitum, the biological system does not work on this suicidal basis.

Inflammatory reactions, by and large, run a regular, and often relatively uneventful, course toward healing. What, then, shuts off the system? Opie (1922) was one of the early workers to address himself to this question, emphasizing the interplay between neutrophil enzymes and antienzymes of the tissue in the modulation of tissue injury. [The subject has been reviewed in recent years by Fritz et al. (1968) and Vogel et al. (1969; see also discussion of endogenous inhibitors of neutrophil constituents in Volume III, Chapter 3 by Cochrane and Janoff and discussion by Lepow (1971).] In recent months it has been possible to obtain what appear to be new insights into this aspect of the problem, based on a small but rapidly proliferating and stimulating literature that as much by accident as by design has fused on three experimental objectives: the respective roles of lysosomes, cyclic AMP, and prostaglandins in the possible servo-mechanisms that are played off against each other during the recovery phase of injury.

Persellin (1969) showed that antiserum prepared in the rabbit to rat peritoneal leukocyte granule (lysosome) membranes retarded the release of enzyme activity from isolated lysosomes. This stabilizing action, isolated in the γ G fraction of antiserum, protected intact rat liver large granules stressed by 30°C incubation and also protected rabbit peritoneal leukocyte granules exposed to Triton X-100. The stabilizing activity could be removed by absorption with homologous and heterologous membrane. It was concluded that since lysosomes are implicated in the induction of various forms of tissue damage, a membrane-reactive antibody capable of stabilizing lysosomes could act to retard the inflammatory process.

In an extension of this work, Persellin also showed that serum from rats with adjuvant arthritis stabilized the membranes of isolated normal rat liver lysosomes (Persellin, 1972). The stabilizer retarded the release of the lysosomal enzymes, acid phosphatase and β-glucuronidase, but not the release of the mitochondrial enzyme, isocitric dehydrogenase. Stabilizing activity in serum paralleled adjuvant disease, being greatest when the inflammation was most intense and subsiding as the arthritis diminished. Activity could be removed from the serum by absorption with isolated membranes; adjuvant arthritis serum did not inhibit enzyme activities. The membrane reactant was neither a corticosteroid nor an antibody but was a large molecular weight substance with charge properties similar to an α globulin. Support for this comes indirectly from the studies of Ward (1966), who showed that lysosomal membrane-stabilizing agents inhibited neutrophil chemotaxis, while those lysosomal membrane-labilizing agents enhanced the chemotactic response of neutrophils.

Prostaglandins seem to be chemotactic for neutrophils but not for macrophages (Kaley and Weiner, 1971a,b) and yet at the same time they may be synthesized in the wake of lysosome destruction. Anderson et al. (1971) injected carageenin suspension subcutaneously into air blebs in the rat and noted, 12 hours later, the appearance of β-glucuronidase and acid phosphatase, plus prostaglandin E_2 in the bleb fluid. They suggested that phospholipases are freed from the lysosomes of leukocytes overactive in the endocytosis of carageenin, and that these attack cell membrane phospholipid to give arachidonic acid, which, in turn, is converted to prostaglandin by freely available tissue enzyme.

The combined effect of five other recent studies provides evidence that prostaglandins and cAMP act as modifiers of motility and lysosomal release, and, in one case, of histamine release, all which would be expected to put a brake on the inflammatory process. Bourne et al. (1972) demonstrated that extracellular histamine stimulates the production of cAMP in human neutrophils and prevents antigenic release of histamine from cells of allergic donors. Weissman et al. (1971a) showed that phagocytosis of undigestible particles causes the selective extrusion of lysosomal enzymes from macrophages and neutrophils and that the process can be modified by cyclic nucleotides, prostaglandin E_1, and colchicine.

Zurier and Quagliata (1971) found that when rats are treated with prostaglandin PGE_1, adjuvant arthritis is prevented and suppressed, supporting earlier studies of Aspinall and Cammarata (1969) and Weissmann et al.

(1971b) concerning the modification of the inflammatory process by prostaglandins, Johnson et al. (1972) showed that dibutyl cAMP or PGE_1 reversibly inhibited motility in fibroblasts. They proposed that cAMP mediates contact inhibition of movement in subconfluent cultures. In confluent cultures of 3T3 cells, movement and also growth are inhibited. It is of interest that Kaley and Weiner (1971b) found that cyclic nucleotides did not have a chemotactic effect on neutrophils.

Along somewhat different lines but with the same objective in mind, Malawista and Bensch (1967) and Bensch and Malawista (1969) found that colchicine and vinblastine inhibit release of lysosomal constituents into the digestion vacuole after ingestion of bacteria, attributing this to a role played by microtubules in the fate of lysosomal granules (Malawista and Bodel, 1967; Malawista, 1968, 1971). In parallel experiments, Weissmann et al. (1971b) demonstrated an inhibition of zymosan particle uptake and bovine serum albumin uptake by macrophages after treatment with colchicine, as noted above, and vinblastine. Further studies by Weissmann's group (1972) provided data suggesting that the release of inflammatory substances from lysosomes is regulated by intracellular cAMP, which activates a protein kinase to control, by means of microtubules, the flow of lysosomes to phagocytic vacuoles or to the cell periphery.

The idea that inflammatory exudates may in fact contain antiinflammatory materials, far from being new, has generated a long and rather uneven literature, but it has received new attention in recent years through studies of the antiinflammatory properties of granuloma pouch exudates (Di Pasquale and Girerd, 1961; Di Pasquale et al., 1963) and of subcutaneously implanted polyester sponges, in rats, reported by two groups (Robinson and Robson, 1964, 1966) and Atkinson and his colleagues (Atkinson and Boura, 1969; Atkinson and Hicks, 1971; Atkinson et al., 1971). Atkinson found that the exudate obtained from sponge implantations possessed both irritant and antiinflammatory activity and suggested that it is possible that the apparent antiinflammatory action of the material may at least be due in part to a counter-irritant mechanism rather than to the presence of a specific antiinflammatory factor.

Looking at this problem from the vantage point of the serum, and in terms of postulated chemotactic factors, rather than in terms of the leukocyte, Berenberg and Ward (1972) produced evidence for the existence in human serum of an inhibitor of such factors. Using in vitro micropore filter techniques and human or rabbit neutrophils as the indicator cells, chemotactic responses of leukocytes to the complement-derived chemotactic factors (C3a, C5a, $C\overline{567}$) and a chemotactic factor from E. coli were studied. The chemotactic inhibitor isolated from human serum blocked the activity of all chemotactic factors tested and was soluble in ammonium sulfate (at 45%

saturation). In sucrose density gradient ultracentrifugation as well as in gel filtration it appeared in a biphasic distribution with activity near the IgC and albumin markers. The inhibitor acted directly on the chemotactic factor rather than on the leukocyte. Evidence for binding of inhibitor to chemotactic factor (C3a) was negative. Demonstration of the inhibitor in normal human serum required fractionation and/or concentration of serum, whereas serum from most patients with agammaglobulinemia (Bruton type) or Hodgkins disease was rich in inhibitor activity. The investigators suggested that the existence in serum of inhibitors of chemotactic factors may represent a control mechanism of these inhibitors. The chemotactic factor inhibitors(s) differed from the anaphylactoxin inactivator in many respects; evidence does not yet permit a conclusive statement about the relationship of these two inhibitors.

In summary, it should be noted that much of the emerging literature on modifying influences in chemotaxis, cited in this section (and excluding the type of mechanism that Berenberg and Ward have uncovered), argues for a viewpoint that extravascular inflammatory foci, whatever their chemotactic character, may, in fact, unloose antiinflammatory mechanisms. Yet a dominant theme in the literature of inflammation is that inflammatory foci have attractant powers for white cells, and it is this chemotactic nature of the lesion that makes it possible to isolate injuries and neutralize them. Here, then, we have a paradox: Inflammatory foci are chemotactic, but they are also antichemotactic. This paradox may be resolved with the discovery that both statements are true. Early, in an inflammatory reaction, there may be chemotactic influences that evoke white blood cells, but later, when these cells are not needed, antichemotactic mechanisms may come into play. If this is a rational thought, then one important goal for workers in the field in the next decade is to analyze the changing chemistry of the inflammatory lesion and to demonstrate subtle alterations, at the molecular level, in the chemotactic and phagocytic properties of cells invading injury sites at different phases of the inflammatory reaction.

VIII. Conclusion

Chemotaxis appears to be an intermediate stage in the basic defense system of small blood vessels. The process starts with endothelial injury and, classically, ends with phagocytosis, but clearly there must be another step having to do with mechanisms that break the chain of events. Whatever the initiating stimulus, a process is set loose in which degranulating cells appear to feed on each other, cannibal-like, creating a mechanism that seems to be equipped to run in only one direction: toward the isolation of injury products.

Yet in fact the system must have built-in controls, possibly several mechanisms regulating a series of checks and balances to make certain that acute inflammatory reactions come to an end.

It was postulated by Grant and his colleagues (1967) that the unloosing of chemotactic materials outside of blood vessels, as in an Artus reaction where the antigen is layered on the tissue instead of being injected into it, could engulf the vessels, altering endothelial membranes, and thereby trapping white cells which, on sticking, could pick up the chemotactic gradient and emigrate into the tissue. Whether the process starts inside or outside the vessel, however, it is conceivable that the type of injury that causes white blood cells to stick may be of a different nature, or different order of magnitude, than the type of injury that causes them to emigrate, a caution emphasized by Florey (1962).

Putting the data together in a somewhat arbitrary and speculative way, one can construct a "flow sheet" of events in inflammation, in which chemotaxis plays a central role:

(1) Endothelial injury sets off the process. This is true in the case of direct assault on the blood vessel, for whatever reason, through such widely disparate stimuli as heat and cold, infection, direct trauma, ionizing radiations, ultraviolet light, antigen–antibody complexes, and noxious experimental solutions. If the injury does not progress beyond the vessel wall, what ensues is thrombosis, not a chemotactic cascade.

(2) White blood cells adhere to injured vessels but they do not emigrate in the absence of extravascular chemotactic effects. If such effects are present, then

(3) Emigration occurs and, in the presence of a suitable stimulus, there is created

(4) A movement of white cells toward attractants (chemotaxis), followed by

(5) Contact and attachment of the cell to the attractant and the subsequent

(6) Ingestion of the phagocytizable material and

(7) Its digestion and destruction, which, in turn, sets up

(8) An expanding pool of inflammatory cells, yielding chemotactic products, drawing in more cells, until

(9) Modifying mechanisms, such as agents that shut off or neutralize hydrolases or neutralize other enzymes that denature protein, take over the assignment and shut down the system, permitting

(10) Repair processes to start the task of reconstruction.

Such a postulate creates more questions than it answers, but there are some internal consistencies. For example, intravascular injury, as with a laser beam that can select a vessel site and confine the simulus to that site, yields no emigration of white blood cells (Grant and Becker, 1965, 1966; Grant, 1974). It is reasonable to assume that most experimental injury, however, is more diffuse, notably stimuli unleashed through intradermal injection, and therefore chemotactic mechanisms created by widespread extravascular cell damage, experimentally, are available to attract the adherent white blood cells. It is permissible to wonder how rigorously such systems mimic biological phenomena. At the same time, the evidence for the chemotactic nature of proteolytic breakdown products, however attractive this concept may be, is by no means clear-cut.

Harris' experiments deny that the products of tissue breakdown are chemotactic but Bessis and Burté demonstrated the chemotactic nature of dead white cells for other living white blood cells. Both sets of experiments were done under rather rigorously controlled *in vitro* circumstances. One conceivable reconciliation of these results could be found in the fact that chemotaxis took place only immediately after the death of the cells in Bessis' system. Possibly, whatever the molecule is that constitutes the attractant, it is easily diffused away, or altered, in injury states. However, this cannot be a wholly satisfactory explanation. Grant achieved what certainly must have been a chemotactic response triggered by the burning of collagen by a laser beam, yet the response took more than 3 hours to evolve, and it is unclear whether the chemotactic cells came from blood vessels or happened to be only extravascular cells in the vicinity of the reaction. On the other hand, this was an *in vivo* system, where many of the ground rules may be different from *in vitro* situations.

One can look at the problem in another way, as many of the experiments described in this monograph imply, by shifting emphasis away from the precise question of whether proteolytic breakdown products are chemotactic or not. Then if one requires that such a construction as that listed in the flow sheet above must, mandatorily, take complement into account, a reasonable entry for this point can be found in the views of Ham and Hurley (1968) and Willoughby *et al.* (1969), who look at the inflammatory reaction largely in terms of vascular permeability; that is, in terms of the result of endothelial injury rather than in terms of the endothelial lesion that presumably triggers the reaction. Such a focus permits one to suggest that in any injury leaked plasma protein can become modified (aggregated) and thus perhaps can be rendered capable of fixing complement, which, in turn, increases vascular permeability and leukocyte emigration, regardless of the avidity, or lack of it, of leukocytes for dead tissue. If valid, such a construction gives one a grasp of immediate events at vascular interfaces but leaves open speculation about the myriad events that occur, their mechanisms largely clouded by imprecise experimental techniques, in the tissues beyond vascular fronts. If one now adds to this hypothesis the assumption that extravascular tissue is drenched in complement, or at least carries enough of it as a source in an inactive state, capable of being fixed, then one can arrange the scheme loosely to make a case for the significance of complement from midstream to the extravascular chemotactic focus.

Yet it is difficult to get around the fact that whereas complement may play a role in some chemotactic reactions, there is a considerable body of evidence that chemotaxis proceeds without difficulty in the absence of complement. Finally, it must be emphasized that agents that seem to incite inflammatory reactions also, under certain conditions, appear to counteract these reactions, a finding calculated to create a fair amount of confusion in the analysis of inflammatory mechanisms. It does, however, keep ajar a door that may open onto a pathway toward an understanding of a process that common sense emphasizes must be shut off if biological tissue is not to devour itself.

IX. Summary

1. Chemotaxis, a phenomenon that results in the focal accumulation of motile cells, is a primordial biological reaction, widespread in the animal and plant kingdoms. It is demonstrated easily in a variety of *in vitro* systems, but its confirmation *in vivo* is made with difficulty. Absolute proof of the phenomenon, by direct observation *in vivo*, has not yet been achieved.

2. In various single cell organisms, chemotaxis can be construed as serving (a) to enable the organism to collect where food is available, (b) to avoid noxious materials, (c) to facilitate the aggregation of organisms so that more complex structures can be created, (d) to facilitate the dispersion of organisms for the optimal use of environmental resources, and (e) to aid in fertilization.

3. In multicellular organisms, highly specialized cells, such as polymorphonuclear leukocytes, have chemotactic potentialities. It is tempting to look on such a phenomenon as a defense mechanism, a viewpoint which has remained virtually unassailed over a century of prodigious biological research.

4. Leukocyte chemotaxis is incited by a wide variety of agents, including bacteria and bacterial filtrates, starch granules, casein, and peptone, none of which seem to require complement, and by an even longer list of material which, when incubated with normal serum, yield chemotactic responses perhaps dependent to a greater or lesser degree on the presence of complement. How often and to what extent the wide disparity in reported results may be a function of the experimental, rather than the biological, system is not clear.

5. In acute inflammatory states, the mounting reaction, to which chemotactic mechanisms make a major contribution, runs in one direction—toward the piling up of degranulating phagocytic cells in a self-perpetuating process that appears to invest tissue with the capacity to devour itself. There are modulating influences at work, however, in the inflammatory process. Some of these moderators may, in fact, be inflammatory agents which, in the evolution of an inflammatory reaction, shift roles and acquire antiinflammatory capacities. If true, this would help to explain how pathological processes are brought back to physiological equilibrium.

6. Leukocyte chemotaxis has been under intense investigation for almost 100 years, but the mechanisms by which attractants and the white blood cell are brought into phase with each other are unknown. Bacterial studies, which show the existence of distinct receptors for various attractants, may offer clues for studying this problem in neutrophils at the cellular level. The system also may be under the control of potentiating compounds, perhaps activated by cellular energy levels.

Acknowledgments

The authors are indebted to the staff of Gilbert J. Clausman, Librarian of the New York University School of Medicine, and in particular to Miss Eleonor Pasmik, Assistant Librarian and Head of Reference, and Mrs. Debra Eisenberg, Assistant Reference Librarian, for yeoman service in chasing down and helping to find and to check references. The authors also would like to acknowledge a debt of gratitude to the National Library of Medicine, MEDLARS Search Unit, for a bibliographic search of the extensive literature on chemotaxis between the years 1960 and 1967, and to the State University of New York (SUNY) Biomedical Communication Network for assistance in retrieval of late 1973 and 1974 references.

One of us (WSR) was a Postdoctoral Fellow in the laboratory of Professor J. P. Trinkaus during the preparation of this article and was supported by USPHS Training Grant HD 00032 to the Biology Department, Yale University.

One of us (LG) was supported in this effort by NIH Grant AM 07501–09.

References

Addison, W. (1843). *Trans. Prov. Med. Surg. Ass.* **11**, 233.
Adler, J. (1966a). *J. Bacteriol.* **92**, 121.
Adler, J. (1966b). *Science* **153**, 708.
Adler, J. (1969). *Science* **166**, 1588.
Adler, J., and Dahl, M. (1967). *J. Gen. Microbiol.* **46**, 161.
Adler, J., and Templeton, B. (1967). *J. Gen. Microbiol.* **46**, 175.
Adler, J., Hazelbauer, G. L., and Dahl, M. M. (1973). *J. Bacteriol.* **115**, 824.
Allen, R. D. (1961). *In* "The Cell" (J. Brachet and A. E. Mirsky, eds.), Vol. 2, pp. 135–216. Academic Press, New York.
Allgower, M., and Block, H. (1949). *Amer. Tuberc. Rev.* **59**, 562.
Allison, F., Jr., Smith, M. R., and Wood, W. B., Jr. (1955). *J. Exp. Med.* **102**, 655.

Alper, C. A., and Rosen, F. S. (1967). *J. Clin. Invest.* **46**, 2021.

Anderson, A. J., Brocklehurst, W. E., and Willis, A. L. (1971). *Pharmacol. Res. Commun.* **3**, 13.

Anderson, B. R., and Van Epps, D. D. (1972). *J. Infec. Dis.* **125**, 353.

Armstrong, J. B., and Adler, J. (1969a). *Genetics* **61**, 61.

Armstrong, J. B., and Adler, J. (1969b). *J. Bacteriol.* **97**, 156.

Armstrong, J. B., Adler, J., and Dahl, M. (1967). *J. Bacteriol.* **93**, 390.

Aspinall, R. L., and Cammarata, P. S. (1969). *Nature (London)* **224**, 1320.

Atkinson, D. C., and Hicks, R. (1971). *Brit. J. Pharmacol.* **41**, 480.

Atkinson, D. C., Boora, A. L., and Hicks, R. (1969). *Eur. J. Pharmacol.* **8**, 348.

Atkinson, D. C., Whittle, B. A., and Hicks, R. (1971). *Eur. J. Pharmacol.* **16**, 254.

Baracchini, O., and Sherris, J. C. (1959). *J. Pathol. Bacteriol.* **77**, 565.

Barkley, D. S. (1969). *Science* **165**, 1133.

Becker, E. L. (1969). *Fed. Proc., Fed. Amer. Soc. Exp. Biol.* **28**, 1704.

Becker, E. L. (1971). *J. Immunol.* **106**, 689.

Becker, E. L. (1972). *J. Exp. Med.* **135**, 376.

Becker, E. L., and Ward, P. A. (1967). *J. Exp. Med.* **125**, 1021.

Becker, E. L., and Ward, P. A. (1969). *J. Exp. Med.* **129**, 569.

Becker, E. L., Davis, A. T., Estensen, R. D., and Quie, P. G. (1972). *J. Immunol.* **108**, 396.

Bell, L. G. E. (1961). *J. Theor. Biol.* **1**, 104.

Bell, L. G. E., and Jeon, K. W. (1962). *Nature (London)* **95**, 400.

Bensch, K. G., and Malawista, S. E. (1969). *J. Cell. Biol.* **40**, 95.

Berenberg, J. L., and Ward, P. A. (1972). *J. Clin. Invest.* **56**, 9a (abstr.).

Berenberg, J. L., Ward, P. A., and Sonenshine, E. E. (1972). *J. Immunol.* **109**, 451.

Berg, H. C. and Brown, D. A. (1972). *Nature (London)* **239**, 500.

Bessis, M., and Burté, B. (1964). *Tex. Rep. Biol. Med.* **23**, 204.

Beyerinck, M. W. (1893). *Zentralbl. Bakteriol., Parasitenk., Infektionskr.* **14**, 827.

Bimpong, C. E., and Clerk, G. C. (1970). *Ann. Bot. (London)* [N. S.] **34**, 617.

Bingley, M., Bell, L. G. E., and Jeon, K. W. (1962). *Exp. Cell Res.* **28**, 208.

Bingley, M. S., and Thompson, C. M. (1962). *J. Theor. Biol.* **2**, 16.

Bonner, J. T. (1947). *J. Exp. Zool.* **106**, 1.

Bonner, J. T. (1970). *Proc. Nat. Acad. Sci. U.S.* **65**, 110.

Bonner, J. T., and Dodd, M. R. (1962). *Biol. Bull.* **122**, 13.

Bonner, J. T., Barkley, D. S., Hall, E. M., Konijn, T. M., Mason, J. W., O'Keefe, G., III, and Wolfe, P. B. (1969). *Develop. Biol.* **20**, 72.

Bonner, J. T., Hall, E. M., Sachsenmaier, W., and Walker, B. K. (1970). *J. Bacteriol.* **102**, 682.

Bonner, J. T., Hirshfield, M. F., and Hall, E. M. (1971). *Exp. Cell Res.* **68**, 61.

Bonner, J. T., Hall, E. M., Noller, S., Oleson, F. B., and Roberts, A. B. (1972). *Dev. Biol.* **29**, 402.

Borel, J. F., and Sorkin, E. (1969). *Experientia* **25**, 1333.

Borel, J. F., Keller, H. U., and Sorkin, E. (1969). *Int. Arch. Allergy Appl. Immunol.* **35**, 194.

Bourne, H. R., Lichtenstein, L. M., and Melmon, K. L. (1972). *J. Immunol.* **108**, 695.

Boyden, S. (1962). *J. Exp. Med.* **115**, 453.

Boyden, S. V., North, R. J., and Faulkner, S. M. (1965). *Complement, Ciba Found.* 1967 pp. 190–213.

Brewer, J. E., and Bell, L. G. E. (1969). *J. Cell Sci.* **4**, 17.

Brier, A. M., Snyderman, R., Mergenhagen, S. E., and Notkins, A. L., (1970). *Science* **170**, 1104.

Brokaw, C. J. (1958a). *J. Exp. Biol.* **35**, 192.

Brokaw, C. J. (1958b). *J. Exp. Biol.* **35**, 197.

Bryant, R. E., DesPrez, R. M., VanWay, M. H., and Rogers, D. E. (1966). *J. Exp. Med.* **124**, 483.

Buckley, I. K. (1963). *Exp. Mol. Pathol.* **2**, 402.

Caner, J. E. Z. (1965). *Arthritis Rheum.* **8**, 757.

Carlile, M. J., and Machlis, L. (1965a). *Amer. J. Bot.* **52**, 478.

Carlile, M. J., and Machlis, L. (1965b). *Amer. J. Bot.* **52**, 484.

Carruthers, B. M. (1966). *Can. J. Physiol. Pharmacol.* **44**, 475.

Carruthers, B. M. (1967). *Can. J. Physiol. Pharmacol.* **45**, 269.

Chambers, R., and Fell, H. B. (1932). *Proc. Roy. Soc., Ser. B* **109**, 380.

Chang, C., and Houck, J. (1970). *Proc. Soc. Exp. Biol. Med.* **134**, 22.

Chang, Y. Y. (1968). *Science* **160**, 57.

Chassy, B. M. (1972). *Science* **175**, 1016.

Cinader, B., Dubiski, S., and Wardlaw, A. C. (1964). *J. Exp. Med.* **120**, 897.

Cinader, B., Jeejeebhoy, H. F., and Koh, S. W. (1971). *J. Exp. Med.* **133**, 81.

Clark, E. R., and Clark, E. L. (1920). *Amer. J. Anat.* **27**, 221.

Clark, E. R., and Clark, E. L. (1922). *Anat. Rec.* **24**, 137.

Clark, E. R., and Clark, L. C. (1930). *Amer. J. Anat.* **46**, 91.

Clark, E. R., and Clark, L. C. (1935). *Amer. J. Anat.* **57**, 385.

Clark, E. R., Clark, E. L., and Rex, R. O. (1936). *Amer. J. Anat.* **59**, 123.

Clark, R. A., and Kimball, H. R. (1971). *J. Clin. Invest.* **50**, 2645.

Clayton, R. K. (1964). *Photophysiology* **2**, 51–77.

Cliff, W. J. (1965). *Quart. J. Exp. Physiol. Cog. Med. Sci.* **50**, 79.

Cliff, W. J. (1966a). *Quart. J. Exp. Physiol. Cog. Med. Sci.* **51**, 112.

Cliff, W. J. (1966b). *J. Exp. Med.* **124**, 543.

Cochrane, C. (1969). *Advan. Immunol.* **9**, 97.

Cochrane, C. G., and Müller-Eberhard, H. J. (1968). *J. Exp. Med.* **127**, 371.

Cochrane, C. G., Müller-Eberhard, H. J., and Aikin, B. S. (1970). *J. Immunol.* **105**, 55.

Cohen, M. H., and Roberston, A. D. J. (1971a). *J. Theor. Biol.* **31**, 101.

Cohen, M. H., and Roberston, A. D. J. (1971b). *J. Theor. Biol.* **31**, 119.

Cohen, S., and Ward, P. A. (1971). *J. Exp. Med.* **133**, 133.

Cohn, Z. A., and Morse, S. I. (1960). *J. Exp. Med.* **111**, 667.

Cohnheim, J. (1882). "Lectures on General Pathology" Vol. 1. New Sydenham Soc., London (translated into English, 1889).

Commandon, J. (1917). *C. R. Soc. Biol.* **80**, 314.

Commandon, J. (1919). *C. R. Soc. Biol.* **82**, 1171.

Cook, A. H., and Elvidge, J. A. (1951). *Proc. Roy. Soc., Ser. B* **138**, 97.

Cook, A. H., Elvidge, J. A., and Heilbron, I. (1948). *Proc. Roy. Soc., Ser. B* **135**, 293.

Cornely, H. P. (1966). *Proc. Soc. Exp. Biol. Med.* **122**, 831.

Cullumbine, H., and Rydon, H. N. (1946). *Brit. J. Exp. Pathol.* **27**, 33.

Dahlquist, F. W., Lovely, P., and Koshland, D. E. (1972). *Nature (London), New Biol.* **236**, 120.

Day, N. K. B., Good, R. A., Finstad, J., Johannsen, R., Pickering, R. J., and Gewurz, H. (1970a). *Proc. Soc. Exp. Biol. Med.* **133**, 397.

Day, N. K. B., Gewurz, H., Johanssen, R., Finstad, J., and Good, R. A. (1970b). *J. Exp. Med.* **132**, 941.

de Haan J. (1917). *Arch. Neer. Physiol.* **2**, 674.

Delaunay, A., Lebrun, J., and Barber, M. (1951). *Nature (London)* **167**, 774.

De Meo, A. N., and Anderson, B. R. (1972). *N. Engl. J. Med.* **286**, 735.

De Shazo, C. V., Henson, P. M., and Cochrane, C. G. (1971). *J. Clin. Invest.* **51**, 50.

De Shazo, C. V., McGrade, M. T., Henson, P. M., and Cochrane, C. G. (1972). *J. Immunol.* **108**, 1414.

DiPasquale, G., and Girerd, R. J. (1961). *Amer. J. Physiol.* **201**, 1155.

DiPasquale, G., Girerd, R. J., Beach, V. L., and Steinetz, B. G. (1963). *Amer. J. Physiol.* **205**, 1080.

Dittrich, H. (1962). Physiology of neutrophils. *In* "Physiology and Pathology of Leucocytes" (H. Brownsteiner and D. Zucker-Franklin, ed.), p. 130. Grune & Stratton, New York.

Dixon, H. M., and McCutcheon, M. (1936). *Proc. Soc. Exp. Biol. Med.* **34**, 173.

Doetsch, R. N., and Hageage, G. J. (1968). *Biol. Rev. Cambridge Phil. Soc.* **43**, 317.

Dryl, S. (1952). *Acta Biol. Exp. (Warsaw)* **16**, 23.

Dryl, S. (1959a). *Acta Biol. Exp. (Warsaw)* **19**, 83.

Dryl, S. (1959b). *Acta Biol. Exp. (Warsaw)* **19**, 95.

Dryl, S. (1961). *Acta Biol. Exp. (Warsaw)* **21**, 75.

Dryl, S. (1963). *Anim. Behav.* **11**, 393.

Dryl, S., and Grebecki, A. (1966). *Protoplasma* **62**, 255.

Dukes, P. D., and Apple, J. L. (1961). *Phytopathology* **51**, 195.

Duthie, E. S., and Chain, E. (1939). *Brit. J. Exp. Path.* **20**, 417.

Dutrochet, M. H. (1824). "Recherches, anatomiques et physiologiques sur la structure intime des animaux et des végétaux, et sur leur motilité." Baillière et Fils, Paris.

Dworkin, M. (1966). *Ann. Rev. Microbiol.* **20**, 75–106.

Ebert, R. H., Sanders, A. G., and Florey, H. W. (1940). *Brit. J. Exp. Pathol.* **21**, 212.

Eckert, R. (1972). *Science* **176**, 473.

Engelmann, T. W. (1881). *Bot. Ztg.* **39**, 441.

Engelmann, T. W. (1883). *Arch. Gesamte Physiol. Menschen Tiere* **30**, 95.

Fleming, R. W., and Williams, F. D. (1968). *Bacteriol. Proc.* p. 29.

Fleming, R. W., Williams, F. D., and Wailes, K. A. (1967). *J. Bacteriol.* **94**, 855.

Florey, H. W. (1962). *In* "General Pathology" (H. W. Florey,), 3rd ed., p. 98. Saunders, Philadelphia, Pennsylvania.

Florey, H. W., and Jennings, M. A. (1970). *In* "General Pathology" (H. W. Florey, ed.), 4th ed., p. 124. Saunders, Philadelphia, Pennsylvania.

Fluegel, W. (1963). *Proc. Minn. Acad. Sci.* **30**, 120.

Fraenkel, G. S., and Gunn, D. L. (1940). "The Orientation of Animals." Oxford Univ. Press, London and New York. (reprinted, Dover, New York, 1961).

Frank, M. M., May, F., Gaither, T., and Ellman, L. (1971). *J. Exp. Med.* **134**, 176.

Fritz, H., Trautschold, I., Haendle, H., and Werle, E. (1968). *Ann. N.Y. Acad. Sci.* **146**, Art. 2, 400.

Gabritchewsky, G. (1890). *Ann. Inst. Pasteur, Paris* **4**, 346.

Gallin, J. I., Clark, R. A., and Kimball, H. R. (1973). *J. Immunol.* **110**, 233.

Gamow, R. I., Böttger, B., and Barnes, F. S. (1971). *Biophys. J.* **11**, 860.

Gerisch, G., Normann, I., and Beug, H. (1966). *Naturwissenschaften* **53**, 618.

Gerisch, G., Malchow, D., Riedel, V., Muller, E., and Every, M. (1972). *Nature (London), New Biol.* **235**, 90.

Gewurz, H., Pickering, R. J., Muschel, L. H., Mergenhagen, S. E., and Good, R. A. (1966). *Lancet* **2**, 356.

Gewurz, H., Page, A. R., Pickering, R. J., and Good, R. A. (1967). *Int. Arch. Allergy Appl. Immunol.* **32**, 64.

Glovsky, M. M., Becker, E. L., and Halbrook, N. J. (1968). *J. Immunol.* **100**, 979.

Glovsky, M. M., Ward, P. A., Becker, E. L., and Halbrook, N. J. (1969). *J. Immunol.* **102**, 1.

Goidl, E. A., Chassy, B. M., Love, L. L., and Krichevsky, M. I. (1972). *Proc. Nat. Acad. Sci. U.S.* **69**, 1128.

Grant, L. (1974). *Microvasc. Res.* (in Press).

Grant, L., and Becker, F. F. (1965). *Proc. Soc. Exp. Biol. Med.* **119**, 1123.

Grant, L., and Becker, F. (1966). *Arch. Pathol.* **81**, 36.

Grant, L., Ross, M. H., Moses, J., Prose, P., Zweifach, B. W., and Ebert, R. H. (1967). *Z. Zellforsch. Mikrosk. Anat.* **77**, 554.

Ham, K. N., and Hurley, J. V. (1968). *J. Path. Bacteriol.* **95**, 175.

Harris, H. (1953a). *J. Pathol. Bacteriol.* **66**, 135.

Harris, H. (1953b). *Brit. J. Exp. Pathol.* **34**, 599.

Harris, H. (1954). *Physiol. Rev.* **34**, 529.

Harris, H. (1960). *Bacteriol. Rev.* **24**, 3.

Harvey, R. L., Kronvall, G., Trour, G. M., Anderson, R. E., and Williams, R. C. (1970). *Proc. Soc. Exp. Biol. Med.* **135**, 453.

Hausman, M. S., Snyderman, R., and Mergenhagen, S. E. (1972). *J. Infec. Dis.* **125**, 595.

Hayashi, H., Yoshida, K., Ozaki, T., and Ushijima, K. (1970). *Nature (London)* **226**, 174.

Hazelbauer, G. L., and Adler, J. (1971). *Nature (London), New Biol.* **230**, 101.

Hazelbauer, G. L., Mesibov, R. E., and Adler, J. (1969). *Proc. Nat. Acad. Sci. U.S.* **64**, 1300.

Hill, J. H., and Ward, P. A. (1969). *J. Exp. Med.* **130**, 505.

Hill, J. H., and Ward, P. A. (1971). *J. Exp. Med.* **133**, 885.

Hirsch, J. G., and Church, A. B. (1960). *J. Exp. Med.* **111**, 309.

Ho, H. H., and Hickman, C. J. (1967). *Can. J. Bot.* **45**, 1983.

Holwill, M. E. J. (1966). *Physiol. Rev.* **46**, 696.

Houck, J., and Chang, C. (1971). *Proc. Soc. Exp. Biol. Med.* **138**, 69.

Houck, J., and Jacob, R. (1959). *Amer. J. surg.* [N. S.] **25**, 244.

Houck, J., and Jacob, R. (1961). *J. Invest. Dermatol.* **36**, 451.

Houck, J., Patel, Y., and Gladner, J. (1967). *Biochem. Pharmacol.* **16**, 1099.

Hurley, J. V. (1963). *Nature (London)* **198**, 1212.

Hurley, J. V. (1964). *Ann. N. Y. Acad. Sci.* **116**, (Art. 3), 918.

Hurley, J. V., and Spector, W. G. (1961a). *J. Pathol. Bacteriol.* **82**, 403.

Hurley, J. V., and Spector, W. G. (1961b). *J. Pathol. Bacteriol.* **82**, 421.

Ingraham, E. S., and Wartman, W. B. (1939). *Arch. Pathol.* **28**, 318.

Ishizaka, T., and Ishizaka, K. (1959). *Proc. Soc. Exp. Biol. Med.* **101**, 845.

Ishizaka, T., and Ishizaka, K. (1960). *J. Immunol.* **85**, 163.

Ishizaka, T., Ishizaka, K, and Borso, T. (1961). *J. Immunol.* **87**, 433

Jacob, R., and Houck, J. (1959). *Surg., Gynecol Obstet.* **109**, 85.

Jahn, T. L., and Bovee, E. C. (1964). *In* "Biochemistry and Physiology of Protozoa" (S. H. Hutner, ed.), pp. 61–129. Academic Press, New York.

Jahn, T. L., and Bovee, E. C. (1965). *Annu. Rev. Microbiol.* **19**, 21.

Jahn, T. L., and Bovee, E. C. (1967). *In* "Research in Protozoology" (T. T. Chen, ed.), Vol. I, pp. 41–200. Pergamon, Oxford.

Jahn, T. L., and Bovee, E. C. (1969). *Physiol. Rev.* **49**, 793.

Jennings, H. S. (1904). "Contributions to the Study of the Behavior of Lower Organisms." Carnegie Institution, Washington, D. C.

Jennings, H. S. (1906). "Behavior of the Lower Organisms." Columbia Univ. Press, New York (reprinted, Indiana Univ. Press, Bloomington, 1962).

Jennings, H. S., and Crosby, J. H. (1901). *Amer. J. Physiol.* **6**, 31.

Jeon, K. W., and Bell, L. G. E. (1962). *Exp. Cell Res.* **27**, 350.

Jeon, K. W., and Bell, L. G. E. (1964). *Exp. Cell Res.* **33**, 531.

Jeon, K. W., and Bell, L. G. E. (1965). *Exp. Cell Res.* **38**, 536.

Johnson, G. S., Morgan, W. D., and Pastan, I. (1972). *Nature (London)* **235**, 54.

Kaley, G., and Weiner, R. (1971a). *Ann. N. Y. Acad. Sci.* **180**, 338.

Kaley, G., and Weiner, R. (1971b). *Nature (London) New Biol.* **234**, 119.

Kaplan, A. P., Kay, A. B., and Austen, K. F. (1972). *J. Exp. Med.* **135**, 81.

Kay, A. B., Stechschulte, D. J., and Austen, K. F. (1971). *J. Exp. Med.* **133**, 602.

Keller, E. F., and Segel, L. A. (1970). *J. Theor. Biol.* **26**, 399.

Keller, E. F., and Segel, L. A. (1971a). *J. Theor. Biol.* **30**, 225.

Keller, E. F., and Segel, L. A. (1971b). *J. Theor. Biol.* **30**, 235.

Keller, H. U. (1966). *Immunology* **10**, 225.

Keller, H. U. (1972). *Agents Actions* **2**, No. 4, 161.

Keller, H. U., and Sorkin, E. (1965a). *Immunology* **9**, 241.

Keller, H. U., and Sorkin, E. (1965b). *Immunology* **9**, 441.

Keller, H. U., and Sorkin, E. (1966). *Immunology* **10**, 409.

Keller, H. U., and Sorkin, E. (1967a). *Experientia* **23**, 549.

Keller, H. U., and Sorkin, E. (1967b). *Proc. Soc. Exp. Biol. Med.* **126**, 677.

Keller, H. U., and Sorkin, E. (1967c). *Int. Arch. Allergy Appl. Immunol.* **31**, 505.
Keller, H. U., and Sorkin, E. (1967d). *Int. Arch. Allergy Appl. Immunol.* **31**, 575.
Keller, H. U., and Sorkin, E. (1968a). *Int. Arch. Allergy Appl. Immunol.* **34**, 513.
Keller, H. U., and Sorkin, E. (1968b). *Experienta* **24**, 641.
Keller, H. U., Borel, J. F., Wilkinson, P. C., Hess, M. W., and Cottier, H. (1972). *J. Immunol. Meth.* **1**, 165.
Ketchel, M. K., and Favour, C. B. (1955). *J. Exp. Med.* **101**, 647.
Ketchel, M. K., Favour, C. B., and Sturgis, S. H. (1958). *J. Exp. Med.* **107**, 211.
Klemperer, M. R., Woodworth, H. C., Rosen, F. S., and Austen, K. F. (1966). *J. Clin. Invest.* **45**, 880.
Konijn, T. M. (1968). *Biol. Bull.* **134**, 298.
Konijn, T. M. (1969). *J. Bacteriol.* **99**, 503.
Konijn, T. M. (1970). *Experientia* **26**, 367.
Konijn, T. M., van de Meene, J. G. C., Bonner, J. T., and Barkley, D. S. (1967). *Proc. Nat. Acad. Sci. U.S.* **58**, 1152.
Konijn, T. M., Barkley, D. S., Chang, Y. Y., and Bonner, J. T. (1968). *Amer. Natur.* **102**, 225.
Konijn, T. M., van de Meene, J. G. C., Chang, Y. Y., Barkley, D. S., and Bonner, J. T. (1969). *J. Bacteriol.* **99**, 510.
Konijn, T. M., and Koevenig, J. L. (1971). *Mycologia* **63**, 901.
Kopp, R. K., and Müller, J. (1965). *Zentralbl. Bakteriol., Parasitenk., Infektionskr. Hyg., Abt. I:Orig.* **198**, 253.
Kopp, R. K., Müller, J., and Lemme, R. (1966). *Appl. Microbiol.* **14**, 873.
Lasfargues, E. (1946). *Rev. Immunol.* **10**, 45.
Leahy, D. R., McLean, E. R., and Bonner, J. T. (1970). *Blood* **36**, 52.
Leber, T. (1888). *Fortschr. Med.* **6**, 460.
Leber, T. (1891). "Die Entstehung der Entzundung." Engelmann, Leipzig.
Lepow, I. H. (1971). *In* "Progress in Immunology" (B. Amos, ed.), p. 579. Academic Press, New York.
Lominski, I., and Lendrum, A. C. (1947). *J. Pathol. Bacteriol.* **59**, 688.
Lotz, M., and Harris, H. (1956). *Brit. J. Exp. Pathol.* **37**, 477.
McCutcheon, M., and Dixon, J. M. (1936). *Arch. Pathol.* **21**, 749.
McCutcheon, M., Wartman, W. B., and Dixon, H. M. (1934). *Arch. Pathol.* **17**, 607.
McCutcheon, M., Coman, D. R., and Dixon, H. M. (1939). *Arch. Pathol.* **27**, 61.
Machlis, L. (1958). *Physiol Plant.* **11**, 181.
Machlis, L. (1969a). *Physiol. Plant.* **22**, 126.
Machlis, L. (1969b). *Physiol. Plant.* **22**, 392.
Machlis, L., and Rawitscher-Kunkel, E. (1963). *Int. Rev. Cytol.* **15**, 97.
Machlis, L., Nutting, Wyn Williams, M., and Rapoport, H. (1966). *Biochemistry* **5**, 2147.
Machlis, L., Nutting, W. H., and Rapoport, H. (1968). *J. Amer. Chem. Soc.* **90**, 1674.
MacInnis, A.J. (1966). *Science* **154**, 216.
McIntyre, J., and Jenkin, C. R. (1969). *Aust. J. Exp. Biol. Med. Sci.* **47**, 625.
Macnab, R. M., and Koshland, D. E. (1972). *Proc. Nat. Acad. Sci. U.S.* **69**, 2509.
McVittie, A., and Zahler, S.A. (1962). *Nature (London)* **194**, 1299.
Malawista, S. E. (1965). *Arthritis Rheum.* **8**, 752.
Malawista, S. E. (1968). *Arthritis Rheum.* **11**, 191.
Malawista, S. E. (1971). *Blood* **37**, 519.
Malawista, S. E., and Bensch, K. G. (1967). *Science* **156**, 521.
Malawista, S. E., and Bodel, P. G. (1967). *J. Clin. Invest.* **46**, 780.
Manten, A. (1948). *Antonie van Leeuwenhoek; J. Microbiol. Serol.* **14**, 65.
Martin, S. P., and Chaudhuri, S. N. (1952). *Proc. Soc. Exp. Biol. Med.* **81**, 286.
Martin, S. P., Pierce, C. H., Middlebrook, G., and Dubos, R. J. (1950). *J. Exp. Med.* **91**, 381.

Menkin, V. (1938a). *J. Exp. Med.* **67**, 129.
Menkin, V. (1938b). *J. Exp. Med.* **67**, 145.
Menkin, V. (1938c). *J. Exp. Med.* **67**, 153.
Mesibov, T., and Adler, J. (1972). *J. Bacteriol.* **112**, 315.
Metchnikoff, E. (1887). *Ann. Inst. Pasteur,* **1**, 321.
Metchnikoff, E. (1892). *In* "Lectures on the Comparative Pathology of Inflammation." Dover, New York, 1968.
Metchnikoff, E. (1893). "Lectures on the Comparative Pathology of Inflammation." Kegal Paul, Trench, Trubner, London.
Miles, I. (1969). *Folia Microbiol. (Prague)* **14**, 560.
Miller, M. E. (1971). *Pediat. Res.* **5**, 487.
Miller, M. E., and Nillson, U. R. (1970). *N. Engl. J. Med.* **282**, 354.
Miller, R. L. (1966a). *Amer. Zool.* **6**, 27.
Miller, R. L. (1966b). *Amer. Zool.* **6**, 443.
Miller, R. L. (1966c). *J. Exp. Zool.* **162**, 23.
Miller, R. L. (1970). *J. Exp. Zool.* **175**, 493.
Miller, R. L., and Brokaw, C. J. (1970). *J. Exp. Biol.* **52**, 699.
Miller, R. L., and Nelson, L. (1962). *Biol. Bull.* **123**, 477.
Mowat, A. G., and Baum, J. (1971a). *N. Engl. J. Med.* **284**, 621.
Mowat, A. G., and Baum, J. (1971b). *J. Clin. Invest.* **50**, 2541.
Müller, D. G. (1967). *Naturwissenschaften* **54**, 496.
Müller, D. G. (1968). *Planta* **81**, 160.
Müller, D. G. (1969). *Naturwissenschaften* **56**, 220.
Müller, D. G., Jaenicke, L., Donike, M., and Akintobi, T. (1971). *Science* **171**, 815.
Müller-Eberhard, H. J. (1968). *Advan. Immunol.* **8**, 1.
Müller-Eberhard, H. J. (1969). *Annu. Rev. Biochem.* **38**, 389.
Müller-Eberhard, H. J. (1971). *Prog. Immunol.* **8**, 1.
Murray, A. W., Spiszman, M., and Atkinson, D. E. (1971). *Science* **171**, 496.
Naitoh, Y., and Kaneko, H. (1972). *Science* **176**, 523.
Nelson, R. A. (1966). *Surv. Ophthalmol.* **11**, 498.
Nelson, R. A., and Lebrun, J. (1956). *J. Hyg.* **54**, 8.
Nilsson, U. R., and Müller-Eberhard, H. J. (1965). *J. Exp. Med.* **122**, 277.
Nossal, R., (1972a). *Exp. Cell Res.* **75**, 138.
Nossal, R. (1972b). *Math. Biosci.* **13**, 397.
Nossal, R., and Chen, S. H. (1973). *Nature (London) New Biol.* **244**, 253.
Oldfield, F. E. (1963). *Exp. Cell Res.* **30**, 125.
Opie, E. L. (1922). *Physiol. Rev.* **2**, 552.
Ozaki, T., Yoshida, K., Ushijima, K., and Hayashi, H. (1971). *Int. J. Cancer* **7**, 93.
Page, A. R., Gewurz, H., Pickering, R. J., and Good, R. A. (1968). *In* "Immunopathology" (P. A. Miescher and P. Graber, eds,). Grune & Stratton, New York.
Pan, P. C., Hill, E. M., and Bonner, J. T. (1972). *Abstr., Annu. Meet., Amer. Soc. Microbiol.* p. 71.
Pannbacker, R. G., and Bravard, L. J. (1972). *Science* **175**, 1014.
Perper, R. J., Sanda, M., Chinea, G., and Oronsky, A. L. (1974a). *J. Lab. Clin. Med.* (in press).
Perper, R. J., Sanda, M., Chinea, G., and Oronsky, A. L. (1974b). *J. Lab. Clin. Med.* (in press).
Persellin, R. H. (1969). *J. Immunol.* **103**, 39.
Persellin, R. H. (1972). *Arthritis Rheum.* **15**, 144.
Pfeffer, W. (1884). *Unters. Bot. Inst. Tübingen* **1**, 363.
Pfeffer, W. (1888). *Unters. Bot. Inst. Tübingen* **2**, 582.
Pfoehl, J. (1898). *Zentralbl. Bakteriol., Parasiten K. Infektimskr.* **24**, 343.
Phelps, P. (1969a). *Arthritis Rheum.* **12**, 189.

Phelps, P. (1969b). *Arthritis Rheum.* **12**, 197.
Phelps, P. (1970a). *Arthritis Rheum.* **13**, 1.
Phelps, P. (1970b). *J. Lab. Clin. Med.* **76**, 622.
Phelps, P., and Stanislaw, D. (1969). *Arthritis Rheum.* **12**, 181.
Policard, A., and Bessis, M. C. R. (1953). *C. R. Soc. Biol.* **147**, 982.
Policard, A., Collet, A., and Martin, J. C. (1961). *C. R. Acad. Sci.* **253**, 41.
Polley, M. J., and Müller-Eberhard, H. J. (1967). *J. Exp. Med.* **126**, 1013.
Rai, P. V., and Strobel, G. A. (1966). *Phytopathology* **56**, 1365.
Ramseier, H. (1969). *J. Exp. Med.* **130**, 1279.
Ramsey, W. S. (1972a). *Exp. Cell Res.* **70**, 129.
Ramsey, W. S. (1972b). *Exp. Cell Res.* **72**, 489.
Ramsey, W. S., and Harris, A. K. (1973). *Exp. Cell Res.* **82**, 262.
Rawitscher-Kunkel, E., and Machlis, L. (1962). *Amer. J. Bot.* **49**, 177.
Riedel, V., and Gerisch, G. (1971). *Biochem. Biophys. Res. Commun.* **42**, 119.
Robertson, A., Drage, D. J., and Cohen, M. H. (1972). *Science* **175**, 333.
Robineaux, R. (1964). *In* "Primitive Motile Systems in Cell Biology" (R. D. Allen and N. Kamiya, eds.), p. 351. Academic Press, New York.
Robinson, B. V., and Robson, J. M. (1964). *Brit. J. Pharmacol. Chemother.* **23**, 420.
Robinson, B. V., and Robson, J. M. (1966). *Britt. J. Pharmacol. Chemother.* **26**, 372.
Rosegger, H. (1932). *Z. Gesamte Exp. Med.* **85**, 712.
Rosen, W. G. (1962). *Quart. Rev. Biol.* **37**, 242.
Rother, K., Rother, U., Müller-Eberhard, H. J., and Nilsson, U. (1966). *J. Exp. Med.* **124**, 773.
Rothert, W. (1901). *Flora (Lena)* **88**, 371.
Rothschild, Lord. (1956). "Fertilization." Methuen, London.
Royle, D. J., and Hickman, C. J. (1964a). *Can. J. Microbiol.* **10**, 151.
Royle, D. J., and Hickman, C. J. (1964b). *Can. J. Microbiol.* **10**, 201.
Runyon, E. J. (1942). *Collec. Net* **17**, 88
Ryan, G. B., and Hurley, J. V. (1966). *Brit. J. Exp. Pathol.* **47**, 530.
Sandberg, A. L., Osler, A. G., Shin, H. S., and Oliveira, B. (1970). *J. Immunol.* **104**, 329.
Sandison, J. C. (1924). *Anat. Rec.* **28**, 281.
Sandison, J. C. (1931). *Anat. Rec.* **50**, 355.
Sandon, H. (1963). "Essays on Protozoology." Hutchinson Educational, London.
Sbarra, H. J., and Karnovsky, M. L. (1959). *J. Biol. Chem.* **234**, 1355.
Schmidt, J. A. (1963). *Z. Naturforsch. B* **18**, 172.
Sevitt, S. (1957). "Burns—Pathology and Therapeutic Applications." Butterworth, London.
Sevitt, S. (1958). *J. Pathol. Bacteriol.* **75**, 27.
Shaffer, B. M. (1956). *J. Exp. Biol.* **33**, 645.
Shaffer, B. M. (1957). *Amer. Natur.* **91**, 15.
Shaffer, B. M. (1962). *Advan. Morphog.* **2**, 109–182.
Sherris, J. C., Preston, N. W., and Shoesmith, J. G. (1957). *J. Gen. Microbiol.* **16**, 86.
Shin, J. L., Snyderman, R., Friedman, E., Mellors, A., and Mayer, M. M. (1968). *Science* **162**, 361.
Smith, J. L., and Doetsch, R. N. (1968). *Life Sci.* **7**, 875
Smith, J. L., and Doetsch, R. N. (1969). *J. Gen. Microbiol.* **55**, 379.
Snyderman, R., Gewurz, H., and Mergenhagen, S. E. (1968). *J. Exp. Med.* **128**, 259.
Snyderman, R., Shin, H. S., Phillips, J. K., Gewurz, H., and Mergenhagen, S. E. (1969). *J. Immunol.* **103**, 413.
Snyderman, R., Phillips, J., and Mergenhagen, S. E. (1970). *Infec. Immunity* **1**, 521.
Snyderman, R., Phillips, J. K., and Mergenhagen, S. E. (1971a). *J. Exp. Med.* **134**, 1131.
Snyderman, R., Shin, H. S., and Hausman, M. H. (1971b). *Proc. Soc. Exp. Biol. Med.* **138**, 387.

Snyderman, R., Wohlenberg, C., and Notkins, A. L. (1972). *J. Infec. Dis.* **126**, 207.

Sorkin, E., Stecher, V. J., and Borel, J. F. (1970a). *Ser. Haemat.* **III**, 131.

Spector, W. G., and Willoughby, D. A. (1963). *Bacteriol. Rev.* **27**, 117.

Spencer, J. A., and Cooper, W. E. (1967). *Phytopathology* **57**, 1332.

Stecher, V. J. (1970). *In* "Mononuclear Phagocytes" (R. van Furth, ed.), p. 133. Blackwell, Oxford.

Stecher, V. J., and Sorkin, E. (1969). *Immunology* **16**, 231.

Stecher, V. J., Sorkin, E., and Ryan, G. B. (1971). *Nature (London) New Biol.* **233**, 95.

Steerman, R. L., Snyderman, R., Leikin, S. L., and Colten, N. R. (1971). *Clin. Exp. Immunol.* **9**, 939.

Strauss, B. S., and Stetson, C. A., (1960). *J. Exp. Med.* **112**, 653.

Symon, D. N., McKay, I. C., and Wilkinson, P. C. (1972). *Immunol.* **22**, 267.

Taubman, S. B., and Lepow, I. H. (1971). *Immunochemistry* **8**, 951.

Taubman, S. B., Goldschmidt, P. R., and Lepow, I. H. (1970). *Fed. Proc., Fed. Amer. Soc. Exp. Biol.* **29**, 434.

Taylor, F. B., Jr., and Ward, P. A. (1967). *J. Exp. Med.* **126**, 149.

Trinkaus, J. P. (1969). "Cells into Organs. The Forces that Shape the Embryo." Prentice-Hall, Englewood Cliffs, New Jersey.

Tsang, N., Macnab, R., and Koshland, D. E. (1973). *Science* **181**, 60.

Turner, P. D. (1963). *Phytopathology* **53**, 1337.

Twitty, V. C. (1944). *J. Exp. Zool.* **95**, 259.

Twitty, V. C., and Niu, M. C. (1948). *J. Exp. Zool.* **108**, 405.

Twitty, V. C., and Niu, M. C. (1954). *J. Exp. Zool.* **125**, 541.

Unanue, E. and Dixon, F. J. (1964). *J. Exp. Med.* **119**, 965.

Vogel, R., Trautschold, I., and Werle, E. (1969). "Natural Proteinase Inhibitors." Academic Press, New York.

von Haller, A. (1757). "A Dissertation on the Motion of the Blood and on the Effects of Bleeding." Whisten & White, London.

von Philipsborn, E. (1925). *Deut. Arch. Klin. Med.* **146**, 5/6.

ven Philipsborn, E. (1928). *Deut. Arch. Klin. Med.* **160**, 5/6.

von Philipsborn, E. (1930). *Deut. Arch. Klin. Med.* **168**, 3/4.

von Philipsborn, E. (1957). *Med. Monatschr.* **11**, 364.

Wagner, R. (1833). "Zur vergleichenden Physiologie des Blutes." Voss, Leipzig.

Wagner, R. (1839). "Erlauterungstafeln zur Physiologie und Entwicklungsgeschichte." Voss, Leipzig.

Walker, W. S., Barlet, R. L., and Kurtz, H. M. (1969). *J. Bacteriol.* **97**, 1005.

Waller, A. (1846). *Phil. Mag.* [3] **29**, 271.

Ward, P. A. (1966). *J. Exp. Med.* **124**, 209.

Ward, P. A. (1967). *J. Exp. Med.* **126**, 189.

Ward, P. A. (1968). *J. Exp. Med.* **128**, 1201.

Ward, P. A. (1971a). *J. Exp. Med.* **134**, 1095.

Ward, P. A. (1971b). *In* "Cellular Interactions in the Immune Response" (S. Korn, G. Cudkowitz, and R. McCluskey, eds.), p. 191. Karger, Basel.

Ward, P. A. (1971c). *In* "Biochemistry of the Acute Allergic Reactions" (K. F. Austen and E. L. Becker, eds.), p. 229. Blackwell, Oxford.

Ward, P. A., and Becker, E. L. (1967). *J. Exp. Med.* **125**, 1001.

Ward, P. A., and Becker, E. L. (1968). *J. Exp. Med.* **127**, 693.

Ward, P. A., and Becker, E. L. (1970a). *Life Sci.* **9**, 355.

Ward, P. A., and Becker, E. L. (1970b). *J. Immunol.* **105**, 1057.

Ward, P. A., and Cochrane, C. G. (1965). *J. Exp. Med.* **121**, 215.

Ward, P. A., and Hill, J. H. (1970). *J. Immunol.* **104**, 535.

Ward, P. A., and Newman, L. J. (1969). *J. Immunol.* **102**, 93.
Ward, P. A., and Zvaifler, N. J. (1971). *J. Clin. Invest.* **50**, 606.
Ward, P. A., and Zvaifler, N. J. (1973a). *J. Immunol.* **111**, 1771.
Ward, P. A., and Zvaifler, N. J. (1973b). *J. Immunol.* **111**, 1777.
Ward, P. A., Cochrane, C. G., and Müller-Eberhard, H. J. (1965). *J. Exp. Med.* **12**, 327.
Ward, P. A., Cochrane, C. G., and Müller-Eberhard, H. J. (1966). *Immunology* **11**, 141.
Ward, P. A., Lepow, I. H., and Newman, L. J. (1968). *Amer. J. Pathol.* **52**, 725.
Ward, P. A., Remold, H. G., and Dävid, J. R. (1969). *Science* **163**, 1079.
Ward, P. A., Remold, H. G., and David, J. R. (1970). *Cell. Immunol.* **1**, 162.
Ward, P. A., Conroy, M. C., and Lepow, I. H. (1971a). *Fed. Proc., Fed . Amer. Soc. Exp. Biol.* **30**, 355 (abstr.).
Ward, P. A., Offen, C. D., and Montgomery, J. R. (1971b). *Fed. Proc., Fed. Amer. Soc. Exp. Biol.* **30**, 1721.
Weibull, C. (1960). *In* "The Bacteria" (I. C. Gunsalus and R. Y. Stanier, eds.), Vol. 1, pp. 153–205. Academic Press, New York.
Weimar, V. (1957). *J. Exp. Med.* **105**, 141.
Weissmann, G., and Dukor, P. (1970). *Advan. Immunol.* **12**, 283.
Weissmann, G., Zurier, R. B., Spieler, P. J., and Goldstein, I. M. (1971a). *J. Exp. Med.* **134**, 1495.
Weissmann, G., Dukor, P., and Zurier, R. B. (1971b). *Nature (London) New Biol.* **231**, 131.
Weissmann, G., Zurier, R. B., Tsung, P., and Hoffstein, S. (1972). *J. Clin. Invest.* **56**, 102a (abstr.).
Wells, H. (1918). "Chemical Pathology." Saunders, Philadelphia, Pennsylvania.
Wessells, N. K., Spooner, B. S., Ash, J. F., Bradley, M. O., Ludeena, M. O., Taylor, E. L., Wrenn, J. T., and Yamada, K. M. (1971). *Science* **171**, 135.
Wharton-Jones, T. (1851). *Guy's Hosp. Rep.* **7**, 1.
Wilhelm, D. C., and Mason, B. (1960). *Brit. J. Exp. Pathol.* **41**, 487.
Wilkinson, P. C., Borel, J. F., Stecher-Levin, V. J., and Sorkin, E. (1969). *Nature (London)* **222**, 244.
Willoughby, D. A., Elizabeth, C., and Turk, J. L. (1969). *J. Pathol.* **97**, 295.
Wissler, J. H. (1972a). *Eur. J. Immunol.* **2**, 73.
Wissler, J. H. (1972b). *Eur. J. Immunol.* **2**, 84.
Wissler, J. H., Stecher, V. J., and Sorkin, E. (1972a). *Eur. J. Immunol.* **2**, 90.
Wissler, J. H., Stecher, V. J., and Sorkin, E. (1972b). *Int. Arch. Allergy Appl. Immunol.* **42**, 722.
Wissler, J. H., Stecher, V. J., Sorkin, E., and Jungi, Th. (1972c). *Commun. 4th Tagung der Gesellschaft fur Immunologie (Abstr.)* p. 61.
Woodin, A. M., and Harris, A. (1973). *Exp. Cell Res.* **77**, 41.
Woodin, A, M., and Wieneke, A. A. (1969). *Brit. J. Exp. Pathol.* **50**, 295.
Woodin, A. M., and Wieneke, A. A. (1970). *J. Gen. Physiol.* **56**, 16.
Yamamoto, S., Yoshinaga, M., and Hayashi, H. (1971). *Immunology.* **20**, 803.
Yoshida, K., Yoshinaga, M., and Hayashi, H. (1968). *Nature (London)* **218**, 977.
Yoshida, K., Ozaki, T., Ushijima, K., and Hayashi, H. (1970). *Int. J. Cancer* **6**, 123.
Yoshinaga, M., Yamamoto, S., Maeda, S., and Hayashi, H. (1971a). *Immunology* **20**, 809.
Yoshinaga, M., Yoshida, K., Tashiro, A., and Hayashi, H. (1971b). *Immunology* **21**, 281.
Yoshinaga, M., Yamamoto, S., Kiyota, S., and Hayashi, H. (1972). *Immunology* **22**, 393.
Zentmyer, G. A. (1966). *Phytopathology* **56**, 907.
Ziegler, H. (1962). *In* "Handbuch der Pflanzenphysiologie" (W. Ruhland, ed.), Vol. 17, Part 2, p. 484. Springer-Verlag, Berlin and New York.
Zigmond, S. H., and Hirsch, J. G. (1973). *J. Exp. Med.* **137**, 387.
Zurier, R. B., and Quagliata, F. (1971). *Nature (London)* **234**, 305.
Zvaifler, N. J. (1969). *J. Clin. Invest.* **48**, 1532.

Addendum

The computer is yielding some 100 major references each year on the subject of chemotaxis. A selection of recent publications is listed below, added in page proof, including a useful and scholarly discussion of the subject in a new monograph by Wilkinson (1974) and experimental evidence for chemotactic activity in dialyzable transfer factor (Gallin and Kirkpatrick, 1974).

Briefly summarized, recent microbial studies cover two theoretical analyses of bacterial chemotaxis (Nossal and Weiss, 1973; Rosen, 1973), a comparison of positive and negative chemotaxis in bacteria (Seymour and Doetsch, 1973), and evidence for the isolation and characterization of a bacterial chemotactic factor from culture filtrates of *E. coli*. (Schiffman *et al.*, 1974). Clinical studies include a report of defective regulation of inflammatory mediators in Hodgkin's disease (Ward and Berenberg, 1974); a report of an apparent inborn error of leukocyte movement (Miller *et al.*, 1973); a postulation of spontaneous chemotaxis in patients with glomerulonephritis and the nephrotic syndrome (Norman and Miller, 1973); and two overviews of various aspects of chemotaxis (Quie, 1973; Stossel, 1974; the last-named forming a part of a review of phagocytosis). Other recent publications are a study of chemotactic activity of leukocytes related to blood coagulation and fibrinolysis (Stecher and Sorkin, 1974); mechanisms of lysosomal enzyme release from human leukocytes; a study that deals with agents that affect microtubule function (Zurier *et al.*, 1974); the regulation of chemotaxis by the anaphylatoxin-related peptide system (Wissler *et al.*, 1973); and a study of the recognition of protein structure in leukocyte chemotaxis (Wilkinson, 1973).

References

Gallin, J. I., and Kirkpatrick, C. H. (1974). *Proc. Nat. Acad. Sci.* USA, **71**, 498.
Miller, M. E., Norman, M. E., Koblenzer, P. J., and Schonauer, T. (1973). *J. Lab. Clin. Med.* **82**, 1.
Norman, M. E., and Miller, M. E. (1973). *J. Pediat.* **83**, 390.
Nossal, R., and Weiss, G. H., (1973). *J. Theor. Biol.* **41**, 143.
Quie, P. G. (1973). *Medicine* **52**, 411.
Rosen, G. (1973). *J. Theor. Biol.* **41**, 201.
Schiffman, E., Showell, H., Corcoran, B., Smith, E., Ward, P. A., Tempel, T., and Becker, E. L. (1974). *Fed. Proc. Abstr.* **33**, No. 3, 631.
Seymour, F. W. K., and Doetsch, R. N. (1973). *J. Gen. Microbiol.* **78**, 287.
Stecher, V. J., and Sorkin, E. (1974). "Antibiotics and Chemotherapy", Vol. 19, p. 1. S. Karger, Basel.
Stossel, T. P. (1974). *New Engl. J. Med.* **290**, No. 13, 717. **290**, No. 14 and 15.
Ward, P. A., and Berenberg, J. L. (1974). *New Engl. J. Med.* **290**, 76.
Wilkinson, P. C. (1973). *Nature (London)* **244**, 512.
Wilkinson, P. C. (1974). "Chemotaxis and Inflammation." Churchill Livingstone, Edinburgh and London.
Wissler, J. H., Stecher, V. J., and Sorkin, E. (1973). Regulation of chemotaxis of leucocytes by the anaphylatoxin-related peptide system. *In* "Proteins and Related Subjects," Protids of Biological Fluids, Vol. 20 (H. Peeters, ed.), Pergamon Press, Oxford, p. 411.
Zurier, R. B., Weissmann, G., Hoffstein, S., Kammerman, S., and Tai, H. H. (1974). *J. Clin. Invest.* **53**, 297.

Chapter 6

PHAGOCYTOSIS

PETER ELSBACH

I. Introduction

The ability to ingest material by engulfment is a property of many cells. Where it involves particulate matter, this activity is called phagocytosis and appears to be limited, at least in a quantitatively important sense to cells of the reticulo-endothelial system (RES) and to other cells, not strictly speaking part of the RES but which are also of mesenchymal origin. In order for phagocytosis to take place a recognition mechanism seems required. In most instances this implies recognition of some measure of foreignness, as in the case of live or nonlive invaders from the external environment, or as a consequence of modification of elements of the organism itself. It is clear that the cellular function of phagocytosis is of prime biological importance, both in health and disease, in ridding the organism of harmful invaders and in allowing it to eliminate altered constituents in a continuous renewal process.

Pinocytosis, a qualitatively similar cellular function, concerns ingestion of soluble material. Both the material ingested and the vesicles through which incorporation takes place are smaller in size. It seems probable that many more cell types are capable of pinocytosis than of phagocytosis. However, much less is known about pinocytosis by animal cells and about its incidence and specific function in individual tissues. This discussion will not be concerned with a detailed consideration of pinocytosis.

In this review we attempt to bring together current views of mechanisms involved in phagocytosis that are based on studies of isolated animal cells, with recent clinical observations on defective cellular host defense. Major emphasis will be placed on investigations, carried out *in vitro*, of metabolic functions of phagocytic cells, and evidence will be considered that has led to a number of widely held concepts concerning the relation between the ordered sequence of events presumed to occur during phagocytosis and certain biochemical activities.

The first edition of *The Inflammatory Process* reviewed some of the advances made in the late fifties and early sixties that have provided new insights into the phagocytic process (see Chapter 6 by Hirsch and Chapter 8 by Cohn in the previous edition). Most prominent among these advances were: (1) the introduction of the concept that degranulation is an integral feature of endocytosis and the demonstration that many of the granules of polymorphonuclear leukocytes and other phagocytic cells are lysosomes. This recognition has given us the most clearly established example, thus far, of an essential biological function for these intracellular organelles and (2) the appreciation of the importance of various metabolic responses for effective phagocytosis, i.e., the apparent need for expenditure of biochemical energy.

Since the appearance of the previous edition no drastically new concepts have developed. Yet, during the past 5 years numerous new observations of great interest have been reported, particularly with regard to the intermediary metabolism of phagocytic cells, that have both deepened and broadened the insights into biochemical mechanisms that may underlie the phagocytic process. Many of these observations have been made on phagocytic cells, obtained from various animal species, which are capable of particle ingestion *in vitro*. The views that have sprung from these studies with respect to the contribution of specific biochemical events to distinct steps in phagocytosis have both been strengthened and modified by recent observations of clinical abnormalities involving cellular host defense mechanisms.

For other aspects of phagocytosis the reader is referred to a number of reviews that have appeared within the past decade. A general review of the subject was written by Hirsch in 1965. The immunological viewpoint of phagocytosis is well represented in the reviews of Rowley (1962) and Austen and Cohn (1963a,b,c). An extensive summary of metabolic findings during phagocytosis by polymorphonuclear leukocytes was contributed by Karnovsky (1962) and more recently by Sbarra *et al.* (1970). Structure and function of monocytes and macrophages were discussed comprehensively by Cohn

(1968) and by Pearsall and Weiser (1970). A synopsis of pinocytosis by mammalian cells, as yet only incompletely studied, also appears in Cohn's review (1968).

II. General Aspects of Phagocytosis

1. PHAGOCYTOSIS AS A CAPABILITY OF DIFFERENT CELL TYPES

Others have reviewed in greater detail than in the ensuing discussion the spectrum of mammalian cells capable of phagocytosis (Mudd *et al.*, 1934; Hirsch, 1965; Cohn, 1968; Pearsall and Weiser, 1970). In brief, it can be said that there are two main classes of phagocytes, those that migrate and those that are fixed in tissues during all or the major portion of their life spans. The former appear capable of seeking and finding the site where their phagocytic function is required and comprise the different types of polymorphonuclear leukocytes and various circulating mononuclear phagocytes. The stationary cells presumably must depend on chance encounter with the foreign materials. A good example of such a sedentary macrophage is the Kupffer cell in the liver.

The study of phagocytosis and its metabolic aspects *in vitro*, with which this review is primarily concerned, requires the use of large numbers of phagocytic cells. Understandably, these are most readily available from the group of migratory phagocytes. Rich sources of neutrophilic polymorphonuclear leukocytes are the blood and sterile peritoneal exudates that can be produced in a number of animal species by injecting various irritants (Stähelin *et al.*, 1956a). Opinions vary as to the extent to which granulocytes from peripheral blood and from peritoneal exudates are similar. There is little doubt that their metabolic properties and responses *in vitro* are qualitatively comparable. Quantitatively, however, differences may exist (Cline, 1970). Unfortunately no systematic studies have been carried out on granulocytes from the two sources using the same animal species. It is uncertain therefore whether species differences, the migration of the leukocytes into the peritoneal cavity in response to an administered irritant, or the much greater heterogeneity of the peripheral blood leukocytes are mainly responsible for observed differences. The advantages of peritoneal exudate granulocytes are considerable; the yields are high (up to 2×10^9 cells from a single rabbit, for instance), the populations are homogeneous (usually more than 90% of the cells are granulocytes), and one does not require potentially damaging techniques to separate leukocytes from red cells. The fear that the migration of the leukocyte into the peritoneal cavity in response to an inflammatory stimulus results in "spent" or already "activated" cells seems unfounded. Observations in our own laboratory (unpublished) have shown that rabbit peritoneal exudate granulocytes maintain their ability to engulf particles and to manifest various metabolic responses for as many as 6 hours after collection. Further, most of the observations on the stimulated metabolism of the engulfing granulocyte have been made on populations of peritoneal cells (Karnovsky, 1962) that were exposed to particles *in vitro*.

The two main sources of mononuclear macrophages in large numbers are again the peritoneal cavity and also the lung. The yields can be markedly enhanced by prior stimulation with mineral oil or casein in the case of the peritoneal cavity (Elberg, 1960; Oren *et al.*, 1963) and with systemic BCG or Freund's adjuvant in the case of the lung (Myrvik *et al.*, 1961a; Leake and Myrvik, 1968). An important source of smaller numbers of macrophages has recently been found in cells obtained from the mouse peritoneal cavity which, in culture, transform from relatively immature mononuclear cells to mature macrophages (Cohn and Benson, 1965a,b,c; Cohn, 1968).

2. CONDITIONS UNDER WHICH PHAGOCYTOSIS TAKES PLACE

In order for phagocytosis to occur a number of requirements must be met. First, contact has to be established between phagocyte and particle. The contact has to be of sufficient duration to allow engulfment to follow. Once the phagocytic vacuole is formed, a complex series of intracellular events may lead to the elimination of the ingested particle. Thus, somewhat arbitrarily, one can distinguish four phases in the process of phagocytosis: (1) chemotaxis, (2) contact and attachment, (3) ingestion, and (4) digestion and/or killing.

Since chemotaxis is discussed in depth in the preceding chapter we will dwell only briefly on some features that are immediately pertinent to our theme. For an earlier review and a more complete discussion of the role of serum factors in phagocytosis, see Austen and Cohn (1963a).

a. CHEMOTAXIS AND CONTACT. Chemotaxis, that is, the migration of the phagocyte toward the particle to be engulfed* under the influence of some attracting force, strictly reasoning, should be considered separate from contact and attachment. The factors, however, that appear of importance to chemotaxis are often also those that govern attachment. It seems reasonable therefore to treat the two together. During the last 5 years the rather nebulous concept of chemotaxis has been under close scrutiny. Until recently, it has not

---

*To our knowledge no information is available concerning the possibility that chemotactic forces can direct microorganisms or other particles to fixed macrophages. However, recent evidence clearly indicates that *E. coli* and probably other bacteria are highly responsive to simple chemotactic agents such as certain sugars and amino acids (Adler, 1969; Hazelbauer and Adler, 1970).

been possible to demonstrate its occurrence in a convincing manner *in vivo*. However, there is now considerable support from *in vitro* studies to indicate that some recognition mechanism accounts for the directed migration of phagocytes toward a number of particles and a variety of molecular species (cytotaxins) (see Chapter 5). Of interest are recent reports that different types of phagocytes may not respond to the same chemotactic agents (Ward, 1968; Wilkinson *et al.*, 1969; Keller and Sorkin, 1968). It has been shown also that subcellular fractions of neutrophils promote migration of mononuclear cells (Ward, 1968) and, according to Borel *et al.* (1969), also of other neutrophils. Evidence reviewed by Ward (1968) suggests that there is an obligatory sequence in the influx of different inflammatory cells into the site of inflammation, neutrophils having to precede mononuclear cells. It has been proposed that the primary phagocytic function of the neutrophil is to deal with microorganisms and that the mononuclear cells serve in a secondary role as scavengers (Pearsall and Weiser, 1970). Thus, the short-lived neutrophils which migrate faster than mononuclear cells (Ward, 1968) would first engage the invading microorganisms and disintegrate in the process, releasing cytotaxins that attract new neutrophils and also macrophages which are to remove dead cells and other debris. It must be emphasized that no concrete evidence is yet available to support this proposed order of events.

Experiments with bacteria have shown that both the migration of neutrophils toward the particles and the subsequent attachment are dependent on serum factors. Some of these are heat-labile, lack specificity, and have tentatively been identified as components of complement, others are heat-stable antibodies that are specific for given bacterial species, and some are heat-labile opsonic substances that appear to be neither antibodies nor components of complement (Hirsch and Church, 1960; Austen and Cohn, 1963a). In the case of microorganisms, the role of these serum factors in promoting chemotaxis and attachment, and in many instances subsequent ingestion, has been attributed entirely to an effect on the surface of the bacteria rather than to a modification of the phagocyte's surface membrane (Vaughan, 1965; Auzins and Rowley, 1963). On the other hand, the studies of Rabinovitch (1967a,b) with glutaraldehyde-treated red blood cells indicate that attachment to cultured mouse peritoneal macrophages occurred in the absence of serum factors and divalent cations, but that engulfment required addition of both serum factors and divalent cations to the incubation medium. Further, the glutaraldehyde-treated red blood cells attached only to macrophages and not to lymphocytes or granulocytes. Thus, in this case as well as in other instances (Elsbach, 1965b; Jones and Hirsch, 1971), attachment can be dissociated from ingestion.

While alteration of the surface of the particle through interaction of surface constituents with serum factors ("opsonization") may indeed be of major importance in determining whether or not attachment and/or engulfment takes place and, in some cases, the rate of ingestion (Ward and Enders, 1933), there is much evidence that the presence of phagocytes in an area of inflammation and the process of phagocytosis itself produces changes in the cell surface. These changes have been inferred from rather crude phenomena that can be observed, such as adhesion to endothelium or other surfaces, aggregation of cells, and inhibition of migration (Bryant *et al.*, 1966). Virtually nothing is known about the chemical or physical nature of the surface alterations that presumably underlie these phenomena. Observations on the binding of immune complexes to phagocytes (Phillips *et al.*, 1969; Messner and Jelinek, 1970) represent a beginning of a more sophisticated evaluation of the molecular interaction that must play a role in modifying the surfaces of both particles and cells so that contact and attachment can take place.

It should be stressed, however, that a number of situations exist where phagocytosis *in vitro* occurs in the absence of serum factors and where recognition of ingestible material is apparently nonspecific. Examples include ingestion of polystyrene beads (Sbarra and Karnovsky, 1959) and the phenomenon of "surface phagocytosis" of encapsulated bacteria that are trapped between phagocytes or against various rough surfaces (Wood *et al.*, 1946).

Strong evidence that chemotaxis is indeed an integral part of host defense mechanisms comes from very recent clinical and laboratory observations. Ward and Schlegel (1969) have reported a child with diminished resistance to infection whose leukocytes manifested decreased ability to migrate in a Boyden chamber compared to cells of normal individuals. The defect appears due to an inhibitor of chemotaxis in the serum of the affected child, since the child's leukocytes behaved normally in the presence of normal serum and since control cells were inhibited in the presence of the child's serum.

Nothing is known about the manner in which the numerous substances that elicit chemotactic responses *in vitro* exert their effect. The study of chemotaxis might benefit from a search for other means of establishing the occurrence of the phenomenon than the counting of cells that migrated through a filter and that represent only a small fraction of the total cell population tested. For example, the enhanced motility that characterizes chemotaxis might be accompanied by stimulation or alteration of biochemical activity. It would also be of interest to know if cytotaxins produce altered surface properties such as changes in net charge.

b. Ingestion and Postphagocytic (Nonmetabolic) Events. The events that follow chemotaxis and attachment lend themselves more readily to experimental observation even though many problems of technique and interpretation remain. Since Metchnikoff's investigations some 6 decades ago, simple light microscopy of stained or unstained preparations of phago-cytes and particles has provided a crude method for assessing engulfment of bacteria and other particles. It is often difficult, if not impossible, how-ever to distinguish between truly intracellular and adherent or superimposed particles. Numerous investigators have attempted to improve the quantit-ative measurement of engulfment. Roberts and Quastel (1963) have used dioxane extraction of washed granulocytes and O.D. readings of the extract to measure uptake of polystyrene or polyvinyl toluene particles. Sastry and Hokin (1966) have tried to assess phagocytosis of polystyrene particles by centrifugation of cell suspensions and measurement of turbidity of the supernatant medium. Several workers have used radioisotopically labeled bacteria or particles to follow uptake (Brzuchowska, 1966; Carpenter, 1966; Carpenter and Barseles, 1967). Michell et al. (1969) have refined this method to measure rates of phagocytosis by determining the radioactivity of monolayers of leukocytes after various times of incubation with ^{32}P-labeled *Salmonella typhimurium* and [1-^{14}C]acetyl or [^{14}C] methyl-labeled starch particles. None of these methods provide a reliable distinction between particles that are firmly stuck to cells or trapped between phagocytes and true intracellular location.

The most convincing evidence of ingestion still appears to be provided by estimates of removal and killing of live bacteria by standard culture techniques. The distinction between extracellular and intracellular survival of microorganisms that can be achieved by the procedure of Maaloe (1946) has been used to great advantage by Cohn and Morse (1959). These and other studies (Rowley, 1962) have established that the limiting factor in killing of many bacterial species (but certainly not all) is the ability of the phagocyte to engulf the organism, killing taking place within minutes after intracellular sequestration. In many instances, therfore, disappearance of viable bacteria from the extracellular fluid and overall bacterial killing run almost parallel.

The electron microscope has afforded another important tool for the appraisal of phagocytosis, since thin sections of cells should reveal with reasonable assurance whether or not particles are inside and surrounded by a membranelike structure. It must be kept in mind, however, that random thin sections cannot distinguish between a particle within a phagocytic vacuole and a particle partly surrounded, but not ingested, by an overlying phagocyte. It may therefore be necessary to include in the morphological evaluation of phagocytosis other intracellular events such as degranulation and fusion of granules with phagocytic vacuoles (Zucker-Franklin and Hirsch, 1964) as further evidence that ingestion has taken place.

Increasing use has been made of the dramatic increases in the metabolic activity of cells engaged in phagocytosis. Of all the foregoing procedures it is probably easiest to follow the conversion of a given isotopically labeled substrate to a product that can be readily measured. In a subsequent section the metabolic concomitants of phagocytosis will be discussed in some detail, and we will also point out the pitfalls of relying solely on metabolic responses as an index of engulfment.

The fate of the ingested particulate matter appears closely linked to the process of degranulation (Robineaux and Frederic, 1955; Hirsch and Cohn, 1960; Daems and Oort, 1962) and the discharge of granule contents into the newly formed phagocytic vacuole or phagosome (Cohn and Hirsch, 1960; Hirsch, 1962; Zucker-Franklin and Hirsch, 1964; Cotran and Litt, 1969; Stossel *et al.*, 1971). The initial morphological and cytochemical studies of degranulation were carried out with neutrophils from various sources and were then extended to several types of macrophages (see Cohn, 1968). The picture that has evolved appears quite clear, has been described extensively in many recent reviews (see Chapter 7 by Hirsch), and will therefore not be discussed here in detail. Briefly, (1) the phagosome is formed by infolding of outer membrane, fusion of the rim of the pouch, and separation of the reconstituted outer membrane from the phagosome, which tends to migrate toward the interior of the cell; and (2) while the phagosome is being formed, or shortly thereafter, granules converge on it, and the lining membranes of both organelles undergo fusion which is followed by dissolution in the area of junction. Thus, the contents of the granules are discharged into the now enlarged digestive vacuole. The granules and their contents, isolated from different phagocytic cells, in particular the polymorphonuclear leukocyte, have been carefully studied. In the neutrophil the granules can be divided into various types with different morphological, physical, biochemical, and cytochemical characteristics (Bainton and Farquhar, 1966, 1968a,b; Wetzel *et al.*, 1967a,b; Baggiolini *et al.*, 1969, 1970b; Michell *et al.*, 1970). In essence, one can distinguish between two categories of granules. The first group corresponds to lysosomes in other tissues and can be subdivided into two classes; one class of large, relatively dense azurophil granules which contain the characteristic acid hydrolases but also myeloperoxidase and lysozyme, and another class of morphologically more heterogeneous granules of low density that also contain acid hydrolases but little or no myeloperoxidase. The second group of smaller, less dense granules resemble so-called specific or secondary granules. These granules are the site of lactoferrin (Baggiolini *et al.* 1970a), of most of the alkaline phosphatase in the cells, and of some lysozyme. It is as yet not clear with which of these granule fractions the various bactericidal substances that have been recognized in granulocytes are associated (Hirsch, 1958, 1958, 1960; Zeya and Spitznagel, 1966, 1968, 1969). The further resolution of the cytoplasmic granules into categories with different properties is of obvious importance in obtaining a clearer insight into the functional role that these various fractions play in the degranulation phenomenon and postphagocytic events in general. In this context, mention should be made of questions that have been raised as to whether degranulation results solely in the discharge of the granule content into the phagocytic vacuole or whether release also occurs into the cytoplasm and to the exterior of the cell. The morphological and histochemical (Zucker-Franklin and Hirsch, 1964; Baehner *et al.*, 1969) evidence for fusion of granule and phagosome is unmistakable. However, Rossi *et al.* (1967) have interpreted their morphological findings as indicating that degranulation also takes place in the cytoplasm. It is pointed out that granule lysis may precede extensive vacuole formation. Weissmann *et al.* (1971) have described experiments that revealed release of lysosomal hydrolases into the medium during phagocytosis and attribute this release to fusion of the phagosome with the outer membrane followed by exocytosis (see also Woodin, 1968). Other investigators have tended to ascribe release of hydrolases to damaged cells. Until very recently, established techniques of cell fractionation did not preserve the fragile phagosomes, so that studies of the redistribution of lysosomal enzymes did not resolve these questions. Stossel *et al.* (1971) have now developed an elegant method for isolation of intact phagosomes. The use of paraffin oil suspensions, stabilized by albumin, as ingestible material offered two important advantages: (1) The liquid particles permitted the phagosomes to remain intact during homogenization and (2) the phagosomes could be easily separated from other cell fractions, because the low density of the ingested oil droplets caused the phagosomes to float on top of a sucrose gradient. Recovery of hydrolases in the phagosome fraction clearly indicated transfer of enzymes from granules to phagocytic vacuoles and not to the soluble fraction.

Although it is possible that the different granule species undergo lysis at different times and in different locations in the cell, this new evidence strongly supports the earliest conclusions that the discharge of the granule content during phagocytosis under reasonably physiological conditions is indeed predominantly into the phagocytic vacuoles.

The fate of the ingested particle has been most intensively examined using live bacteria. As mentioned earlier, many bacterial species lose their ability to multiply shortly after ingestion and, by this criterion, are considered to have been killed. By the same criterion, a number of micro-organisms, notably the mycobacteria, retain their viability even after prolonged residence within phagocytic cells. Relatively little is known about the factors that determine whether or not a given microorganism is susceptible to the bactericidal and degradative effects of phagocytosis. It appears that the physical–chemical nature of the bacterial cell wall is a major determinant. For example, the waxy coat of mycobacteria is thought to provide a potent barrier to bactericidal substances and hydrolytic enzymes.

In the case of bacteria that are readily killed by both granulocytes and macrophages only a beginning has been made in assessing which of the multiple intracellular agents that can affect bacterial structure and function are responsible for killing and/or digestion and in what order these agents exert their effects. Not only are there differences in the contents of bactericidal substances and catabolic enzymes of various types of phagocytes (Rowley, 1962; Cohn, 1968) that are capable of disposing of the same microorganisms, but in addition different bacterial species appear to show different susceptibility to the spectrum of bactericidal compounds (Zeya and Spitznagel, 1968).

The relationship between bacterial killing and the action of lytic enzymes on bacterial structure is not well understood. Cohn's observations (Cohn, 1963a,b), and work currently being carried out in our laboratory (Elsbach et al., 1972), indicate that the rate of killing of various bacterial species is much more rapid than the degradation of isotopically labeled bacterial constituents such as proteins, nucleic acids, and lipids. Further, this degradation is usually incomplete and often reaches a plateau between 1 and 2 hours after the labeled bacteria were presented to the suspension of phagocytes. It is unknown whether the incomplete degradation reflects fragmented and incompletely digested bacteria or whether complete structural dissolution of bacteria can occur without extensive hydrolysis of all or most of the bacterial macromolecules. Morphological evidence with regard to rate and extent of digestion of different microorganisms by various phagocytes is relatively limited (North and Mackaness, 1963; Ayoub and White, 1969; Leake et al., 1971). It is also unclear at present whether the degradation that takes place follows killing or whether killing can only occur after some initial breakdown of the bacterial cell wall has provided access to bactericidal substances. Cohn (1963a) has reported that acid extracts of granules of polymorphonuclear leukocytes are highly bactericidal and cause release of acid-soluble material without carrying out significant breakdown of bacterial macromolecules. These findings suggest that killing is associated with a permeability change but not necessarily with hydrolysis of structural components. On the other hand, we have found that addition of whole homogenates of rabbit peritoneal granulocytes to *E. coli* not only causes killing but is also associated with degradation of bacterial constituents (Elsbach et al., 1972; Patriarca et al., 1972; Elsbach et al., 1973).

Cohn (1963a) has concluded that leukocytic hydrolases play a major role in degradation of bacterial macromolecules, although autolysis may contribute to breakdown. Experiments in our laboratory indicate that *E. coli* boiled for 10 minutes or treated with deoxycholate exhibit marked hydrolysis of previously labeled bacterial lipids. It therefore appears that the complement of bacterial degradative enzymes may indeed be of considerable importance in the intracellular breakdown that follows death. It will be of great interest to dissect out the relative roles of leukocyte and bacterial enzymes in postphagocytic events.

III. Metabolism during Phagocytosis

Fenn (1921), Ponder (1927, 1928), and Mudd *et al.* (1934) proposed that engulfment of particles by phagocytic cells could be explained entirely by physical determinants of surface interactions and that phagocytosis did not require expenditure of energy. Subsequent studies showed that *in vitro* incubation conditions had to remain within certain limits of pH, temperature, osmotic, and ionic composition of the medium (Mudd *et al.*, 1934; Greendyke *et al.*, 1963). Although such limits could be imposed by physical as well as biochemical requirements of the phagocytic event, these findings suggested the possibility of a metabolic involvement.

It was not until 1956 that Stähelin and co-workers (1956a,b,c) provided convincing evidence of enhanced metabolic activity during ingestion of particles. These investigators showed a marked increase in oxygen uptake by guinea pig peritoneal exudate leukocytes, incubated with heat-killed myco-bacteria. Cohn and Morse and a number of investigators in Karnovsky's laboratory (for review, see Karnovsky, 1962) examined various aspects of intermediary metabolism of leukocytes obtained from rabbit or guinea pig peritoneal exudates, and came to the conclusion that phagocytosis required expenditure of metabolic energy. Mononuclear phagocytes (peripheral blood, peritoneal, and lung macrophages) and eosinophils also manifest heightened metabolic activity during phagocytosis (Cline and Lehrer, 1968; Oren *et al.*, 1963; Cline *et al.*, 1968), and interference with energy-yielding pathways in these cells inhibits phagocytic activity. It is important to bear in mind that different types of phagocytic cells rely on different metabolic pathways as a source of energy. Polymorphonuclear leukocytes possess few mitochondria, and Krebs cycle activity probably provides less than 20% of ATP produced during catabolism of glucose (Beck, 1958), most energy therefore stemming from the Embden Meyerhof pathway. By contrast, both peritoneal and lung macrophages contain numerous mitochondria, and ATP production in these cells derives mainly from oxidative phosphorylation. Comparative studies with the various types of phagocytic cells and the use of various inhibitors of intermediary metabolism (Oren *et al.*, 1963) undoubtedly have greatly supported the concept that engulfment of particles requires metabolic energy. In particular, the findings that inhibitors of oxidative metabolism inhibit ingestion by macrophages but have no effect on granulocytes, whereas inhibitors of glycolysis abolish phagocytic activity by granulocytes and only partially inhibit macrophages, appear to confirm the belief that specific pathways serve the energy needs of engulfment.

However, interpretation of experiments with substances that inhibit biological activity of whole cells is often exceedingly difficult. Numerous chemicals and biologically occurring agents have been examined for their effect on phagocytosis and other functions of phagocytic cells without sufficient realization that few inhibitors are highly specific for single biochemical steps or events. Most compounds that have been used to inhibit a given enzymatic activity can be shown to act also on other biochemical reactions and cellular functions not necessarily related to the presumed primary mode of action. For example, the agents iodoacetate and NaF are often used to inhibit glycolysis. The inhibition by iodoacetate of the enzyme 3-phosphoglyceraldehyde dehydrogenase and by NaF of enolase in the glycolytic cycle has been established clearly (Fruton and Simmonds, 1958). These agents effectively reduce or abolish glucose uptake and lactate production and therefore can deprive the granulocyte of its main source of energy. They also interfere with K^+ and Na^+ transport and cause swelling, however (Elsbach and Schwartz, 1959). Woodin (1962) has pointed out that such effects could secondarily result in inhibition of phagocytosis and that this inhibition need not be due to a direct action on energy metabolism. Further, iodoacetate and NaF inhibit a number of other reactions in cell-free preparations of granulocytes, including lipase activity (Elsbach and Rizack, 1963). In contrast to earlier studies, it has been reported recently that ingestion and bacterial killing could proceed in the presence of NaF in concentrations that prevented uptake and utilization of glucose (Bodel and Malawista, 1969). Such divergent observations with respect to the dependence of ingestion on glycolysis need clarification by further work. A problem in this regard has been the fact that granulocytes contain large stores of glycogen and the enzymatic apparatus to break these down (Scott, 1968; Stossel et al., 1970). It has not been possible therefore to effectively deplete the granulocyte of glucose.

The possibility has been considered that lipids may provide energy during phagocytosis. Evidence has been presented that indicates that complex lipids such as triglycerides and the major circulating phospholipids cannot be incorporated as such (Elsbach, 1965a,b). However, both leukocytes and macrophages incorporate free fatty acid into cell lipids in vitro (Elsbach, 1963, 1964, 1965a,b). Fatty acid uptake is appreciable and is dependent on concentration in the medium. Engulfment of particles, however, does not stimulate esterification of fatty acid nor their oxidation (Elsbach, 1963; Sastry and Hokin, 1966). Further, when leukocyte lipids are labeled during prior incubation with carboxyl-labeled ^{14}C fatty acid, $^{14}CO_2$ production is the same during subsequent incubation in the presence and absence of particles, even though loss of fatty acid from endogenous labeled triglycerides is greater during phagocytosis than at rest (Elsbach and Farrow, 1969).

Although we have pointed out some remaining uncertainties, it must be stressed, particularly in the case of polymorphonuclear leukocytes, that there is now virtually unanimous acceptance of the concept that the complex series of biochemical responses known to accompany the encounter between granulocyte and particle can be divided into two main categories: those that are linked to the process of engulfment and those that relate to the formation or release of bactericidal and degradative agents. Table I summarizes these metabolic events, their presumed relation to either ingestion or killing (digestion), and additional evidence in support of the belief that two distinct sets of metabolic responses exist.

The association of engulfment with glycolysis has been considered earlier. In addition, a small stimulation of Krebs cycle activity during phagocytosis has been attributed to the ingestion phase. Evidence which suggests that ingestion is also associated with increased net synthesis of phospholipid will be reviewed later.

The postphagocytic events of degranulation and of killing and/or digestion of ingested microorganisms by polymorphonuclear leukocytes are accompanied by a many-fold stimulation of O_2 consumption (CN^- insensitive), of CO_2 production [which can be accounted for by direct oxidation of glucose via the hexose monophosphate shunt (HMPS)], and by an increase in

TABLE I

GRANULOCYTE METABOLISM

		Stimulation during phagocytosis	
	Normal	CGD[a]	Colchicine[b] Vinblastine[c] Hydrocortisone[d]
Ingestion Glucose utilization Lactate production Krebs cycle activity Lecithin synthesis (from lysolecithin)[e]	Yes	Yes	Yes
Killing (digestion) O_2 Consumption (oxidase activity) HMPS Activity H_2O_2 Production	Yes	No	No

[a]CGD, Chronic granulomatous disease.
[b]Malawista and Bodel (1967).
[c]Malawista (1971).
[d]Mandell et al. (1970).
[e]Elsbach (1968).

H_2O_2 production. The observation by several workers that engulfment is not impaired in a nitrogen atmosphere, but that killing of several bacterial species is reduced (Sbarra and Karnovsky, 1959; Selvaraj and Sbarra, 1966; Mc-Ripley and Sbarra, 1967a), provided until recently the most convincing indication that in granulocytes the two sets of metabolic responses served separate functions. The identification of chronic granulomatous disease as a clinical syndrome of decreased resistance to infection due to abnormal phagocyte function has done much to strengthen this view (Good et al., 1968). In this disorder, the patients' leukocytes can ingest normally but manifest impaired killing; glycolysis and lactate production are normal but engulfment results in no stimulation of O_2 consumption and CO_2 production, and several species of ingested microorganisms exhibit prolonged intracellular survival.

1. POSSIBLE MECHANISMS OF INCREASED RESPIRATION BY GRANULOCYTES DURING PHAGOCYTOSIS

The very dramatic increase in O_2 consumption observed during phagocytosis of various inert particles and microorganisms by granulocytes has prompted an intensive search for the mechanism of this response. Numerous reports have appeared and have been discussed in recent reviews (Karnovsky, 1968; Sbarra et al., 1970). We will therefore limit this discussion to highlighting the major findings that have led to an as yet unresolved controversy concerning the cellular and/or biochemical events that underlie the increase in respiration.

There is little doubt that increased O_2 consumption, CO_2 production, and H_2O_2 formation are biochemically linked to each other in some fashion (Iyer et al., 1961; McRipley and Sbarra, 1967b; Reed, 1969). It is also clear that the paucity of mitochondria in granulocytes and also the CN^- insensitivity of almost all the respiratory burst implicates pathways other than the cytochrome system.

A case has been made for activation of a CN^--insensitive NADH oxidase as the primary event after ingestion. This would explain both an increase in O_2 uptake and in H_2O_2 production (Cagan and Karnovsky, 1964; Baehner and Karnovsky, 1968). The increase in HMPS activity as measured by $^{14}CO_2$ production from $1\text{-}^{14}C$* glucose must then be explained by some mechanism of transhydrogenation to account for formation of oxidized NADP. Transhydrogenation can be brought about directly by the enzyme transhydrogenase $(NAD + NADPH \Longleftrightarrow NADP + NADH)$. This enzyme has been identified in human leukocytes (Silber et al., 1963), but its activity appears too low to allow sufficient NADP to be formed in the reaction (Evans and Kaplan,

---

*The limited oxidation of glucose via pyruvate and Krebs cycle justifies the oversimplification of equating $^{14}CO_2$ production from $1-^{14}C$ glucose with HMPS activity (Katz and Wood, 1960).

1966). Transhydrogenation can also take place in several coupled reactions. One such proposed mechanism involves an NADPH requiring lactate dehydrogenase in guinea pig leukocytes with acid pH optimum (Karnovsky *et al.*, 1966). However, this activity is absent in rat leukocytes (Reed, 1969). In this animal species it is thought that H_2O_2 itself can stimulate the HMPS and that a glutathione peroxidase and glutathione reductase complete the cycle (Reed, 1969) Table II, scheme I) (Holmes *et al.*, 1970).

Other investigators deny the primary importance of an NADH oxidase and believe that activation of a granule-associated CN^--insensitive NADPH oxidase operates in the cycle (Iyer and Quastel, 1963; Rossi and Zatti, 1964, 1966; Zatti and Rossi, 1966; Rossi *et al.*, 1969; Paul and Sbarra, 1968; Strauss *et al.*, 1969). One way in which this enzyme might participate in the enhanced O_2 consumption and CO_2 and H_2O_2 production is indicated in Table II, scheme II (Holmes *et al.*, 1970). According to this scheme, glutathione reductase activity would increase within 15 seconds after addition of particles to a leukocyte suspension and set the cycle in motion (Strauss *et al.*, 1969). To complicate matters further, divergent results have been obtained by the different investigators with respect to intracellular localization, particle engulfment, degranulation, CN^- sensitivity, pH optimum, and affinity for substrate of the two pyridine nucleotide oxidases (Reed and Tepperman, 1969). Other controversial aspects of the functional significance of these oxidases will be discussed later in the context of the metabolic abnormalities of leukocytes in chronic granulomatous disease.

TABLE II

TWO POSSIBLE REACTION SEQUENCES EXPLAINING LINKED STIMULATION OF O_2 CONSUMPTION, CO_2 PRODUCTION, AND H_2O_2 FORMATION

I $2\ NADH + 2\ H^+ + 2\ O_2 \xrightarrow{\text{NADH oxidase}} 2\ NAD^+ + 2\ H_2O_2$ \hfill (1)

$2\ H_2O_2 + 4\ GSH \xrightarrow[\text{peroxidase}]{\text{glutathione}} 2\ GSSG + 4\ H_2O$ \hfill (2)

$2\ GSSG + 2\ NADPH + 2\ H^+ \xrightarrow[\text{reductase}]{\text{glutathione}} 2\ NADP^+ + 4\ GSH$ \hfill (3)

$G\text{-}6\text{-}P + 2\ NADP^+ \xrightarrow{\text{HMPS}} 2\ NADPH + 2\ H^+ + CO_2$ \hfill (4)

II $2\ GSSG + 2\ NADPH + 2\ H^+ \xrightarrow[\text{reductase}]{\text{glutathione}} 2\ NADP^+ + 4\ GSH$ \hfill (1)

$G\text{-}6\text{-}P + 2\ NADP^+ \xrightarrow{\text{HMPS}} 2\ NADPH + 2\ H^+ + CO_2$ \hfill (2)

$NADPH + H^+ + O_2 \xrightarrow{\text{NADPH oxidase}} NADP^+ + H_2O_2$ \hfill (3)

$H_2O_2 + 2\ GSH \xrightarrow[\text{peroxidase}]{\text{glutathione}} GSSG + H_2O$ \hfill (4)

2. Biological Significance of Increased H_2O_2 Production

The increased production of H_2O_2, a by product of enhanced pyridine nucleotide oxidase activity during phagocytosis, has been shown to fulfill an important role in the leukocyte's microbicidal capabilities (Klebanoff, 1970). It is in particular the work of Klebanoff and his collaborators and McRipley and Sbarra that has revealed the bactericidal, (Klebanoff *et al.*, 1966; Klebanoff, 1967, 1968; McRipley and Sbarra, 1967a,b), fungicidal (Lehrer, 1969), and virucidal (Belding *et al.*, 1970) properties of the combination H_2O_2, leukocyte myeloperoxidase, and an oxidizable substance such as iodide (but also other anions). The observation of decreased intracellular killing by leukocytes of several species of ingested microorganisms during anaerobiosis and in the presence of inhibition of peroxidase further implicates the importance of both production of H_2O_2 and peroxidase (McRipley and Sbarra, 1967a,b). This antimicrobial activity can be shown to be associated with iodination of bacteria within the phagocytic vacuole (Klebanoff and White, 1969; Pincus and Klebanoff, 1971). The H_2O_2-requiring reaction occurs most actively at acid pH presumed to prevail in the immediate environment of the engulfed particle (Klebanoff, 1967; Rous, 1925 ; Mandell, 1970).

Antimicrobial activity of H_2O_2 in conjunction with ascorbic acid at neutral pH *in vitro* (in the absence of phagocytes) has also been reported (Ericsson and Lundbeck, 1955a,b). Recently, Miller (1969) has suggested that this bactericidal activity at neutral pH is mediated by formation of free radicals. These would then alter the bacterial envelope and render the bacteria more susceptible to lysis by agents such as lysozyme.

The evidence of the very significant role of the H_2O_2–myeloperoxidase–halogen system in bacterial killing has been further strengthened by recent clinical observations (see further).

3. Other Microbicidal Factors

It has been firmly established that many other factors contribute to the overall bactericidal capabilities of the phagocyte in addition to those related to oxidative metabolism and H_2O_2 production. Both granulocytes and macrophages contain lysozyme (the latter in quantities that vary with the source) (Myrvik *et al.*, 1961b) and a large array of other degradative lysosomal enzymes (Dannenberg *et al.*, 1963a,b; Dannenberg and Bennett, 1964; Bainton and Farquhar, 1966, 1968a,b; Elsbach and Rizack, 1963; Elsbach and Kayden, 1965; Baggiolini *et al.*, 1969, 1970a,b) that undoubtedly contribute to the demise of intracellular bacteria.

Phagocytin, a basic protein which is bactericidal, also resides in the granule fraction of the polymorphonuclear leukocyte (Hirsch, 1956). Recently, a group of other granule-associated cationic proteins have been described (Zeya and Spitznagel, 1966, 1968, 1969). These investigators propose that each of the bactericidal protein fractions may be specific for different bacterial species (Zeya and Spitznagel, 1969). None of these basic proteins has been found in macrophages (Zeya and Spitznagel, 1969).

The drop in pH observed almost 50 years ago by Rous (1925) within the phagocytic vacuole of granulocytes may potentiate bactericidal activity in several ways, for example, by enhancing activity of acid hydrolases and by inhibiting bacterial metabolism. It is uncertain whether the pH drop also occurs in macrophages. A popular concept is that in granulocytes H^+ ions accumulate because of the increased lactate production that accompanies phagocytosis. In turn, this lactate accumulation is explained by the low Krebs cycle activity in this cell that does not permit the increased pyruvate to be oxidized. Since macrophages contain many mitochondria, no lactate should accumulate. However, this reasoning may well be too simple. There is no biochemical evidence that enough lactate accumulates to cause a drop in pH, since lactate formed rapidly diffuses out of the cell (Wurster *et al.*, 1971). On the other hand, lactate as well as other acid metabolites may accumulate in amounts too small to detect chemically, producing a pH drop in discrete areas in the cell in both granulocytes and macrophages. An understanding of the mechanism of intracellular pH changes must therefore await techniques for their detection, perhaps at interphases, in the microanatomy of a phagocyte.

4. FORMATION AND BREAKDOWN OF CELLULAR MEMBRANES DURING PHAGOCYTOSIS

The dramatic morphological alterations during phagocytosis involving both outer and intracellular membranes (Hirsch, 1962; Zucker-Franklin and Hirsch, 1964) have led several investigators to seek evidence that the concomitant increased energy production serves for synthesis of new membrane needed to accomodate the ingested particles. Almost all the work in this area has focused on metabolism of lipids. As in other studies of membrane biochemistry, it is easier to examine constituents that for practical purposes may be considered to be restricted to membranes, i.e., lipids, than to investigate molecular species that are ubiquitous in the cell, such as proteins. In the latter case, much more rigorous fractionations of cell constituents are necessary. To our knowledge only one study of $[^{14}C]$ leucine incorporation into acid precipitable material of resting and phagocytizing guinea pig leukocytes has been reported (Sbarra and Karnovsky, 1960). Since no attempt was made to isolate membrane proteins, it is not surprising that no difference was found in the amount of radioactivity incorporated into total protein by the two populations of granulocytes. Clearly, therefore, pertinent studies of protein synthesis must be carried out along with appropriate fractionation and isolation of (plasma) membrane preparations. Unfortunately, progress in this latter area has been limited by the difficulties encountered in obtaining good yields of reasonably pure membrane preparations (Woodin and Wieneke, 1966a).

5. INCORPORATION OF SIMPLE BUILDING BLOCKS INTO LIPIDS OF PHAGOCYTES

On the other hand, lipid metabolism by resting and engulfing phagocytes has been extensively investigated. Initially, incorporation of $[^{14}C]$ acetate, ^{32}Pi, and $[^{14}C]U$-glucose was followed as an index of lipid synthesis by rabbit, guinea pig, and human granulocytes (Elsbach, 1959; Sbarra and Karnovsky, 1960; Buchanan, 1960; Marks et al., 1960). Although these precursors were incorporated to a greater extent during phagocytosis than at rest, it was uncertain whether increased labeling reflected increased net synthesis of membrane lipids. In fact, there were several reasons to doubt this: (1) the increased incorporation of $[^{14}C]$acetate was much more pronounced in leukocyte triglyceride than into phospholipids; (2) circumstantial evidence suggested that acetate incorporation into leukocyte lipids occurred by chain elongation of preexisting fatty acids rather than by *de novo* synthesis (Elsbach, 1959). The subsequent demonstration by Majerus and Lastra (1967) that mature leukocytes lack acetyl-CoA carboxylase proved that this was indeed the case; and (3) increased incorporation of ^{32}Pi into phospholipids of engulfing leukocytes only led to increased specific activity of phosphatidic acid and phosphatidyl inositol, minor components of the leukocyte's phospholipids (Karnovsky and Wallach, 1961; Sastry and Hokin, 1966).* One comparative study of ^{32}Pi incorporation into phosphatides showed increased labeling during phagocytosis by peritoneal but not by alveolar macrophages (Oren et al., 1963). It is thus apparent that these tracer studies had not revealed convincing evidence of increased net synthesis of membrane lipid from simple building blocks.

New membrane lipid might also derive from preexisting lipids in the extracellular fluids. Virtually all mammalian cells that have been studied are capable of incorporating free fatty acids bound to albumin into complex cellular lipids. This also is true for leukocytes and macrophages (Day and Fidge, 1962; Day, 1967; Elsbach, 1963, 1964, 1965a,b; Evans and Mueller, 1963). The extent of incorporation of fatty acids is dependent on their concentration in the medium and can reach very appreciable amounts of added

---

* The interested reader is referred to the publication of Sastry and Hokin (1966) for an examination of biochemical mechanisms that may account for increased ^{32}P labeling of these two phospholipid species.

lipids under reasonably physiological conditions (Elsbach, 1964). However, during phagocytosis of heat-killed streptococci (Elsbach, 1963), or of polystyrene particles (Sastry and Hokin, 1966) by polymorphonuclear leukocytes, no stimulation of fatty acid incorporation was observed.

Uptake of triglycerides and diacylphosphatides by phagocytic cells appears very different from the avid incorporation and metabolism of fatty acids. When labeled triglycerides or phospholipids are incubated with rabbit granulocytes, small amounts of radioactive lipid are found in association with the washed cells (Elsbach, 1962, 1965a,b). However, in contrast to the findings with free fatty acids, this association appears to be physical in nature rather than dependent on active metabolism. It was concluded that the labeled complex lipids, including chylomicra, particles large enough to be ingested by a phagocytosis-like process, adhered to the cell surface without entering the metabolic pathways of the cell or actually becoming part of the cell membrane. A comparison was also made of uptake of labeled triglycerides, mixed phospholipids, or chylomicra by resting granulocytes and by cells actively engaged in phagocytosis of heat-killed bacteria. Even during engulfment no evidence was found of metabolic utilization of these labeled complex lipids. In this context it is of interest that a suspension of chylomicra had no detectable effect on respiration in contrast to a marked stimulation of O_2 uptake by leukocytes engulfing heat-killed bacteria (Elsbach, 1965a).

Similar experiments with alveolar macrophages yielded results that differed from those obtained with granulocytes. Although exogenous phospholipids again appeared not to enter the metabolic pathways of the macrophages, these cells not only incorporated free fatty acids but also metabolized $1\text{-}^{14}C$ fatty acid-labeled triglycerides as well as chylomicra present in the incubation medium (Elsbach, 1965b). The findings indicated that the utilization of the labeled triglycerides did not reflect incorporation of the intact molecules, but was, in fact, due to hydrolysis of triglycerides prior to entry, most likely on the surface of the cells, with subsequent incorporation of the hydrolyzed fatty acids.

It thus appeared that of the lipid species examined in these studies only free fatty acids were incorporated into cell lipids by a process that required biochemical activity. Further, not only was it unlikely that a phagocytosis-like process accounted for such selectivity in uptake of lipids, but, in fact, engulfment of particles by granulocytes caused no detectible increase in incorporation of any of these lipid species, not even free fatty acids.

6. Utilization of Lysocompounds for Synthesis of Cellular Phospholipids

In none of the earlier studies of lipid metabolism discussed thus far had the possibility been considered that lysocompounds (monoacyl phosphatides) in the extracellular environment might serve as precursors of membrane lipids.

Both lysolecithin and lysophosphatidylethanolamine have been identified as naturally occurring circulating lysophosphatides. (Phillips, 1957; Newman *et al.*, 1961; Misra, 1965; Switzer and Eder, 1965). The physiological significance of lysolecithin has been most extensively investigated. This compound represents roughly 10 % of plasma phospholipids in several animal species and occurs almost exclusively in association with albumin (Switzer and Eder, 1965). Lands (1960) and Erbland and Marinetti (1965) have demonstrated in liver homogenates that pathways exist for the direct conversion of lysolecithin to lecithin. Subsequently, numerous investigators have shown that many tissues and cell types, including plants and bacteria, contain enzyme(s) that carry out the transfer of a fatty acid (in most instances from a fatty acyl-CoA derivative) to lysolecithin (reviewed by van Deenen, 1965).

Stein and Stein (1966) injected radioisotopically labeled lysolecithin complexed to albumin intravenously into rats and showed that the direct acylation of lysolecithin is not only of significance in the turnover of endogenous phospholipids but also in providing the whole animal with an extracellular source of an essential membrane phospholipid of many mammalian tissues, as demonstrated by the accumulation of labeled lecithin in these tissues. Even though lysolecithin constitutes only a relatively small portion of the circulating phospholipids, the enzyme lecithin-cholesterol-acyl transferase in cell-free plasma ensures a mechanism for the repletion of plasma lysolecithin (Glomset, 1962).

The possibility that lysocompounds participate in membrane phospholipid turnover during phagocytosis has prompted a search for enzymes concerned with their metabolism. In a series of studies it has been shown that homogenates of rabbit peritoneal granulocytes and alveolar macrophages acylate both lysolecithin and lysophosphatidylethanolamine to the respective diacyl derivatives (Lands, 1960; Elsbach, 1966, 1967). In addition, granulocyte homogenates convert lysolecithin to lecithin in a reaction in which a fatty acid from one lysolecithin molecule is transferred to another (Erbland and Marinetti, 1965). In contrast to Land's pathway, most active in the microsomal fraction at physiological pH, this latter reaction does not require added ATP and CoA, manifests an acid pH optimum, and is fully active in a high-speed supernatant fraction (Elsbach *et al.*, 1965; Elsbach, 1967). Lysophosphatidylethanolamine is not a substrate in this reaction.

Since both granulocytes and macrophages contain phospholipase A activity (Elsbach and Rizack, 1963; Elsbach *et al.*, 1965; Elsbach, 1966), these cells contain the enzyme components of a diacyl–monoacyl phosphatide cycle. It is conceivable that such a cycle would participate in the phenomena of membrane lysis and fusion, as seen in engulfing granulocytes during formation of the phagocytic vacuole and when granules fuse with the vacuole followed by lysis in the area of junction and discharge of the granule contents (Zucker-Franklin and Hirsch, 1964). The operation of the cycle implies that naturally occurring membrane-lytic lysocompounds are formed, but that these products can also be reutilized for synthesis of major membrane constituents. The physiological significance of such a cycle involving the membrane phospholipids of phagocytes has not been established. It must be emphasized that the cytosol of both granulocytes and macrophages contains lysophospholipases that degrade lysophosphatides to nonlytic water-soluble products by removal of the remaining fatty acid (Elsbach *et al.*, 1965; Elsbach, 1966, 1967). It has not been possible, moreover, to demonstrate more rapid degradation of previously labeled leukocyte or macrophage phospholipids with accumulation of monoacyl phosphatides during phagocytosis (Elsbach, 1968; Elsbach *et al.*, 1972; Franson *et al.*, 1973).

More clearcut results have been obtained with respect to conversion of medium lysolecithin and lysophosphatidylethanolamine complexed to albumin into the respective diacyl derivatives by intact granulocytes and macrophages (Elsbach, 1968). Since this conversion involves a single biochemical step, the amount of diacyl phosphatide synthesized from the monoacyl compound can be reasonably accurately determined from the specific radioactivity of the substrate in the medium. By converting lysolecithin to lecithin, granulocytes add, on the average, 5% to their lecithin content in 30 minutes (Elsbach, 1968). Macrophages convert comparable amounts of lysolecithin to lecithin per cell, but because these cells are far larger and contain much more lecithin, the percent contribution to lecithin content is considerably less than for the granulocyte. The effect of ingestion of particles on incorporation of medium lysolecithin into lecithin of granulocytes and macrophages is shown in Fig. 1, which presents the mean values of at least four paired experiments at each time interval in the absence and presence of polystyrene or zymosan particles. It is evident that addition of particles markedly stimulates lecithin synthesis from lysolecithin. This stimulation is up to twofold with polystyrene and up to threefold with zymosan particles. Phosphatidylethanolamine synthesis from lysophosphatidylethanolamine is similarly increased during phagocytosis. By contrast, degradation of these two lysophosphatides is the same in the absence and presence of particles. This suggests that their increased use for synthesis of diacyl compounds is not merely the consequence of increased availability of substrate during engulfment nor necessarily a reflection of a general stimulation of metabolism. The increase in lecithin synthesis by granulocytes can be accounted for entirely by acylation of lysolecithin (Lands, 1960). In intact leukocytes, no evidence has been obtained for operation of the pathway: 2 lysoleci-

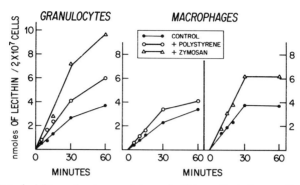

Fig. 1. Effect of addition of various particles on lecithin synthesis from medium lysolecithin by granulocytes and alveolar macrophages. Lysolecithen biosynthetically labeled with 32p was added to the incubation mixture complexed to serum albumin. Each value represents the mean of at least four paired experiments at each time interval: the details of the procedures used were described by Elsbach (1968). Reproduced with permission of the American Society for Clinical Investigation, Inc.

thin ⟶ lecithin + glycerylphosphorylcholine (Elsbach, 1968). The stimulation of lecithin synthesis following addition of particles is not affected by inhibition of protein synthesis with puromycin or cycloheximide (P. Elsbach, unpublished observations) and is not seen with broken cell preparations. Homogenates of granulocytes previously incubated with particles are no more active than homogenates of resting cells.

It has been concluded that the increased formation of two major phospholipids during phagocytosis represents net addition, because increased synthesis occurs without concomitantly increased degradation of cellular lipids and without loss into the extracellular medium (Elsbach, 1968).

Human peripheral blood leukocytes also convert approximately twice as much lysolecithin to lecithin during phagocytosis as they do at rest (Elsbach et al., 1969).

It is tempting to postulate that this first evidence of net phospholipid synthesis during phagocytosis is indicative of increased formation of membrane, presumably needed for engulfment of particles. This hypothesis, reasonable as it may appear, is not easily proved, however. Such proof requires at least that less phagocytosis takes place when acylation is reduced and that any circumstances that interfere with acylation also result in decreased engulfment.

The inherent limitations of experiments in which various inhibitory agents are used have already been discussed. It is of interest nonetheless to compare the effects of a number of substances that have been employed in the past to assess the apparent dependence of ingestion by different types of phagocytes

on the major energy-yielding pathways, on both uptake of particles (Oren
et al., 1963) and on acylation of lysolecithin (Elsbach, 1971). Table III shows
that NaF and iodoacetic acid (IAA) inhibit most of the usual stimulation of
acylation of lysolecithin by granulocytes in parallel with their effects on
phagocytosis, whereas inhibitors of oxidative metabolism affect neither
lecithin synthesis nor engulfment by these cells. On the other hand, engulfment
by alveolar macrophages is inhibited not only by NaF or IAA but also by
interference with oxidative phosphorylation (KCN, DNP, or N_2 atmosphere).
The extent of inhibition of the stimulation of acylation during ingestion of
polystyrene particles is roughly comparable to that of engulfment. Colchicine
which is reported to have no effect on ingestion by granulocytes but to inhibit
intracellular killing (Malawista and Bodel, 1967) has no effect on acylation.

Wurster *et al.*, (1971) have examined the effect of the morphine analog
levorphanol on a wide variety of metabolic functions of resting and engulfing
granulocytes. Levorphanol reversibly inhibits uptake of polystyrene particles
and uptake and killing of *E. coli* (Zucker-Franklin *et al.*, 1971) and also
reversibly inhibits acylation of lysocompounds (Wurster *et al.*, 1971).

More conclusive evidence that exogenous lysocompounds are a requirement for effective engulfment and vacuole formation is lacking. Uptake of
microorganisms and particles such as zymosan requires the presence of serum,
which means that albumin and attached lysolecithin are also present. Uptake
of polystyrene particles is reported to proceed well in the absence of serum or
albumin (Sbarra and Karnovsky, 1959). A careful morphological comparison
of ingestion by granulocytes incubated in balanced salt solution with or with-

TABLE III

INHIBITION OF LECITHIN SYNTHESIS AND PHAGOCYTOSIS BY VARIOUS AGENTS

	Granulocytes		Macrophages	
	Lecithin synthesis (%)	Inhibition of phagocytosis	Lecithin synthesis (%)	Inhibition of phagocytosis
Control	54		63	
+ particles	100		100	
+ particles + IAA	59	+ + +	60	+ + +
+ particles + NaF	64	+ + +	83	+ + +
+ particles + KCN	131	0	70	+ +
+ particles + N_2	100	0	47	+ +
+ particles + DNP	93	0	84	+ +
+ particles + colchicine	120	0		

[a]The following final concentrations were used: IAA, iodoacetate—(0.001 M); NaF—
(0.02 M); KCN—(0.02 M); DNP, 2,4-dinitrophenol—(0.02 M); colchicine—(0.00003 M).

out albumin has not been carried out to our knowledge, but such a study is complicated by the fact that some metabolic responses of leukocytes incubated in the absence of protein may be reduced (P. Elsbach, unpublished observations).

7. Lipid-Splitting Enzymes and Their Possible Relevance to the Phagocytic Process

The existence in phagocytic cells of lipid-splitting activities has been referred to earlier in this review. Only a few attempts have been made to determine whether or not these degradative enzymes serve a specific function during phagocytosis. For example, cholesterol esterase activity has been found in macrophages (Day, 1967), but its physiological significance has not yet been examined.

Exceedingly active lipases* (triglyceride acylhydrolases) have been identified in homogenates of rabbit granulocytes and alveolar macrophages (Elsbach and Rizack, 1963; Elsbach and Kayden, 1965; Elsbach, 1965a,b). In both cell types the pH optimum of hydrolysis with respect to various triglyceride substrates is acid, and in granulocytes the activity is to a large extent associated with the granule fraction. Granulocytes contain sizable stores of triglycerides (approximately 20% of total cell lipids) (Elsbach, 1959). Recently, Elsbach and Farrow (1969) have shown that during ingestion of polystyrene particles by granulocytes whose triglycerides and phospholipids had previously been labeled with [1-^{14}C]fatty acid a flux of radioactive fatty acid takes place from triglyceride to lecithin. It may be recalled that uptake and esterification of medium free fatty acid by granulocytes are not enhanced during phagocytosis. Thus it appears that cellular triglyceride provides fatty acid needed for the increased acylation of medium lysolecithin by engulfing leukocytes. The most likely explanation of the transfer of fatty acid from triglyceride to lecithin is that activation of the acid lipase results in release of fatty acid which is then reesterified. The operation of the lipase in intact leukocytes toward endogenous triglyceride can indeed be demonstrated at acid ambient pH when loss of triglyceride radioactivity is matched by the accumulation of fatty acid radioactivity (Elsbach and Farrow, 1969). Since at more physiological pH no fatty acid accumulates, the possibility of a direct acyl transfer from triglyceride to lysolecithin without mediation of a lipase, although less likely, cannot be excluded.

Production of $^{14}CO_2$ from granulocyte lipids labeled with [1-^{14}C] fatty acid is the same at rest and during phagocytosis. It appears, therefore, that

---

*We do not consider here a number of esterases of unknown biological significance that have been described in granulocytes and macrophages (Rossiter and Wong, 1949; Cohn and Wiener, 1963; Dannenberg et al., 1963a,b).

oxidation of hydrolyzed fatty acids does not contribute toward meeting the increased energy demands of phagocytosis (Elsbach and Farrow, 1969).

Homogenates of rabbit peritoneal granulocytes and alveolar macrophages also contain acid phospholipase A and neutral lysophospholipase activities (Elsbach et al., 1965; Elsbach, 1966, 1967). The hypothetical significance of a diacyl–monoacyl phosphatide cycle has already been discussed in the preceding section. Whereas alveolar macrophages rapidly degrade previously labeled lecithin, intact leukocytes manifest a very slow turnover of their major phospholipids, including lecithin. Ingestion of polystyrene particles does not detectably affect cellular phospholipid breakdown by either phago-cyte (Elsbach, 1968; Elsbach et al., 1972). With regard to endogenous phospholipid therefore, the phospholipase A has no obvious function during phagocytosis. Since at least part of the phospholipase A activity is associated with the granule fraction in the leukocyte, it has been suggested that this hydrolase aids in bacterial digestion (Elsbach and Rizack, 1963). Evidence that bacterial lipid undergoes partial degradation during phago-cytosis has been presented by Cohn (1963a). He assumed that this degradation was due to action of the leukocyte's enzymes. This assumption seems not unreasonable, especially since recent studies in our laboratory have shown that phosphatidylethanolamine and phosphatidylglycerol, major phos-pholipids of several bacterial species, are readily broken down by leukocyte homogenates (Elsbach et al., 1972; Patriarca et al., 1972). The granule fraction is particularly active. However, it must be borne in mind that many microorganisms used in studies of phagocytosis in vitro contain their own complement of phospholipase. E. coli, for example, has been shown to contain phospholipase A and lysophospholipase activities (Okuyama and Nojima, 1969; Fung and Proulx, 1969; Proulx and Fung, 1969). Certain strains of E. coli also contain phospholipase C activity (Proulx and van Deenen, 1967a,b). We have found that heat killing of E. coli may result in accelerated breakdown of previously labeled bacterial lipid (Patriarca et al. 1972). The products released are those of degradation by phospholipase A. Under these circumstances it is clearly difficult to determine whether any bacterial lipid breakdown during killing is due to activation of the organism's own phospholipases, to those of the leukocytes, or to a com-bined action.

Little information is available concerning the relationship between the composition of the cell envelope of a given microorganism and its susceptibil-ity to the bactericidal action of phagocytes. The notable resistance of myco-bacteria to intracellular killing and the unusual lipid composition of their cell envelope supports the notion that lipids are important in this context.

Of interest is that virtually complete killing of a number of microorganisms is accompanied by only partial digestion of various bacterial macromolecular constituents labeled with ^{32}P (Cohn, 1963a). In our own studies, degradation of [^{14}C] glycerol- or [1-^{14}C] palmitate-labeled lipids of *E. coli* incubated with granulocytes is less than 15% in 1 hour and then reaches a plateau, whereas bacterial survival falls at least 1 log in 30 minutes (Elsbach *et al.*, 1972; Patriarca *et al.*, 1972).

Such findings indicate not only that digestion of ingested and killed bacteria by polymorphonuclear leukocytes may be very incomplete but also that bacterial killing requires no extensive degradation of the lipids of the bacterial envelope. This does not mean of course that an enzymatic attack on the envelope is less than essential for effective killing, even if only a small portion of its macromolecules is involved.

8. Metabolic Effects of Several Agents on Phagocytes and Their Relevance to Phagocytosis

Earlier in this section we discussed the prevalent concept that the metabolic responses that accompany phagocytosis follow an ordered sequence in which one can separate, on the one hand, those biochemical alterations that appear to subserve ingestion and, on the other hand, those that follow ingestion and that have been designated as "postphagocytic" events. The latter include the respiratory burst. Indeed, studies of inborn errors of leukocyte metabolism, to be discussed below, tend to support the evidence presented earlier. Nevertheless, in the light of a growing number of recent observations, there is now ample reason to question the view that the biochemical aspects of the postphagocytic events must necessarily follow the formation of the phagocytic vacuoles. Numerous substances, among which are microbial products and other naturally occurring compounds, several surfactants, and pharmacological agents, elicit metabolic responses that may be indistinguishable from those that occur during phagocytosis. The property that these different substances appear to have in common is a direct or indirect effect on the surface of the cell. Among bacterial products that affect the metabolism and function of leukocytes, leucocidin, streptolysin O, and endotoxin have been studied most intensively. Leucocidin, an extracellular product of staphylococcus, has multiple effects on granulocytes (for review of the voluminous work of Woodin and Wieneke, see Woodin, 1968; Woodin and Wieneke, 1970). Addition of highly purified preparations of leucocidin to suspensions of granulocytes results in a selective release of granule protein (i.e., a number of lysosomal enzymes) into the surrounding medium, increased $^{14}CO_2$ production from [1-^{14}C]glucose, increased incorporation of ^{32}Pi into phospholipids (specifically triphosphoinositide), and increased permeability to cations. The nature of the interaction between leucocidin and leukocytes seems highly complex. The fact that leucocidin is not appreciably taken up by the leukocyte while being inactivated in the medium and the dependence of its action on Ca^{2+} provide the strongest support for Woodin's contention that the effect is on the outer membrane. The effect of streptolysin O is so clearly similar to that of leucocidin that the mode of action of the streptococcal toxin on leukocytes and macrophages is likely to be the same (Hirsch *et al.*, 1963; Woodin and Wieneke, 1964, 1966b; Zucker-Franklin, 1965). *E. coli* endotoxin is another bacterial product that induces a respiratory burst, increased direct oxidation of glucose via the hexose monophosphate shunt, and enhanced incorporation of $^{32}P_i$ into acidic phospholipids in leukocytes and mononuclear phagocytes (Strauss and Stetson, 1960; Graham *et al.*, 1967).

The detergents deoxycholate and digitonin also produce these changes in phagocytes, but other surface active agents such as the neutral detergents Triton X-100 and Tween-80 and a number of cationic detergents do not or actually depress respiration. Some negatively charged surfactants exhibit minimal or less stimulatory effects than deoxycholate and digitonin (Graham *et al.*, 1967). The polyene antibiotics nystatin and amphotericin, substances known to interact with cell surfaces, have no effect on respiration by leukocytes (Graham *et al.*, 1967). No pattern has emerged that suggests particular molecular configurations or physical chemical properties that determine whether or not these diverse compounds exert metabolic and/or structural effects.

Rossi *et al.* (1971) have reported that antibodies against guinea pig leukocytes stimulate respiration, H_2O_2 formation, and hexose monophosphate shunt activity of these cells without affecting glycolysis. Marked cytotoxicity and only transient metabolic stimulation was apparent in the presence of complement, but not after heat treatment of the immune serum and not when isolated globulin was added to the cells. The cytotoxic effects of complement and immuneserum suggest that antibodies directed at the leukocytes were present, even though red cell ghosts were not removed during preparation of the immune serum. Pertinent is the demonstration by Messner and Jelinek (1970) of cell-surface receptors on human neutrophils, for human γ G antibodies directed at bacterial antigens. These observations complement previous studies of others showing such receptor sites, but with different specificities, on mononuclear phagocytes (for review, see Messner and Jelinek, 1970). The studies of Rossi *et al.* (1971) indicate that the presence of antibodies not directed at leukocyte antigens produces no metabolic effects.

Although a number of the observations under discussion are suggestive of a surface effect, it must be recognized that high concentrations of the various substances have been used. The physical- chemical state of many of these agents, in most of the experimental conditions used, is not known. It is conceivable therefore that finely particulate matter rather than soluble material was presented to the cell suspensions. Cline (1970) has proposed that the respiratory stimulation seen with endotoxin can be explained by ingestion of such particles. On the other hand, some of the metabolic changes that occur in cells treated with surface-active agents are associated with drastic fine structural changes that strongly suggest serious cell damage. This is particularly noticeable in the case of digitonin (Graham *et al.*, 1967), streptolysin O (Hirsch *et al.*, 1963; Zucker-Franklin, 1965), and leucocidin (Woodin, 1968). Other agents that produce similar metabolic responses can exert their effects without recognizable morphological alterations. These include deoxycholate, endotoxin (Graham *et al.*, 1967), and isolated anti-leukocyte globulin (Rossi *et al.*, 1971). In some cases the respiratory stimulation occurs without impairment of glycolysis, for example, in the presence of antibody (Rossi *et al.*, 1971); in other instances glycolysis is inhibited, as noted on treatment of granulocytes with saponin (Zatti and Rossi, 1966) or phospholipase C (Patriarca *et al.*, 1970). These diverse metabolic and structural consequences of different agents may reflect differences in mode of action; e.g., isolated and primary effects on the cell surface as opposed to passage of a given substance through the cell membrane with additional effects on cytoplasm and/or intracellular organelles such as lysosomes.

In none of the studies reviewed here has the ability been examined of the phagocyte to ingest particles or to kill microorganisms in the presence of or following exposure to the various agents. The extent to which granulocytes or other phagocytes are capable of carrying out bacterial killing would provide an index of the overall functional integrity of the phagocyte and presumably of the nonspecific damaging effect of the agent examined. It has also not been reported whether or not any of the effects are reversible.

Despite the obvious difficulties in interpretation of studies of this kind, one important conclusion must be drawn; namely, an increase in respiration and associated metabolic responses can follow many and very different stimuli inflicted on phagocytes. Several of such stimuli represent severe trauma to the cell. Therefore, the ability of a phagocytic cell to mount a respiratory response cannot categorically be accepted as evidence that phagocytosis has taken place. Conversely, the failure to exhibit increased respiration need not mean that ingestion has not occurred.

In addition to investigations of leukocyte metabolism as affected by agents which elicit responses that mimic those seen during phagocytosis, we must also consider a rapidly increasing number of studies on phagocytosis itself in which pharmacologically and physiologically active substances have been examined.

The antiinflammatory drugs colchicine, phenylbutazone, and several steroid hormones appear to modify the phagocytic process *in vitro*. Malawista and Bodel (1967) have described an uncoupling effect of colchicine on ingestion and respiratory stimulation. Removal and killing of streptococci by normal and colchicine-treated leukocytes were indistinguishable, whereas increasing concentrations of colchicine correspondingly produced increasing inhibition of the respiratory response. In addition, colchicine appeared to reduce degranulation and release of acid phosphatase from the granule fraction during phagocytosis. Similar observations have been made on the pharmacological agent vinblastine (Malawista, 1971).

Phenylbutazone inhibits not only the respiratory stimulation and H_2O_2 production by engulfing leukocytes but also inhibits glycolysis and, presumably as a consequence of the latter, particle uptake (Strauss et al., 1968).

Release of lysosomal enzymes and bactericidal activity are also decreased in the presence of phenylbutazone; these effects are thought to be independent of the impaired uptake, since the drug also reduces bactericidal activity of homogenized leukocytes. The cells in these experiments were obtained from guinea pig peritoneal exudates.

Hydrocortisone in high concentrations (2.1 mM) has been reported to impair intracellular killing without affecting ingestion by human polymorphonuclear leukocytes (Mandell et al., 1970). Since reduction of nitrobluetetrazolium (Baehner and Nathan, 1968), O_2 consumption, H_2O_2 production, and oxidation of NADH were all inhibited by hydrocortisone, the authors attribute the decreased intracellular killing to a direct inhibitory effect of the steroid on NADH oxidase (Yielding and Tomkins, 1959). No impairment of degranulation was observed. Somewhat similar (preliminary) findings have been reported for estrogens (Bodel et al., 1970). Kvarstein and Stomorken (1971) have reported parallel inhibition of uptake of latex particles and of the respiratory response of human peripheral blood leukocytes (and platelets), by exceedingly high concentrations of acetylsalicylic acid, phenylbutazone, colchicine, and hydrocortisone.

It has been speculated that the clinical effects of these drugs may be related to these in vitro observations. In none of the above studies has it been mentioned whether or not the effects were reversible on washing away the drug.

Morphine analogs, also in high concentrations (2 mM), inhibit ingestion of polystyrene particles and killing of microorganisms by rabbit peritoneal granulocytes. Synthesis of major phospholipids from lysocompounds in the medium is markedly decreased and the usual stimulation of hexosemonophosphate shunt activity and of the reduction of nitrobluetetrazolium are eliminated (Elsbach et al., 1970; Wurster et al., 1971; Zucker-Franklin et al., 1971). All effects are completely reversible after removal of the drug. The nonnarcotic enantiomorphs have identical inhibitory effects, and morphine antagonists do not protect (Wurster et al., 1971).

The effects of X irradiation on leukocyte function and phagocytosis have been reviewed recently by Sbarra *et al.* (1970). Numerous other agents, hormones, and metabolities have been studied for their effects on leukocyte metabolism and function. These investigations will not be reviewed here, because they do not have specific relevance to phagocytosis and its accompanying events or because they have been considered in other chapters.

A potentially important new finding is a partially characterized inhibitor of phagocytosis, which is released by alveolar macrophages incubated *in vitro*. The inhibitory substance is a heat-stable glycoprotein (Ulrich and Zilversmit, 1970). The investigators speculate that such inhibitory substances, perhaps in concert with opsonins, may act as regulators of the rate and extent of engulfment. They also raise the possibility that the glycoprotein is derived from the cell surface of the phagocyte and represents a binding site for foreign particles. When released into the extracellular environment, reduction of uptake would not only result from loss of binding sites, but the material might also coat the particles and thus render these less foreign and less prone to adherence to the macrophage. Apparently no information is as yet available concerning such inhibitors derived from leukocytes or active against phagocytosis by leukocytes.

Finally, the well-established role of delayed hypersensitivity in promoting phagocytic and bactericidal activities (Mackaness, 1970; Simon and Sheagren, 1971) has assumed new significance in the studies of Nathan *et al.* (1971). Antigenically stimulated lymphocytes release a factor that enhances peritoneal macrophage adherence, phagocytosis, spreading, motility, and HMPS activity.

IV. Clinical Abnormalities of Cellular Host Defense

The better understanding that has been gained in the past decade of determinants of leukocyte behaviour during phagocytosis has led to the recent recognition, description, and in several instances the tentative identification of pathophysiological mechanisms of a rapidly increasing number of defects in cellular host defense. Conversely, the observations on patients and on phagocytes, obtained from such individuals, that perform abnormally *in vitro* have aided greatly in clarifying relationships between specific events in phagocytosis and certain cellular as well as noncellular functions. In theory, decreased resistance to infection may be due to abnormalities in any of the steps in the overall process of phagocytosis. Most of the defects that are currently known appear to be inborn errors of metabolism, a few are acquired, or, as discussed in the preceding section, perhaps are induced by administration of various drugs.

1. Decreased Resistance to Infection Because of Impaired Contact between Phagocytes and Microorganisms

Animal studies have shown that migration of leukocytes out of the circulation toward the site of invasion by microorganism may be impaired when the osmolality of the plasma is elevated (Austen and Cohn, 1963c; Ainsworth and Allison, 1970). It is not known whether the increased susceptibility to infection of patients in diabetic acidosis and under other conditions in which the composition of the body fluids is altered can be attributed to hypertonicity or is due to other factors such as disturbances in acid-base balance or a compromised circulation (Brayton et al., 1970). Mowat and Baum (1971) have shown decreased chemotaxis of leukocytes from patients with diabetes mellitus, apparently unrelated to levels of insulin, glucose, CO_2, and urea nitrogen in the blood. Chemotaxis in vitro was restored to normal by treatment of diabetic leukocytes with insulin, provided glucose was present in the medium.

Several cases of congenitally diminished resistance to bacterial infections have been described very recently in which leukotactic activity as determined in the Boyden chamber (Boyden, 1962) was reduced, apparently in each case because of a different humoral defect. Since in each instance phagocytic activity in vitro was also impaired, uncertainty remains concerning the relevance of diminished chemotactic responsiveness of the patient's leukocytes in vitro to their increased susceptibility to infections.

Ward and Schlegel (1969) have reported a 4-year-old boy with recurrent severe cutaneous and respiratory infections, whose leukocytes showed only 10–20% of the chemotactic activity exhibited by the leukocytes of the parents and other normal individuals. Leukocytes of the patient's healthy brother showed a somewhat reduced chemotactic responsiveness in vitro. The patient's leukocytes also showed impaired migration in a Rebuck skin window (Rebuck and Crowley, 1955). Thus, the in vivo findings appear to correspond to those in vitro. While the defect in leukotaxis seemed nonselective, impaired phagocytosis and bactericidal activity in vitro was selective for certain gram-negative bacteria and was not manifest with respect to the gram-positive organism Staphylococcus aureus and Serratia marcescens. The latter is noteworthy because, if substantiated, this finding would provide a sharp distinction with the well-established susceptibility of patients with chronic granulomatous disease to infections with these two bacterial species. Further, in this same study, leukocytes of two patients with chronic granulomatous disease showed normal chemotactic responsiveness. The mechanism of impaired chemotaxis remains unknown. However, the demonstration, on the one hand, that washing of the patient's leukocytes and resuspension in normal serum largely restored leukotaxis and, on the other hand, that leukocytes from normal individuals showed dose-dependent inhibition of chemotaxis in the patient's serum is consistent with the authors' postulate of the presence of an inhibitor in this serum. The meaning of impaired reduction of the dye nitrobluetetrazolium (NBT) (Baehner and Nathan, 1968) by the patient's leukocytes on incubation with polystyrene particles is unclear, especially in view of the reported effectiveness of killing of *Staphylococcus aureus* and *Serratia marcescens*. Intracellular killing of these organisms presumably requires increased H_2O_2 production linked to metabolic responses that also lead to enhanced reduction of NBT (the relevance of this test to the metabolism of the granulocyte is discussed later in this section).

Two other case reports (Miller and Nilsson, 1970; Alper *et al.*, 1970a,b) indicate that increased susceptibility to infection may be associated with abnormalities of the complement system and concomitantly reduced chemotaxis.

Miller and Nilsson (1970) have described a family with an abnormality of the fifth component of complement (C5) in 17 relatives. In one of these, a 7-month-old girl, there was an associated increased susceptibility to mainly gram-negative bacterial infections. *In vitro* the patient's leukocytes exhibited both decreased chemotactic responsiveness and decreased phagocytosis of yeast particles when incubated in serum deficient in C5, but not in the presence of normal serum. Addition of purified C5 corrected the functional impairment of the patient's leukocytes, and infusion of fresh normal plasma caused improved handling of infections. Since no quantitative deficiency of C5 could be demonstrated, it is proposed that the C5 produced is abnormal. This possibility is supported by the finding that C5 isolated from family members could not restore the reduced phagocytic activity, in contrast to C5 from other individuals. No explanation is offered for the fact that only 1 of 17 relatives with defective C5 showed evidence of increased susceptibility to infection. Thus, insufficient information is as yet available to permit the conclusion that C5 deficiency or an abnormal C5 *per se* can account for the multiple infections observed in this one child.

Another instance of an abnormal component of complement (C3) associated with increased susceptibility to infection has been carefully studied by Alper *et al.* (1970a,b). The patient, a young adult with Klinefelter's syndrome, had suffered since infancy from numerous infections with both gram-positive and gram-negative organisms. Humoral antibody production, cellular immunity, and leukocyte function all were normal and so were the concentrations of the components of complement C1, C2, C4, C5, and C6. However, the concentration of C3 was markedly reduced as determined by immunochemistry and undetectible by agarose electrophoresis. Further electrophoretic studies revealed that most of the immunochemically reactive C3 was in the form of an inactive product (C3b) (Alper *et al.*, 1970b). Leukocyte function *in vitro*, including phagocytosis and chemotaxis, was restored by normal serum but not by purified C3. The abnormality in the patient is therefore not merely the result of a lack of C3. The authors suggest that the inborn error concerns a deficiency of an inhibitor of a protease that has C3 as substrate. Of interest is that serum of this patient corrected the defect in phagocytosis of the patient of Miller and Nilsson (1970) and vice versa, clearly establishing that the two defects are different.

2. DECREASED RESISTANCE TO INFECTION BECAUSE OF IMPAIRED INGESTION

To our knowledge no specific abnormalities in the ability of phagocytes to ingest microorganisms have as yet been identified. That defective antibody production and agammaglobulinemia are associated with increased incidence of infection is well established. The role of antibodies in the surface inter-action between phagocyte and bacteria *in vitro* has been reviewed briefly in an earlier section. However, to what extent the decreased ability of individuals with congenital or "acquired" agammaglobulinemia to resist infection is due to defective phagocytosis *in vivo* or to factors not related to cellular defense mechanisms is not entirely clear. The firmest evidence that leukocyte function may be impaired when globulin is deficient is provided by the *in vitro* study of Mickenberg *et al.* (1970) that showed decreased phagocytic, bactericidal, and metabolic activities of peripheral blood leukocytes from three patients with "acquired" hypogammaglobulinemia. All parameters of leukocyte function were corrected by normal serum, γ-globulin, or purified IgG.

In line with these results, Douglas *et al.* (1970b) have described transiently impaired neutrophil bactericidal activity *in vitro* against opsonized *Staphylococcus aureus* and *Serratia marcescens* in association with a mixed cryoglobulin and antiglobulin. In this 75-year-old patient, clinical improvement coincided with diminished circulatory cryoglobulin and recovery of neutrophil bactericidal activity. On the other hand, the same group of investigators (Douglas *et al.*, 1970a) report normal phagocytosis and bactericidal activity by leukocytes obtained from patients with "acquired" agammaglobulinemia. No details were given however concerning the absence or presence of opsonizing factors and the organisms examined. Since some bacterial species require added opsonins for *in vitro* ingestion whereas others do not, these studies need not contradict those of Mickenberg *et al.* (1970).

It is obvious that these observations represent only the beginning of a much needed evaluation of the role of abnormal globulin levels in defective cellular host defense.

3. DECREASED RESISTANCE TO INFECTION BECAUSE OF IMPAIRED KILLING OF INGESTED ORGANISMS

Earlier in this chapter we discussed the various bactericidal factors that are currently recognized. Several more or less distinct clinical entities of increased susceptibility to bacterial infection have recently been described that appear related to absence or defectiveness of one or more of these bactericidal systems.

Increased susceptibility to infection may be related to congenital abnormalities in the antimicrobial activity provided by myeloperoxidase (of leukocytes) or catalase [in rabbit alveolar macrophages (Gee et al., 1970)], in conjunction with H_2O_2, and an oxidizable halogen (Klebanoff, 1971).

Lehrer and Cline (1969) and Salmon et al. (1970) have described a patient with systemic candidiasis whose neutrophils and monocytes had no detectable myeloperoxidase. In vitro the patient's leukocytes not only failed to kill candida albicans but also killed Staphylococcus aureus and Serratia marcescens at a slower rate than normal leukocytes, even though ingestion was unaffected. All other aspects of cellular or humoral immune responses were normal. [For an extensive review of cellular immunity in relation to chronic mucocutaneous candidiasis, see Kirkpatrick et al. (1971).]

It must be recognized, however, that several isolated as well as related individuals have been described in the world literature (see Lehrer and Cline, 1969) with myeloperoxidase-deficient neutrophils and mononuclear cells, as determined by histochemistry, without any evidence of decreased resistance to infection.

The enzyme deficiency is thought to be transmitted as an autosomal recessive characteristic.

Failure to enhance production of H_2O_2, when myeloperoxidase activity is normal, may also lead to diminished bacterial killing after ingestion. The most dramatic example of such a disorder is fatal chronic granulomatous disease of childhood. This congenital disorder, first recognized as a clinical entity in 1957 (Berendes et al., 1957), has elicited an intensive search for the underlying mechanism(s). Since several reviews of the clinical features and the metabolic abnormalities of the leukocytes of patients with chronic granulomatous disease have appeared recently (Good et al., 1968; Sbarra et al., 1970), our discussion will be restricted to those developments that cast new light on the disease and phagocytosis in general.

Briefly, ingestion in vitro by leukocytes of patients with chronic granulomatous disease is normal but subsequent killing of certain bacterial species is markedly impaired. The prolonged survival of intracellular organisms such as Staphylococcus aureus, E. coli, Serratia marcescens, and Paracolon hafnia has been shown to be related, at least in part, to the leukocyte's inability to produce increased amounts of H_2O_2 as part of the characteristic respiratory response to phagocytosis (Holmes et al., 1966, 1967; Quie et al., 1967; Baehner and Nathan, 1966).

The detection of the disease has been greatly aided by a simple test in which the reduction is followed of the dye nitrobluetetrazolium (NBT) with formation of blue formazan by resting and phagocytizing leukocytes (Baehner and Nathan, 1968). Whereas normal leukocytes manifest easily recognizable and measurable reduction of the dye during phagocytosis, leukocytes of patients with chronic granulomatous disease fail to show significant reduction of NBT.

Chronic granulomatous disease has been described mainly as a sex-linked inherited leukocyte defect, but several females with the disease have now been reported (Quie *et al.*, 1969; Baehner and Nathan, 1968, Douglas *et al.*, 1969; Holmes *et al.*, 1970). As expected, in the sex-linked variety, isolated leukocytes of the female carriers of the disease manifest diminished reduction of NBT, because the leukocyte population consists of normal as well as abnormal cells. Leukocytes of the parents of afflicted girls, on the other hand, exhibit no abnormality in the test. Thus, in these instances an autosomal recessive inheritance of the disorder is postulated.

Chandra *et al.* (1969) have suggested that transmission of the disease in boys may not be sex-linked, because lowered bactericidal activity and reduction of NBT was found in the fathers as well as in the mothers. It is speculated that the greater rarity of the disease in females can be explained by assuming sex modification of the autosomal recessive inheritance, with a more severe manifestation of the defect in the female, causing death *in utero*. Since there is no evidence that chronic granulomatous disease causes any clinical abnormalities other than those attributable to impaired cellular host defense against certain bacterial species, it seems unlikely that the defect would be lethal *in utero*. At this time the evidence in support of sex-linked transmission in most of the cases of chronic granulomatous disease in boys appears strong. The mere fact that the disease occurs in girls, however, implies that other mechanisms of genetic transmission are likely to exist, as also pointed out by Douglas *et al.* (1969).

The NBT test appears useful not only in detecting patients with chronic granulomatous disease, carriers, and possibly other disorders of intracellular killing, but also in distinguishing bacterial from nonbacterial febrile illnesses (Park *et al.*, 1968).

While the correlation between the occurrence of the cyanide insensitive respiratory burst that accompanies phagocytosis with the reduction of NBT suggests that the two phenomena are linked in some fashion, the mechanism of the dye reduction is unknown. Question concerning a close relationship between the reduction of NBT and the increased respiratory and associated activities is also raised by the observations of Ward and Schlegel (1969) on a patient with circulating inhibitor of chemotaxis (see above). Granulocytes from this patient, apparently capable of normal H_2O_2 production and intracellular killing, showed impaired reduction of NBT.

Several recent observations seem to support the concept that the impaired bactericidal activity of leukocytes from patients with chronic granulomatous disease is a consequence of an inability to produce increased amounts of H_2O_2.

Klebanoff and White (1969) and Pincus and Klebanoff (1971) have used iodination of ingested bacteria as an index of the antimicrobial activity of myeloperoxidase, acting in concert with H_2O_2 and the oxidation of halogen. They found no iodination of *Serratia marcescens* and of heat-killed *Lactobacillus acidophilus* after ingestion by neutrophils from patients with chronic granulomatous disease or with myeloperoxidase deficiency. Iodination was apparent however when live *L. acidophilus* were engulfed. The explanation for the improved iodination and killing of live *L. acidophilus* and clinically also of other microorganisms such as pneumococci appears to lie in the capability of these organisms to generate H_2O_2 in excess of their capacity to degrade or use it. Hence, *L. acidophilus* contribute to their own demise by furnishing the H_2O_2 that the defective leukocyte cannot produce.

Further, the interesting experiments of Baehner *et al.* (1970) have demonstrated that introduction of a H_2O_2 generating system into the leukocytes of a patient with chronic granulomatous disease partially repairs the metabolic and bactericidal defects. This was achieved by presenting the leukocytes with polystyrene particles coated with glucose oxidase. Oxidation of ^{14}C formate and $1-^{14}C$ glucose to $^{14}CO_2$ was markedly stimulated by the coated particles. Concomitantly killing of *Staphylococcus aureus* and *Serratia marcescens* was appreciably enhanced (Johnston and Baehner, 1970).

An intensive search for the mechanism(s) underlying the defect in leukocyte function in chronic granulomatous disease is under way. Quie *et al.* (1967), on the basis of electron microscopic observations, have proposed that diminished degranulation during phagocytosis accounts for impaired killing and the lack of metabolic responses. Other morphological observations (Kauder *et al.*, 1968; Elsbach *et al.*, 1969; Douglas, 1970) have revealed normal degranulation. Moreover, subcellular distribution of several granule enzymes and histochemical evidence of peroxidase activity within phagocytic vacuoles were the same for normal leukocytes and leukocytes with chronic granulomatous disease (Baehner *et al.*, 1969). While abnormalities in degranulation, too subtle to detect by the techniques used in these studies, cannot be excluded, a primary metabolic defect appears more probable at this time then one involving the transfer of granule contents to phagosomes.

Earlier in this review we alluded to the controversy that exists with respect to the enzyme(s) responsible for the stimulated O_2 uptake by normal phagocytizing leukocytes. This controversy is also apparent in the speculation concerning any enzymatic abnormalities that might explain the failure of granulocytes of patients with chronic granulomatous disease to mount a respiratory response. It may be useful to refer again to the two biochemical schemes shown in Table II (Holmes *et al.*, 1970). Either scheme could account for the stimulation of O_2 consumption of the HMPS and H_2O_2 production during phagocytosis. The schemes differ in the enzymatic step presumed to initiate the sequence and also in the inclusion of an NADH as opposed to an NADPH oxidase. Baehner and his associates believe that a deficiency of NADH oxidase represents a major, if not the crucial, defect in chronic granulomatous disease. In support of this contention, this group found low to absent NADH oxidase activity in homogenates of the abnormal leukocytes (Baehner and Karnovsky, 1968, Nathan *et al.*, 1969). Holmes *et al.* (1967), presumably also in cases of sex-linked transmission of chronic granulomatous disease, found normal levels of NADH oxidase, however. These divergent findings have as yet not been reconciled. Since enzymatic activity assayed in broken cell preparations need not reflect activity in the intact cell, the effect of hydrocortisone on normal intact human leukocytes, as described by Mandell *et al.* (1970), may be pertinent. The steroid in high concentration (2.1 mM) did not interfere with ingestion of bacteria but inhibited O_2 consumption, H_2O_2 production, NADH oxidase activity, and intracellular killing, thus mimicking the *in vitro* behavior of leukocytes from patients with chronic granulomatous disease. These findings, by analogy, might implicate NADH oxidase in the metabolic defect. It must be obvious, however, that a deficiency or inhibition of any one enzymatic activity in the reaction sequence depicted in the two schemes would interfere with the expression of all their biochemical concomitants. In this context the partial repair of the metabolic defect by the introduction of glucose oxidase into the abnormal cells (Baehner *et al.*, 1970) merely indicates that the cycle will operate once set in motion. In fact, it appears that more than one enzyme deficiency can give rise to the metabolic defects of chronic granulomatous disease; Holmes *et al.* (1970) have reported diminished glutathione peroxidase activity in leukocytes of two female patients with chronic granulomatous disease.

As expected, leukocytes totally or nearly totally deficient in glucose-6-phosphate dehydrogenase (G6PD) show the same metabolic and bactericidal defects *in vitro* that are manifested by chronic granulomatous disease leukocytes (Cooper *et al.*, 1970; Baehner *et al.*, 1971). Despite the *in vitro* similarities, however, the clinical consequences of the defective leukocyte metabolism are not clearly established. In only one instance of total G6PD deficiency has an increased susceptibility to infection been inferred and this was in a 52-year-old lady who died of an overwhelming *E. coli* sepsis, but who apparently had led a normal life until her final illness. It follows, therefore, that the effectiveness of the combined host defenses cannot be as readily predicted by dissection of granulocyte function alone, as the earlier studies of chronic granulomatous disease had suggested. Whether or not an individual with an abnormality in leukocyte metabolism will be prone to infection must depend on additional factors that have not yet been identified. This is also apparent from the case report by Moellering and Weinberg (1970), who described persistent salmonella infection in the mother of three sons who died of typical chronic granulomatous disease. This patient represents the first recognized instance of a female carrier with decreased resistance to infection. Despite the ability of approximately 40 % of the patient's granulo-cyte population to reduce NBT during phagocytosis *in vitro* and normal sensitivity of the microorganism to antibiotics, the patient continued to harbor *Salmonella enteritidis*. This is particularly noteworthy because this type of salmonella ordinarily is of low virulence in man. The authors suggest that facultative intracellular parasites such as *Salmonella, M. tuberculosis, Brucella*, and *Listeria monocytogenes* can survive in hosts such as this patient because they find residence in long-lived macrophages and monocytes with the same bactericidal defect that characterizes a large portion of the granulocytes (Davis *et al.*, 1968; Nathan *et al.*, Rodey *et al.*, 1969). In these abnormal macrophages such organisms might also be protected against antibiotics and humoral antibacterial factors.

4. IN CONCLUSION

During the last decade our insight into the process of phagocytosis has deepened considerably. Isolated clinical observations of inborn defects in phagocyte metabolism have aided in large measure in assigning specific functions to various biochemical concomitants of phagocytosis. The initial enthusiasm generated by striking correlations between metabolic findings and abnormalities in bactericidal activity *in vitro*, on the one hand, and increased susceptibility to infection, on the other, must be dampened somewhat by the growing realization that a complex polymorphism in the phagocyte's intricate antimicrobial armamentarium must exist to account for the apparent incon-sistencies in the observations reviewed here.

The relative rarity of seriously impaired cellular host defense against infection may well be due to a "large overkill capacity for most organisms owing to the level and variety of its systems. Only when leukocyte function is compromised, as in chronic granulomatous disease, does the antibacterial effect become dependent upon the level of activity of one or other of these antibacterial systems" (Klebanoff and White, 1969).

It seems quite possible, in the light of observations such as those of Moellering and Weinberg (1970), that thus far unrecognized genotypic differences in the array of antimicrobial factors possessed by a given in-dividual's phagocytes play at least as important a role in predisposing to infection with certain microbes as random encounter between host and potential pathogen.

Addendum

Since the completion of this manuscript numerous publications dealing with phagocytic cells and phagocytosis have appeared. Exhaustive treatment of this literature is not possible but I have added what I consider particularly pertinent to some of the areas that were highlighted in this chapter.

The central role of cyclic nucleotides as regulatory substances of many biological processes apparently does not include phagocytosis. Manganiello *et al.* (1971) have established that the elevated $3',5'$-adenosine monophosphate levels of peripheral blood leukocyte suspensions are attributable to increased levels in mononuclear cells. Levels in homogeneous suspensions of phagocytizing granulocytes and alveolar macrophages are not elevated. On the other hand, various agents, added *in vitro* to leukocyte suspensions, that alter intracellular levels of cyclic nucleotides do affect motility, ingestion, and degranulation (Zurrier *et al.*, 1973).

Work on the phagocytosis-stimulatory tetrapeptide "tuftsin" (Nishioka *et al.*, 1972) continues. This small peptide is split off a γ globulin, which itself has stimulatory activity, by a membrane-associated enzyme. Dr. Najjar's group (Constantopoulos and Najjar, 1973) now shows that membrane sialic acid is required for stimulation by tuftsin.

The mechanism of the striking respiratory burst that accompanies phagocytosis and that underlies the increased production of H_2O_2 is still uncertain and continues to be debated hotly. Patriarca *et al.* (1971a,b) have submitted further evidence that NADPH oxidase rather than NADH oxidase is the key enzyme in the reaction sequence. Karnovsky (1973) in an admirable review of the controversy and of the metabolic defect of chronic granulomatous disease puts normal and abnormal leukocyte function and metabolism in perspective.

Matters are complicated further by the findings of DeChatelet *et al.* (1972) of a NAD kinase in leukocytes, and of Babior *et al.* (1973) who report increased production of superoxide (O_2^-) during phagocytosis by leukocytes. Superoxide is a highly reactive compound which may be microbicidal by itself or after its conversion to H_2O_2 $(2\,O_2^- + 2\,H^+ \longrightarrow O_2 + H_2O_2)$.

Of considerable interest is a histochemical study by Jensen and Bainton (1973) of the pH changes within the phagocytic vacuoles of neutrophils. Ingested yeast particles stained with pH-sensitive dyes seem to show that there is an initial (within 3 minutes) drop in pH to 6.5, followed after 7–15 minutes by a drop to approximately 4.0. It should be noted that the pH changes within the phagosomes of a given cell were not uniform.

An important set of observations on lipids and membranes in relation to phagocytosis has been presented by Werb and Cohn (1972). Cultured mouse peritoneal macrophages reconstitute their plasma membrane lipids *after* ingestion of particles. This reconstitution must take place in order to permit a second ingestion to follow.

Elsbach *et al.* (1972) have found that most of the increment in cellular ^{32}P lecithin, derived from acylation of medium ^{32}P lysolecithin during phagocytosis of paraffin particles by rabbit granulocytes, is in the subsequently isolated phagosome fraction. This is also the case when cellular lecithin is prelabeled before phagocytosis. These findings give direct evidence that this mechanism of net phospholipid synthesis can provide new membrane lipid for formation of the phagocytic vacuole.

Further evidence has been provided indicating that the molecular degradation of ingested and killed bacteria is quite incomplete (Elsbach *et al.* 1973). In fact it appears that certain Gram negative organisms (*Escherichia coli*) may retain so much structural integrity that the biochemical apparatus can continue to carry out integrated biosynthetic activity for at least 1 hour after almost all organisms have been killed.

In a recent review of intraleukocytic microbicidal defects, Klebanoff (1971) wrote: "The designation of Chediak-Higashi syndrome as a neutrophil dysfunction syndrome associated with an intraleukocytic microbicidal defect must await further study." Since this time a number of new observations have been made. Among these are those of Clark and Kimball (1971), Root *et al.* (1972), and Stossel *et al.* (1972); showing chemotactic sluggishness but also retarded killing of some ingested bacterial species and possibly a selective degranulation defect. It appears therefore that at least part of the increased occurrence of infections in this syndrome may be caused by defective intraleukocytic microbicidal activity.

An intriguing report by Miller *et al.* (1972) suggests that the extent of stimulation of O_2 consumption accompanying phagocytosis of bacteria may relate to virulence. Whereas relatively nonvirulent strains of *Salmonella typhi* produced the familiar increased rate of O_2 consumption, ingestion of virulent *Salmonella typhi* did not cause enhanced O_2 uptake.

References

Adler, J. (1969). *Science* **166**, 1589.

Ainsworth, S. K., and Allison, F. (1970). *J. Clin. Invest.* **49**, 433.

Alper, C. A., Abramson, N., Johnston, R. B., Jr., Jandl, J. H., and Rosen, F. S. (1970a). *N. Engl. J. Med.* **282**, 349.

Alper, C. A., Abramson, N., Johnston, R. B., Jr., Jandl., and Rosen, F. S. (1970b). *J. Clin. Invest.* **49**, 1975.

Austen, K. F., and Cohn, Z. A., (1963a). *N. Engl. J. Med.* **268**, 933.

Austen, K. F., and Cohn, Z. A., (1963b). *N. Engl. J. Med.* **268**, 944.

Austen, K. F., and Cohn, Z. A., (1963c). *N. Engl. J. Med.* **268**, 1056.

Auzins, I., and Rowley, D. (1963). *Aust. J. Exp. Biol. Med. Sci.* **41**, 539.

Ayoub, E. M., and White, J. G. (1969). *J. Bacteriol.* **98**, 728.

Babior, B. M., Kipnes, R. S., and Curnutte, J. T. (1973). *J. Clin. Invest.* **52**, 741.

Baehner, R. L., and Karnovsky, M. L. (1968). *Science* **162**, 1277.

Baehner, R. L., and Nathan, D. G. (1966). *Blood* **28**, 1010.

Baehner, R. L., and Nathan, D. G. (1968). *N. Engl. J. Med.* **278**, 971

Baehner, R. L., Karnovsky, M. J., and Karnovsky, M. L. (1969). *J. Clin. Invest.* **48**, 187.

Baehner, R. L., Nathan, D. G., and Karnovsky, M. L. (1970). *J. Clin. Invest.* **49**, 856.

Baehner, R. L., Johnston, R. B., and Nathan, D. G. (1971). *J. Clin. Invest.* **50**, 4a.

Baggiolini, M., Hirsch, J. G., and DeDuve, C. (1969). *J. Cell Biol.* **40**, 529.

Baggiolini, M., De Duve, C., Masson, P. L., and Heremans, J. F. (1970a). *J. Exp. Med.* **131**, 559.

Baggiolini, M., Hirsch, J. G., and De Duve, C. (1970b). *J. Cell. Biol.* **45**, 586.

Bainton, D. F., and Farquhar, M. G. (1966). *J. Cell Biol.* **28**, 277.

Bainton, D. F., and Farquhar, M. G. (1968a). *J. Cell Biol.* **39**, 286.

Bainton, D. F., and Farquhar, M. G. (1968b). *J. Cell Biol.* **39**, 299.

Beck, W. (1958). *Ann. N. Y. Acad. Sci.* **75**, 4

Belding, N. E., Klebanoff, S. J., and Ray, C. G. (1970). *Science* **167**, 195.

Berendes, H., Bridges, R. A., and Good, R. A. (1957). *Minn. Med.* **40**, 309.

Bodel, P., and Malawista, S. E. (1969). *Exp. Cell Res.* **56**, 15.

Bodel, P., Dillard, G. M., Kaplan, S., and Malawista, S. (1970). *J. Clin. Invest.*.**49**, 10a.

Borel, J. F., Keller, H. U., and Sorkin, E. (1969). *Int. Arch. Allergy Appl. Immunol.* **35**, 194.

Boyden, S. (1962). *J. Exp. Med.* **115**, 453.

Brayton, R. G., Stokes, P. E., Schwartz, M. S., and Louria, D. G. (1970). *N. Engl. J. Med.* **282**, 123.

Bryant, R. E., DesPrez, R. M., VanWay, M. H., and Rogers, D. E. (1966). *J. Exp. Med.* **124**, 483.

Brzuchowska, W. (1966). *Nature (London)* **212**, 210.

Buchanan, A. A. (1960). *Biochem. J.* **75**, 315.

Cagan, R. H., and Karnovsky, M. L. (1964). *Nature (London)* **204**, 255.

Carpenter, R. R. (1966). *J. Immunol.* **96**, 922.

Carpenter, R. R., and Barseles, P. B. (1967). *J. Immunol.* **94**, 884.

Chandra, R. K., Cope, W. A., and Soothill, J. F. (1969). *Lancet* **2**, 71.

Clark, R. A., and Kimball, H. R., (1971). *J. Clin Invest.* **50**, 2645.

Cline, M. J. (1970). In "Regulation of Hematopoiesis" (A.S. Gordon, ed.), Vol. II, pp. 1045. Appleton, New York.

Cline, M. J., and Lehrer, R. I. (1968). *Blood* **32**, 423.

Cline, M. J., Hanifin, J., and Lehrer, R. I. (1968). *Blood* **32**, 922.

Cohn, Z. A. (1963a). *J. Exp. Med.* **117**, 27.

Cohn, Z. A. (1968b). *J. Exp. Med.* **117**, 43.

Cohn, Z. A. (1968). *Advan. Immunol.* **9**, 163.

Cohn, Z. A., and Benson, B. (1965a). *J. Exp. Med.* **121**, 153.

Cohn, Z. A., and Benson, B. (1965b). *J. Exp. Med.* **121**, 279.

Cohn, Z. A., and Benson, B. (1965c). *J. Exp. Med.* **121**, 835.

Cohn, Z. A., and Hirsch, J. G. (1960). *J. Exp. Med.* **112**, 1015.

Cohn, Z. A., and Morse, S. I. (1959). *J. Exp. Med.* **110**, 419.

Cohn, Z. A., and Wiener, E. (1963). *J. Exp. Med.* **118**, 991.

Constantopoulos, A., and Najjar, V. A. (1973). *J. Biol. Chem.* **248**, 3819.

Cooper, M. R., De Chatelet, L. R., Lavia, M. F., McCall, C. E., Spurr, C. L., and Baehner, R. L. (1970). *J. Clin. Invest.* **49**, 21a.

Cotran, R. S., and Litt, M. (1969). *J. Exp. Med.* **129**, 1291.

Daems, W. T., and Oort, J. (1962). *Exp. Cell Res.* **28**, 11.

Dannenberg, A. M., and Bennett, W. E. (1964). *J. Cell Biol.* **21** 1.

Dannenberg, A. M., Burstone, M. S., Walter, P. C., and Kinsley, J. W. (1963a). *J. Cell Biol.* **17**, 465.

Dannenberg, A. M., Walter, P. C., and Kapral, F. A. (1963b). *J. Immunol.* **90**, 448.

Davis, W. C., Huber., V., Douglas, S. D., and Fudenberg, H. H. (1968). *J. Immunol.* **10**, 1093.

Day, A. J. (1967). *Advan. Lipid Res.* **5**, 185.

Day, A. J., and Fidge, N. H. (1962). *J. Lipid Res.* **3**, 333.

DeChatelet, L. R., McCall, C. E., Cooper, M. R. and Shirley, P. S. (1972). *J. Reticuloendothel. Soc.* **12**, 387.

Douglas, S. D. (1970). *Blood* **35**, 851.

Douglas, S. D., Davis, W. C., and Fudenberg, H. (1969). *Amer. J. Med.* **46**, 901.

Douglas, S. D., Goldberg. L. S., and Fudenberg, H. H. (1970a). *Amer. J. Med.* **48**, 48.

Douglas, S. D., Lahav, M., and Fudenberg, H. H. (1970b). *Amer J. Med.* **49**, 274.

Elberg, S. S. (1960). *Bacteriol. Rev.* **24**, 67.

Elsbach, P. (1959). *J. Exp. Med.* **110**, 969.

Elsbach, P. (1962). *Nature* (*London*) **195**, 383.

Elsbach, P. (1963). *Biochim. Biophys. Acta* **70**, 157.

Elsbach, P. (1964). *Biochim. Biophys, Acta* **84**, 8.

Elsbach, P. (1965a). *Biochim. Biophys. Acta.* **98**, 402.

Elsbach, P. (1965b). *Biochim. Biophys. Acta* **98**, 420.

Elsbach, P. (1966). *Biochim. Biophys. Acta* **125**, 110.

Elsbach, P. (1967). *J. Lipid Res.* **8**, 359.

Elsbach, P. (1968). *J. Clin. Invest.* **47**, 2217.

Elsbach, P., and Farrow, S. (1969). *Biochim. Biophys. Acta* **176**, 438.

Elsbach, P., and Kayden, H. J. (1965). *Amer. J. Physiol.* **209**, 765.

Elsbach, P., and Rizack, M. A. (1963). *Amer. J. Physiol.* **205**, 1154.

Elsbach, P., and Schwartz, I. L., (1959). *J. Gen. Physiol.* **42**, 383.

Elsbach, P., van den Berg, J. W. O., van den Bosch, H., and van Deenen, L. L. M. (1965). *Biochim. Biophys. Acta* **106**, 338.

Elsbach, P., Zucker-Franklin, D., and Sansaricq, C. (1969). *N. Engl. J. Med.* **280**, 1319.

Elsbach, P., Wurster, N., Lebow, S., Pettis, P., and Simon, E. J. (1970). *J. Clin. Invest.* **49**, 27a.

Elsbach, P., Goldman, J., and Patriarca, P. (1972). *Biochim. Biophys. Acta* **280**, 33.

Elsbach, P., Patriarca, P., Pettis, P., Stossel, T. P., Mason, R. J., and Vaughan, M. (1972). *J. Clin. Invest.* **51**, 1910.

Elsbach, P., Pettis, P., Beckerdite, S., and Franson, R. (1973). *J. Bacteriol.* **115**, 490.

Erbland, J. F., and Marinetti, G. V. (1965). *Biochim. Biophys. Acta* **105**, 139.

Ericsson, Y., and Lundbeck, H. (1955a). *Acta Pathol. Microbiol. Scand.* **37**, 493.

Ericsson, Y., and Lundbeck, H. (1955b). *Acta Pathol. Microbiol. Scand.* **37**, 507.

Evans, A. E., and Kaplan, N. O. (1966). *J. Clin. Invest.* **45**, 1268.

Evans, W. H., and Mueller, P. S. (1963). *J. Lipid Res.* **4**, 39.

Fenn, W. O. (1921). *J. Gen. Physiol.* **4**, 373.

Franson, R., Beckerdite, S., Wang, P., Waite, M., and Elsbach, P. (1973). *Biochim. Biophys. Acta* **296**, 365.

Fruton J. S., and Simmonds, S. (1958). "General Biochemistry." Wiley, New York.

Fung, C. K., and Proulx, P. R. (1969). *Can. J. Biochem.* **47**, 37.

Gee, J. B. L., Vassallo, C. L., Bell, P., Kaskin, J., Basford, R. E., and Field, J. B. (1970). *J. Clin. Invest.* **49**, 1280.

Glomset, J. A. (1962). *Biochem. Biophys. Acta* **65**, 128.

Good, R. A., Quie, P. G., Windhorst, D. B., Page, A. R., Rodey, G. E., White, J., Wolfson, J. J., and Holmes. B. H. (1968). *Semin. Hematol.* **5**, 215.

Graham, R. C., Jr., Karnovsky, M. J., Shafer, A. W., Glass, E. A., and Karnovsky, M. L. (1967). *J. Cell Biol.* **32**, 629.

Greendyke, R. M., Brierty, R. E., and Swisher, S. N. (1963). *Blood* **22**, 295.

Hazelbauer, G. L., and Adler, J. A. (1970). *Nature* (*London*), *New Biol.* **230**, 101.

Hirsch, J. G. (1956). *J. Exp. Med.* **103**, 589.

Hirsch, J. G. (1958). *J. Exp. Med.* **108**, 925.

Hirsch, J. G. (1960). *Bacteriol. Rev.* **24**, 133.

Hirsch, J. G. (1962). *J. Exp. Med.* **116**, 827.

Hirsch, J. G. (1965). *Annu. Rev. Microbio.* **19**, 339.

Hirsch, J. G., and Church, A. B. (1960). *J. Exp. Med.* **111**, 309.

Hirsch, J. G., and Cohn, Z. A. (1960). *J. Exp. Med.* **112**, 1005.

Hirsch, J. G., Bernheimer, A. W., and Weissmann, G. (1963). *J. Exp. Med.* **118**, 223.

Holmes, B., Quie, P. G., Windhorst, D. B., and Good, R. A. (1966). *Lancet* **1**, 1225.

Holmes, B., Page, A. R., and Good, R. A. (1967). *J. Clin. Invest.* **46**, 1422.

Holmes, B., Park, B. H., Malawista, S. E., Quie, P. G., Nelson, D. L., and Good, R. A. (1970). *N. Engl. J. Med.* **283**, 217.

Iyer, G. Y. N., and Quastel, J. H. (1963). *Can. J. Biochem. Physiol.* **41**, 427.

Iyer, G. Y. N., Islam, M. F., and Quastel, J. H. (1961). *Nature (London)* **192**, 535.

Jensen, M. S., and Bainton, D. F. (1973). *J. Cell. Biol.* **56**, 379.

Johnston, R. B., Jr., and Baehner, R. L. (1970). *Bloo.* **35**, 350.

Jones, T. C., and Hirsch, J. G. (1971). *J. Exp. Med.* **133**, 231.

Karnovsky, M. L. (1962). *Physiol. Rev.* **42**, 143.

Karnovsky, M. L. (1968). *Semin. Hematol.* **5**, 156.

Karnovsky, M. L. (1973). *Fed. Proc.* **32**, 1527.

Karnovsky, M. L., and Wallach, D. F. H. (1961). *J. Biol. Chem.* **236**, 189.

Karnovsky, M. L., Shafer, A. W., Cagan, R. H., Graham, R. C., Karnovsky, M. J., Glass, E. A., and Saito, K. (1966). *Trans. N. Y. Acad. Sci.* [2] **28**, 778.

Katz, J., and Wood, H. G. (1960). *J. Biol. Chem.* **235**, 2165.

Kauder, E., Kahle, L. L., Moreno, H., and Partin, J. C. (1968). *J. Clin. Invest.* **47**, 1753.

Keller, H. U., and Sorkin, E. (1968). *Int. Arch. Allergy Appl. Immunol.* **34**, 513.

Kirkpatrick, C. H., Rich, R. R., and Bennett, J. E. (1971). *Ann. Intern. Med.* **74**, 955.

Klebanoff, S. J. (1967). *J. Exp. Med.* **126**, 1063.

Klebanoff, S. J. (1968). *J. Bacteriol.* **95**, 2131.

Klebanoff, S. J. (1970). *In* "Biochemistry of the Phagocytic Process: Localization and the Role of Myeloperoxidase and the Mechanism of Halogenation Reaction" (J. Schultz, ed.) North-Holland Publ., Amsterdam.

Klebanoff, S. J. (1971). *Ann. Rev. Med.* **22**, 39.

Klebanoff, S. J., and White, L. R. (1969). *N. Eng. J. Med.* **280**, 460.

Klebanoff, S. J., Clem, W. H., and Luebke, R. G. (1966). *Biochim. Biophys Acta* **117**, 63.

Kvarstein, B., and Stormorken, H. (1971). *Biochem. Pharmacol.* **20**, 119.

Lands, W. E. M. (1960). *J. Biol. Chem.* **235**, 2233.

Leake, E. S., and Myrvik, Q. N. (1968). *RES. J. Reticuloendothel. Soc.* **5**, 33.

Leake, E. S., Evans, D. G., and Myrvik, Q. N. (1971). *RES, J. Reticuloendothel. Soc.* **9**, 174.

Lehrer, R. I. (1969). *J. Bacteriol.* **99**, 361.

Lehrer, R. I., and Cline, M. J. (1969). *J. Clin. Invest.* **48**, 1478.

Maaloe, O. (1964). "On the Relation between Alexin and Opsonin." Munksgaard, Copenhaggen.

Mackaness, G. B. (1970). *In* "Infectious Agents and Host Reactions" (S. Mudd, ed.), pp. 62–67. Saunders, Philadelphia, Pennsylvania.

Manganiello, V., Evans, W. H., Stossel, T. P., Mason, R. J., and Vaughan, M. (1971). *J. Clin Invest.* **50**, 2741.

McRipley, R. J., and Sbarra, A. J. (1967a). *J. Bacteriol.* **94**, 1417.

McRipley, R. J., and Sbarra, A. J. (1967b). *J. Bacteriol.* **94**, 1425.

Majerus, P. W., and Lastra, R. R. (1967). *J. Clin. Invest.* **46**, 1596.

Malawista, S. E. (1971). *Blood* **37**, 519
Malawista, S. E., and Bodel, P. T. (1967). *J. Clin. Invest.* **46**, 786.
Mandell, G. L. (1970). *Proc. Soc. Exp. Biol. Med.* **134**, 447.
Mandell, G. L., Rubin, W., and Hook, E. W. (1970). *J. Clin. Invest.* **49**, 1381.
Marks, P. A., Gellhorn, A., and Kidson, C. (1960). *J. Biol. Chem.* **235**, 2579.
Messner, R. P., and Jelinek, J. (1970). *J. Clin. Invest.* **49**, 2165.
Michell, R. H., Pancake, S. J., Noseworthy, J., and Karnovsky, M. L. (1969). *J. Cell Biol.* **40**, 216.
Michell, R. H., Karnovsky, M. J., and Karnovsky, M. L. (1970). *Biochem. J.* **116**, 207.
Mickenberg, I. D., Root, R. K., and Wolff, S. M. (1970). *J. Clin. Invest.* **49**, 1528.
Miller, M. E., and Nilsson, U. R., (1970). *N. Engl. J. Med.* **282**, 354.
Miller, T. E. (1969). *J. Bacteriol.* **98**, 949.
Miller, R. M., Garbus, J., and Hornick, R. B. (1972). *Science* **175**, 1010.
Misra, U. K. (1965). *Biochim. Biophys. Acta* **106**, 371.
Moellering, R. C., and Weinberg, A. N. (1970). *Ann. Intern. Med.* **73**, 595.
Mowat, A. G., and Baum, J. (1971). *N. Engl. J. Med.* **284**, 621.
Mudd, S., McCutcheon, M., and Lucké, B. (1934). *Physiol. Rev.* **14**, 210.
Myrvik, Q. N., Leake, E. S., and Fariss, B. (1961a). *J. Immunol.* **86**, 128.
Myrvik, Q. N., Leake, E. S., and Fariss, B. (1961b). *J. Immunol.* **86**, 133.
Nathan, C. F., Karnovsky, M. L., and David, J. R. (1971). *J. Exp. Med.* **133**, 1377.
Nathan, D. G., Baehner, R. L., and Weaver, D. K. (1969). *J. Clin. Invest.* **48**, 1895.
Newman, H. A. I., Liu, C. T., and Zilversmit, O. G. (1961). *J. Lipid Res.* **2**, 403.
Nishioka, K., Constantopoulos, A., Satoh, P. S., and Najjar, V. A. (1972). *Biochem. Biophys. Res. Commun.* **47**, 172.
North, R. J., and Mackaness, G. B. (1963). *Brit. J. Exp. Pathol.* **44**, 601.
Okuyama, H., and Nojima, S. (1969). *Biochim. Biophys. Acta* **176**, 120.
Oren, R., Farnham, A. E., Sato, K., Milofsky, E., and Karnovsky, M. L. (1963). *J. Cell Biol.* **17**, 1487.
Park, B. H., Fikrig, S. M., and Smithwick, E. M. (1968). *Lancet* **2**, 532.
Patriarca, P., Zatti, M., Cramer, R., and Rossi, F. (1970). *Life Sci., Part I* **9**, 841.
Patriarca, P., Cramer, R., Marussi, M., Rossi, F., and Romeo, D. (1971a). *Biochim. Biophys. Acta* **237**, 335.
Patriarca, P., Cramer, R., Moncalvo, S., Rossi, F., and Romeo, D. (1971b). *Arch. Biochem. Biophys.* **145**, 255.
Patriarca, P., Beckerdite, S., and Elsbach, P. (1972). *Biochim. Biophys. Acta* **260**, 593.
Patriarca, P., Beckerdite, S., Pettis, P., and Elsbach, P. (1973). *Biochim. Biophys. Acta* **280**, 45.
Paul, B. B., and Sbarra, A. J. (1968). *Biochim. Biophys. Acta* **156**, 168.
Pearsall, N., and Weiser, R. S. (1970). "The Macrophage." Lea & Febiger, Philadelphia, Pennsylvania.
Phillips, G. B. (1957). *Proc. Nat. Acad. Sci. U.S.* **43**, 566.
Phillips-Quagliata, J. M., Levine, B. B., and Uhr, J. W. (1969). *Nature (London)* **222**, 1290.
Pincus, S. H., and Klebanoff, S. J. (1971). *N. Engl. J. Med.* **284**, 744.
Ponder, E. (1927). *Protoplasma* **3**, 611.
Ponder, E. (1928). *J. Gen. Physiol.* **11**, 757.
Proulx, P. R., and Fung, C. K. (1969). *Can. J. Biochem.* **47**, 1125.
Proulx, P. R., and van Deenen, L. L. M. (1967a). *Biochim. Biophys. Acta* **125**, 591.
Proulx, P. R., and van Deenen, L. L. M. (1967b). *Biochim. Biophys. Acta* **1144**, 171.
Quie, P. G., White, J. G., Holmes, B., and Good, R. A. (1967). *J. Clin. Invest.* **46**, 668.
Quie, P. G., Kaplan, E. L., Page, A. R., Gruskay, F. L., and Malawista, S. (1969). *N. Engl. J. Med.* **278**, 976.

Rabinovitch, M. (1967a). *Exp. Cell Res.* **46**, 19.
Rabinovitch, M. (1967b). *Proc. Soc. Exp. Biol. Med.* **124**, 396.
Rebuck, J. W., and Crowley, S. H. (1955). *Ann. N. Y. Acad. Sci.* **59**, 757.
Reed, P. W. (1969). *N. Biol. Chem.* **244**, 2459.
Reed, P. W., and Tepperman, J. (1969). *Amer. J. Physiol.* **216**, 223.
Roberts, J., and Quastel, J. H. (1963). *Biochem. J.* **89**, 150.
Robineaux, J., and Frederic, J. (1955). *C. R. Soc. Biol.* **149**, 486.
Rodey, G. E., Park, B. H., Windhorst, D. B., and Good, R. A. (1969). *Blood* **33**, 813.
Root, R. K., Rosenthal, A. S., and Balestra, D. J. (1972). *J. Clin. Invest.* **51**, 649.
Rossi, F., and Zatti, M., (1964). *Brit. J. Exp. Pathol.* **65**, 548.
Rossi, F., and Zatti, M. (1966). *Biochim. Biophys. Acta* **113**, 395.
Rossi, F., Mazzocchi, G., Zatti, M., and Meneghelli, V. (1967). *Sperimentale* **117**, 63.
Rossi, F. Zatti, M., M., and Patriarca, P. (1969). *Biochim. Biophys. Acta* **184**, 201.
Rossi, F., Zatti, M., Patriarca, P., and Cramer, R. (1971). *RES, J. Reticuloendothel. Soc.* **9**, 67.
Rossiter, R. J., and Wong, E. (1949). *J. Biol. Chem.* **180**, 935.
Rous, P. (1925). *J. Exp. Med.* **41**, 399.
Rowley, D. (1962). *Advan. Immunol.* **2**, 241.
Salmon, S. E., Cline, M. J., Schultz, J., and Lehrer, R. I. (1970). *N. Engl. J. Med.* **282**, 250.
Sastry, P. S., and Hokin, L. E. (1966). *J. Biol. Chem.* **241**, 3354.
Sbarra, A. J., and Karnovsky, M. L. (1959), *J. Biol. Chem.* **234**, 1355.
Sbarra, A. J., and Karnovsky, M. L. (1960). *J. Biol. Chem.* **235**, 2224.
Sbarra, A. J., Paul, B., Strauss, R., and Mitchell, G. W., Jr. (1970). *In* "Regulation of Hematopoiesis" (A. S. Gordon, ed.), Vol. II, pp. 1081–1108. Appleton, New York.
Scott, R. B. (1968). *J. Clin. Invest.* **47**, 344.
Selvaraj, R. J., and Sbarra, A. J. (1966). *Nature (London)* **211**, 1272.
Silber, R., Huennekens, M., and Gabrio, B. W. (1963). *J. Clin. Invest.* **42**, 1908.
Simon, H. B., and Sheagren, J. N. (1971). *J. Exp. Med.* **133**, 1377.
Stähelin, H., Suter, E., and Karnovsky, M. L. (1956a). *J. Exp. Med.* **104**, 121.
Stähelin, H., Suter, E., and Karnovsky, M. L. (1956b). *J. Exp. Med.* **104**, 137.
Stähelin, H., Suter, E., and Karnovsky, M. L. (1956c). *J. Exp. Med.* **105**, 265.
Stein, Y., and Stein, O. (1966). *Biochim. Biophys. Acta* **116**, 95.
Stossel, T. P., Murad, F., Mason, R. J., and Vaughan, M. (1970). *J. Biol. Chem.* **245**, 6228.
Stossel, T. P., Pollard, T. D., Mason, R. J., and Vaughan, M. (1971). *J. Clin. Invest.* **50**, 89a.
Stossel, T. P., Root, R. K., and Vaughan, M. (1972). *N. Engl. J. Med.* **286**, 120.
Strauss, B. S., and Stetson, C. A. (1960). *J. Exp. Med.* **112**, 653.
Strauss, R. R., Paul, B. B., and Sbarra, A. J. (1968). *J. Bacteriol.* **96**, 1982.
Strauss, R. R., Paul, B. B., Jacobs, A. A., and Sbarra, A. J. (1969). *Arch. Biochem. Biophys.* **135**, 265.
Switzer, S., and Eder, H. A. (1965). *J. Lipid Res.* **6**, 506.
Ulrich, F., and Zilversmit, D. B. (1970). *Amer. J. Physiol.* **218**, 1118.
van Deenen, L. L. M. (1965). *In* "Progress in Chemistry of Fats and other Lipids" (R. T. Holman, ed.), Vol. VIII, Pt. 1. Pergamon Press, Oxford.
Vaughan, R. B. (1965). *Brit. J. Exp. Pathol.* **46**, 71.
Ward, H. K., and Enders, J. F. (1933). *J. Exp. Med.* **57**, 527.
Ward, P. A. (1968). *J. Exp. Med.* **128**, 1201.
Ward, P. A., and Schlegel, R. J. (1969). *Lancet* **2**, 344.
Weissmann, G., Dukor, P., and Zurier, R. B. (1971). *Nature (London), New Biol.* **231**, 131.
Werb, Z., and Cohn, Z. A. (1972). *J. Biol. Chem.* **247**, 2439.
Wetzel, B. K., Horn, R. G., and Spicer, S. S. (1967a). *Lab. Invest.* **16**, 349.
Wetzel, B. K., Spicer, S. S., and Horn, R. G. (1967b). *J. Histochem. Cytochem.* **15**, 311.

Wilkinson, P. C., Borel, J. F., Stecher-Levin, V. J., and Sorkin, E. (1969). *Nature* (*London*) **222**, 244.

Wood, W. B., Smith, M. R., and Watson, B. (1946). *J. Exp. Med.* **84**, 387.

Woodin, A. M. (1962). *Biochem. Soc. Symp.* **22**, 126.

Woodin, A. M. (1968). *Biol. Basis Med.* **2**, 373–396.

Woodin, A. M., and Wieneke, A. A. (1964). *Biochem. J,* **90**, 498.

Woodin, A. M., and Wieneke, A. A. (1966a). *Biochem. J.* **99**, 493.

Woodin, A, M., and Wieneke, A. A. (1966b). *Exp. Cell Res.* **43**, 319.

Woodin, A. M., and Wieneke, A. A. (1970). *In* "Calcium and Cellular Function" (A. Cuthbert, ed.), pp. 183. Macmillan, New York.

Wurster, N., Elsbach, P., Simon, E. J., Pettis, P., and Lebow, S. (1971). *J. Clin. Invest.* **50**, 1091.

Yielding, K. L., and Tomkins, G. M. (1959). *Proc. Nat. Acad. Sci. U.S.* **45**, 1730.

Zatti, M., and Rossi, F. (1966). *Experientia* **22**, 758.

Zeya, H. I., and Spitznagel, J. K. (1966). *J. Bacteriol.* **91**, 750.

Zeya, H. I., and Spitznagel, J. K. (1968). *J. Exp. Med.* **127**, 927.

Zeya, H. I., and Spitznagel, J. K. (1969). *Science* **163**, 1069.

Zucker-Franklin, D. (1965). *Amer. J. Pathol.* **47**, 419.

Zucker-Franklin, D., and Hirsch, J. G. (1964). *J. Exp. Med.* **120**, 569.

Zucker-Franklin, D., Elsbach, P., and Simon, E. J. (1971). *Lab. Invest.* **25**, 415.

Zurrier, R. B., Hoffstein, S., and Weissman, G. (1973). *Proc. Nat. Acad. Sci. U.S.* **70**, 844.

Part II

INFLAMMATORY PROCESS AT THE CELL LEVEL

Chapter 7

NEUTROPHIL LEUKOCYTES

I. Introduction

Over 100 years ago, in the early days of microscopic anatomy, it was discovered that blood and tissues of animals contained large numbers of cells that resembled in many regards free living amoebae. These cells were capable of locomotion and showed a tendency to engulf foreign material from their environment. Originally they were thought to function as simple scavengers, and it was generally held that they were responsible for spreading infections by engulfing and transporting microbes in the tissues. In the late 1800's Metchnikoff performed his classic studies on these amoeboid cells and gave them the name phagocytes (eating cells). Metchnikoff's great contribution, for which he was awarded the Nobel Prize, was the discovery that phagocytes were not mere scavengers, but rather constituted one of the principal agencies of defense against microbial invaders. He demonstrated that phagocytes engulf and promptly kill most common bacteria, and that those microbes capable of producing disease in the normal animal are, by and large, those resisting engulfment by phagocytes or those able to survive in their cytoplasm (Metchnikoff, 1893).

Phagocytes of vertebrates may be divided into two general classes on the basis of their nuclear structure: (a) polymorphonuclear cells with a nuclear apparatus divided into two or more lobes connected by thin strands and (b) mononuclear cells possessing a single oval or kidney-shaped nucleus.

I shall discuss in this chapter the commonest type of blood phagocyte, the neutrophil. Mononuclear phagocytic cells are considered elsewhere in this volume (see Chapter 8). My aim will not be a comprehensive review of the literature on neutrophils, for this literature has over the years grown so voluminous as to render such a task virtually impossible and largely pointless. Rather I shall attempt a general summary of the current state of knowledge on biology of these cells.

Whenever possible, references will be made to recent reviews on selected aspects of neutrophil structure or function rather than to the very large numbers of original papers on these various topics.

II. Terminology and Morphology

A. Terminology

The cell under discussion has a variety of names, most of which reflect some prominent feature of its structure or function, and none of which is, in fact, entirely suitable. Polymorphonuclear leukocyte or granulocyte are not sufficiently specific designations, since they apply equally well to neutrophils, eosinophils, and basophils. Similarly lacking in precision is the name microphage, a term used by Metchnikoff for the polymorphonuclear phagocytic cell in blood or tissues to distinguish it from its larger mononuclear relative, the macrophage. Neutrophilic leukocyte or neutrophil would be entirely satisfactory terms were it not for the fact that in certain species, such as rabbit and guinea pig, the cytoplasmic granules are in fact eosinophilic, thus requiring in these instances a different designation, namely, heterophil or pseudo-eosinophil. Functionally and from other points of view these hetero- phils correspond to neutrophils of other species; they are in fact readily distinguishable from the true eosinophils. The term neutrophil will be employed since this name, more than any other, indicates clearly the specific type of cell.

B. Morphology

The appearance of neutrophils after fixation and staining with mixed dyes of the Romanovsky type is well known to most readers and need not be illustrated or discussed extensively here. The cells measure approximately 10 μm in diameter. The nucleus stains darkly and is divided into several sausage-shaped lobes, connected to one another by very thin strands of nuclear material. The cytoplasm is not basophilic. The cytoplasm contains large numbers (50–200) of granules which vary in size and in staining pro- perties depending on the species. Granules of human, horse, and rodent neutrophils are very small, nearly at the limit of resolution of the light micro- scope (0.2 μm), and stain tan or faintly pink. Guinea pig and rabbit cells have larger round granules (~ 0.5 μm) which are distinctly acidophilic in staining behavior. Avian cells have still larger granules of a bioblate spheroid shape. Early studies on histochemical reactivity of neutrophils (reviewed by Wach- stein, 1955) showed positive diffuse reactions for glycogen and dehydrogenase and granular reactions for peroxidase, acid phosphatase and alkaline phos- phatase. These chemical reactions have now been extended to include other enzymes at both light and electron microscopic levels (Ackerman, 1968; Wetzel et al., 1967b; Bainton and Farquhar, 1968a,b; Bainton et al., 1971).

Figure 1 shows the appearance of living neutrophils migrating on glass slides as viewed by phase contrast and by Nomarski interference microscopy. The cells range from 10 to 15 μm in diameter. The shape of the moving cell changes constantly; the leading edge usually takes the form of a broad, smooth, or slightly ruffled pseudopod with a clear, granule-free layer of cyto- plasm at the periphery. Commonly at the trailing portion there is a constric- tion into a taillike structure, often with thin strands extending from it. Nuclear lobes appear homogeneous under phase optics or may show peri- pheral darkening.

The unusual nuclear shape of neutrophils is one of the most striking features of these cells. The molecular mechanism for development and main- tenance of a nucleus divided into oval or sausage-shaped lobes connected by thin strands is completely unknown. Metchnikoff (1893) originally suggested

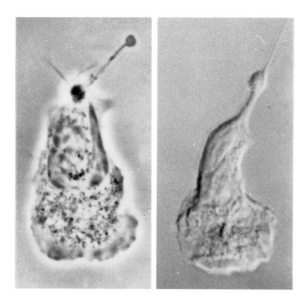

Fig. 1. Neutrophils migrating in a glass slide-coverslip preparation, as viewed by phase contrast (left) and by Nomarski interference (right) microscopy. The cells were moving from top to bottom. The leading edge is a slightly ruffled, broad pseudopod with a peripheral layer of clear, granule-free cytoplasm. Granules are seen in the central region of the cells. Nuclear lobes are located toward the rear, and the trailing edge takes the form of a constricted taillike structure, sometimes with thin strands extending from it. Magnification × 2000.

that this unique nuclear structure was developed during the course of evolution by animals possessing a circulatory system, the polymorphous nucleus facilitating passage of these cells through the capillary wall.

Few or no cytoplasmic structures other than granules are seen in neutrophils under the phase microscope. Most of these granules are usually gathered in the center of the cell, nestled in the area between the nuclear lobes, forming a radiating pattern about the centrosphere region. Granules appear to be fixed in the cytoplasm; they show Brownian motion only in a newly formed pseudopod or in damaged cells with some degree of cytoplasmic liquifaction.

There have been several studies on ultrastructural features of neutrophils in recent years (Bessis and Thiery, 1961; Bainton and Farquhar, 1966; Wantanabe et al., 1967; Daems, 1968; Hirsch and Fedorko, 1968; Bainton et al., 1971). The appearance of a human neutrophil as observed by electron microscopy after fixation in glutaraldehyde and osmium tetroxide is shown in Fig. 2. Nuclear structures often appear multiple as a result of thin sectioning through more than one lobe. Abundant heterochromatin is seen at the periphery of the nuclear lobes. Cytoplasmic granules are round or rod-shaped

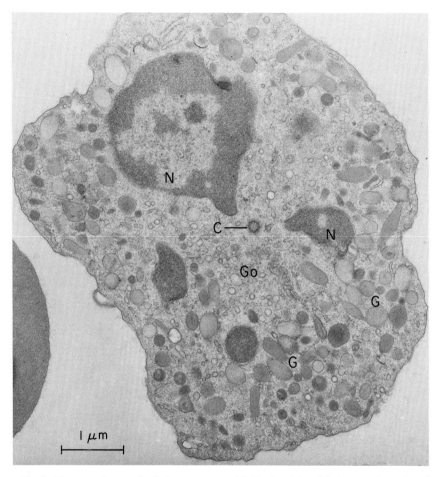

Fig. 2. Electron micrograph of a human neutrophil. Nuclear lobes (N) show condensation of dense staining material at the periphery. Cytoplasmic granules (G) appear as dense homogeneous structures of a round or rod shape, with considerable variation in size and electron opacity. A small Golgi complex (Go) consisting of tiny vesicles and flattened saccules is seen surrounding the centriole (C). A few small mitochondria are visible. Endoplasmic reticulum is sparse. Magnification × 11,620.

membrane-bounded structures with a homogeneous, electron dense matrix. In human neutrophils, these cytoplasmic granules vary widely in size and electron opacity (see Fig. 2), whereas in rabbit cells, two distinct classes of granules are seen (see Fig. 3; also see Horn and Spicer, 1964; Bainton and Farquhar, 1966). One of the notable features of neutrophil ultrastructure is the rarity of organized cytoplasmic structures other than the granules. In

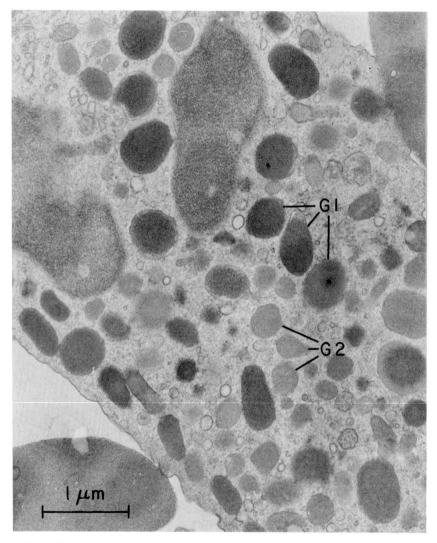

Fig. 3. Electron micrograph of a rabbit polymorphonuclear leukocyte showing the two classes of cytoplasmic granules. The azurophil or primary granules (G1) are large (0.5–0.8 μm) and very electron opaque, whereas the specific or secondary granules (G2) are smaller (0.3–0.5 μm) and less dense.

suitable preparations, abundant glycogen deposits are seen in the cytoplasm (Scott and Still, 1968; Wanson and Tielemans, 1971). Little or no smooth or rough endoplasmic reticulum is present, ribosomal aggregates are not seen, and mitochondria are small in size and few in number. A small Golgi apparatus is frequently found.

III. Formation, Distribution, and Fate of Neutrophils

A. Production of Neutrophils from Marrow Stem Cells

The life history of neutrophils is now well understood, largely as a result of studies employing radiolabeling procedures in the past decade (see reviews by Boggs, 1967; Athens, 1969; Cronkite and Vincent, 1970; Perry, 1970; Metcalf and Moore, 1971). In the adult mammal, neutrophils are produced mainly in the bone marrow. They arise from a population of stem cells that have not yet been identified with certainty, but probably are small mononuclear cells that differ from lymphocytes in detailed aspects of their nuclear and cytoplasmic morphology (van Bekkum et al., 1971). Techniques have been devised in recent years that enable the enumeration of these stem cells and evaluation of their growth potential (reviewed by Rickard et al., 1970; McCulloch and Till, 1971; Metcalf and Moore, 1971). They are pleuripotential, i.e., capable of giving rise to granulocytic, monocytic, or erythroid cell lines. At any given time a significant proportion of the stem-cell population is in a nonreplicating "G_0" state; the rate of neutrophil production is determined, at least in part, by regulatory mechanisms that act on this dormant stem-cell population. Maturation proceeds through the well-recognized myeloblast, promyelocyte, myelocyte, and metamyelocyte stages to "Stab" or juvenile forms and finally the mature marrow neutrophils. The morphology in stained smears of these immature granulocytes is covered in several hematology textbooks and needs no further description here. The ultrastructure of maturing rabbit granulocytes has been studied by Bainton and Farquhar (1966), and by Wetzel et al. (1967a); human neutrophil development has also been investigated by electron microscopy (Scott and Horn, 1970; Bainton et al., 1971). The main morphological features of this maturation process are illustrated diagramatically in Fig. 4. Progranulocytes have a large oval nucleus with preponderance of euchromatin and prominent nucleoli; their cytoplasm contains abundant ribosomal clusters as well as cisternae of rough endoplasmic reticulum. The large primary or azurophil granules formed at this stage bud from the concave face of the Golgi apparatus. Myelocytes have a more mature but still active nucleus; at this stage the azurophil granules are no longer being made, but secondary or specific

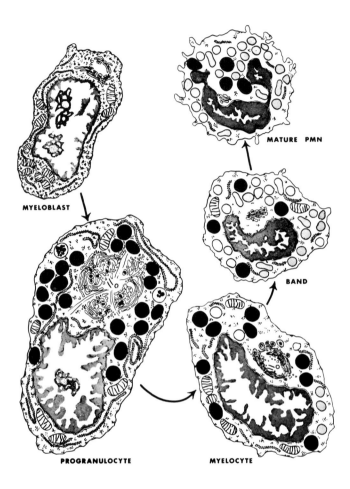

Fig. 4. Schematic representation of the various stages in marrow maturation of rabbit polymorphonuclear leukocytes (after Bainton and Farquhar, 1966). Promyelocytes (progranulocytes)
have a large euchromatic nucleus with prominent nucleolus, abundant rough endoplasmic
reticulum, many large electron-opaque azurophil granules, and a prominent Golgi complex with
azurophil granules budding from the concave face. Production of azurophil granules ceases
prior to the myelocyte stage, and the number of these large granules per cell is then reduced as
they are divided between daughter cells during division in the myelocyte stage. Myelocytes show
a less active nucleus; at this stage the smaller, less electron-opaque specific or secondary granules
are formed by budding from the outer, convex Golgi face. During maturation between myelocyte
and segmented neutrophil stages, endoplasmic reticulum and mitochondria atrophy or disappear,
the Golgi complex becomes much less prominent, and the nucleus becomes progressively more
heterochromatic and undergoes segmentation.

granules are formed by budding from the convex Golgi face. More will be said below about these two distinct granule types which differ not only in their morphogenesis but also in content.

These proliferative stages (myeloblast, promyelocyte, and myelocyte) involve four or more cell divisions and have an overall duration of approximately 6 days. Kinetic data suggest that the rate of production of granulocytes is regulated by changes in the cell cycle time and number of mitoses in the myelocyte stage, as well as by the rate of stem-cell proliferation. This regulation is achieved by feedback controls that are under active study at present.

Maturation from metamyelocytes to fully segmented neutrophils takes about 6 days, during which time most of the cytoplasmic organelles other than granules atrophy or disappear and the nucleus becomes progressively heterochromatic and segmented. The mature neutrophils of the rabbit contain many more specific than azurophil granules, but the azurophils are larger, so that the overall volumes of these two granule compartments is nearly equal. In general, the specialized functional properties of neutrophils develop during the maturation phase in the bone marrow (Brandt, 1967). A summary of the kinetic features and stages of neutrophil production in the marrow is shown in Fig. 5.

B. Distribution and Fate of Mature Neutrophils

The overall distribution of neutrophils and the duration of their sojourn in various body compartments are depicted in Fig. 6. The bone marrow contains a large reserve pool of mature granulocytes (approximately 80×10^{10} in man) that can be rapidly mobilized in times of need. Neutrophils from the marrow enter the bloodstream and are carried to all parts of the body. In the bloodstream of man, there are about 60×10^9 neutrophils, half of which are marginated and half of which are circulating at any given time. These neutrophils leave the blood and move into tissues in random fashion with a mean half-time in the circulation of 6–7 hours. Emigration into tissues involves sticking of neutrophils to vascular endothelium, followed by crawling between adjacent endothelial cells (Marchesi, 1961; see Volume II, Chapter 7 for detailed discussion). Nothing is yet known of the mechanism by which neutrophils separate the overlapping adherent endothelial cells or penetrate the underlying basement lamina.

The size of the tissue pool of neutrophils is not known accurately. They survive in tissues for a few days at most; they are end cells incapable of reproduction or rejuvenation. In order that the system by kept in balance, approximately 10^{11} neutrophils must disappear from a man's tissues each day. There is no known leukocyte graveyard to handle this 100 ml of packed cells

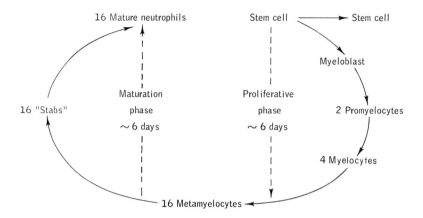

Fig. 5. A summary of the kinetic features and various stages of neutrophil production in the bone marrow (see Cronkite and Vincent, 1970).

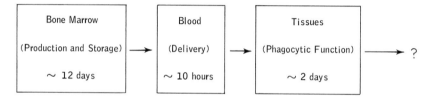

Fig. 6. The flow of neutrophils and the duration of their sojourn in various body compartments.

daily. Probably most of these disappearing neutrophils pass into the outside world through various mucous membranes, especially in the intestine.

IV. The Nature of Neutrophil Granules

One of the most distinguishing features of neutrophils is the abundance of cytoplasmic granules, a feature giving rise to the alternate name, granulocyte. The ultrastructure, cytochemistry, and function of these neutrophil granules has recently been reviewed (Spicer and Hardin, 1969). Neutrophil granules were first isolated in reasonably pure form a little more than 10 years ago (Cohn and Hirsch, 1960a). A list of some of the substances that have been demonstrated to be localized in these granules is presented in Table I. As mentioned above, rabbit leukocyte granules appear to be of two types: (a) the larger, more electron-opaque granules, called azurophilic or primary, which are produced from the concave face of the Golgi complex in promyelocytes; and (b) the smaller, less dense secondary or specific granules that bud from the convex face of the Golgi in myelocytes. A distinction between these two types

TABLE I

NEUTROPHIL GRANULE CONSTITUENTS

Enzymatic	Proteases:	Cathepsin, leukoprotease, collagenase, elastase, histonase
	Carbohydrases:	Lysozyme, β-glucuronidase, β-galactosidase, α-glucosidase, α-mannosidase, N-acetyl β-glucosaminidase
	Lipases:	Acid lipase, phospholipase, sphingomyelinase, glucocerebrosidase
	Miscellaneous:	Ribonuclease, deoxyribonuclease, nucleotidase, peroxidase, oxidases, esterases, aryl sulfatase, acid phosphatase, alkaline phosphatase
Nonenzymatic		Mucopolysaccharides, lactoferrin, cationic proteins

of granules has also been made by cytochemical techniques. The azurophil granules in immature cells react positively for various typical lysosomal hydrolases, such as acid phosphatase and arylsulfatase, and they also give strong reactions for peroxidase. The specific granules react positively for alkaline phosphatase but not for acid hydrolases or peroxidase (Wetzel et al., 1967b; Bainton and Farquhar, 1968a,b). Entirely similar results have been obtained in studies on human neutrophil granulogenesis and histochemical reactivity (Bainton et al., 1971).

The physical separation by rate density or by isopycinic sedimentation in sucrose gradients of the two major rabbit polymorphonuclear leukocyte granule populations has also recently been accomplished (Baggiolini et al., 1969, 1970a). The larger (0.5–0.8 μm), more dense (1.26) granules contain peroxidase as well as various typical lysosomal hydrolases and some lysozyme. The smaller (0.25–0.4 μm), less dense (1.23) granules contain little or no peroxidase or acid hydrolases, but are rich in alkaline phosphatase, lysozyme, and the iron-binding protein lactoferrin (Baggiolini et al., 1970b).

Neutrophil granules contain at least two classes of nonenzymatic substances, namely, mucopolysaccharides and cationic proteins. Both sulfated and nonsulfated polysaccharides have been found (Horn and Spicer, 1964; Fedorko and Morse, 1965; Dunn and Spicer, 1969; Olsson, 1969); the sulfated mucosubstances are located in the azurophil granules, at the rim of these structures in promyelocytes, and distributed centrally in the azurophil granules of more mature cells. Cationic proteins also are found in neutrophil granules, on the basis of both cytochemical (Spitznagel and Chi, 1963; Dunn and Spicer, 1969) and granule separation (Zeya and Spitznagel, 1968a,b) studies. These substances appear to be located mainly in the large azurophil granules of rabbit cells (Zeya and Spitznagel, 1971).

Thus, the azurophil granules qualify as primary lysosomes; they are membrane-bounded structures containing acid hydrolases which have not yet reacted with their substrates. They differ morphologically from primary lysosomes in other cell types, which in most cells are represented by Golgi vesicles, and they differ furthermore in their content of peroxidase and lysozyme, two enzymes not typical of lysosomal hydrolases. The cationic proteins of azurophil granules probably exert antibacterial effects in the phagocytic vacuole (see below). The granule mucopolysaccharides probably form a ground substance within the granules, perhaps binding to the enzymes or the cationic proteins to stabilize them or maintain them in a latent state.

The specific granules are clearly not lysosomes by the usual definitions. The lysozyme that they contain may serve to degrade bacterial cell wall components, but no clear functions are established for the alkaline phosphatase and lactoferrin in them.

One group of investigators has presented evidence for a third population of small granules containing acid hydrolases in mature rabbit polymorphonuclear leukocytes (Wetzel et al., 1967a,b). The existence of these so-called tertiary granules continues to be disputed; no firm conclusion can be drawn at present in this dispute, which has been extensively discussed in the recent literature (see Bainton and Farquhar, 1966; Wetzel et al., 1967b; Baggiolini et al., 1970a; Bainton et al., 1971).

V. Metabolism of Neutrophils

The carbohydrate metabolism of neutrophils has been studied extensively and the findings recently reviewed (Karnovsky, 1962, 1968; Karnovsky et al., 1970). The cell utilizes glucose as an energy source and stores a reserve supply of this nutrient, in the form of glycogen, in its cytoplasm. Even under aerobic conditions, neutrophils derive most (in excess of 90 %) of their energy from glycolysis, not respiration. Neutrophil functions such as phagocytosis depend on glycolysis; the cells function well in an anaerobic environment or in the presence of respiration inhibitors such as cyanide, but cell performance is blocked completely by addition of a glycolysis inhibitor, say iodoacetate, to the medium. From the teleologic point of view, this ability of neutrophils to perform their duty in the absence of oxygen may be highly advantageous, for example by enabling them to control bacterial proliferation or help clean up debris in necrotic tissue devoid of a blood supply.

Studies on use by neutrophils of glucose radiolabeled on specific carbon atoms show that these cells utilize the hexosemonophosphate shunt for degradation of sugar. Under normal conditions, over 90% of glucose degradation occurs in the standard glycolytic pathway and less than 10% via the shunt.

During phagocytosis the rates of glucose uptake and lactic acid production increase 25–50%, and the hexosemonophosphate shunt is strikingly stimulated with as much as a tenfold increase in the oxidation of [1-^{14}C] glucose to carbon dioxide (Sbarra and Karnovsky, 1959). Oxygen uptake also increases two- to threefold during phagocytosis (Baldridge and Gerard, 1933). The increased utilization of oxygen in this situation is cyanide insensitive and appears to be caused largely by the activation of cytoplasmic oxidases, especially NADH oxidase, during phagocytosis (Cagan and Karnovsky, 1964).

Hydrogen peroxide is produced in the course of metabolism of neutrophils (Iyer et al., 1961; Paul and Sbarra, 1968; Zatti et al., 1968) probably as a result of the action of cytoplasmic oxidases such as NADH oxidase or D-amino acid oxidase. The production of peroxide is stimulated two- to threefold following phagocytosis, in parallel with the increase in oxygen uptake.

A probable pathway linking the increases in oxygen uptake, peroxide production, and shunt activity following uptake of particles is the following (see Karnovsky et al., 1970): Phagocytosis activates an NADH oxidase, leading to oxygen utilization and peroxide production; the peroxide operates through a glutathione cycle (Reed, 1969), and/or an ascorbic acid oxidation–reduction system (De Chatelet et al., 1972), to oxidize NADPH to NADP. The NADP so generated then drives the shunt.

Neutrophils also exhibit active metabolism and turnover of lipids of various types, and the turnover of neutral lipids and of phosphatides increases markedly during phagocytosis (see Chapter 6 for detailed discussion). This accelerated lipid metabolism accompanying particle ingestion may reflect general metabolic stimulation of the cell during activity or may be based on specific events such as synthesis of new cell membrane following phagocytosis.

Mature neutrophils show essentially no incorporation of labeled precursors into deoxyribonucleic acid and little ribonucleic acid synthesis, in keeping with their nondividing state and low level of protein biosynthesic activity. The cells do have an amino acid pool in their cytoplasm, and this pool includes a concentration of taurine much higher than that found in plasma (McMenamy et al., 1960). The origin and possible function of taurine in leukocytes is not known.

VI. Physiology of Neutrophils

In an inflammatory reaction resulting from, for instance, introduction of bacteria into tissues, neutrophil function involves a sequence of steps as follows: (A) sticking of blood leukocytes to capillary endothelium in the inflamed area, (B) locomotion, (C) emigration through the vessel wall into tissues, (D) attraction to the microbes, or chemotaxis, (E) engulfment of the invading bacteria, or phagocytosis, (F) degranulation, (G) bactericidal action, and (H) digestion or egestion of the engulfed particles. Let us consider each of these steps from the point of view of neutrophil physiology.

A. Margination: Sticking of Neutrophils to Vascular Endothelium

This phenomenon is discussed in detail elsewhere (see Volume II, Chapter 7). It is a poorly understood process, involving changes in surface properties of endothelial cells and perhaps also of the leukocytes. We shall limit our discussion here to the little information that is available concerning the surface properties of neutrophil membranes and the factors involved in adhesion of neutrophils to one another or to foreign structures. In serum or physiological salt solutions the net surface charge of neutrophils is negative. Microelectrophoresis experiments (Ruhenstroth-Bauer et al., 1962) indicate that neutrophils in the marrow reserve are more electronegative than are those in the circulation and indicate furthermore that this negative surface charge is caused in part by the presence of sialic acid in or on the cell membrane.

Neutrophils show a striking tendency under certain conditions to stick to foreign surfaces such as glass or to stick to one another to form clumps. Factors involved in these adhesion reactions have received considerable attention (Tullis, 1953; Brittingham, 1958; Garvin, 1961; Allison et al., 1963). Divalent cations are required for sticking, and at least in some situations plasma proteins, and fibrinogen in particular, seem to play a role.

B. Neutrophil Locomotion

One of the most striking properties of leukocytes is their ability to crawl about on blood vessel walls, in tissues, or on foreign surfaces such as glass. The cells do not usually move for long distances in a straight line, but rather tend to change direction every 20 μm or so by sending out a new pseudopod in random fashion; the path of a single cell commonly forms a zig-zag pattern. Rate of neutrophil locomotion varies depending on the physicial and chemical nature of the environment. Under ideal conditions they can travel 35–40 μm/ minute (cited by Dittrich, 1962). The mechanism by which locomotion is accomplished by neutrophils remains a mystery. Use of the term amoeboid to describe the locomotion paints a suitable word picture but does not clarify the mechanism. Locomotion has been studied intensively in amoebae for many years, and many theories have been proposed to explain it—snail or snakelike crawling, continuous movement in an over-and-over fashion of the membrane, gel–sol transformation at the leading edge with expulsion forward from normal intracellular tension or from contractile activity at the rear end of the cell, and, most recently, organized cytoplasmic streaming. All these have been put forth as the mechanism underlying amoeboid locomotion, but none can as yet be considered established (Weiss, 1961; Allen, 1961). In any event, locomotion in neutrophils may have a basis different from that in amoebae. Cytoplasmic streaming with formation of a fountain zone at the forward end of the moving cell should be readily detectable in neutrophils since the cytoplasmic granules are well visualized in cells under phase-contrast conditions. Observations on this point, however, show no cytoplasmic streaming; neutrophil granules generally maintain their position during locomotion.

C. Emigration from Bloodstream into Tissues

The ability of neutrophils to penetrate through tiny openings has long been remarked. This activity is seen in impressive form when these cells are observed crawling through capillary walls, as discussed in detail in Volume II, Chapter 7 and is reviewed briefly here to preserve continuity in our discussion of neutrophil physiology. Observation of neutrophil emigration in living tissue under the light microscope shows gradual passage of the cell through the capillary or venule; the leukocyte is markedly constricted at the vessel wall, i.e., it appears to be squeezing itself through a tiny opening in the wall. Frequently this passage of neutrophils is not accompanied by escape from the capillary of other formed elements such as erythrocytes or platelets nor is there grossly detectable expulsion of blood fluid. The mechanism of this emigration has been studied by electron microscopy. Usually leukocytes emigrate by penetrating the junction between endothelial cells (Marchesi and Florey, 1960; Marchesi, 1961; Florey and Grant, 1961), although in some situations passage through endothelial cells in vacuoles has also been seen (Williamson and Grisham, 1961).

D. Chemotaxis

The phenomenon of chemotaxis—directed locomotion toward or away from substances or particles in the environment—has been studied in phagocytic cells for more than 70 years. Present state of knowledge on the phenomenon is reviewed in Chapter 5. Although some of the results in the literature may well reflect technical artifacts rather than true chemotaxis (reviewed by Harris, 1954, 1959), the phenomenon is nevertheless real. Direct observation or camera lucida recording of neutrophil movements show clearly that once within a certain range, usually 100 μm or less, of an attractive object such as a clump of bacteria the random pattern of movement disappears and the cell proceeds in a reasonably straight line toward its intended victim or meal. The basis for this primitive sensory response is not known (McCutcheon, 1955). Most investigators have proposed the existence of a chemical concentration gradient surrounding the chemotactic particle, the directed movement of the neutrophil then being caused by a system of unknown nature by which the cell detects and responds to this gradient. Concentration gradients, if they do exist, might be set up by substances diffusing from the particles into the medium or by adsorption of chemicals from the medium into the particles. Also possible, but unsupported by experimental evidence, is a mechanism whereby a single neutrophil first encounters the particle by chance and then, as a result of this encounter, liberates into the area some chemical messenger to call other leukocytes to the scene.

Extensive observations have been made on chemotaxis using the Millipore chamber (Boyden, 1962) in recent years. Agents that exert an impressive chemotactic influence in this system include substances produced by certain bacteria, complement components, and factors released by cells (Ward et al., 1965; Sorkin et al., 1970; Ward, 1971; Zigmond and Hirsch, 1973).

Many studies have been made in which accumulation of neutrophils at a given site is interpreted as chemotaxis. Such accumulation can result from emigration, followed by random migration and immobilization, without involving true directed locomotion or chemotaxis.

Obviously our understanding of chemotaxis is grossly inadequate. Particularly notable is the absence of any information, or even hypothesis, concerning possible mechanisms whereby factors in the environment alter neutrophil physiology so as to produce directed movement. The relative importance of chemotaxis *in vivo* has not been clearly established, but such a response, even if limited to a short range, can obviously serve a very important role in facilitating contact neutrophils and microbes in tissues.

E. Phagocytosis

Direct observation of phagocytosis under the microscope is a fascinating process to behold. When contact is established between a neutrophil and a suitably appetizing small particle, the particle appears to pass directly through the cell membrane into the cytoplasm. With larger objects, such as the *Bacillus megaterium* shown in the picture sequence in Fig. 7, the neutrophil flows slowly about the bacteria until complete ingestion has been accomplished. The cell flows in and about structured objects such as clumps of bacteria; cell membrane and bacteria seem to unite closely, and extracellular fluid is not visibly engulfed. Chemical studies, however, suggest that

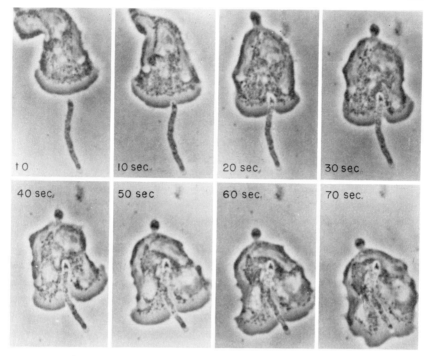

Fig. 7. Sequences from a motion picture of a neutrophil engulfing a chain of *B. megaterium,* as viewed by phase-contrast microscopy. Morphological features of phagocytosis and the rate of the process are illustrated. Approximately × 1500.

some of the surrounding medium is, in fact, taken into the leukocyte along with the particles, a process termed "piggy back" phagocytosis (Sbarra *et al.,* 1962).

Detailed morphology of the phagocytic process is illustrated in the electron micrographs shown in Fig. 8 and in the drawings of Fig. 9. The cell sends out small armlike projections, filopodia, which are closely apposed to the particle. These arms meet and fuse at the distal edge of the particle, and the resulting pouch containing the ingested material is drawn into the cell. Little is known about the cytoplasmic agencies responsible for the micropseudopod formation or the determinants of the membrane fusion by which the bacterium is translocated inside the cell. Phagocytosis (cell eating) thus differs from pinocytosis (cell drinking) in the nature of the initiating cell response (evagination *vs.* invagination) as well as in the size and content of the internalized pouch.

Recent studies on phagocytosis in macrophages (Rabinovitch, 1967, 1968) have demonstrated that it is a process with at least two distinct stages, attachment and ingestion. These two stages certainly exist also in the case of neutrophil phagocytosis; the determinants for these two stages differ, one from another, and also differ depending on the nature of the particle.

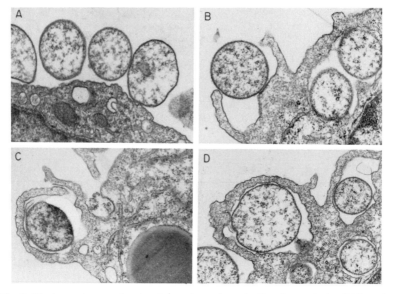

Fig. 8. Electron micrographs showing various stages in the phagocytosis of *Mycoplasma pulmonis* by mouse macrophages. Panel A shows the mycoplasmas near or attached to the plasma membrane. In B and C the cell is sending out micropseudopods, which fuse to enclose the microorganism as seen in panel D. Approximately × 12,000.

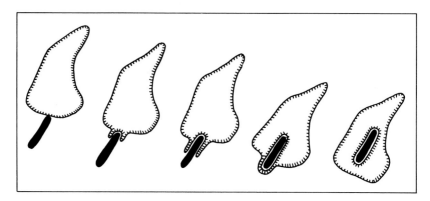

Fig. 9. A series of drawings illustrating the mechanism by which phagocytosis is accomplished. The cell extends micropseudopods to surround the particle; these fuse and the particle is drawn into the cell, lying in a pouch lined by membrane derived from the cell surface.

Ordinarily both bacteria and neutrophils have a negative net surface charge and would be expected to repel one another on the basis of electrostatic forces. Some type of physical or chemical bond must be established between cell membrane and particle to be ingested; no information on this point is available.

Serum substances, of either antibody or complementlike nature (Hirsch and Strauss, 1964; Smith and Wood, 1969) and collectively termed opsonins, act on the surface of many bacteria, presumably by simple adsorption, to render them susceptible to phagocytosis. In the absence of serum, ingestion of most microbes by neutrophils proceeds slowly or not at all. In addition to its opsonizing effect on the bacteria, serum also seems to promote cell function. This beneficial effect of serum on cells may be due to colloid osmotic effects, to binding and inactivation of toxic substances present in trace amounts in the environment, or to other activities as yet undefined.

Other features of the environment exert profound influence on the course of phagocytosis. The rate of particle uptake is highest under somewhat hypotonic conditions (approximately 0.5 % NaCl) and is slowed or completely blocked if conditions are sufficiently hypertonic, say 2 % NaCl. Divalent cations appear to be required for phagocytosis, since any of a variety of calcium-chelating agents prevent ingestion. Neutrophils engulf particles efficiently over a pH range from 6 to 8 and, as mentioned previously, are not dependent on oxygen in the environment for this function. In carbohydrate-free media, neutrophils continue to engulf suitable objects for an hour or so, probably utilizing endogenous stores of glycogen for their energy source. After exhaustion of these stores, activity ceases, but addition of glucose to the medium results in return of function and resynthesis of glycogen in the cell.

The physical nature of the environment also influences strikingly the phagocytic function of neutrophils. As discussed by Wood (1951), leukocytes can take in encapsulated, unopsonized microbes provided the surfaces on which they act or the cell densities are such that the cells can trap the bacteria in corners or between cells. This phenomenon, termed surface phagocytosis, may be considerable importance in tissues, where many rough surfaces or corners are probably to be found.

F. Neutrophil Degranulation

As indicated above, bacteria ingested by neutrophils are contained in a pouch formed by plasma cell membrane taken in during phagocytosis. Digestive enzymes and antibacterial substances of the neutrophil are confined within the membrane-bound azurophil and specific granules of the cell. If, then, the neutrophil is to carry out its function of killing and digesting engulfed organisms, we should expect to see degranulation following phagocytosis. Such a phenomenon was, in fact, reported first by Robineaux and Frederic (1955) and has since been studied more thoroughly by others (Hirsch and Cohn, 1960; Sbarra *et al.*, 1961). In the upper portion of Fig. 10 are shown a normal neutrophil with abundant granules, and, in contrast, a neutrophil degranulated following the ingestion of many bacilli. De-

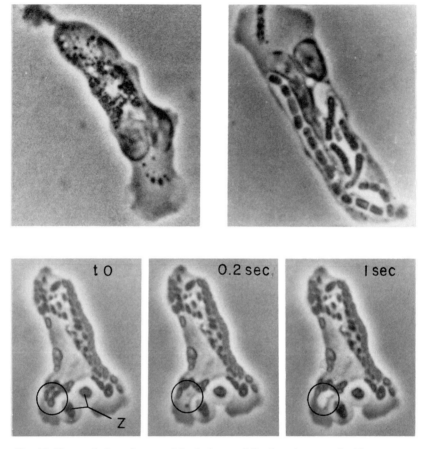

Fig. 10. Degranulation of neutrophils during or following phagocytosis. The upper row shows, on the left, a normal rabbit neutrophil with abundant granules. At right is a similar cell which has ingested numerous microorganisms; cytoplasmic granules have virtually disappeared. Magnification × 1500. The three photographs below demonstrate the morphological and temporal features of lysis of two granules, in the circled areas, during an early stage of phagocytosis of yeast cell walls (Zymosan, Z). Chicken neutrophil. Magnification × 1000.

granulation accompanying particle ingestion by neutrophils has also been confirmed by histochemical demonstration of phosphatases in the phagocytic vacuoles (Horn et al., 1964) and by biochemical studies showing transfer of hydrolytic enzymes from a granule-bound state to a soluble form following phagocytosis (Cohn and Hirsch, 1960b) or transfer to phagocytic vacuoles containing mineral oil–protein emulsions that facilitate their recovery (Stossel et al., 1971).

Cinemicrophotographic studies (Hirsch, 1962) and electron microscope observations (Lockwood and Allison, 1963; Zucker-Franklin and Hirsch, 1964; Horn et al., 1964) have established the mechanism underlying the degranulation reaction. When the membranes of the granules and those surrounding the ingested particle come into contact, they fuse with resulting discharge of hydrolases and bactericidal substances directly into the phagocytic pouch and addition of the granule membrane to the pouch membrane. Both azurophil and specific granules participate in this degranulation response. The specific granules appear generally to coalesce within 3–5 minutes after phagocytosis, whereas the azurophil granules fuse on the average somewhat later (5–10 min) (Bainton, 1973). The sequence of photographs in the lower portion of Fig. 10, made from a phase-contrast motion picture study, shows detailed morphological and temporal features of granule lysis in a chicken neutrophil during ingestion of a yeast preparation. Fusion of membranes surrounding the granule and the phagocytic pouch and discharge of granules directly into the pouch are illustrated in the electron micrograph shown in Fig. 11 and the diagram in Fig. 12.

Neutrophil eating and digestion are thus similar in many regards to these same processes in man or other animals. The cell ingests food in a pouch or stomach and then discharges digestive enzymes into this pouch rather than into the cytoplasm. This mechanism thus provides a means for controlled granule lysis and furthermore probably explains how the neutrophil can degrade engulfed material without at the same time digesting its own cytoplasmic and nuclear structures.

G. Bactericidal Action of Neutrophils

As originally demonstrated by Metchnikoff, most common bacteria are taken in by neutrophils and rapidly killed within the cell; only a few types of microbes, such as tubercle bacilli and brucellae, are not susceptible to killing in this situation. Death of microorganisms soon after engulfment by neutrophils has been established by many different techniques, perhaps the most direct and elegant being that of Wilson et al. (1957). Mixtures of leukocytes and streptococci were observed and photographed under phase-contrast microscopy in thin coverslip preparations. At any chosen time following phagocytosis, neutrophils in the preparation could be disrupted, without damage to the bacteria, by passing an electric current through the preparation, and then observations were continued for many hours to see whether growth of the streptococcal chains liberated from the leukocytes occurred. Streptococci which resided inside neutrophils for less than 5 minutes almost always survived and grew, whereas those organisms held within neutrophils for 15 minutes or longer were usually dead.

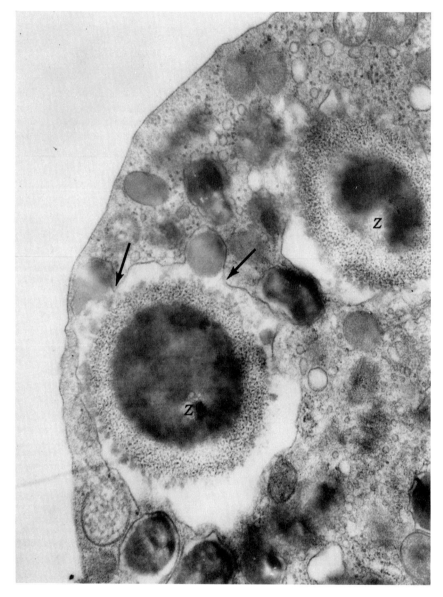

Fig. 11. Electron micrograph showing detailed features of a rabbit neutrophil soon after engulfment of zymosan (Z) particles. At the points indicated by arrows, membranes surrounding the granules are continuous with the membrane lining the phagocytic vacuole. Granule contents are thus discharged directly into the vacuole. Magnification × 32,000. (From Zucker-Franklin and Hirsch, 1964.)

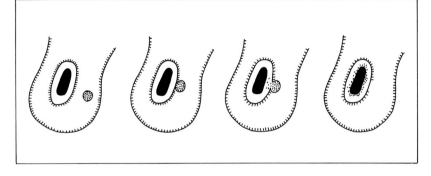

Fig. 12. A series of diagrams illustrating the mechanism by which granule contents are transferred to the phagocytic pouch. The limiting membranes of the granules fuse with the pouch membrane. Contents of the granule are thus discharged into the pouch, and the granule membrane becomes a part of the pouch membrane.

What accounts for death of bacteria inside neutrophils? Ordinary digestive enzymes, such as proteinases, cannot be held responsible since bacteria generally thrive in the presence of these substances (Salton, 1953). Numerous antibacterial chemicals or conditions have been demonstrated in neutrophils in the past decade (see Table II and review by Klebanoff, 1971).

As mentioned earlier, neutrophils produce large quantities of lactic acid in the course of their glycolytic metabolism. Studies employing indicator vital dyes or introduction of microelectrodes indicate that the pH surrounding engulfed particles may be as low as 4–5 (Ishilawa, 1935; Sprick, 1956; Mandell, 1970). The vacuolar pH reaches these low levels within about 10 minutes after phagocytosis (Jensen and Bainton, 1973). This degree of acidity, especially when accompanied by the presence of organic acids (Dubos, 1950, 1953), is lethal to many types of microbes. Acidity of the phagocytic vacuole, similar to the acidity of the stomach juices in man, may thus exert an antibacterial effect. Acid cannot however account completely

TABLE II

BACTERICIDAL AGENTS IN PHAGOLYSOSOMES

Organic acids
Lysozyme
Cationic proteins
Hydrogen peroxide
Peroxidase—peroxide—halide
Lactoferrin

for microbial death in neutrophils, since many bacteria which survive at acid pH, for example, coliforms, are rapidly killed in these cells.

Studies by Iyer *et al.* (1961) indicated indirectly that neutrophils in the course of their metabolism produce significant amounts of hydrogen peroxide, and peroxide has recently been measured directly in these cells by Paul and Sbarra (1968). More information is needed about stability of the H_2O_2 produced and about its possible transfer to the phagocytic vacuole; however, it appears probable that in some situations bactericidal action within neutrophils may be exerted by peroxide (McRipley and Sbarra, 1967; Paul *et al.*, 1970a).

Hydrogen peroxide also participates in a more complex antibacterial mechanism, the peroxidase-mediated bactericidal system studied extensively by Klebanoff (1967, 1968). As mentioned above, the azurophil granules contain large amounts of myeloperoxidase. This enzyme, or peroxidases from other sources, acts in the presence of peroxide and a suitable co-factor such as halide ions or thiocyanate to kill microorganisms. If a halide participates in the reaction, then halogenation of the bacteria takes place. Iodide is much more effective than chloride in this halogenation reaction. The reaction is thus entirely similar to peroxidase-mediated halogenation in the thyroid gland. Peroxide participating in this reaction may diffuse into the phagocytic vacuole from its probable site of metabolic production in the cytoplasm, or in some instances peroxide may be generated in sufficient quantities directly in the phagocytic vacuole as a result of bacterial metabolism (Mandell and Hook, 1969).

Other metabolic products that may exert antibacterial action under some circumstances inside leukocytes include aldehydes (Paul *et al.*, 1970b) and ascorbic acid (Ericsson and Lundbeck, 1955; Miller, 1969; De Chatelet *et al.*, 1972).

Antibacterial proteins associated with neutrophil granules appear to be of three different types in terms of molecular nature and granule distribution. The first of these to be recognized was lysozyme, an aminopolysaccharidase discovered by Fleming (1922). Lysozyme is present in large amounts in neutrophils—approximately 2 mg of lysozyme per gram wet weight of packed cells—and is found in both azurophil and specific granules. Lysozyme degrades bacterial cell walls and causes death and lysis of the few species of bacteria in which the cell wall substrate is available to enzymatic attack. Acting along with other agents such as acid, cation chelators, or antibody and complement (Amano *et al.*, 1954; Repaske, 1956), lysozyme kills other types of microbes as well. Whether lysozyme acts in neutrophils primarily as an antibacterial agent or as a digestive enzyme remains to be established; perhaps both activities are operative, at least in some situations.

Polymorphonuclear leukocytes also contain a group of bactericidal cationic proteins, first extracted from cells and granules in a crude form called "phagocytin" (Hirsch, 1960). This material was subsequently purified and separated into at least six cationic fractions each of which displays a characteristic spectrum of antimicrobial activity (Zeya and Spitznagel, 1968a). The cationic granule proteins are located mainly in the azurophil granules (Zeya and Spitnagel, 1971). They are highly effective at acid pH and are present in cells at concentrations much higher than those required for killing bacteria *in vitro*. The mechanism of their antibacterial action is not entirely clear, but probably involves damage to the bacterial membrane (Zeya and Spitznagel, 1968b).

The third type of leukocyte antibacterial protein is lactoferrin, localized to the specific granules of rabbit cells. Lactoferrin is a protein with strong affinity for iron, even at acid pH. It displays antibacterial properties *in vitro* (Masson, 1970). The mechanism of its antibacterial action and the probability that it has this action in the phagocytic vacuole remain to be established.

Thus, polymorphonuclear leukocytes have available several different mechanisms for killing microorganisms they engulf. Some of these agencies are preformed and stored in the granules, ready for delivery to the phagocytic vacuole at time of need. Others are generated by metabolic events associated with the phagocytic act and presumably diffuse into the vacuole. It is difficult or impossible to establish which specific mechanism is the one primarily responsible for killing a particular species of microorganism under a particular set of circumstances. In some instances, genetically determined deficiencies of some of these mechanisms occur and have been studied (see section on abnormal neutrophils below).

Many of these antibacterial systems are active under conditions similar to those that probably obtain *in vivo*, but it remains nevertheless possible that other factors, yet to be discovered, play a major role in intracellular bactericidal action. In this vein it is worth mentioning that many mononuclear phagocytic cells (see Chapter 8) engulf and kill a wide variety of microorganisms effectively despite the fact that they contain little or no peroxidase, cationic proteins, lactoferrin, or lysozyme and in some instances they produce little or no hydrogen peroxide. Also, certain metabolic bactericidal steps can be inhibited in normal neutrophils *in vitro* with little or no detectable impairment of bactericidal action. For example, high concentrations of colchicine block the hexosemonophosphate shunt, and high concentrations of ascorbic acid block intraleukocytic iodination by the myeloperoxidase system; in both of these circumstances cells show normal phagocytic and bactericidal activity (De Chatelet *et al.*, 1971; McCall *et al.*, 1971b).

H. Digestion or Egestion of Engulfed Particles by Neutrophils

The fate of particles taken in by neutrophils varies depending on the nature of the particle. Inert materials such as carbon or polystyrene may be ingested and remain essentially unchanged over the course of many hours within the cell. Most bacteria engulfed by neutrophils are slowly degraded. Morphological changes in gross appearance or staining properties of the ingested microbes are usually seen after 30–60 minutes, and the process goes on to fragmentation or complete digestion over the course of several hours.

Cohn (1963) has studied the degradation within neutrophils of various types of bacteria labeled with ^{14}C or ^{32}P. Macromolecular componenents such as proteins, nucleic acids, and complex lipids are broken down within an hour into smaller molecules, eventually to be excreted or to be utilized by the neutrophil for its own metabolic and synthetic processes. The somatic O antigen of some coliform bacteria is rapidly attacked within neutrophils (Walsh and Smith, 1951; Cohn, 1962). The attack results in loss of immuno-genicity; in other words the degraded antigen no longer stimulates production of antibodies on injection into animals. The fate of other types of antigens within neutrophils has not yet been studied. Neutrophils contain enzymes capable of degrading polymers of various types and are thus well equipped for the digestion of various types of biological materials (see Table I).

Bacteria or other particles are sometimes engulfed by neutrophils and then at a later time passed out of the cell into the medium, a process called egestion by Wilson (1953). Egestion may be the equivalent of regurgitation of unwanted food in higher forms or may represent some sort of defecation process. Egestion appears to be a rare occurrence in neutrophils observed under various conditions *in vitro* and *in vivo*.

VII. Neutrophil Functions

A. Role of the Neutrophil in Host Resistance to Infectious Disease

The role of the neutrophil as an essential agency for protection of the host against microbial invaders is established beyond doubt and is perhaps best evidenced from the overall point of view by the enormous increase in susceptibility of sepsis of persons afflicted with agranulocytosis, a clinical condition in which neutrophils are conspicuously absent. In many other situations featured by lowered host resistance, for example, following massive X irradiation or excessive levels of certain adrenal cortical steroids, neutrophil availability or function is also disturbed, along with other host-resistance mechanisms such as antibody formation.

It must be emphasized that neutrophil function in host resistance to microbial invaders involves multiple steps and activities: production from marrow stem cells, maturation, release into the circulation, sticking to vessel walls, locomotion, emigration into tissues, response to chemotaxis, phagocytosis, degranulation, and finally antibacterial action and digestion. Abnormality or interference anywhere along the line may result in functional deficiency. A few examples may help to emphasize this point.

Production of neutrophils in the bone marrow is intermittently inadequate in a condition called cyclic neutropenia; the basis for this disorder may well be overaction of the feedback regulatory mechanism that controls normal neutrophil function with a mild fluctuation on a 20-day cycle (Page and Good, 1957; Lund et al., 1967; see also Cronkite and Vincent, 1970). Neutrophil production can also be suppressed or blocked by cytotoxic drugs or by X irradiation, with a resulting fall in levels of circulating and tissue neutrophils several days later, after depletion of the marrow pool of non proliferating maturing or mature neutrophils.

A maturation arrest in the myelocyte stage of neutrophil production appears to occur in some forms of chronic granulocytic leukemia, with production and delivery to the bloodstream of large numbers of the immature cells. Increased susceptibility to infection may be present in this situation, since the myelocytes are functionally as well as morphologically immature (Brandt, 1967).

Circulating blood levels of mature, functionally normal neutrophils (Hirsch and Church, 1961) are elevated when large doses of cortisone are administered, yet host resistance is low. The best evidence indicates that margination and emigration of neutrophils is impaired in this situation and thus a suppressed or delayed inflammatory cell response to challenge may well account, at least in part, for the heightened susceptibility to infection (reviewed by Germuth, 1956).

The high susceptibility to certain forms of bacterial sepsis of the renal medulla seems to be correlated with delayed or inadequate influx of neutrophils in the inflammatory response to microbial lodgement (Rocha and Fekety, 1964). The high salt concentration of peritubular fluids may well impair neutrophil emigration or phagocytic capacity in this situation (Chernew and Braude, 1962). In addition, ammonia produced in the kidney may inactivate the fourth component of complement and thus interfere with chemotactic mechanisms or opsonic activity dependent on complement (Beeson and Rowley, 1959).

B. *Function of Neutrophils Involving Phagocytosis of Objects Other Than Microbes*

We have thus far discussed neutrophil function only as it relates to the role of these cells in eliminating microbial invaders. They are also capable of engulfing, digesting, and transporting suitably appetizing inanimate particles in tissues. Neutrophils are, for instance, attracted to antigen–antibody precipitates and, at least in some cases, ingest and digest these complexes, thus serving a homeostatic function in protecting the host from the damaging effects of some immune complexes.

Foreign, nonmicrobial matter introduced into mammalian tissues by injury may be engulfed by neutrophils and either digested or eliminated from the body by carriage into respiratory or intestinal excretions. If the neutrophil cannot break down or transport such foreign matter in this scavenger role, the ingested material is released into tissues on death of the cell to be engulfed again by other neutrophils or by mononuclear phagocytes.

C. *Role of the Neutrophil in the Production of Inflammation, Necrosis, and Fever*

Neutrophils also serve some functions in which their phagocytic capacity is not primarily involved. For example, the neutrophil is one of the featured actors on the stage of the inflammatory reaction, serving in this situation not only as a phagocyte, but also to determine the production or severity of the inflammation itself. In other words, this cell appears in some instances to be responsible for damage or death not only to foreign invaders but also to the host tissue. This aspect of neutrophil function, considered at length elsewhere in this treatise (see Volume III, Chapter 3), is perhaps best exemplified in the Arthus or Shwartzman reactions. These reactions run their typical course only if neutrophils accumulate in the area; in the neutropenic animal no reaction, or one much reduced in intensity, occurs (Stetson and Good, 1951; Humphrey, 1955; Horn and Collins, 1968). Originally it was proposed that local vascular and tissue injury might be caused directly or indirectly by accumulation of toxic concentrations of lactic acid consequent to neutrophil infiltration (Thomas and Stetson, 1949; Stetson, 1951). More recently, emphasis has been placed on the possible role in inflammation and necrosis of leukocyte granule autolytic enzymes or cationic proteins released into tissues (Janoff and Zweifach, 1964; Golub and Spitznagel, 1965; reviewed by Weissmann, 1967). Degranulation of neutrophils in the Arthus reaction has been demonstrated by electron microscopy (Daems and Oort, 1962). The participation of neutrophils in local tissue damage thus seems beyond question. However, it remains to be demonstrated that acid hydrolases of the azurophil granules exert significant effects in the neutral or nearly neutral tissue environment. The neutrophil constituents or products responsible for inflammation need to be studied further; they may be metabolic products, enzymes with neutral pH optima, or non enzymatic materials such as cationic peptides.

The release of neutrophil granule constituents into tissue spaces may occur from intact cells by a process analogous to secretion when granule and plasma membranes fuse without prior formation of a phagocytic vacuole. This occurs normally in the course of uptake of large particles (Baehner and Karnovsky, 1969) and also occurs when leukocytes contact appetizing material in a noningestible form such as antigen–antibody complexes in an artificial membrane (Hawkins and Peeters, 1971; Hensen, 1971).

Neutrophils play a central role in inflammatory lesions of metabolic as well as immunological origin, as exemplified by the acute attack of gout. The acute inflammation of gout involves deposition of urate crystals, emigration of neutrophils into the joint, phagocytosis of urate crystals, cytoxic effects of intracellular urate on the phagocytic vacuolar membrane with damage and death of leukocytes, and release of factors chemotactic for neutrophils (Phelps and McCarty, 1966; Phelps, 1969). This vicious cycle leads to progressive accumulation of neutrophils and neutrophil products and to progressive inflammation, unless the cycle is interrupted by appropriate drug therapy (Phelps, 1970).

The action of neutrophils on host tissues is not limited to the local site of their accumulation; they also play an important role in initiating some of the general host reactions to inflammation or sepsis. This type of function of neutrophils is illustrated by studies during recent years of the mechanisms underlying the production of fever, a topic considered in detail in another section (see Volume III, Chapter 11). Suffice it to state here that endogenous pyrogen—a direct-acting fever-producing substance—can be derived from neutrophils (Beeson, 1948), and evidence available at present indicates strongly that these cells play a major role in the pathogenesis of fever arising in various clinical and experimental laboratory situations.

VIII. Abnormal Neutrophils

A. Congenital Abnormalities

Several congenital anomalies of neutrophil structure or function have been described in man and animals. Discussion of many of these conditions will be found in other chapters of this book and in recent reviews (Perry *et al.*, 1968; Zucker-Franklin, 1968; Davidson, 1968; Douglas *et al.*, 1969; Nathan and Baehner, 1970; Windhorst, 1970; Klebanoff, 1971).

Defective nuclear maturation occurs in the so-called Pegler-Huet neutrophils, in which the mature cells exhibit an incompletely segmented bilobed nucleus of dumbbell or peanut shape. Neutrophil nuclear hypersegmentation also occurs as an inherited abnormality. Neither of these conditions is associated with defective cell function.

Inherited abnormalities in neutrophil cytoplasmic structures also occur. Crescent-shaped blue-staining cytoplasmic inclusions, called Döhle bodies, are seen in neutrophils of persons with the May-Hegglin anamoly. Under the electron microscope these Döhle bodies appear as foci of rough endoplasmic reticulum; there appears to be a local defect in clearance, by autophagy or otherwise, of this structure during maturation in the marrow. The cells function normally. In the Alder-Reilly abnormality, neutrophils, and other blood cells also, show heavy azurophil granulation, perhaps associated with storage of abnormal polysaccharides.

In some lipid-storage diseases, the blood neutrophils exhibit, as do other cells, an inability to degrade certain types of phospholipids. Thus in Gaucher's disease, neutrophils show a very low level of glucocerebroside-cleaving activity, and neutrophils from patients afflicted with Niemann-Pick's disease are unable to degrade sphingomyelin normally (Kampine *et al.*, 1967). White blood cells are particularly easy to obtain as a "biopsy" representative of nucleated cells, and their use for investigation and diagnosis of other general cellular congenital deficiencies holds much promise.

The Chediak-Steinbrinck-Higashi syndrome is an inherited disorder producing giant granules in various leukocytes, associated with increased susceptibility to infections, and giant granules in melanocytes, producing partial albinism (reviewed by Padgett, 1968). The disease occurs in mink and cattle as well as in man. The giant granules in neutrophils have a heterogeneous appearance, often showing internal membrane lamellae; they contain acid hydrolases as demonstrated by histochemistry (White, 1966). The defect seems to be in formation or in stability of the neutrophil azurophil granules (Davis *et al.*, 1971). Neutrophil function in this condition is abnormal, but not strikingly so. The afflicted cells contain apparently normal granules as well as the giant granules. Current evidence indicates that the giant granules do not readily fuse with phagocytic vacuoles, whereas the small granules do so normally (Padgett, 1967). The cells may have a limited capacity then for normal antibacterial function, and defects in function may occur only under conditions of a large demand placed on the individual cell.

Several genetically determined deficiencies of neutrophil metabolism have now been detected. These deficiencies are not accompanied by morphological abnormalities and may or may not be accompanied by defects in cell function. The most thoroughly studied of this group of conditions is chronic granulomatous disease (CGD) of childhood. This is an inherited disease, or group of diseases, characterized by recurrent sepsis and widespread granulomatous inflammation (Berendes *et al.*, 1957). Neutrophils from these patients are normal in number and morphology and in general display normal functions such as locomotion and phagocytosis. They fail, however, to kill certain bacteria that they have ingested (Holmes *et al.*, 1966; Quie *et al.*, 1967). Initially it was proposed that defective degranulation might account for the cellular malfunction, but subsequent studies have demonstrated that degranulation occurs in these cells (Kauder *et al.*, 1968; Baehner *et al.*, 1969), although additional studies need to be done on the possibility that degranulation may be disturbed in its overall timing or in relation to the normal sequence of specific and azurophil discharge. Further studies on neutrophils of CGD patients revealed a metabolic defect; the burst of oxygen consumption and shunt activity normally occurring after phagocytosis is absent in these cells (Holmes *et al.*, 1967). As discussed above, in the normal cell this oxygen uptake is at least in part a reflection of activation of a NADH oxidase, a reaction which produces hydrogen peroxide and which acts, probably through the glutathione cycle, to generate NADP which drives the hexosemonophosphate shunt. With all of these responses turned off or damped, various types of deficiencies may arise to account for the impaired antibacterial function of the CGD cells, but most workers believe that the most important deficiency in this regard is the lessened or absent production of hydrogen peroxide, a substance capable of acting on its own or in conjunction with myeloperoxidase and halides or other cofactors to kill bacteria. Strong support for the concept of a peroxide deficiency being of primary importance is the fact that CGD cells kill normally a variety of microorganisms that generate peroxide and not catalase, in which case apparently the microbe provides the missing factor (peroxide) that leads to its own destruction (Mandell and Hook, 1969). Further evidence of a defective peroxidase mediated antibacterial system in CGD neutrophils is their failure to halogenate ingested bacteria under appropriate conditions (Klebanoff and White, 1969). NADH oxidase has been reported to be low in CGD cells (Baehner and Karnovsky, 1968), and the proposal made that this is the primary defect, but this finding has been disputed (Holmes *et al.*, 1970), and the issue is not yet settled. Others have reported subnormal activities in CGD cells of NADPH oxidase (Zatti and Rossi, 1965), glucose 6-phosphate dehydrogenase (Bellanti *et al.*, 1970), or glutathione peroxidase (Holmes *et al.*, 1970). It is of interest that other peroxide-generating systems, such as D-amino acid oxidases present in neutrophils (Cline and Lehrer, 1969), are normal in CGD neutrophils (Eckstein *et al.*, 1971); perhaps the peroxide generated by these other systems is not sufficient in quantity or does not reach the phagocytic vacuole.

If the dye nitrobluetetrozolium (NBT) is included in the medium of a phagocytosis system containing normal neutrophils, some of the dye enters the cell during particle ingestion and then is reduced to the insoluble colored form as a consequence of the metabolic responses to the phagocytic event (Baehner and Nathan, 1966). In the case of CGD cells, this reduction of NBT does not occur or is markedly less than in normal cells (Nathan *et al.*, 1969; Baehner and Nathan, 1968). The NBT reaction thus provides a simple and reliable diagnostic test for CGD; the reaction is also being studied in various other known or suspected neutrophil abnormalities. It is important to keep in mind that the NBT test is, at the current stage of its development, somewhat empirical; cell damage or phagocytosis are required for the dye to enter the cell, and the precise mechanism of its reduction by cell metabolic events is yet to be established.

Another genetically determined disease of neutrophils is the absence of peroxidase (Lehrer and Cline, 1969). Only a small number of patients with this disease have thus far been reported. Although one of them was afflicted with recurrent candidiasis, in general they seem to be quite healthy. Their neutrophils show a delayed but not markedly suppressed bactericidal action on staphylococci (Klebanoff, 1970). The fact that these patients do not suffer from recurrent serious bacterial infections would imply that the myeloperoxidase-mediated antibacterial system is not essential for adequate host resistance. Evidently the other antibacterial mechanisms in the neutrophil can take the place of the peroxidase system in this instance. There is in fact evidence suggesting that these other systems may be more active than normal in the cells lacking peroxidase (Klebanoff, 1970).

Initial reports on patients with a congenital deficiency of neutrophil glucose 6-phosphate dehydrogenase suggest that their cells are incapable of killing catalase-positive microorganisms normally (Cooper *et al.*, 1972). This appears not to be the case in all instances, however. It has been possible to block this enzyme and the hexosemorphate shunt with colchicine (De Chatelet *et al.*, 1971) in normal cells, with no resulting impairment of bactericidal activity, indicating that an intact shunt is not required for this activity.

Congenital defects also occur in mechanisms that regulate neutrophil production or function, an example being a condition called periodic neutropemia in man and in the "grey collie." In this condition severe neutropemia and often associated infections occur approximately every 20 days (Page and Good, 1957; Lund *et al.*, 1967). Another example not yet completely investigated is a syndrome termed "lazy leukocytes" in which neutrophils are apparently produced in normal numbers and are capable of normal phagocytic and bactericidal function but lack one or more receptors or other agencies necessary for chemotactic responses (Miller *et al.*, 1971).

B. Acquired Neutrophil Abnormalities

The major diseases of the neutrophil system, such as leukemia or agranulocytosis, produce in severe cases marked reduction or even absence of mature functioning neutrophils in blood and tissues, with resulting marked susceptibility to infection. There are also relatively minor changes in neutrophils that accompany various conditions. One of the best examples is the so called "toxic granulation" of neutrophils recognized to occur in association with cases of overwhelming sepsis or some kinds of intoxication. These "toxic" granules have now been shown to be the neutrophil azurophil granules, modified in their staining reactions apparently as a result of abnormal maturation or other conditions. "Toxic" granules appear identical to normal azurophil granules under the electron microscope, and they stain as do azurophil granules in immature myeloid cells; azurophil granules in normal cells stain as "toxic" granules if the staining time is extended markedly (McCall *et al.*, 1969). These toxic neutrophils apparently function nearly as well as normal cells (McCall *et al.*, 1971a).

Another example of an acquired neutrophil abnormality is the deficiency, or apparent total absence, of alkaline phosphatase seen in mature neutrophils of patients with chronic myelogenous leukemia or paroxysmal nocturnal hemoglobinuria. Adequate studies have not yet been done to establish whether or not this cytochemical alteration is accompanied by ultrastructural abnormalities, such as the absence of specific granules, or by abnormalities in some aspects of cell function.

References

Ackerman, G. A. (1968). *Lab. Invest.* **19**, 290.
Allen, R. D. (1961). *In* "The Cell" (J. Brachet and A. E. Mirsky, eds.), Vol. 2, pp. 135–216. Academic Press, New York.
Allison, F., Jr., Lancaster, M. G., and Crosthwaite, J. L. (1963). *Amer J. Pathol.* **43**, 775.
Amano, T., Inai, S., Seki, Y., Kashiba, S., Fujikawa, J., and Nishimura, S. (1954). *Med. J. Osaka Univ.* **4**, 401.
Athens, J. W. (1969). *Nat. Cancer Inst., Monogr.* **30**, 135.
Baehner, R. L., and Karnovsky, M. L. (1968). *Science* **162**, 1277.
Baehner, R. L., and Karnovsky, M. L. (1969). *J. Clin. Invest.* **48**, 187.
Baehner, R. L., and Nathan, D. G. (1966). *Blood* **28**, 1010.

Baehner, R. L., and Nathan, D. G. (1968). *N. Engl. J. Med.* **278**, 971.

Baehner, R. L., Karnovsky, M. J., and Karnovsky, M. L. (1969). *J. Clin. Invest.* **48**, 187.

Baggiolini, M., Hirsch, J. G., and de Duve, C. (1969). *J. Cell Biol.* **40**, 529.

Baggiolini, M., Hirsch, J. G., and de Duve, C. (1970a). *J. Cell Biol.* **45**, 586.

Baggiolini, M., de Duve, C., Masson, P., and Heremans, J. F. (1970b). *J. Exp. Med.* **131**, 559.

Bainton, D. F. (1973). *J. Cell Biol.* **58**, 249.

Bainton, D. F., and Farquhar, M. G. (1966). *J. Cell Biol.* **28**, 277.

Bainton, D. F., and Farquhar, M. G. (1968a). *J. Cell Biol.* **39**, 286.

Bainton, D. F., and Farquhar, M. G. (1968b). *J. Cell Biol.* **39**, 299.

Bainton, D. F., Ullyot, J. L., and Farquhar, M. G. (1971). *J. Exp. Med.* **134**, 907.

Baldridge, C. W., and Gerard, R. W. (1933). *Amer. J. Physiol.* **103**, 235.

Beeson, P. B. (1948). *J. Clin. Invest.* **27**, 524.

Beeson, P. B., and Rowley, D. (1959). *J. Exp. Med.* **110**, 685.

Bellanti, J. A., Cantz, B. E., and Schlegel, R. J. (1970). *Pediat. Res.* **4**, 405.

Berendes, H., Bridges, R. A., and Good, R. A. (1957). *Minn. Med.* **40**, 309.

Bessis, M., and Thiery, J. (1961). *Int. Rev. Cytol.* **12**, 199.

Boggs, D. R. (1967). *Semin. Hematol.* **4**, 359.

Boyden, S. (1962). *J. Exp. Med.* **115**, 453.

Brandt, L. (1967). *Scand. J. Hematol., Suppl.* **2**, 102.

Brittingham, T. E. (1958). *Proc. Soc. Exp. Biol. Med.* **99**, 252.

Cagan, R. H., and Karnovsky, M. L. (1964). *Nature (London)* **204**, 255.

Chernew, I., and Braude, A. I. (1962). *J. Clin. Invest.* **41**, 1945.

Cline, M. J., and Lehrer, R. I. (1969). *Proc. Nat. Acad. Sci. U.S.* **62**, 756.

Cohn, Z. A. (1962). *Nature (London)* **196**, 1066.

Cohn, Z. A. (1963). *J. Exp. Med.* **117**, 27.

Cohn, Z. A., and Hirsch, J. G. (1960a). *J. Exp. Med.* **112**, 983,

Cohn, Z. A., and Hirsch, J. G. (1960b). *J. Exp. Med.* **112**, 1015.

Cooper, M. R., De Chatelet, L. R., McCall, C. E., La Via, M. F., Spurr, C. L., and Baehner, R. L. (1972). *J. Clin. Invest.* **51**, 769.

Cronkite, E. P., and Vincent, P. C. (1970). *In* "Hemopoetic Cellular Proliferation" (F. Stohlman, ed.), p. 221. Grune & Stratton, New York.

Daems, W. T. (1968). *J. Ultrastruct. Res.* **24**, 343.

Daems, W. T., and Oort, J. (1962). *Exp. Cell Res.* **28**, 11.

Davidson, W. M. (1968). *Semin. Hematol.* **5**, 255.

Davis, W. C., Spicer, S. S., Greene, W. B., and Padgett, G. A. (1971). *Lab. Invest.* **24**, 303.

De Chatelet, L. R., Cooper, M. R., and McCall, C. E. (1971). *Infec. Immunity* **3**, 66.

De Chatelet, L. R., Cooper, M. R., and McCall, C. E. (1972). *Antimicrob. Chemother.* **1**, 12.

Dittrich, H. (1962). *In* "The Physiology and Pathology of Leukocytes" (R. Braunsteiner and D. Zucker-Franklin, eds.), pp. 130–151. Grune & Stratton, New York.

Douglas, S. D., Davis, W. C., and Fudenberg, H. H. (1969). *Amer. J. Med.* **46**, 901.

Dubos, R. J. (1950). *J. Exp. Med.* **92**, 41.

Dubos, R. J. (1953). *J. Exp. Med.* **98**, 145.

Dunn, W. B., and Spicer, S. S. (1969). *J. Histochem. Cytochem.* **17**, 668.

Eckstein, M. R., Baehner, R. L., and Nathan, D. G. (1971). *J. Clin. Invest.* **50**, 1985.

Ericsson, Y., and Lundbeck, H. (1955). *Acta Pathol. Microbiol. Scand.* **37**, 493.

Fedorko, M. E., and Morse, S. I. (1965). *J. Exp. Med.* **121**, 39.

Fleming, A. (1922). *Proc. Roy. Soc., Ser.* **93**, 306.

Florey, H. W., and Grant, L. H. (1961). *J. Pathol. Bacteriol.* **82**, 13.

Garvin, J. E. (1961). *J. Exp. Med.* **114**, 51.

Golub, E. S., and Spitznagel, J. K. (1965). *J. Immunol.* **95**, 1060.

Harris, H. (1954). *Physiol. Rev.* **34**, 529.

Harris, H. (1959). *Bacteriol. Rev.* **24**, 3.

Hawkins, D., and Peeters, S. (1971). *Lab. Invest.* **24**, 483.

Hensen, P. M., (1971). *J. Exp. Med.* **134**, 114s.

Hirsch, J. G. (1960). *J. Exp. Med.* **111**, 323.

Hirsch, J. G. (1962). *J. Exp. Med.* **116**, 827.

Hirsch, J. G., and Church, A. B. (1961). *J. Clin. Invest.* **40**, 794.

Hirsch, J. G., and Cohn, Z. A. (1960). *J. Exp. Med.* **112**, 1005.

Hirsch, J. G., and Fedorko, M. E. (1968). *J. Cell Biol.* **38**, 615.

Hirsch, J. G., and Strauss, B. (1964). *J. Immunol.* **92**, 145.

Holmes, B., Quie, P. G., Windhorst, D. B., and Good, R. A. (1966). *Lancet* **1**, 1225.

Holmes, B., Page, A. R., and Good, R. A. (1967). *J. Clin. Invest.* **46**, 1422.

Holmes, B., Park, B. H., Maliwista, S. E., Quie, P. G., Nelson, D. L., and Good, R. A. (1970). *N. Engl. J. Med.* **283**, 217.

Horn, R. G., and Collins, R. D. (1968). *Lab. Invest.* **18**, 101.

Horn, R. G., and Spicer, S. S. (1964). *Lab. Invest.* **13**, 1.

Horn, R. G., Spicer, S. S., and Wetzel, B. K. (1964). *Amer. J. Pathol.* **45**, 327.

Humphrey, J. H. (1955). *Brit. J. Exp. Pathol.* **36**, 268.

Ishilawa, A. (1935). *Z. Klin. Pathol. Hematol. (Jap.)* **4**, 305.

Iyer, G. Y. N., Islam, D. M. F., and Quastel, J. M. (1961). *Nature (London)* **192**, 535.

Janoff, A., and Zweifach, B. W. (1964). *J. Exp. Med.* **120**, 747.

Jensen, M. S., and Bainton, D. F. (1973). *J. Cell Biol.* **56**, 379.

Kampine, J. P., Brady, R. O., Kanfer, J. N., Feld, M., and Shapiro, D. (1967). *Science* **155**, 86.

Karnovsky, M. L. (1962). *Physiol. Rev.* **42**, 143.

Karnovsky, M. L. (1968). *Semin. Hematol.* **5**, 156.

Karnovsky, M. L., Simmons, S., Noseworthy, J., and Glass, E. A. (1970). *In* "Formation and Destruction of Blood Cells" (T. J. Greenwalt and G. A. Jamieson, eds.), p. 207. Lippincott, Philadelphia, Pennsylvania.

Kauder, E., Kahle, L. L., Moreno, H., and Partin, J. C. (1968). *J. Clin. Invest.* **47**, 1753.

Klebanoff, S. J. (1967). *J. Exp. Med.* **126**, 1063.

Klebanoff, S. J.(1968). *J. Bacteriol.* **95**, 2131.

Klebanoff, S. J. (1970). *Science* **169**, 1905.

Klebanoff, S. J. (1971). *Annu. Rev. Med.* **22**, 39.

Klebanoff, S. J., and White, L. R. (1969). *N. Engl. J. Med.* **280**, 460.

Lehrer, R. I., and Cline, M. J. (1969). *J. Clin. Invest.* **48**, 478.

Lockwood, W. R., and Allison, F. (1963). *Brit. J. Exp. Pathol.* **54**, 593.

Lund, J. E., Padgett, G. E., and Ott, R. L. (1967). *Blood* **29**, 452.

McCall, C. E., Katayama, I., Cotran, R., and Finland, M. (1969). *J. Exp. Med.* **129**, 267.

McCall, C. E., Caves, J., Cooper, R., and De Chatelet, L. (1971a) *J. Infec. Dis.* **124**, 68.

McCall, C. E., De Chatelet, L. R., Cooper, M. R., and Ashburn, P. (1971b). *J. Infec. Dis.* **124**, 194.

McCulloch, E. H., and Till, J. E. (1971). *Amer. J. Pathol.* **65**, 601.

McCutcheon, M. (1955). *Ann. N.Y. Acad. Sci.* **59**, 941.

McMenamy, R. H., Lund, C. C., Neville, G. J., and Wallach, D. F. H. (1960). *J. Clin. Invest.* **39**, 1675.

McRipley, R. J., and Sbarra, A. J. (1967). *J. Bacteriol.* **94**, 1425.

Mandell, G. L. (1970). *Proc. Soc. Exp. Biol. Med.* **136**, 447.

Mandell, G. L., and Hook, E. W. (1969). *J. Bacteriol.* **100**, 531.

Marchesi, V. T. (1961). *Quart. J. Exp. Physiol. Cog. Med. Sci.* **46**, 115.

Marchesi, V. T., and Florey, H. W. (1960). *Quart. J. Exp. Physiol. Cog. Med. Sci.* **45**, 343.

Masson, P. (1970). "La Lactoferrine," Thesis, Université Catholique de Louvain, Editions Arscia, Bruxelles..

Metcalf, D., and Moore, M. A. S. (1971). In "Hemopoeitic Cells, Frontiers of Biology," Vol. 24. North-Holland Publ., Amsterdam.

Metchnikoff, E. (1893). "Lectures on the Comparative Pathology of Inflammation" (translated by F. A. Starling and E. H. Starling). Kegan, Paul, Trench, Truber, London.

Miller, M. E., Oski, F. A., and Harris, M. B. (1971). Lancet 1, 665.

Miller, T. E. (1969). J. Bacteriol. 98, 949.

Nathan, D. G., and Baehner, R. L. (1970). In "Blood Cells as a Tissue" (W. L. Holmes, ed.), p. 157. Plenum, New York.

Nathan, D. G., Baehner, R. L., and Weaver, D. K. (1969). J. Clin. Invest. 48, 1895.

Olsson, I. (1969). Exp. Cell Res. 54, 314.

Padgett, G. A. (1967). Blood 29, 906.

Padgett, G. A. (1968). Advan. Vet. Sci. 12, 239.

Page, A., and Good, R. A. (1957). AMA J. Dis. Child. 94, 623.

Paul, B. B., and Sbarra, A. J. (1968). Biochim. Biophys. Acta 156, 168.

Paul, B. B., Strauss, R. R., Jacobs, A. A., and Sbarra, A. J. (1970a). Infec. Immunity 1, 338.

Paul, B. B., Jacobs, A. A., Strauss, R. R., and Sbarra, A. J. (1970b). Infec. Immunity 2, 414.

Perry, S. (1970). In "Formation and Destruction of Blood Cells" (T. J. Greenwalt and G. A. Jamieson, eds), p. 194. Lippincott, Philadelphia, Pennsylvania.

Perry, S., Godwin, H. A., and Zimmerman, T. S. (1968). J. Amer. Med. Ass. 203, 937 and 1025.

Phelps, P. (1969). Arthritis Rheum. 12, 197.

Phelps, P. (1970). Arthritis Rheum. 13, 1.

Phelps, P., and McCarty, D. J. (1966). J. Exp. Med. 124, 115.

Quie, P. G., White, J. G., Holmes, B., and Good, R. A. (1967). J. Clin. Invest. 46, 668.

Rabinovitch, M. (1967). Exp. Cell Res. 46, 19.

Rabinovitch, M. (1968). Semin. Hematol. 5, 134.

Reed, P. W. (1969). J. Biol. Chem. 244, 2459.

Repaske, R. (1956). Biochim. Biophys. Acta 22, 189.

Rickard, K. A., Shadduck, R. K., Morley, A., and Stohlman, F. (1970). In "Hemopoeitic Cellular Proliferation" (F. Stohlman, ed.), p. 238. Grune & Stratton, New York.

Robineaux, J., and Frederic, J. (1955). C. R. Soc. Biol. 149, 486.

Rocha, H., and Fekety, F. R., Jr. (1964). J. Exp. Med. 119, 131.

Ruhenstroth-Bauer, G., Fuhrmann, G. F., Granzer, E., Kübler, W., and Rueff, F. (1962). Naturwissenschaften 49, 363.

Salton, M. J. R. (1953). J. Gen. Microbiol. 9, 512.

Sbarra, A. J., and Karnovsky, M. L. (1959). J. Biol. Chem. 234, 1355.

Sbarra, A. J., Bardawil, W. A., Shirley, W., and Gilfillan, R. F. (1961). Exp. Cell Res. 24, 609.

Sbarra, A. J., Shirley, W., and Bardawil, W. A. (1962). Nature (London) 194, 255.

Scott, R. B., and Still, W. J. S. (1968). J. Clin. Invest. 47, 353.

Scott, R. E., and Horn, R. G. (1970). Lab. Invest. 23, 292.

Smith, M. R., and Wood, W. B. (1969). J. Exp. Med. 130, 1209.

Sorkin, E., Borel, J. F., and Stecher, V. J. (1970). In "Mononuclear Phagocytes" (R. van Furth, ed.), p. 397. Blackwell, Oxford.

Spicer, S. S., and Hardin, J. H. (1969). Lab. Invest. 20, 488.

Spitznagel, J. K., and Chi, H. Y. (1963). Amer. J. Pathol. 43, 697.

Sprick, M. G. (1956). Amer. Rev. Tuberc. Pulm. Dis. 74, 552.

Stetson, C. A. (1951). J. Exp. Med. 93, 489.

Stetson, C. A., and Good, R. A. (1951). J. Exp. Med. 93, 49.

Stossel, T. P., Pollard, T. D., Manson, R. J., and Vaughan, M. (1971). J. Clin. Invest. 50, 1745.

Thomas, L., and Stetson, C. A. (1949). *J. Exp. Med.* **89**, 461.

Tullis, J. L. (1953). *In* "Blood Cells and Plasma Proteins. Their State in Nature" (J. L. Tullis, ed.), Academic Press, New York.

van Bekkum, D. W., van Noord, M. J., Maat, B., and Dicke, K. A. (1971). *Blood* **38**, 547.

Wachstein, M. (1955). *Ann. N.Y. Acad. Sci.* **59**, 1052.

Walsh, T. E., and Smith, C. A. (1951). *J. Immunol.* **66**, 303.

Wanson, J. C., and Tielemans, L. (1971). *J. Cell Biol.* **49**, 817.

Ward, P. A. (1971). *Amer. J. Pathol.* **64**, 521.

Ward, P. A., Cochrane, C. G., and Müller-Eberhard, H. J. (1965). *J. Exp. Med.* **122**, 327.

Watanabe, I., Donahue, S., and Hoggatt, N. (1967). *J. Ultrastruct. Res.* **20**, 366.

Weiss, P. (1961). *Exp. Cell Res., Suppl.* **8**, 260.

Weissmann, G. (1967). *Annu. Rev. Med.* **18**, 97.

Wetzel, B. K., Spicer, S. S., and Horn, R. G. (1967a). *Lab. Invest.* **16**, 349.

Wetzel, B. K., Spicer, S. S., and Horn, R. G. (1967b). *J. Histochem. Cytochem.* **15**, 311.

White, J. G. (1966). *Blood* **28**, 143.

Williamson, J. R., and Grisham, J. W. (1961). *Amer. J. Pathol.* **39**, 239.

Wilson, A. T. (1953). *J. Exp. Med.* **98**, 305.

Wilson, A. T., Wiley, G. G., and Bruno, P. (1957). *J. Exp. Med.* **106**, 777.

Windhorst, D. (1970). *Advan. Intern. Med.* **16**, 329.

Wood, W. B., Jr. (1951). *Harvey Lect.* **47**, 72.

Zatti, M., and Rossi, F. (1965). *Biochim. Biophys. Acta* **99**, 557.

Zatti, M., Rossi, F., and Patriarca, P. (1968). *Experientia* **24**, 669.

Zeya, H. I., and Spitznagel, J. K. (1968a). *J. Exp. Med.* **127**, 927.

Zeya, H. I., and Spitznagel, J. K. (1968b). *J. Bacteriol.* **91**, 755.

Zeya, H. I., and Spitznagel, J. K. (1971). *Lab. Invest.* **24**, 229.

Zigmond, S. H., and Hirsch, J. G. (1973). *J. Exp. Med.* **137**, 387.

Zucker-Franklin, D. (1968). *Semin. Hematol.* **5**, 109.

Zucker-Franklin, D., and Hirsch, J. G. (1964). *J. Exp. Med.* **120**, 569.

Chapter 8

THE METABOLISM AND PHYSIOLOGY OF THE MONONUCLEAR PHAGOCYTES

RALPH M. STEINMAN AND ZANVIL A. COHN

I. Introduction

Since the first edition of *The Inflammatory Process*, considerable progress has been made in defining the life history, turnover, metabolism, and functional roles of the mononuclear phagocytes. These topics have been the subject of a number of reviews and texts. These include general reviews by Cohn (1968), Nelson (1969), and Pearsall and Weiser (1970). In addition, specific advances by a number of workers can be found in *The Mononuclear Phagocytes* (1970) and in a volume of *Seminars in Hematology* (Miescher and Jaffé, 1970). These sources point out much of the recent information on this class of cell and should be consulted by any serious student of the subject.

The purpose of this chapter is to review our current knowledge concerning the properties of the large mononuclear phagocytes of the blood and tissues. Studies of these cells have accumulated over the last 75 years and have resulted in a vast literature which is scattered throughout the fields of cytology, immunology, hematology, microbiology, and biochemistry. Much of the earlier data were concerned with morphology, staining reactions, and organ distribution, and it has only been in the last decade that a concerted effort has been made to examine their functional capacities in more detail. In most instances their similarities have been stressed, and possible differences in phagocytes obtained from different sites and under varying degrees of stimulation have not been exploited.

The early history of the mononuclear phagocytes is intimately associated with the histological investigations of von Recklinghausen (1863), Ranvier (1900), Marchand (1898), Ziegler (1890), and Gravitz (1890). It was, however, Metchnikoff (1905) who fully realized their capabilities and in a series of brilliant comparative studies related the phagocytic function of the amoebocytes of Metazoa to the macrophages of the vertebrates. In this work he clearly outlined their importance in the defense reactions of the host to infectious agents and other forms of inflammatory stimuli. Somewhat later, Goldmann (1909), Tschaschin (1913), and Kiyono (1914), employing the methods of vital staining, extended these observations and illustrated the widespread occurrence and organ localization of these cells. The technique of vital staining, employing dyes such as pyrrhol blue, isanim blue, trypan blue, lithium carmine, and neutral red, was of great importance in differentiating this system of phagocytes from other cells, such as the fibroblast which did not segregate dyes as readily. The outcome of these investigations led to the concept of a widely distributed group of cells, whose functional similarities were drawn together in the descriptive term reticuloendothelial system (RES) (Aschoff, 1924). Continuing interest in the RES has been concerned with their phagocytic properties, quantitation of particle uptake, the variety of factors which influence this property, and their relation to immune mechanisms. Because of the difficulty in classifying and isolating homogeneous populations of mononuclear phagocytes, their intrinsic metabolic properties have only recently been investigated. With employment of the newer cytological and biochemical techniques, it is now partially feasible to describe properties of macrophages and compare them with other phagocytic cells. This information will be discussed in this as well as other chapters of this three volume treatise.

II. Life History

The identification of a cell as belonging to the mononuclear phagocytes depends on a number of criteria. These include active phagocytosis, morphological criteria such as active membrane ruffling, and, finally, evidence concerning the cell's life history. The functional criteria are more evident in the more mature macrophages, whereas studies of lineage and differentiation are required for the progenitors of the macrophage. A recent text on the *Mononuclear Phagocytes* was partially devoted to this question and the cells involved are outlined in Table I.

Through the use of tritiated thymidine labeling and careful kinetic studies, the origin and fate of the mononuclear phagocytes has largely been elucidated. These more recent studies have clarified the progenitors of the tissue macrophage and have gone a long way to nullify many of the earlier observations based on stained smears and static morphological criteria. In general, these cells have a distinct lineage and pattern of differentiation which sets them apart from the lymphocytes and fibroblasts. In this chapter, we will deal with three populations of mononuclear phagocytes which are present within bone marrow, blood, and tissues, namely, the promonocyte, monocyte, and macrophage.

A. The Bone Marrow Compartment

The first clear evidence that tissue macrophages arose from bone marrow precursors stems from investigation on X-irradiated recipients which had received allogeneic bone marrow cells (Balner, 1963; Goodman, 1964; Virolainen, 1968). A month or more after the adoptive transfer, the free macrophages of the peritoneal cavity were found to be of donor origin. This impression was substantiated by the elegant experiments of Volkman and Gowans (1965a,b) and Volkman (1966). In this instance, the transfer of bone marrow cells labeled with thymidine gave rise to tissue macrophages which were also labeled. In addition, it could be shown that shielding one long bone

TABLE I

MONONUCLEAR PHAGOCYTES

Stem cell ⎫
   ↓   ⎬   Bone marrow
Promoncyte ⎭

   ↓

Monocyte   Blood
   ↓
Macrophage   Tissues

Liver (Kupffer cells)
Lung (alveolar macrophages)
Connective tissue (histiocytes)
Bone marrow (histiocytes)
Spleen (free and fixed macrophages)
Serous cavities (pleural and peritoneal macrophages)
Granulomata (epitheliod and giant cells)

Not included

Endothelial cell
Fibroblast
Lymphocyte
Dendritic cell of germinal centers
Reticular cell

prior to irradiation allowed the subsequent production of blood monocytes and tissue macrophages. These studies also presented evidence that the spleen was not an important source of mononuclear phagocyte precursors.

Following these observations, van Furth and Cohn (1968) provided more direct information concerning the nature of the bone marrow precursor in the mouse. These studies depended on a method for culturing the bone marrow precursor and studying its labeling pattern after *in vivo* and *in vitro* exposure to tritiated thymidine. The success of the procedure was in large measure related to the property of glass adherence which is expressed by the *promonocyte*. Following the parenteral administration of tritiated thymidine, the earliest mononuclear phagocyte which is labeled is the promonocyte. These cells begin to exhibit label within a few hours and 24 hours after a single pulse, about 70 % are labeled. Such cells, when cultured *in vitro*, subsequently take on the properties of macrophages (van Furth and Cohn, 1968).

A second set of experiments indicated that the promonocyte was capable of synthesizing DNA *in vitro* and of dividing. Addition of [^{3}H]thymidine results in the labeling of more than 50 % of the cultured cells. From this type of data, van Furth and Diesselhoff-Den Dulk (1970) and van Furth *et al.* (1970) have calculated that the promonocyte has an average generation time of 9.7 hours and a DNA synthesis time of 6.8 hours. The promonocyte can therefore be considered a rapidly dividing cell which gives rise to the blood monocyte.

The precursor of the promonocyte has not as yet been identified. It is quite possible that it arises, as do many other blood cells, from a multipotential stem cell. In this regard, the cultivation of bone marrow cells in soft agar gives rise to both granulocyte and macrophage colonies. Many other properties of the promonocyte still remain obscure. These include the influence of inflammatory stimuli on their rate of division, their pool size in the marrow, and the possibility that under conditions of stress this immature member of the mononuclear phagocytes may be released into the circulation. In any event, it is quite apparent that the promonocyte represents only a minor population of cells in the bone marrow ($< 1 \%$) and that there is no appreciable reserve pool of more adult cells in the marrow. In this regard, their life history differs markedly from the granulocytic series.

B. Peripheral Blood Compartment

The division of the promonocyte gives rise to the *monocyte*, which, after a short maturation phase (+ hours) in the marrow, is released into the peripheral blood. This is a more functionally active cell which, under normal steady-state conditions, does not divide (van Furth and Cohn, 1968). Following a single pulse of [^{3}H]thymidine, labeled blood monocytes appear in the circulation at a rate of about 2% per hour, reaching a peak of labeling at 48 hours (60%). This is quite a rapid influx and exceeds the labeling pattern of granulocytes, lymphocytes, and erythroid elements. It implies that the monocyte is released into the circulation shortly after the division of the promonocyte.

Once in the circulation, the monocyte represents only a small percentage of the blood-borne white cells. In most instances this rarely exceeds $8-10 \%$ of the total white count, although in certain bacterial and viral infections or in cases of granulocytopenia this level may be doubled. Their intravascular life span has thus far been studied only in small laboratory rodents. In the mouse (van Furth and Cohn, 1968), under steady-state conditions, labeled monocytes disappear from the circulation in an exponential fashion. This suggests that random emigration is occurring in all small vessels, and no evidence has accrued that an important marginated pool exists in the intravascular compartment.

When equally labeled cohorts of cells are examined, the disappearance from the circulation occurs with a half-life of 22 hours and an average transit time of 32 hours. This figure is appreciably longer than the half-life of neutrophilic or heterophilic leukocytes. The half-life of the monocyte in the rat's circulation has been reported to be somewhat longer (Whitelaw, 1966), but this is based on a heterogeneous population of labeled cells. Almost nothing is known about the turnover of monocytes in the blood of primates and man.

Under unusual situations of disease and stress, cells with the appearance of typical macrophages may appear in the circulation in small numbers. These may enter via the thoracic duct, although other portals may also exist. In this regard, the macrophages of the liver (Kupffer cells) may be dislodged and circulate for brief periods.

C. Emigration and Chemotaxis

The emigration of monocytes from the intravascular to extravascular compartment was clearly described by Ebert and Florey (1939) some 30 years ago. Employing the rabbit ear chamber, direct observations under the phase-contrast microscope revealed the path of monocytes through the vessel wall and their emergence into the perivascular connective tissue. The mechanism by which diapedesis took place was clarified by Marchesi and Florey (1960) 20 years later. Under the electron microscope, monocytes insert pseudopods between the endothelial cells of postcapillary venules, penetrate the basement membrane, and move through the intercellular spaces. Following this process they appear unchanged at the ultrastructural level. This presumably takes place in all capillary beds. In addition, monocytes may attach themselves to the walls of sinusoids, i.e., liver, where they mature into macrophages without leaving the intravascular compartment.

The mechanism underlying the emigration of monocytes in noninflammatory situations is unknown. Presumably this is related, at least in part, to the special attributes of the vascular endothelium. Under inflammatory conditions, following the release of vasoactive amines, the intercellular spaces between adjacent endothelial cells may be widened and influence the migration of monocytes.

The directed movement of mononuclear phagocytes has been described in a number of in vitro situations (Harris, 1954; Ward, 1968; Sorkin et al., 1970). Most recent investigators have employed the Boyden chamber in which cells migrate through Millipore filters. In most instances, the effects of agents on the rate of motility and directionality have not been clearly separated. However, a directional response can be demonstrated by manipulating the concentration of chemotactic factor on each side of the chamber. With this method, Ward (1968) has described a heat-stable factor in rabbit serum exposed to immune complexes. This factor does not require the presence of $C'(5,6,7)$ for its generation and in this regard differs from a similar product which is highly chemotactic for neutrophils. Soluble bacterial products as well as agents in lysed neutrophils have chemotactic activity. Organophosphorus inhibitors block chemotaxis, but inhibition profiles differ from those examined with neutrophils. Sorkin *et al.* (1970) has described a chemotactic factor in normal sera, with a molecular weight of approximately 200,000. This is active for macrophages, whereas a smaller component of normal sera (5,000–30,000 MW) stimulates neutrophils. This suggests a degree of specificity of the two cell types to exogenous stimuli.

There is no information concerning the ability of the above factors to influence emigration. Conceivably, they may modify the direction of movement once the monocyte is in the extravascular space and their eventual accumulation at inflammatory sites. From the studies of Spector and Willoughby (1963), monocytes leave the circulation quite early in the inflammatory response and during the major egress of neutrophils. Their numbers, however, are masked by the preponderance of short-lived granulocytes. The same authors have also described subsequent waves of monocyte migration, late in inflammation, at a time when neutrophils cease entering the lesion.

D. Origin and Turnover of the Inflammatory Macrophage

It is now quite clear that the vast majority of macrophages which accumulate in inflammatory areas are of monocyte origin. This appears to be the case irrespective of the site in the body and includes the skin, serous cavities, parenchymatous organs, or central nervous system (see van Furth, 1970a,b). Two examples will serve to illustrate the type of information on which this statement is based.

The first concerns a mild, nonspecific inflammatory response in the skin as described by Volkman and Gowans (1965a,b) and also by Spector *et al.* (1965). It is quite likely, if not certain, that it would also apply to other specific immunological reactions of both acute and delayed types. In these experiments, blood monocytes are labeled by the parenteral administration of tritiated thymidine and in addition may contain a cytoplasmic marker in the form of a phagocytized particulate. Following the labeling procedure or during it, coverslips are implanted in the subcutaneous tissue and act as inflammatory agents. Thereafter, coverslips are removed and examined by autoradiography and microscopy. From such studies it is clear that the macrophages which adhere to the coverslips exhibit labeling patterns similar to that seen in the circulating monocyte. In addition, the administration of thymidine to animals already harboring coverslips results in the labeling of insignificant numbers of cells. These data indicate that the macrophages arise from circulating monocytes and do not divide at the site during early stages of the lesion (1–3 days). This statement should be modified when older (+4 days) sites are examined, as studied by Spector and Ryan (1970). In this case, there was evidence that division of macrophages took place in older lesions and could result in a significant increase in cell numbers.

Similar data have been obtained in the peritoneal cavity of prelabeled mice (van Furth and Cohn, 1968). Following the intraperitoneal administration of calf serum as a mild irritant, large numbers of labeled monocytes entered the cavity and could account for the increased numbers of cells in the inflammatory exudate. Again, no evidence for *in situ* division was evident.

Although it seems quite certain that monocytes are the direct precursors of the macrophages which accumulate in acute lesions, increasing evidence suggests that the situation in chronic reactions is more complex. In part, this depends on the nature of the inducing agent as described by Spector and his colleagues (Spector and Lyke, 1966; Spector, 1967; Spector and Willoughby, 1968). The introduction of Freund's adjuvant into the skin results in the usual emigration of monocytes and their maturation into macrophages. This is followed by a cessation of emigration and the continual division of the macrophages, a process which may last as long as 3 months. It appears therefore that the long-term maintenance of this type of granuloma is dependent on mitotic activity. In contrast, the use of carrageenin evokes a similar lesion but a much reduced incidence of *in situ* labeling. This suggests the presence of a long-lived macrophage population, which is reinforced by cells from the circulation. It is apparent that further studies are indicated, in a variety of granulomatous responses, before a coherent picture emerges of the mitotic potential of the inflammatory macrophage.

E. Origin and Turnover of the Tissue Macrophage

As noted in Table I, macrophages are present throughout the body and are enriched in certain parenchymatous organs. Actually, rather little is known about the turnover of many of these cells under steady-state conditions, and their origin is assumed to be the blood monocyte in most instances examined. Direct evidence does, however, exist for the Kupffer cell, alveolar macrophage, and for the resident cells of the peritoneal cavity.

In the absence of exogenous stimuli, the Kupffer cells lining liver sinusoids divide infrequently and exhibit a very low level of thymidine uptake (North, 1969a,b; van Furth, 1970a,b). In the mouse, following a short pulse of isotope, less than 2% of the Kupffer cells are labeled. Thereafter, the number of labeled cells increases, reaching a peak at 84 hours of 7%. This is the result of the influx of labeled monocytes from the circulation and indicates that the normal tunover of Kupffer cells is on the order of 60 days. The situation is quite different during the development of cellular immunity following infection with *Listeria* (North, 1969b). As delayed hypersensitivity develops and in the presence of a committed lymphocyte population, actively phagocytic Kupffer cells exhibit striking DNA synthesis and presumably divide. The importance of this dividing population is unclear, since at the same time, blood monocytes are rapidly entering the interstitial granuloma, the site of bacillary multiplication.

Alveolar macrophages of a number of species appear to have their origin from a bone marrow-derived cell which is presumably the monocyte. Some of these experiments employed karyotypic markers (Pinkett et al., 1966; Virolainen, 1968) in adoptive transfer experiments. The necessity of sampling only a dividing population restricted the interpretations, since morphology could not be adequately evaluated. Nevertheless, more than 50% were thought to be of bone marrow origin. Other studies using a thymidine label indicate the low rate of division of the alveolar macrophage (Bowden et al., 1969; van Furth, 1970a,b; Shorter et al., 1964). Employing the labeling index of 6% at 60 hours after a pulse, it has been calculated that alveolar macrophages have a turnover time of 50 days under normal conditions. Pulmonary infections and other stimuli would evoke a more rapid influx of blood-borne cells and probably shorten this value.

Within the peritoneal cavity of most species there is a resident population of macrophages that exhibits a gradual increase in numbers with advancing age and weight. This is a particularly prominent cell in the mouse peritoneum, and 5×10^6 macrophages can easily be harvested from most strains of animals. Under steady-state conditions, these cells are nondividing and are maintained at a rather constant number. From labeling studies (van Furth and Cohn, 1968), these cells turnover at approximately 0.1–0.2% per hour and it requires 30–40 days for complete replacement.

It is apparent that the longevity of tissue macrophages is dependent on a variety of factors. These probably include their site in the body, whether or not they are in contact with a vascular bed, their proximity to portals of egress, i.e., airways, and the particle load to which they are exposed. In addition, under inflammatory conditions the nature of the stimulus plays an important role. Toxic macromolecules and viable microorganisms might be expected to injure a proportion of cells and require a constant replacement with new cells. In general, we are quite ignorant of the eventual fate of macrophages in the normal host. Some may be continually lost through the respiratory and digestive tracts and others may suffer a fate similar to that of other effete cells, namely, phagocytosis and digestion by other macrophages.

F. The Influence of Irradiation and Drugs

In view of the recent understanding of the kinetics and pool sizes of the mononuclear phagocytes, it is not surprising that their response to X-irradiation and antiinflammatory drugs has not been advanced to a level similar to that of the lymphocyte and granulocyte. However, a few studies have been illuminating and indicate that further work is both important and necessary for a clear understanding of the inflammatory process.

Following the exposure of small rodents to sublethal doses of X-irradiation, the production of circulating monocytes is promptly curtailed (Volkman and Gowans, 1965a,b; van Furth and Cohn, 1968). This is apparently the result of irradiation damage to bone marrow precursors such as the promonocyte. Within 24 to 48 hours, and in conjunction with the loss of other white cells and platelets, the number of blood monocytes falls to low levels and requires a number of weeks to be replenished. Little information is available about a direct toxic effect of ionizing irradiation on the circulating monocyte. Since this cell is not actively dividing, it is probable that the depletion of blood monocytes is the result of both decreased production and a normal or accelerated emigration into the tissues. Macrophages already present in the tissues are quite resistant to ionizing radiation and their numbers remain constant at least during the initial phases of the reaction. Certain authors have described a reduction in functional activities following X rays, but these must be interpreted with care, since they were performed *in vivo* and could represent the reduction in pool size. In preliminary studies (unpublished observations), peritoneal macrophages from mice receiving 550 rads were more fragile under *in vitro* conditions but were still able to phagocytize and kill an inoculum of bacteria.

Recently, Thompson and van Furth (1970) have examined the influence of large doses of corticosteroids on the dynamics of mononuclear phagocytes. They found, as did previous investigators (Cohn, 1962a,b), that steroids decreased the number of cells which entered an inflammatory lesion in the peritoneal cavity but did not influence the number of resident macrophages. The same dose of hydrocortisone acetate rapidly depleted the peritoneal lymphocyte population, which coexists with the macrophages. Of particular interest, these authors describe a marked rapid reduction in circulating monocytes in the absence of any clearcut evidence for a decreased labeling of bone marrow precursors. They speculate on the sequestration of monocytes and a possible lytic effect. In any event, a depleted circulating pool would obviously influence the number of cells arriving at an inflammatory reaction and thereby add to the woes of both steroid-treated animals and patients in terms of enhanced susceptibility to infection.

Although considerable efforts have been expended in developing immunosuppressive regimens, little information has accrued on the cellular events underlying their mechanism of action. In particular, the influence of agents such as 6-mercaptopurine on the production rates and turnover of mononuclear phagocytes has not been examined in detail. Studies by Hurd and Ziff (1968) and Latta and Gentry (1958) have documented a reduction in monocytes in both rabbits and mice. This was associated with a reduced number of inflammatory macrophages in skin sites. Unfortunately, there is no information concerning the state of bone marrow precursors and the formation of more mature members of the system. In contrast, cyclophosphamide (Ziff *et al.*, 1970) does not appear to reduce the circulating level of monocytes. The important problems facing the immunosuppressed grafted patient require more farreaching experiments in both man and animals.

III. Morphology

The distinction between various classes of lymphocytes, monocytes, and macrophages has been in large measure based on simple morphological criteria. Because the distinction among these cell types is important in understanding the inflammatory process, the unique features of mononuclear phagocytes will be discussed in detail and the reliability of these structural features compared under different methods of fixation and staining. In general, it is usually possible to differentiate among these cells either at the light or electron microscopic level.

A. Monocyte: Light and Phase Microscopy

The structural features of the blood monocyte have been reviewed in the past (Cohn, 1965; Low and Freeman, 1958). Following the usual Romanovsky stains and methanol fixation, the cell exhibits an indented nucleus and a moderate amount of bluish gray cytoplasm, which contains azurophilic granules. Peroxidase staining has been used to distinguish the monocytes from larger lymphocytes. However, it is not clear what proportion of blood monocytes exhibits positively stained granules in the cytoplasm, and there may be species differences. This cytochemical technique appears to differentiate a portion of the positive monocytes from negative lymphoid cells, but may not adequately reflect the total number of monocytes in the circulating blood.

A more satisfactory method of identifying monocytes is to observe the surface membranes of live preparations under phase-contrast microscopy. Under conditions in which the cells adhere to and spread out on glass surfaces, monocytes have distinctive ruffled membranes which are continually in motion and which are involved in the formation of phase-lucent pinocytic vacuoles. Lymphoid cells under the same conditions are quite different in appearance, without ruffled membranes, and contain mitochondria which are considerably thicker and/or less elongate than in the monocytic series. In addition, phase-contrast microscopy reveals a modest number of spherical phase-dense cytoplasmic granules in monocytes which are absent in lymphoid cells.

The distinctions between "mononuclear cells" becomes much more difficult in paraffin-embedded tissue sections. Although nuclear morphology and chromatin pattern of the nuclei are occasionally of benefit, no clear cut distinction can be made in the usual preparation, such as that employed to study delayed hypersensitivity reactions. The task is somewhat easier when monocytes have matured into larger macrophages. More recently, investigators have turned to 0.5–1.0 μm sections of material fixed and embedded for electron microscopy and stained with Romanovsky or other basic dyes (Dvorak et al., 1970). This method is advantageous in revealing more clearcut cytoplasmic and nuclear staining and often the existence of the ruffled surface of phagocytic cells, but unfortunately it still cannot be used to identify with security all the cells present in inflammatory reactions.

B. Monocyte: Electron Microscopy

The electron microscopic appearance of blood monocytes has been described in a variety of species and the basic features are similar for both man and lower forms (Fedorko and Hirsch, 1970; Nichols et al., 1971). The nucleus contains one or more nucleoli, and condensed peripheral chromatin (Fig. 1). Little glycogen is seen in the cytoplasm. There is a moderate amount of rough-surfaced endoplasmic reticulum consisting of short, flat cisternae devoid of electron-dense material. Some free ribosomes are normally observed, although polysomes are unusual. Scattered through the cytoplasm are slim mitochondria. In the hof of the nucleus, there is a well-developed Golgi zone with associated centrioles. There are numerous smooth membrane-bounded vesicles, which in some cases appear to be budding from the stacks of Golgi membranes. One occasionally observes linear arrays of fibrils in the perinuclear region, the nature and function of which is unclear. A few microtubules can be seen in the peripheral cytoplasm following appropriate fixation. The cell surface contains microvilli, and in most cases there are electron-lucent micropinocytic vesicles in the cell periphery. Some pinosomes are surrounded by spiked projections and are termed coated vesicles.

The other important cytoplasmic organelle of the monocyte is the membrane-bounded dense body which corresponds to the azurophil granule seen in Romanovsky stains. The recent work of Nichols et al. (1971) has greatly clarified the nature of these granules. Mononuclear phagocytes, similar to their polymorphonuclear counterparts, develop a group of primary lysosomes while in the bone marrow and, in some species, continue to do so during their circulation in the bloodstream. The granules contain hydrolytic, acid pH-optimum enzymes, and peroxidase, which, in turn, are synthesized

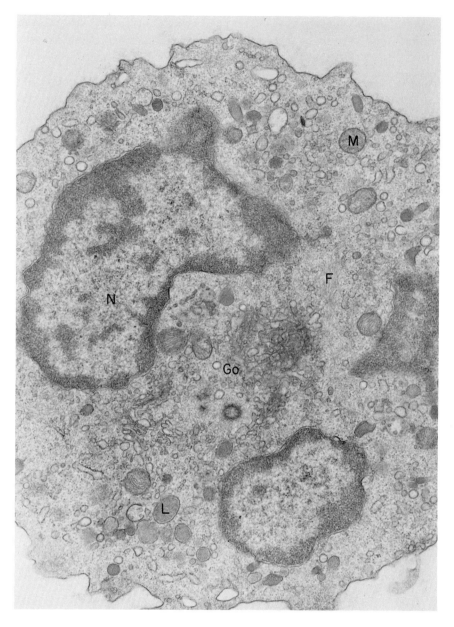

Fig. 1. An electron micrograph of a monocyte. × 16,000. The indented nucleus (N) exhibits peripheral heterochromatin, and nucleoli are not apparent. Within the cytoplasm, the saccules and vesicles of the Golgi apparatus (Go) are centrally located in the "hof" of the nucleus and surround a centriole. Mitochondria (M) are scattered through the cytosol. Occasional dense granules or lysosomes (L) are evident but are outnumbered by electron-lucent vesicles of pinocytic origin. A network of filaments (F) is often observed in the nuclear area.

in the rough endoplasmic reticulum and packaged in the Golgi. The resulting storage granules usually are not utilized until the monocyte emigrates into the tissues and undergoes an endocytic event accompanied by degranulation. The tissue macrophage may resume the production of lysosomal hydrolases in accordance with environmental stimuli (see Section IV). However, it does not package them as storage granules. The synthesis of peroxidase cannot be detected histochemically in tissue macrophages of certain species, e.g., rabbit (Nichols *et al.*, 1971) and mouse (van Furth *et al.*, 1970) peritoneal cells, but may occur in others, e.g., rat (Robbins *et al.*, 1971) and guinea pig (Cotran and Litt, 1970) peritoneal cells and rat Kupffer cells (Widmann *et al.*, 1972). The differentiation of peroxidase from catalase histochemically cannot be made with certainty and this confuses the interpretation of these data.

C. Promonocyte

The precursor to the blood monocyte, the promonocyte, has now been identified in glass-adherent populations prepared from cell suspensions of mouse bone marrow (van Furth *et al.*, 1970; Fedorko and Hirsch, 1970). Stained smears provide little assistance in identifying the promonocyte, except that this çell has relatively few azurophilic granules in comparison to the abundant numbers in immature granulocytes (which initially may be present in these preparations). Under phase-contrast optics, however, one observes many adherent mononuclear cells with a high nuclear-to-cytoplasmic ratio and a ruffled border. These cells are able to endocytose suitable test materials. Both of the latter criteria are of great value in distinguishing the cell as an immature member of the monocytic series, although membrane ruffling and the capacity to endocytose seem less well developed than in the more mature monocytes and macrophages. The nucleus of the promonocyte may be as large as 10–12 μm. It can be elongate or indented and contains one or two large nucleoli and dispersed chromatin. The Golgi zone is well developed and consists of stacks of lamellae, smooth surfaced vesicles, and a pair of centrioles. There are a few flat cisternae of rough endoplasmic reticulum and abundant unattached polysomes. The typical morphological features of endocytosis in mononuclear phagocytes are beginning to develop in the promonocyte. There are a few membrane-bound electron-dense bodies and micropinocytic vesicles, and the cell surface contains scattered microvilli. Cells with these same structural features have been identified by Nichols *et al.* (1971) in bone marrow smears from rabbit, guinea pig, and man.

D. Macrophage: Light and Phase Microscopy

The morphology of the tissue macrophage is much more heterogeneous. Much of the heterogeneity in structure appears to be related to previous endocytic events and the resulting sensitivity of ingested materials to intracellular hydrolysis. When compared to the monocyte, the macrophages are larger ($20–100\mu$m) and contain greater numbers of cytoplasmic dense bodies and mitochondria. In stained sections their nuclei are less condensed than lymphoid cells and vary from spherical to deeply indented structures. The cytoplasm is light blue or even slightly eosinophilic, and ingested debris are often seen. A similar picture is obtained when stained smears are prepared from exudates.

A more informative examination can be made with isolated cells which are allowed to spread on glass surfaces and viewed with phase-contrast microscopy. When observed in the living state (Robineaux and Pinet, 1960; Cohn and Benson, 1965c), the activity of the peripheral membrane is marked and of considerable importance in identifying the cell type. This is typified by slow undulations and ruffles which are continuous and result in a wavelike action moving in a centripetal fashion. Such ruffles can also be seen in glutaraldehyde-fixed preparations and appear to be the origin of many phase-lucent pinocytic vesicles (Figs. 2a and 2b). Long, slim mitochondria extend into the pseudopods and are intermingled as well with spherical dense granules in the perinuclear region. This area contains an assortment of dense granules and lucent vacuoles, which may be scattered randomly or arranged in a rosette about the Golgi complex. Lipid droplets are often present in the cytoplasm. Large phagosomes are common and contain an array of particulates ranging from crystalloids to relatively intact cells.

E. Macrophage: Electron Microscopy

The ultrastructure of macrophages has been described in a variety of tissue sites including the Kupffer cell (Novikoff and Essner, 1960), alveolar macrophage (Karer, 1958), peritoneal macrophage (North, 1966), and cells from spleen and lymph nodes (Weiss, 1964). The overall structure is basically similar in all tissues and varies from the blood monocyte in terms of the mass and contents of the cytoplasm (Fig. 3). In general, the Golgi apparatus, situated in the nuclear hof, is more highly developed and contains multiple stacks of lamellae and numerous tiny, smooth surfaced vesicles. The rough endoplasmic reticulum is found most abundantly at the cell periphery and on that side of the nucleus opposite to the Golgi complex. There is often marked variation in the amount of rough ER contained in cells from different sources and even among the same population. Dense cytoplasmic granules are usually prominent and may be quite variable in composition. Alveolar macrophages, especially in animals exposed to respiratory irritants, typically reveal exuberant development of dense bodies.

Many, if not all, of the dense granules are thought to be secondary lysosomes and are probably derived from fusion of the various components of the vacuolar apparatus, i.e., endocytic vacuoles, primary lysosomes budding

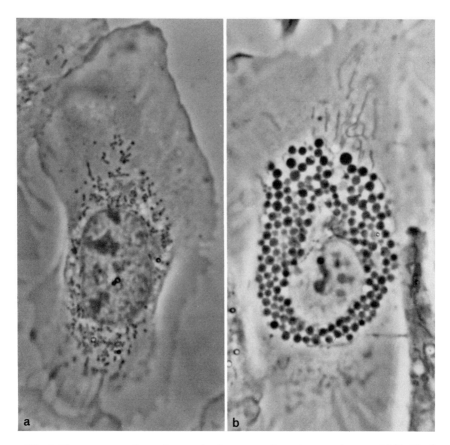

Fig. 2. Phase-contrast photomicrograph of mouse peritoneal macrophages. × 2,040. Fixed with 1.25 % glutaraldehyde. (a) Cell obtained from the unstimulated peritoneal cavity which was allowed to spread on a cover slip for 60 minutes. Pseudopods have been extended, and slight ruffling has occurred. The majority of phase-dense organelles clustered about the nucleus are mitochondria. (b) Twenty-four hours after cultivation in 50 % calf serum marked changes have taken place. The cell area is now increased and filamentous mitochondria have migrated into the pseudopods. The perinuclear area is now engorged with phase-dense granules which represent secondary lysosomes. The clear zone adjacent to the nuclear "hof" is the location of the Golgi complex.

Fig. 3. Electron micrograph of a rabbit alveolar macrophage. × 13,500. The cytoplasm (upper) is filled with a morphologically heterogeneous population of lysosomes (L), arranged in a rosette about the Golgi apparatus (Go). The vesicular compartments of the Golgi are most prominent in this section. Rough-surfaced endoplasmic reticulum is arranged about the cell periphery and pinocytic vesicles are also present. Higher magnification (lower) of perinuclear region illustrating the association of lysosomes (L) and Golgi (Go) saccules. The lysosomes vary considerably in electron density. N, nucleus.

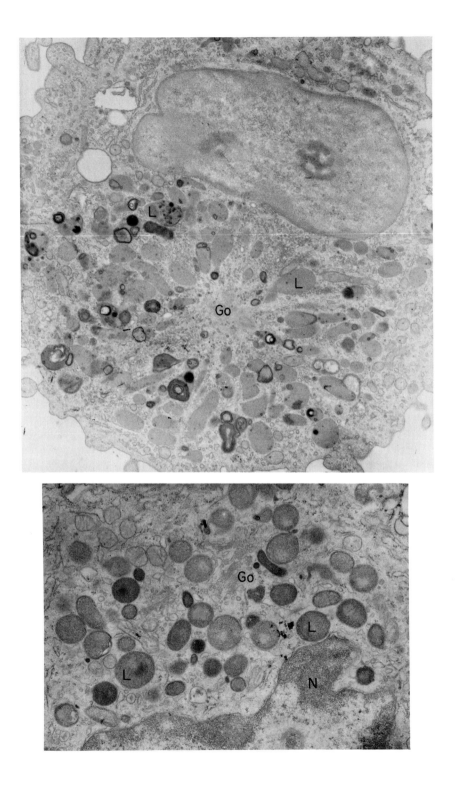

from the Golgi, and other secondary lysosomes (see Section IV). Multivesicular bodies and membrane-bound myelin figures are also seen and may have two possible origins. The first is a heterophagic event in which membrane-containing structures are engulfed by the cell, and the second is an autophagic process which can also be induced experimentally by chloroquin (Fedorko et al., 1968a,b) and Tris buffer (Steinman and Cohn, 1972a). In autophagy, a portion of the macrophage cytoplasm, including mitochondria, endoplasmic reticulum, etc., is enveloped by a pinocytic vacuole or lysosome and surrounded and subsequently degraded within a membrane-bounded structure. In other cases, it appears that small invaginations of the vacuole wall occur, pinch off, and result in multivesicular bodies. It, therefore, appears that both heterophagic and autophagic phenomena can lead to the same morphological end result. Unless one can employ appropriate markers and follow the life history of these organelles, it is difficult, if not impossible, to state their origin with certainty.

Microtubules and microfilaments have been observed in macrophages. A full description of their relative numbers, orientation, and distribution is not available at this time. Clusters of microtubules are found in the centriolar area (Bhisey and Freed, 1971a) and are also seen in pseudopods running longitudinally in association with similarly oriented mitochondria (J. G. Hirsch and Z. A. Cohn, unpublished observations). Low concentrations of colchicine disrupt the polarization of cytoplasmic organelles in macrophages such that pseudopods retract, mitochondria are distributed randomly, and endocytic vacuoles no longer flow centripetally (Bhisey and Freed, 1971b). Presumably these effects are secondary to drug-induced disruption of microtubules. Little is known about macrophage microfilaments or the effects of cytochalasin, a drug known to alter microfilaments in other systems. Preliminary observations by Reaven and Axline (1973) reveal that cultivated macrophages do have a system of microfilaments that lies beneath the cell surface and is sensitive to cytochalasin B.

F. Epithelioid and Giant Cells

Epithelioid and giant cells arise from inflammatory macrophages. The highly phagocytic macrophage undergoes nuclear and cytoplasmic changes during the course of a granulomatous response or under in vitro culture conditions (Sutton and Weiss, 1966; Dumont and Shelden, 1965; Gusek, 1964; Wanstrup and Christensen, 1966). In many cases the nucleus becomes elongated, a response which may reflect the tight packing of cells in the granuloma and subsequent elongation of the cytoplasm. Slim cytoplasmic extensions are formed, and these are tightly intertwined with adjacent epithelioid cells. In addition, the cytoplasm contains more mitochondria and fewer dense bodies.

The giant cell of the granuloma appears to result from the fusion of pre-existing macrophages. Following fusion the nuclei become oriented in a peripheral fashion and the cytoplasmic organelles are mixed in the central zone (Hirsch *et al.*, 1966). This results in multicentric Golgi complexes and a corresponding increase in mitochondria and other cytoplasmic organelles. This reorganization has been followed by phase-contrast cinematography and can be prevented by colchicine, implying that the organization of giant cell organelles is dependent on intact microtubules (Gordon and Cohn, 1970). The factors involved in the induction of giant cell formation are not resolved nor have specific functions been related to the syncytium.

IV. Maturation

Beginning with the first definable member of the mononuclear phagocytes, the promonocyte, there is an overall scheme of maturation or differentiation which eventually leads to the formation of highly active tissue macrophages. The morphological and chemical events underlying this sequence will be reviewed in this section, and it will be apparent that many gaps exist in our knowledge. Much of this information came initially from observations on cell populations in intact animals, although more recently it has been possible to reproduce and analyze these events in a tissue culture environment.

A. Morphological Observations

Since many of the details concerning the structure of these cells have been described in other sections of this chapter, only those modifications linked with functional changes will be reviewed. As one progresses from the pro-monocyte to macrophage, nuclear size decreases, nucleoli become small and rudimentary, and progressively larger amounts of heterochromatin are observed. These alterations are in keeping with the decreased mitotic potential of the series and the fixation of the macrophage in a prolonged G_0 state. These changes are reversible, however, and in the presence of conditioned medium (Virolainen and Defendi, 1967), or when placing the G_0 nucleus in the cytoplasm of a dividing cell by induced viral fusion (Harris, 1966; Gordon and Cohn, 1970, 1971a,b), nuclear changes are reversed and DNA synthesis is initiated. Perhaps the most striking alterations occur in the content and distribution of cytoplasmic organelles. Initially the monocyte contains a few azurophilic granules derived from the Golgi apparatus and in some species containing peroxidase (Nichols *et al.*, 1971; van Furth *et al.*, 1970). Following the conversion to macrophages, these granules are lost and are no longer synthesized by the macrophage. They are, however, replaced by a new population of organelles, quite heterogeneous in ultrastructure and characterized by a limiting unit membrane and large amounts of acid hydrolases. These organelles have been identified as lysosomes (Cohn and Wiener, 1963a) and arise as the result of endocytic activity (Cohn and Fedorko, 1969). They contain, therefore, in addition to digestive enzymes, a wide spectrum of extracellular molecules to which the cell is exposed. Because these materials are both taken up and digested at different rates, their accumulation in the digestive vocuoles has a marked influence on the untrastructure of the granule matrix. The number and size of secondary lysosomes in mature macrophages is quite variable for similar reasons.

Another corollary of maturation is the development of the Golgi complex and the formation of multiple stacks of smooth membraned sacs and associated vesicles in the perinuclear region. The appearance of a highly developed Golgi apparatus is correlated with the formation of lysosomes. It is thought likely that the Golgi vesicle is the primary lysosome of the macrophage, which carries newly synthesized hydrolytic enzymes from their origin in the rough ER to endocytic or autophagic vacuoles. The evidence for this statement will be presented in a later section.

Other alterations involve the system of microfilaments and microtubules present in the cytoplasm. With increasing maturity and particularly in macrophages which are adherent to surfaces, larger numbers of microtubules are present and radiate from the centrioles into the thinner projections of pseudopods. Furthermore, small bands of microfilaments are seen beneath the plasma membrane in both an oriented and nonoriented state (Reaven and Axline, 1973). The function of these filaments has not been clarified at this time.

Finally, there are modifications in the plasma membrane associated with advancing differentiation. Structurally, the plasma membrane shows no changes when visualized in thin sections of osmium fixed cells. What is quite apparent, however, is an increased activity of the membrane which is expressed as an increasing number of surface projections. These increase the surface area of the cell and are often associated with the formation of pinocytic or phagocytic vacuoles.

B. Biochemistry of Maturation

Little detailed information has accrued on the biochemistry of the promonocyte, largely because of our inability to harvest and purify these cells in sufficient quantities. Most of this section will therefore deal with properties of the isolated monocyte and modification in its energy producing pathways and synthetic capabilities as it becomes a macrophage.

Monocytes and macrophages derive energy from both respiratory and glycolytic pathways. Early studies by Vanotti (1961) and Frei *et al.* (1961) using mixed populations of blood leukocytes indicated that monocytes had a relatively high rate of aerobic glycosis. This exceeded that of polymorphonuclear leukocytes by a factor of 1.5 and was approximately threefold greater than lymphocyte glycolysis. More recently, Bennett and Cohn (1966) evaluated glucose utilization and lactate production in isolated homogeneous populations of horse monocytes maintained in a tissue culture environment. As these cells matured into typical macrophages, in the absence of cell division, there was a twofold increase in lactate formation. Under the same conditions, the levels of a constitutive mitochondrial enzyme, cytochrome oxidase, also doubled after 72 hours of cultivation. Although no detailed studies on the oxygen consumption of isolated monocytes has been reported, it seems likely that comparable changes would also take place during maturation.

Most investigators studying carbohydrate metabolism of the macrophage have employed relatively pure populations of cells obtained from induced peritoneal exudates or alveolar macrophages from bronchial lavages (Stahelin *et al.*, 1956; Oren *et al.*, 1963; West *et al.*, 1968). In general, all these cells exhibit active glycolytic and respiratory pathways, the rates of which are higher than polymorphonuclear luekocytes. When compared, the alveolar macrophage was more active on a cell basis and its rate of oxygen consumption was threefold greater than cells obtained from the peritoneal cavity. Glucose utilization through the hexose monophosphate shunt pathway was minimal and accounted for less than 2% of the total.

In interpreting these experiments, consideration should be given to cytoplasmic mass and the relative enrichment in organelles. For example, the alveolar macrophage is a much larger cell than the oil- or glycogen-induced peritoneal cell and is particularly enriched in its apparent number of mitochondria. In view of its close contact with high oxygen environments, it is possible that this factor might influence the formation of mitochondria and therefore the metabolic properties of the population. Other examples of the adaptive response of mononuclear phagocytes to their micro environments will be outlined in subsequent sections.

C. Lysosomal Enzymes

Perhaps the most extensively studied enzymatic correlate of maturation are the intracellular levels of acid hydrolases. These enzymes, packaged within membrane systems, are of critical importance in the degradation of ingested material and are therefore related to many of the roles these cells play in body economy. Table II outlines certain enzymes that are associated with macrophage lysosomes. The list is less extensive than that described for rat liver, probably because the assays have not been carried out. It should be pointed out that many of these enzymes are present in multiple molecular forms and that none have been purified and adequately characterized in terms of substrate specificity. As described by Axline (1968), the acid phosphatases of the rabbit alveolar macrophages are present as five distinct forms on acrylamide gels. Approximately 60% of the activity can be released from the lysosomes by physical means, and these turn out to be of lower molecular weights. The remainder can only be solubilized with surfactants and suggests that they are more firmly bound to the lysosomal membrane.

The typical acid hydrolases are localized to membrane-bounded dense bodies of the cell and exhibit the property of latency. Enzymatic activity is markedly enhanced by agents which disrupt the integrity of the lysosomal membrane, thereby allowing the interaction of substrates with their respective enzymes. By means of differential centrifugation, the majority of the lysosomal enzymes are pelleted in the large granule fraction where they are mixed with mitochondria (Cohn and Weiner, 1963a). These organelles can be separated from mitochondria by means of isopycnic sucrose gradient centrifugation. This is particularly easy in the alveolar macrophage, where secondary lysosomes are quite dense. Gradients from these cells, employing the large granule fraction as starting material, exhibit two main protein peaks. The peak that equilibrates at a sucrose density of approximately 1.19 contains mitochondria and the bulk of mitochondrial enzymes, such as cytochrome oxidase. In contrast, a denser peak at 1.25 is the locus of six acid hydrolases and contains the electron-dense granules seen in the intact cell. Not all macrophage populations contain such dense lysosomes. For example, casein- or peptone-induced mouse or rabbit peritoneal macrophages contain lysosomes which overlap in density with mitochondria and cannot be readily separated (Z. A. Cohn, unpublished). This is in large part

TABLE II

ACID HYDROLASES OF MACROPHAGES

Acid Phosphatase	β-N-Acetyl glucosaminidase
"Acid Nucleotidase"	Cholesterol esterase
Acid Ribonuclease	Lipase
Acid Deoxyribonucleose	
Arylsulfatase	Cathepsin D
β-Galactosidase	BPN Hydrolase (? cathepsin D)
α-Glucosidase	Lysozyme
β-Glucuronidase	Hyaluronidase

caused by the storage of exogenous materials within the lysosome which alters their density (de Duve and Wattiaux, 1966).

The localization of enzymes within the lysosome can also be inferred from cytochemical studies. Although a less extensive armamentarium of techniques is available, many authors have commented on the discrete localization of acid phosphatase and arylsulfatase at both the light and electron microscopic level. The majority of the reaction product is found within the confines of the secondary lysosomes or digestive bodies, although, as we will discuss later, portions of the Golgi complex are often positive. Reaction product is rarely seen over the endoplasmic reticulum, plasma membrane, or mitochondria.

A number of studies employing both cytochemical (Weiss and Fawcett, 1953; Dannenberg *et al.*, 1963; Dannenberg and Bennett, 1964) and biochemical techniques (Suter and Hullinger, 1960; Cohn and Wiener, 1963a; Myrvik *et al.*, 1961) have documented that the level of lysosomal enzymes differs among macrophage populations and that in general the level is greater in the more mature or "activated" cells. A comparison with blood monocytes (Bennett and Cohn, 1966) is even more striking and suggests that an increase in hydrolases is a concomitant of maturation. To examine this question in more detail, studies were performed with homogeneous populations of cells maintained under tissue culture conditions. For this purpose one could employ isolated blood monocytes or the rather immature mononuclear phagocyte found in the unstimulated mouse peritoneal cavity (Bennett and Cohn, 1966; Cohn and Benson, 1965a). Because of the relative ease with which one could obtain the mouse peritoneal cell, most experiments were performed with this cell type. Table III illustrates the influence of *in vitro* cultivation on the hydrolase levels of mouse peritoneal cells under optimum conditions. It is apparent that marked increases occur and that these take place in the absence of appreciable cell division. Since this rise in total enzyme level occurs under conditions in which total cell protein is also increasing, the specific activity (units/mg protein) is about twofold less. It should be pointed out that this type of experiment is very difficult to carry out with either guinea pig or rabbit exudate cells because large numbers of macrophages are lost during *in vitro* cultivation.

The accumulation of intracellular digestive enzymes requires ongoing protein synthesis (Cohn and Benson, 1965b) and is largely the result of new enzyme formation. However, modifications in the degradation of hydrolases may also play some role. Under these conditions the level of hydrolases is clearly related to the extent of pinocytic activity (Cohn and Benson, 1965c). The more extensive the formation of pinocytic vesicles, the higher the levels of hydrolases. This was not the result of nonspecific nutritional effects of serum and could be reproduced by adding inducers of pinocytosis to in-

TABLE III

PERCENT INCREASES IN TOTAL MACROPHAGES ACID
HYDROLASES FOLLOWING 72 HOURS *IN VITRO*
CULTIVATION[a]

Enzyme	% Increase
Acid phosphatase	2000–3500
Cholesterol esterase	1000–1200
β-Glucuronidase	600–900
Cathepsin D	500–800
β-N-Acetyl glucosaminidase	500–700
β-Galactosidase	300–600
Acid ribonuclease	300–500
Aryl sulfatase	400–600

[a]Cultivated in 50% newborn calf serum, TC No. 199.

inactive sera (Cohn and Parks, 1967b). Similarly, depressing pinocytic activity to low levels leads to a loss in total enzyme activity (Cohn and Benson, 1965c) without significant extracellular release of enzymes. These results suggested a significant turnover of lysosomal enzymes and differential rates of their intralysosomal inactivation.

The correlation between pinocytic activity and hydrolase levels suggested at least two possibilities. The first was that exogenous substrates controlled digestive enzyme levels, and the second that the interiorization of plasma membrane might play a significant role. To distinguish between these possibilities, Axline and Cohn (1970) employed the phagocytosis of larger particles. Macrophages were then allowed to ingest equal numbers of a digestible (RBC) and nondigestible particle (polystyrene) of equal diameter. This ensured that approximately the same amount of plasma membrane was interiorized to form the phagocytic vacuoles after a 1-hour pulse. The results indicated that the ingestion of erythrocytes led to a significant increase in hydrolases, whereas no alteration was observed after phagocytosis of latex. This suggests that the uptake of digestible macromolecules in some way stimulates the accumulation of digestive enzymes. There is as yet no suggestion that specific substrate-mediated induction takes place. In fact, the phagocytosis of aggregated proteins leads to an increase in a variety of hydrolases not related to their intracellular fate.

These studies suggest that the content of lysosomal enzymes in the macrophage is adaptively controlled by their endocytic activity. The more high molecular weight substrates entering the cell by bulk transport, the higher the intracellular level of digestive enzymes. Presumably, under *in vivo* conditions, macrophages may be able to undergo repeated cycles of hydrolase formation and destruction in response to environmental stimuli. Such activity is of obvious benefit to the host in terms of one of its longer lived phagocytic cells.

D. Lysosome Formation and the Intracellular Distribution of Hydrolases

During maturation of the macrophage and as acid hydrolases accumulate within the cell, there is a concomitant increase in the number of cytoplasmic granules or dense bodies which have the properties of lysosomes (Fig. 2). In this section we will review the evidence concerning the origin of these structures as well as the flow and redistribution of newly synthesized enzymes within the cell.

Studies on the origin of the digestive granule or secondary lysosome come from combined morphological and cytochemical observations (Cohn and Benson, 1965c) on living cultured macrophages. Under the phase-contrast microscope, it was apparent that soon after explanting macrophages they began to extend pseudopods and spread out on the glass surface. In the presence of high levels of calf serum, pinocytosis was induced and phase-lucent vesicles could be seen arising from the peripheral cytoplasm. These vesicles flowed toward the perinuclear region and were seen to congregate in the peri-Golgi area. During the centripetal movement of vesicles, they sometimes fused with one another to yield larger phase-lucent vacuoles, and a similar process continued in the Golgi zone. By means of time-lapse cinematography, it was possible to follow the fate of newly formed pinosomes. Within a period as short as 90 minutes, only those pinocytic vesicles in the Golgi region underwent modifications in density. The end result was a spherical phase-dense granule which was somewhat smaller than the initial lucent vesicle. With more prolonged cultivation, a larger population of these granules accumulated in the centrosphere region, and it was apparent that pinosomes were continually fusing with these structures. When cells were stained for acid phosphatase, a lysosomal marker, none of the more peripherally located lucent vesicles contained reaction product. In contrast, the denser granules in the centrosphere area were uniformly positive. Similar observations have been made with the electron microscope on static material, and the morphological and cytochemical conclusions were similar (Cohn et al., 1966). This indicated that endocytic vesicles formed from the plasma membrane were being converted to secondary lysosomes or digestive bodies in the vicinity of the Golgi apparatus. Enzymes of a lysosomal nature were presumably transferred at this cytoplasmic site.

The mechanism by which enzyme transfer occurred was revealed by electron microscopy and concomitant autoradiography (Cohn et al., 1966; Hirsch et al., 1968). Particular interest was focused on the Golgi region in view of the prior findings of Novikoff *et al.* (1964). Examination of thin sections of cultured macrophages showed the presence of a large Golgi zone composed of multiple stacks of smooth surfaced membranes or saccules and large numbers of small vesicles which appeared to be budding from the ends of the saccules. In many instances the tiny Golgi vesicles were seen in the act of fusing with the electron-lucent pinocytic vacuoles which had been previously marked with an electron-dense colloid. Interactions with other membrane-bounded organelles such as mitochondria and endoplasmic reticulum were never seen. This suggested that the Golgi vesicle might be the primary lysosome of the macrophage, an organelle carrying newly synthesized hydrolases that was a carrier between the point of synthesis and the digestive body.

Two other pieces of information indicate that this is probably the case. The first comes from electron microscopic cytochemistry in which reaction product for acid phosphatase is prominent in the saccules and vesicles of the Golgi complex and suggests that packaging of enzymes takes place in this site (Nichols *et al.*, 1971). The second comes from autoradiographic techniques following short pulse-chase experiments with tritiated leucine. Under conditions in which the amount of incorporated amino acid remains constant, there are marked shifts in the intracellular localization of newly synthesized protein. Grains are first seen over the rough surfaced endoplasmic reticulum (RER), the site of synthesis. With time into the chase period, grains disappear over the RER and accumulate in the Golgi region. Thereafter, the majority of grains are localized over the dense granules or secondary lysosomes. This suggested an intracellular flow of newly synthesized protein from the RER, through the Golgi complex, and eventually segregation in the secondary lysosome.

In addition to the formation of secondary lysosomes through the conversion of endocytic or heterophagic vacuoles, the macrophage also demonstrates formation through autophagy. In this case, portions of the macrophage cytoplasm may be segregated within membrane systems and exposed to digestive enzymes. This may occur in two forms, depending on the size of the object which is surrounded, i.e., micro- and macroautophagy. Under supposedly normal or physiological circumstances, autophagic vacuoles may be occasionally observed *in vivo* and after *in vitro* cultivation. Under the electron microscope, they exhibit a peripheral unit membrane and may contain all sorts of cytoplasmic organelles, i.e., mitochondria, lipid droplets, and endoplasmic reticulum, as well as cytochemically demonstrable acid hydrolases. The extent to which autophagy occurs in the macrophage may be influenced by the use of drugs. Perhaps the best studied example comes from the work of Fedorko *et al.* (1968a,b) on the effects of the antimalarial agent chloroquine. Exposure of cells to microgram quantities of chloroquine is followed by the rapid fusion of preexisting secondary lysosomes to form large lucent vacuoles containing acid hydrolases. Certain evidence suggests that Golgi-derived vesicles also take part in this initial reaction. The membrane of the newly formed "toxic vacuoles" is rather flexible and in many instances can be seen to invaginate deeply into the vacuole. During this process, cytosol and cytoplasmic organelles enter the confines of the vacuole and are then trapped when the pedicle pinches off. This leaves a double-membraned structure which is rapidly transformed to a typical autophagosome on destruction of the inner membrane. The contents of the autophagic vacuole are then degraded by the contained hydrolases, at a rate determined by the nature of the substrates.

Evidence presented by Hirsch et al. (1968) suggest that "microautophagy" may be the mechanism underlying the formation of multivesicular bodies. In this instance, tiny invaginations of endocytic vacuole membrane take place, resulting in the transient presence of vesicles within the larger vacuole. This process could, depending on its extent, result in the transfer of significant amounts of cytosol constituents into digestive bodies and probably adds to the heterogeneous composition of secondary lysosomes.

Figure 4 reviews some of the pathways for the formation of primary and secondary lysosomes in macrophages and points out the extensive membrane fusions which can occur and which serve to mix exogenous and endogenous substrates with hydrolytic enzymes.

V. Endocytosis

The ability of macrophages to interiorize exogenous molecules of both soluble and particulate nature is highly developed and sets them apart from many other tissue cells with similar, but less pronounced, activities. In fact, it is this ability, recognized for the past century, which has distinguished them from other members of the immune system and allowed earlier cytologists a convenient handle through their use of vital dyes, colloids, and particulates. In contrast to the other "professional phagocyte," the neutrophilic leukocyte, the macrophage has a much wider spectrum of molecules which it can take up. In particular, it can ingest particles smaller than 0.1 μm as well as soluble molecules, whereas the neutrophil is ineffective in this size range. Figure 5 schematically outlines the endocytic activity of macrophages and the range of molecules which it can sequester and concentrate in its cytoplasm. The term pinocytosis or "cell drinking" is employed to characterize the uptake of soluble molecules and phagocytosis or "cell

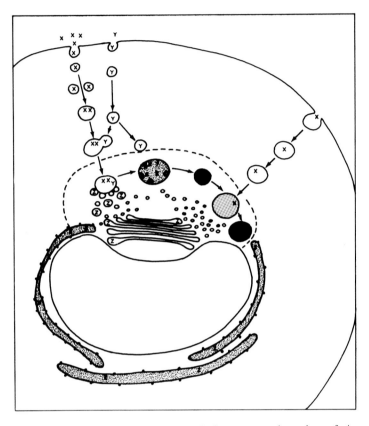

Fig. 4. A schematic representation of endocytosis, lysosomes, and membrane fusions which occur in the macrophage. Exogenous molecules (X) and (Y) are sequestered within vacuoles, derived from the plasma membrane, and transferred into the perinuclear area (---). Newly synthesized proteins, including hydrolytic enzymes (Z), are produced in the cisternae of the rough endoplasmic reticulum, transferred to the Golgi complex, and packaged into Golgi-derived vesicles or primary lysosomes. Fusion of primary lysosomes with endocytic vacuoles mixes hydrolases and exogenous substrates, giving rise to the digestive body or secondary lysosome. These structures may become more condensed. The secondary lysosome may continue to accept exogenous substrates derived from pinocytosis or may fuse with a larger phagocytic vacuole, converting it into a digestive body.

eating" for the uptake of particles. In certain instances this is a somewhat arbitrary definition, and the exact size of molecules, which distinguishes the two processes, is uncertain. For the purposes of this discussion, inert colloids with particles smaller than 100 Å will serve as the dividing line. Reviews by Rabinovitch (1968) and North (1970c) should be consulted for a more comprehensive view of the field.

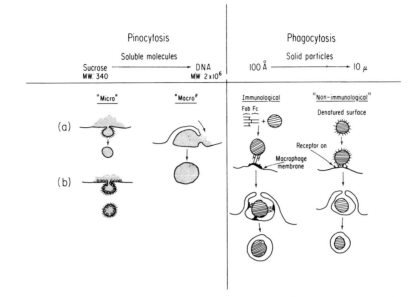

Fig. 5. A schematic representation of endocytic mechanisms in the macrophage. During the process of pinocytosis, exogenous molecules too large to penetrate the plasma membrane are interiorized by vesicle formation. These may be as small as sucrose or as large as DNA. "Micro" pinocytosis refers to the formation of tiny coated vesicles. These vesicles as well as those derived by "Macro" pinocytosis may encompass all molecules in the cell's environment, (a) or if these are bound to the plasma membrane, (b) they are selectively interiorized. Macro-pinocytosis is the most evident form in macrophages and requires the active motion or motility of the cell surface.

Two examples of phagocytosis dependent on separate surface receptors are illustrated on the right. Under "Immunological" recognition, an erythrocyte is coated with IgG molecules which bind to its surface through the Fab piece. The Fc piece is free to interact with receptors on the macrophage plasma membrane. This stimulates interiorization although not necessarily by means of cell-surface extensions as illustrated. The "Non-Immunological" series exemplifies the binding of denatured surfaces, i.e., damaged or aldehyde-treated RBC, to the macrophage membrane.

A. Pinocytosis

The process of pinocytosis was first described by Warren Lewis (1931) in his studies of cultured monocytes and subsequently observed in many other cell types. Very little can be added to his morphological description of the mechanism by which macrophages interiorize fluid-filled droplets. Of particular significance were his observations that phase-lucent vesicles arose from areas of membrane movement or ruffling and then moved centripetally into the perinuclear region. This is the predominant form of pinocytic vesicle formation as seen under the light microscope and the one about which we have the most information. In addition, under the electron microscope, tiny pits or caveolae are formed which give rise to smaller pinosomes, which are similar in structure to the pinocytic vesicles described in endothelial cells (Bruns and Palade, 1968). The control of this type of "micropinocytosis" in the macrophage is unclear and will not be considered in this chapter.

1. ENERGY REQUIREMENTS

Employing cultivated mouse macrophages, studies have been conducted on the metabolic determinants of the process (Cohn, 1966). These have used morphological criteria for assessing pinocytosis and are based on the number of newly formed vesicles. It should be pointed out that the uptake of labeled macromolecules can also be used as an index of pinocytic activity. These procedures vary in large measure on whether or not the compound is bound to the plasma membrane prior to interiorization, whereas the vesicle count method gives an estimate of the interiorization of membrane. From this work it is evident that pinocytosis is a temperature- and energy-dependent process. Although the "Q_{10}" of vesicle formation is approximately 3.0, complete obliteration of pinocytosis requires temperatures of 4°C or less. When the temperature is again raised to 37°C, vesicle formation is usually initiated promptly. The energy requirements for the process have thus far been studied only in the cultivated mouse macrophage. Agents which inhibit the respiratory chain, e.g., anaerobiosis, cyanide, and antimycin A, reduce activity in a dose-dependent fashion with maximum inhibition of 90%. Similar results are obtained with inhibitors of oxidative phosphorylation. Vesicle formation is also inhibited by high levels of fluoride and iodoacetate, but to a smaller extent. In addition, there appears to be a requirement for ongoing protein synthesis. Concentrations of puromycin and cycloheximide, which inhibit amino acid incorporation by at least 75%, depress vesicle formation after a lag period of 15–30 minutes. It is not clear whether or not these proteins are needed for the formation of new plasma membrane.

Some of the above pinocytic inhibitors are known blockers of mitochondrial energy production and suggest an important role of this organelle in pinocytic activity. This possibility is reinforced by direct observations of the process in living cells. One is struck by the peripheral orientation of mitochondria in pseudopods, often in close proximity to the undulating membrane. It is almost always in areas rich in mitochondria that vesicle formation is initiated. From unpublished observations, the maintenance and orientation of mitochondria in macrophage pseudopods is associated with the presence of cytoplasmic microtubules. Agents such as colcemid and vinblastine, which depolymerize peripheral microtubules, produce a retraction of mitochondria into the central cell body. At this time, membrane ruffling and pinocytic activity ceases in the peripheral cytoplasm. Similarly, inhibitors of respiration and oxidative phosphorylation also decrease membrane undulations and pinocytic activity. It seems likely, therefore, that membrane movement is a critical determinant of pinocytic activity in the macrophage.

2. INDUCTION OF PINOCYTOSIS

Studies by Cohn and Parks (1967a,b,c) have categorized a number of exogenous molecules which stimulate the pinocytic activity of mouse macrophages. These represent what appear to be both nonspecific and specific molecules which under *in vitro* situations are capable of increasing the formation of pinocytic vesicles. It should be pointed out that we have no clear idea of the factors which regulate pinocytosis under *in vivo* conditions. Some of the agents to be described are found in inflammatory environments and may play a concerted role in stimulating macrophages.

A large number of anionic molecules have the ability to induce vesicle formation. Some of these are outlined in Table IV. In contrast, neutral

TABLE IV

MACROANIONIC INDUCERS OF PINOCYTOSIS

Compound	Minimal effective concentration (μg/ml)	Maximal stimulating effect (control = 1.0)
Albumin	1,200	14
Albumin (defatted)	50,000	2
Fetuin	500	12
Fetuin (minus sialic acid)	6,500	1.3
β-Lactoglobulin	10,000	6
Bovine γ-globulin	10,000	4
Polyglutamic acid	10	17
Polylysine	—	1.2
L-Glutamic acid	1,200	6.5
L-Aspartic acid	1,200	7.2
Dextran (2×10^6 MW)	50,000	1.5
Dextran-SO$_4$ (2×10^6 MW)	0.1	22
Dextran-SO$_4$ (5×10^6 MW)	10	16
Ficoll	50,000	4
Hyaluronic acid	3	10
Chondroitin sulfate C	4	11
Heparin	10	10
RNA (yeast)	100	12
DNA (thymus)	2	12

macromolecules are relatively ineffective and produce only a small degree of stimulation at high concentrations. Cationic agents such as polylysine and DEAE dextran are quite toxic, but at concentrations which do not lyse cells they are without stimulatory effects. These agents do, however, bind to the macrophage membrane (Seljelid *et al.*, 1973) or may complex anionic molecules in the environment. Such complexes formed either in the medium or on the cell surface may then be ingested by phagocytosis. In general, the pinocytosis-inducing properties of anions is a function of molecular weight; the higher the molecular weight, the more potent the compound.

A second class of agents produce marked increases in vesicle formation and result in increased spreading of the macrophage on glass surfaces. Adenosine, as well as its 5′-mono-, di-, and triphosphates, exert such an effect (Cohn and Parks, 1967b). It seems probable that the phosphorylated compounds are initially dephosphorylated to the nucleoside and then enter the cell. Their subsequent fate is not clearly known; however, rephosphorylation is likely to occur, and intracellular high energy intermediates may then exert an influence on both spreading and vesicle formation.

A third class of agents functions on an immunological basis (Cohn and Parks, 1967c). Antibodies directed against macrophage membrane constituents, in the absence of hemolytic complement, have a markedly stimulatory effect on both membrane ruffling and pinocytic vesicle formation. Linear dose–response relationships exist, but at high levels of antibody, pinocytosis is progressively inhibited. When complement is present in the system, lysis of the membrane occurs rapidly. This influence of plasma membrane-directed antibody on the stimulation of pinocytosis should be kept in mind when dealing with cells such as the lymphocyte. Macrophages cultured in the presence of low levels of antibody exhibit more extensive secondary lysosome formation and increased levels of intracellular hydrolytic enzymes, presumably as the result of increased substrate interiorization.

B. Phagocytosis

The process of particle ingestion may be separated into two distinct phases. The first encompasses a group of specific and nonspecific interactions of the particle to the external surface of the plasma membrane and will be referred to as "attachment." The second phase involves the interiorization of the particle and includes membrane fusion and the formation of the phagocytic vacuole or phagosome. In some instances these phases can be clearly separated (Rabinovitch, 1967a,b).

Macrophages, because of their location in the organism, are constantly exposed to a number of "physiological" particles and clearly serve an important role on the basis of their phagocytic activity. Such particles include chylomicra, effete erythrocytes, and many other injured or dead cells. In addition, under pathological situations they encounter a wide variety of foreign materials which are recognized and engulfed.

1. METABOLIC REQUIREMENTS

Other chapters in this volume will detail the biochemical requirements and consequences of phagocytosis. In this section we wish to compare the requirements of phagocytosis and pinocytosis in the mouse macrophages, the only cell in which this comparison has as yet been made. It is clear that agents which interfere with respiration and oxidative phosphorylation have only a minor influence on the phagocytic activity of this cell (Cohn, 1970) although pinocytic activity is markedly depressed. In contrast, agents which interfere with glycolysis, including fluoride, iodoacetate, and 2-deoxyglucose, have significant inhibitory activity. Trypsinization of the cell surface interferes with pinocytic activity, reduces the ruffling movement of the membrane, but does not influence the uptake of erythrocytes or bacteria. Membrane motility therefore appears to be of less consequence to the uptake of particles and suggests a more prominent role for plasma membrane receptors in this process.

2. CELL SURFACE RECEPTORS

A large number of studies have now documented that the macrophage surface can distinguish different types of particles (Berken and Benacerraf, 1966; Lo Buglio *et al.*, 1967; Huber *et al.*, 1968; Lay and Nussenzweig, 1968; Rabinovitch, 1968). At the present time at least three binding sites which behave as functional receptors have been categorized. The first recognizes the Fc portion of IgG and is apparently responsible for the attachment of cytophilic antibody to macrophage surfaces. It is a particularly useful receptor in that it is expressed for long periods by cultivated cells and is resistant to the action of trypsin. Little is known about its topography on the plasma membrane or its chemical determinants; however, recent studies on isolated macrophage membranes suggest a more direct approach to this problem (Nachman *et al.*, 1971a,b). This receptor is expressed in macrophage–melanoma cell heterokaryons (Gordon and Cohn, 1971c) for some time. However, the phagocytic activity of the heterokaryons is subsequently lost as the result of "masking" by a melanoma-derived protein. Trypsinization of the heterokaryons removes this substance and their phagocytic activity returns to normal levels (Gordon and Cohn, 1971c). In these instances, immunoglobulin-coated erythrocytes can be shown to bind tightly to the macrophage surface and binding requires an intact Fc piece. It is possible that after an antigen–antibody interaction conformational changes occur which are then recognized by the macrophage receptors (Uhr, 1965). Further studies of this question are required. Of some interest are the recent studies of Rabinovitch (1969) pointing out that the Fc receptor is not present on cultured fibroblasts and indicating that the ingestion by "non-professional phagocytes" is in fact inhibited by the presence of immunoglobulin-coated particles.

A second class of receptors recognized complement components as described by Lay and Nussenzweig (1968). In this instance and in those of Rabinovitch (1967b), complement markedly enhances the ingestion of IgM-coated erythrocytes. In contrast, IgG coated RBC do not appear to require C'. Finally, Rabinovitch (1967a) has described receptors which recognize the surface of denatured particles such as aldehyde-treated red cells. These receptors appear to be less specific and may be found on a wider spectrum of phagocytic cells (Rabinovitch, 1969).

The dissociation of receptors has been reemphasized by the recent observations of Holland et al. (1972) In this case, antimembrane antibodies (IgG) bind to the macrophage surface and selectively inhibit receptors. For example, the Fc receptor is almost completely blocked and the cell is unable to ingest opsonized particles. However, it is quite capable of phago-cytizing aldehyde-treated red cells or polystyrene particles. Such approaches, employing specific antibodies as probes, should give us a better under-standing of membrane mosaicism and the mechanisms of phagocytosis in the macrophage.

3. Postphagocytic Events

Once the particle has been enclosed within a portion of the plasma mem-brane and the phagosome has formed, it then migrates into the central cell body. Here it may fuse with preexisting secondary lysosomes, and hydrolytic enzymes come in contact with the ingested particle (Cohn and Wiener, 1963b). The process of degranulation can be followed cytochemically by tracing enzymes such as acid phosphatase or by fractionation procedures in which the phagolysosomes can be isolated (Stossel et al., 1971). One example of the process is illustrated in Fig. 6, showing the fusion of a thoro-trast-filled secondary lysosome with a phagosome containing a polystyrene particle. Although the mechanism of membrane fusion is unknown, it is clear that there is specificity in the reaction. This is evidenced by the lack of fusion with either smooth or rough surfaced endoplasmic reticulum, mito-chondria, or lipid droplets. Fusion may take place with Golgi-derived vesicles which in this cell represent primary lysosomes.

Evidence from studies with bacteria and viruses (Silverstein, 1970) indicate that . viable microorganisms follow pathways similar to inert particles. Recent studies of Armstrong and D'Arcy Hart (1971) suggest

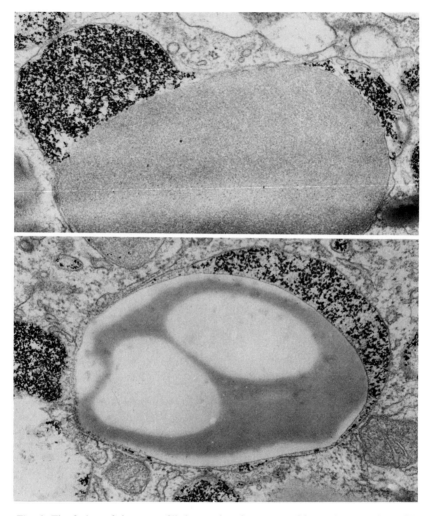

Fig. 6. The fusion of thorotrast-filled secondary lysosomes with a polystyrene latex-filled phagocytic vacuole. The upper micrograph illustrates the initial fusion process and continuity of membranes. The lower is somewhat later, and electron-dense thorotrast particles are migrating about the plastic particle.

that fusion with lysosomes may not always be a consequence of the phagocytic process. Employing cultivated mouse macrophages, they noted that virulent tubercle bacilli enclosed in a phagosome fail to fuse with preexisting secondary lysosomes. The evidence came from electron microscopic examination in which ferritin-labeled lysosomes did no discharge their contents into the phagocytic vacuole, nor did acid phosphatase activity appear in this structure. In contrast, dead or altered bacilli, as well as less virulent strains, underwent the usual cycle of events. This study points out another variable in the host–parasite interaction which deserves future consideration with other systems.

4. Intracellular Digestion

From the preceding section it should be clear that endocytized molecules, too large to permeate the plasma membrane, are segregated and concentrated within the membranes of secondary lysosomes. In this locus they are exposed to a wide variety of hydrolytic enzymes, which act in concert and are capable of degrading most biologically active molecules. Since the levels of these enzymes vary quite markedly, it is not surprising that there is a wide disparity in the rate of intracellular digestion. The extent of intralysosomal hydrolysis by macrophages is often underestimated, and it is only when a given enzyme is missing, as in an inborn error, does this become apparent. It should be realized, however, that most of the turnover of the constituents of blood cells, altered tissue cells, extracellular constituents, and perhaps plasma proteins is the result of mononuclear phagocyte activity.

Once a macromolecule is present within a digestive body, there does not appear to be a metabolic requirement for its degradation. Studies by Ehrenreich and Cohn (1967) were unable to demonstrate an effect of inhibitors of oxidative phosphorylation, glycolysis, or respiration on the degradation of iodinated albumin. Presumably, the lysosomal enzymes function in an acid milieu. The production and maintenance of a sufficiently high hydrogen ion concentration may very well be the result of metabolism, but this as yet has not been clearly demonstrated. A reduction in ambient temperature to 4°C does inhibit intralysosomal digestion and is easily reversed under *in vitro* conditions.

Most studies on the fate of pinocytized macromolecules have dealt with labeled proteins (Ehrenreich and Cohn, 1967, 1968a,b). Iodinated albumin which is taken up by the macrophage is degraded to small building blocks. Examination of the extracellular digestion products reveals the presence of monoiodotyrosine and free iodide, which presumably results from deiodination. No larger peptides or intact molecules are excreted into the cells' environment. Similar studies performed with [^{3}H]leucine-labeled hemoglobin (prepared in reticulocytes) gave identical results. In this case labeled leucine was the sole extracellular product. When nondigestible molecules are evaluated, i.e., [^{3}H]Dextran sulfate, 2×10^6 MW; [^{14}C]Inulin, cell-bound radioactivity remains constant for as long as 3 days of cultivation. In addition to illustrating the lack of degradation of these polysaccharides, it points out that bulk export of these macromolecules is not taking place to any significant extent. Experiments with nondigestible particles such as polystyrene and colloidal gold have given similar results and argue against any appreciable exocytosis in the cultivated macrophage.

The degradation of isotopically labeled bacteria and viruses have also been followed within the confines of both rabbit and mouse macrophages (Cohn, 1963a,b; Silverstein, 1970). Depending in part on the nature of the organism, extensive hydrolysis of microbial macromolecules may take place within the phagosome. In the case of susceptible bacteria, killing occurs rapidly and is followed by degradation. It is not at all clear whether or not hydrolases play any role in the initial bactericidal event. The initial lesion, however, appears to be in the bacterial membrane and is followed by the release of its acid soluble pool of small molecular weight metabolites. Later, hydrolysis of nucleic acids, proteins, and lipids takes place and acid soluble constituents are released into the medium. Depending on the nature of the extracellular milieu, some of the degradation products may be utilized by the macrophage for the synthesis of macromolecules. As mentioned in Section VI,B,2, the protein coat of many viruses may be stripped off within the confines of the phagosome (Silverstein, 1970). The viral genome, either DNA or double-stranded RNA, may then be released into the cytosol and initiate replication. However, when coated with antibody globulin, the virion is retained in the phagolysosome, and both the nucleic acid and proteins are digested. In general, highly organized molecules such as DNA are digested more slowly.

Studies by Cohn and Ehrenreich (1969) and Ehrenreich and Cohn (1969) have examined the nature of molecules which are able to permeate through the lysosomal membrane and enter the cytosol. For this purpose, nondigestible peptides containing D-amino acids and oligosaccharides have been employed. From this work it appears that most disaccharides with molecular weights above 300, i.e., sucrose, are taken up by pinocytosis, concentrated within lysosomes, and unable to freely diffuse through the membrane. In this case, as with β-glucosides, the macrophage lysosome does not contain a hydrolytic enzyme capable of splitting the glycosidic linkage. However, such enzymes when added to the cells' environment are pinocytized enter the sucrose filled vacuole, and then split the disaccharide to glucose and fructose residues. The monosaccharides, then, are able to penetrate the membrane and enter the ground cytoplasm. Similar studies with peptides indicate that tripeptides are retained within the lysosome, whereas most dipeptides and all amino acids escape quite readily. The dividing line occurs at a molecular weight of approximately 220. This suggests that the intralysosomal hydrolysis of proteins is quite extensive and only small molecular weight, nonimmunogenic molecules interact with cytosol constituents.

The escape of constituents from lysosomes probably depends on a variety of factors other than molecular weight and molal volume. For example, it seems that the heme moiety of hemoglobin is probably capable of entering the cytosol (Pimstone *et al.*, 1971) since the heme oxygenase necessary for its conversion to bilirubin is a microsomal enzyme.

Certain rather large planar molecules such as cholesterol may be exchanged across plasma and lysosomal membranes (Werb and Cohn, 1971a,b). Free cholesterol bound to serum lipoproteins is accepted by receptors on the macrophage plasma membrane and rapidly equilibrates with all cholesterol-containing cytomembranes, primarily of lysosomal origin. In contrast, cholesterol esters are not exchanged and presumably have to enter the cell by bulk transport. Once cholesterol esters are within macrophage lysosomes, they may be degraded by acid cholesterol esterases to free cholesterol. The cholesterol may then be exchanged back to the plasma membrane and be picked up by serum lipoproteins (Werb and Cohn, 1972). Under no circumstance thus far studied is the cholesterol molecule further modified, and the formation of bile acids has not been described.

VI. Macrophages and Host Defense

The participation of macrophages in host defense has continued to receive considerable attention since the original contributions of Metchnikoff (1905). Similar to polymorphonuclear leukocytes, mononuclear phagocytes have an intrinsic ability to interiorize and to inactivate a variety of noxious agents. Also, the numbers of both types of phagocytic cell at a given site can be increased during inflammatory responses by mechanisms that are being elucidated. However, in contrast to neutrophilic leukocytes, macrophages may develop enhanced resistance with time. This acquisition of resistance at the cellular level may be mediated by both immunologically specific and nonspecific factors. These influences will be reviewed in general terms, and then we shall consider the more specific details whereby macrophages are involved in antibacterial, antiviral, and anticellular defenses.

The resistance of macrophages to a given noxious agent may be modulated by nonimmunological factors, examples of which can be found in an inflammatory site. Thus, the introduction of serum into the peritoneal cavity results in an influx of young monocytes, the differentiation of the resident macrophages into a more "activated" state with enhanced cytoplasmic mass and organelles, and with increased microbicidal capacity (Mackaness and Blanden, 1967).

Much more attention has been given to the influence of specifically sensitized lymphocytes on the enhancement of macrophage resistance. Thymus-independent or B lymphocytes give rise to specific antibodies which serve as opsonins for the interiorization of noxious agents. Thymus-derived or T lymphocytes apparently do not secrete antibodies, but may play a major role in the development of macrophage defense. The evidence is more indirect and is generally inferred from the following constellation of findings. (1) The particular agent can be killed during a primary exposure by macrophages, but resistance is expressed more effectively and/or more quickly following a second exposure to the agent. (2) Resistance can be adoptively transferred to an unimmunized host by sensitized lymphoid cells as opposed to immune serum. Presumably the transferred cells are not functioning by the local production of antibodies. (3) Establishment and/or transfer of resistance is correlated with the appearance of a positive-delayed skin test to the antigens of the specific agent. The existence of delayed-type hypersensitivity depends on thymus-derived lymphocytes (see Volume III, Chapter 1).

The role of the macrophage in the delayed skin reaction has therefore been studied as a prototype for the interaction of macrophages and lymphocytes in the acquisition of host defense. Bloom and Bennett (1970) have reviewed this area concisely and their conclusions are still applicable. Histologically, a positive delayed skin response to an antigen involves the influx of numerous monocytes into the site of antigen inoculation. The migration and/or subsequent function of monocytes in the skin site appears to be mediated by sensitized lymphocytes, which themselves represent a tiny fraction at best of the inflammatory cells. In animals sensitized by adoptive transfer of lymphoid cells, the unsensitized recipient bone marrow provides the phagocytic cells that subsequently move into the skin site (Lubaroff and Waksman, 1968).

Several *in vitro* correlates of delayed skin reactivity have been discovered (see Volume III, Chapter, 7). In most, sensitized lymphocytes release soluble mediators which, in turn, may alter the macrophage. At this time only the macrophage inhibitory factor (MIF) has been purified and studied in purified macrophage populations *in vitro* (Nathan *et al.*, 1971). These preliminary observations suggest that MIF enhances the adherence of guinea pig peritoneal macrophages and may lead to enhanced phagocytosis of certain test materials. The elucidation of the mechanisms underlying the proposed lymphocyte–macrophage interaction in host defenses represents an exciting, but untapped, area for cell biologists.

A. Antibacterial Defense

1. INTRINSIC MICROBICIDAL ACTIVITY

Several *in vitro* studies have shown that freshly harvested tissue macrophages can inactivate a wide variety of gram-positive and gram-negative bacteria following uptake into the cell (Whitby and Rowley, 1959; Mackaness, 1960; Cohn, 1963a). Macrophages may vary in their killing capacity depending on the source of the cells (Pavillard and Rowley, 1962) and maturation of the animal (Karthigasu *et al.*, 1965); e.g., the fetal rat and chicken are unable to kill gram-negative bacteria even in the presence of specific antibodies and adequate phagocytosis.

Many of the bactericidal mechanisms found in polymorphonuclear leukocytes (see Chapter 7) are not present in mononuclear phagocytes. Macrophages do not possess the cationic proteins (phagocytin) which are found in granulocyte granules and which are bactericidal in cell-free systems (Hirsch, 1956). The production of hydrogen peroxide, and/or its utilization by myeloperoxidase, is considered to be important in granulocyte killing (Klebanoff, 1968) and may explain why these cells only kill under aerobic conditions. Alveolar macrophages do produce H_2O_2 (Gee *et al.*, 1970; Vogt *et al.*, 1971), but this has not been demonstrated in macrophages from other sources. In addition, myeloperoxidase is not detectable in many tissue macrophages, especially after cultivation *in vitro* (van Furth *et al.*, 1970). Finally, several workers (Nakae *et al.*, 1967; Cline, 1970; Thalinger and Mandell, 1971) have noted that macrophages may kill many types of bacteria under anaerobic conditions.

Although many bacteria are killed within the lysosomes of mononuclear phagocytes, it has yet to be established that lysosomal hydrolases are involved directly. One would expect that lysozyme, which is present in alveolar and peritoneal macrophages of several species (Myrvik *et al.*, 1961; Brumfitt and Glynn, 1961; Ramseier and Suter, 1964), may affect gram-positive organisms. However, it is conceivable that most instances of bacterial killing in macrophages result from some nonhydrolytic alteration of the bacterial surface, e.g., by a surface-active agent that irreversibly alters permeability and/or transport. It is known that a significant percentage of many bacteria are killed within 10 minutes of entry into the cell, whereas detectable digestion of bacterial macromolecules begins later (Cohn, 1963a,b). The discrepancy between bacterial kill and digestion is especially evident in the case of opsonized organisms where the delay may be as long as 2 or 3 hours. It was also observed that shortly after entry into the cell the bacteria lose their pool of acid-soluble metabolites, suggesting a rapid alteration in the cell membrane. A possibly relevant observation is that administration of Triton WR-1339 renders mice (Cornforth *et al.*, 1951) and their cultivated macrophages (Mackaness, 1954) more resistant to tuberculosis. This material is a detergent known to segregate within liver lysosomes (Wattiaux *et al.*, 1963), but its localization within macrophages has not been studied.

2. Effects of Opsonins

Several types of opsonin have been described that enhance bacterial ingestion and subsequent killing (reviewed by Suter and Ramseier, 1964). By far the most important is specific antibacterial antibodies. Many virulent bacterial strains, e.g., *Staph aureus*, possess surface antiphagocytic principles which are neutralized by antibody (Mackaness, 1960; Cohn, 1962a,b). A recent illustrative infection is that of mouse peritoneal macrophages by *Mycoplasma pulmonis* (Jones and Hirsch, 1971). These organisms attach to and proliferate on the surface of the phagocytes. Within minutes after addition of specific antibody, ingestion and rapid killing occurs. In contrast, alveolar macrophages from the same mice are able to ingest and kill the mycoplasmas in the absence of antibody.

Immune sera may effect the bacteria–macrophage interaction in ways other than opsonization. Several workers have reported that the presence of immune serum can protect macrophages, especially in immunized animals, from the cytotoxicity of intracellular parasites (Fong *et al.*, 1957; Gelzer and Suter, 1959; Vickrey and Elberg, 1971). The virulent parasites themselves continue to divide. Immunologically specific and nonspecific factors have been found in the antisera studied.

3. EFFECTS OF IMMUNE CELLS

A variety of organisms, *e.g., Mycobacterium tuberculosis, Listeria monocytogenes, Brucella abortus, Salmonella typhi,* and *Pasteurella tularensis,* have been found to survive and even proliferate within the confines of the macrophage. The development of host defense to these facultative intracellular parasites has been most extensively studied by Mackaness and his colleagues and has been reviewed elsewhere (Mackaness and Blanden, 1967; Mackaness, 1970). Resistance involves both immunologically specific and nonspecific factors, and these have been especially well studied in Listeria infection in mice. During a primary infection, Listeria multiply for some 3 to 4 days in parenchymal organs, especially liver and spleen (Mackaness, 1962). Host resistance then develops and is nonspecific in that it can be expressed against other intracellular parasites. If animals which have recovered from Listeria are reinfected, resistance can now be established more rapidly (2 days) and to much higher inocula. Again, the acquired defense can be directed against other antigenically unrelated microbes (Fong *et al.*, 1957; Elberg *et al.*, 1957; Howard, 1961; Mackaness, 1964a,b; Blanden *et al.*, 1966), and even fungi (Gentry and Remington, 1971) and viruses (Remington and Merigan, 1969). However, only Listeria reinfection can induce the accelerated buildup of resistance in animals previously infected with Listeria (Mackaness, 1964a).

The acquisition of host resistance to facultative organisms is largely mediated through specifically sensitized lymphocytes. This can be demonstrated by adoptive transfer experiments. Transfer of Listeria-immune serum does not confer resistance to unprimed syngeneic recipients, but transfer of Listeria-immune lymphoid cells does (Mackaness, 1969). The responsible cell must be a lymphocyte because of its specificity requirements (Mackaness, 1969), its sensitivity to antilymphocyte globulin (Mackaness and Hill, 1969), its ability to circulate in thoracic duct lymph (McGregor *et al.*, 1971), and its nonstickiness to glass (Mackaness, 1969). McGregor and co-workers (1971; Koster and McGregor, 1971; Koster *et al.*, 1971) have characterized this lymphocyte further in the rat. It does not recirculate extensively in thoracic duct, is short lived, and egresses into inflammatory exudates regardless of the nature of the inflammatory stimulus. Transfer of resistance with immune lymphoid cells has been demonstrated as well in several other facultative microbial infections (Sever, 1960; Allen, 1962; Saito *et al.*, 1962; Miki and Mackaness, 1964).

Even though lymphocytes may mediate the acquisition of host resistance to facultative organisms, they are not bactericidal by themselves (Mackaness, 1969; Howard *et al.*, 1971). *In situ* studies suggested that killing occurs within macrophages (reviewed by Lurie, 1965), and *in vitro* studies confirmed this (Suter, 1953; Pomales-Lebron and Stinebring, 1957; Holland and Pickett, 1958; Mackaness, 1962; Gentry and Remington, 1971; Sato *et al.*, 1961; Berthong and Hamilton, 1959). The most critical population of phagocytes *in situ* is that supplied by the bone marrow into the parenchymal foci where organisms are multiplying. North (1969a) has pulse labeled the bone marrow phagocyte precursor pool with thymidine prior to Listeria infection. He was then able to follow the influx of labeled monocytes into infective foci. In a primary infection, neutrophilic leukocytes first invade the foci. Monocytes supersede them by day 3 to 4, which is the time that the host begins to overcome the Listeria. The neutrophilic phase is bypassed during reinfection, and the infective foci are almost immediately infiltrated with macrophages. The influx of phagocytes can be blocked by whole-body X irradiation (Tripathy and Mackaness, 1969), vinblastine (North, 1970b), and steroids (North, 1971). Finally, adoptive transfer of sensitized lymphoid cells into bone marrow-suppressed animals does not establish resistance (Tripathy and Mackaness, 1969), presumably because there is no macrophage precursor pool in the recipients.

Recovery from Listeria is also associated with a proliferation of resident tissue macrophages both in infected organs, e.g., liver Kupffer cells, and in sterile areas, e.g., the peritoneal cavity. As much as 10–20 % of these normally resting cells (G_0) can be induced to divide during infection (North, 1969b, 1970a). However, recovery from the doses of Listeria studied can occur in the absence of this proliferation of tissue macrophages. Local hepatic irradiation was used to block Kupffer cell mitosis (North, 1970a). The normal curves of Listeria growth and death were not altered, however, because the influx of new monocytes from the bone marrow was unimpeded.

In addition to changes in the numbers of macrophages, the infected host may undergo important changes in the individual cell's bactericidal capacity.

It has long been apparent that phagocytic cells undergo striking morphological and histochemical changes at the site of infection (Lurie, 1965;
Dannenberg, 1968). Even in sterile tissues, e.g., the peritoneal cavity in
animals infected with sublethal doses of Listeria, the isolated macrophages
are larger, have many more lysosomes and mitochondria, attach to and
spread on glass more avidly, and phagocytize three times as many test polystyrene particles/30 minutes than an equivalent number of cells from un-
infected mice (North, 1969a). The microbicidal activity of purified populations
of peritoneal macrophages was beautifully demonstrated by Mackaness
(1962). He used a low multiplicity of infection so that a few of the macrophages contained but a single organism. Plaques were then formed in a
macrophage monolayer, secondary to bacterial replication. More than 90 %
of the infected cells from normal animals yielded plaques versus less than
10 % in immune animals, even though the latter originally ingested 10 times
as many organisms. The peritoneal cells acquired enhanced resistance at the
same time as the host, i.e., at day 3 to 4 of a primary infection. Blanden *et al.*
(1966) tried to determine if the cellular resistance, similar to the host's, could
be directed against other intracellular parasites. A peritoneal cavity assay
system was used. Opsonized Salmonella or Listeria were injected intraperitoneally into normal Listeria-immune and Salmonella-immune animals.
Ten minutes later the peritoneal cells were harvested, separated from extracellular organisms by centrifugation, and followed for bacterial kill in
suspension culture. The peritoneal cells from animals infected with either
organism killed both Listeria and Salmonella more rapidly (80 % *vs.* 0 % in 10
minutes) and more effectively (final kill of 95 % *vs.* 55 %) than normal cells.
In these studies it is difficult to decide if the individual macrophages have
undergone a qualitative change in the microbicidal activity or whether the
observations resulted from increased numbers of cells, increased size of the
cells, or differences in uptake of organisms.

Several groups have attempted to study the activation of macrophages *in
vitro* by sensitized lymphocytes (Patterson and Youmans, 1970; Howard *et
al.*, 1971; Gentry and Remington, 1971; Krahenbuhl and Remington, 1971;
Simon and Sheagren, 1971). The most clear cut of these studies is that of
Simon and Sheagren, who examined the influence of specific antigen on
mixed populations of peritoneal exudate macrophages and lymphocytes
obtained from normal and immune animals. The immunized donors all had
positive delayed skin reactivity to one of the three antigens used. The peritoneal cells were cultivated for 24 hours in the presence of specific or nonspecific antigen. The antigen and nonadherent cells were then washed off,
leaving a constant number of macrophages. Serum-opsonized Listeria were
then added for 30 minutes, the extracellular organisms were washed away,
uptake was determined in some cultures by colony counts of lysed cells and
direct counts of stained cells, and other cultures were followed for 5 hours to

assess bacterial kill. Organisms administered over a wide range of infectivity (30–300 Listeria added per macrophage) were killed, if previously the immune exudate cells had been exposed to the specific sensitizing antigen. In contrast, Listeria proliferated in cultures of normal cells plus antigen or immune cells plus nonspecific antigen. Preliminary observations suggested that immune lymphocytes and antigen could activate normal macrophages. Current speculation is that antigen–stimulated lymphocytes may release a soluble mediator that enhances the macrophages's antimicrobial capacity. Other more nonspecific interpretations are possible. One involves antigen-induced lymphocyte proliferation. Since considerable cell death occurs in replicating lymphoid cells *in situ*, e.g., in germinal centers (Odartchenko *et al.*, 1967) and thymus, the resulting large load of dying cells may induce quantitative changes in the macrophages that are expressed as an increased killing ability. This possibility seems relevant because other nonspecific stimuli may enhance macrophage killing, e.g., serum (Mackaness and Blanden, 1967) and glycogen (Patterson and Youmans, 1970).

B. Antiviral Resistance

Several kinds of host defense mechanisms have been described for viral infections: local tissue factors (reviewed by Baron, 1967), antiviral antibodies, interferon, macrophage resistance, and defenses mediated by sensitized lymphocytes. The relative importance of each factor varies with the particular virus in question, and, in many instances, has yet to be clearly defined. In this section, we shall review the evidence that macrophages participate in viral resistance and then describe some of the mechanisms that may be involved. A more detailed review of many of the topics discussed here has already been published (Silverstein, 1970).

1. CLEARANCE OF VIRUS BY PHAGOCYTIC CELLS

It is clear that the widespread distribution of monocytes and macrophages enables them to interact early with virus introduced from a variety of routes (reviewed by Mims, 1964). Experimentally, the intravenous mode of virus inoculation has been the most extensively studied, and rightfully so, since many viral infections have an associated viremia prior to the onset of widespread organ damage (Fenner, 1948, 1949). The intravascular clearance of virus particles resembles that observed for other particulate materials that are taken up by phagocytic cells of the reticuloendothelial system. The rapid uptake of virus into mononuclear phagocytes, especially the liver Kupffer cells, can be substantiated with fluoresceinated, specific antisera. Eclipse of viral antigens then ensues; however, further details on the result of this initial encounter between virus and macrophage cannot readily be obtained *in situ.*

2. *In Vivo* and *In Vitro* Correlates

Several *in vitro* studies reveal a striking correlation between host viral resistance and that exhibited by macrophages *in vitro.* Bang and Warwick (1957) noted that a virulent strain of Newcastle Disease virus grew in chicken macrophage cultures, whereas the avirulent did not. These same authors (1960) and Kantock *et al.* (1963) demonstrated that mouse hepatitis virus (MHV) proliferates in hepatic and peritoneal macrophages isolated from mouse strains that were genetically susceptible to MHV *in vivo.* Virus did not grow in macrophages taken from resistant strains. Age-induced resistance of adult mice to the extracranial inoculation of herpes simplex is associated with a similar age difference in the resistance of peritoneal macrophages *in vitro* (Johnson, 1964; Hirsch *et al.*, 1970). The susceptibility of different species to various viruses also correlates with macrophage susceptibility *in vitro.* Thus, vaccinia (cowpox) causes extensive disease in rabbits and replicates in rabbit monocytes and macrophages *in vitro* (Beard and Rous, 1938). However, this same virus does not overcome mice and does not grow in tissue cultures of mouse peritoneal macrophages (Nishmi and Niecikowski, 1963; Silverstein, 1970). At this time, no instance is known to the authors where a virus produces widespread disease *in situ*, but at the same time is unable to replicate in that animal's macrophages *in vitro*, following uptake into the cell.

In two instances, observations are available on the mechanisms whereby unstimulated peritoneal macrophages may halt the growth of virus *in vitro*. In the case of vaccinia infection (Silverstein, 1970), the virion enters the cytoplasm, probably by escaping from the endocytic vacuole. One early function of the virus is expressed, i.e., thymidine kinase formation, but another, release of viral DNA from the viral core, does not occur (S. C. Silverstein, unpublished). As a result, virus does not replicate. The replication of herpes simplex virus in mouse peritoneal macrophages proceeds further than that seen in vaccinia (Stevens and Cook, 1971). Both viral DNA and protein synthesis occurs in infected cells, but adequate virus assembly does not ensue. In electron micrographs, the virions of infected cells contain cores of relatively low electron density, and these abortive particles rarely contain an outer membrane. In both herpes simplex (Stevens and Cook, 1971) and vaccinia (Nishmi and Niecikowski, 1963) infection *in vitro*, the host macrophage itself is killed by an as yet undefined mechanism (reviewed by Silverstein, 1970). Other cell types are killed by these viruses as well, but only after proliferation of infective particles has occurred. In spite of the observed death of macrophages, the lack of growth of virus in the cell type that captures much of the infecting virus load must be an important means of host defense.

3. Macrophages and Interferon

Macrophages may participate in host resistance mediated by interferons. The interferons are species specific proteins which are produced in most cell types following viral infection and which then impede viral replication in other cells [possible modes of interferon action are considered by Joklik and Merigan (1966) and Marcus and Salb (1967)]. Macrophages produce large amounts of interferon following induction by virus or other substances and may even secrete small amounts of interferon spontaneously (Smith and Wagner, 1967). It is also possible that macrophages may be the site of action for interferons produced by other cells. A relevant example might include interferons secreted by sensitized lymphocytes following antigen stimulation (Green et al., 1969). Some authors have noted that cultivated macrophages from immunized animals may be more resistant to virus than unimmunized cells (Steinberger and Rights, 1963; Glasgow, 1966). The cell suspensions studied in these instances (spleen and peritoneal exudate) were heterogeneous, and interferon released by reactive lymphocytes may have enhanced macrophage defense.

4. Macrophages and Antibodies

Although antiviral antibodies (presumably of IgM class) may be directly lytic to membrane-bound virions in the presence of complement (Berry and Almeida, 1968), most neutralizing antibodies must exert their influence at the cellular level (reviewed by Svéhag, 1968). Two general mechanisms have been proposed. The first relates to the effect of antibody on adsorption of virus to the target cell. Serum-neutralizing antibody impedes the adsorption and uptake of Newcastle Disease virus to HeLa cells (Silverstein and Marcus, 1964) and of vaccinia to L cells (Dales and Kajioka, 1964). Antibody may work similarly on other fibroblastic and epithelial cell types. Preliminary evidence in the macrophage (S. C. Silverstein, unpublished observations) suggests that antibodies can serve as opsonins and enhance interiorization of labeled vaccinia twofold. The mode of action of antiviral secretory IgA (reviewed by Rossen et al., 1971) has not yet been studied in vitro. It is possible that IgA blocks adsorption to the epithelial cells of body surfaces and enhances uptake in lining macrophages, e.g., alveolar macrophages in the lung.

Neutralizing antibodies also affect the fate of virus once inside the cell. The studies of Mandel suggest that in poliovirus infection of HeLa cells antibodies may work primarily at this level. Mandel (1967a) observed that adsorption of virus was not blocked if low concentrations of antibody were used or if the viral–antibody complexes were allowed to form in the cold for more than a day prior to their administration to the cells. However, the antibody still neutralized virus infectivity for target cells, which Mandel

(1967b) attributes to enhanced degradation of neutralized virus. More detailed evidence for a similar process has been obtained in the case of vaccinia infection of L cells (Dales and Kajioka, 1964) and of macrophages (Silverstein, 1970). In both cell types, free vaccinia is endocytosed but seems to escape the phagocytic vacuole. Virus replication does not occur in macrophages, but the host macrophage or L cell is killed. Antibody-coated virus is also interiorized in phagocytic vacuoles, but now fusion of vacuole with preexisting lysosomes occurs. The virus macromolecules are then thoroughly degraded to the building block level, and the host cell survives.

5. CELLULAR IMMUNITY

Specifically sensitized lymphocytes may be involved in virus–host defense. We have previously cited the possible roles of lymphoid cells in synthesizing interferon and specific antiviral antibodies and thus influencing the fate of virus in mononuclear phagocytes. Still other types of lymphocyte–macrophage interaction are suggested by Blanden's studies of acquired immunity to Ectromelia virus or mouse pox (1970, 1971a,b).

There are two periods in which Ectromelia appears in phagocytic cells following the inoculation of virus, either intravenously or subcutaneously. The first involves the initial clearance of virus from the blood by sinusoidal lining cells, as in liver and spleen (Mims, 1959a). Viral antigens are eclipsed in phagocytes, but the yield of infectious particles per phagocytic cell has not been well characterized. Roberts (1964) demonstrated that viral antigens are produced in peritoneal macrophages following eclipse *in vitro*. This does not prove that infectious virions are being produced however, as was demonstrated for herpes simplex by Stevens and Cook (1971).

Whatever the result of the initial viral–macrophage interaction may be, it is clear that Ectromelia reappears in the parenchyma of infected organs (Mims, 1959b; Blanden, 1970). Viral multiplication continues for several days to produce areas of parenchymal necrosis (Blanden, 1971b). In the majority of animals (80% under the experimental conditions studied), viral resistance then develops, associated with an influx of mononuclear cells, including phagocytes, into the infectious foci, e.g., at day 4 following intravenous infections and day 5 after subcutaneous infection. This second phase in the interaction of macrophages, or more precisely mononuclear cells, with virus appears to be the critical one for host recovery.

Simultaneous with the onset of recovery, positive delayed skin reactions to viral antigens appeared (Blanden, 1970). Positive immediate skin tests, serum neutralizing antibodies, and interferon production by infected organs all occurred later, e.g., 3–5 days after onset of recovery in the case of subcutaneously inoculated Ectromelia. Delayed hypersensitivity is probably mediated by thymus-derived lymphocytes (see Volume III, Chapter 1). Further evidence that sensitization of thymus–derived lymphocytes might be important in the mediation of recovery was obtained by infecting animals pretreated with antithymocyte serum (Blanden, 1970). The initial clearance, eclipse, and reappearance of virus was identical in treated animals and controls. However, virus multiplication never stopped and delayed skin sensitivity did not appear. In contrast, the treated animals developed normal immediate hypersensitivity and neutralizing antibodies and had enhanced splenic interferon production.

Adoptive transfer experiments were performed to prove that the acquisition of resistance to Ectromelia was secondary to cell- rather than humoral-mediated immunity. Mice were inoculated intravenously with Ectromelia. Twenty-four hours later they were given spleen cells from syngeneic donors immunized 6 days previously with virus. Twenty-four hours after immune spleen cell transfer the titre of liver and spleen plaque-forming units had fallen dramatically from control levels of 6.4 and 5.1 to log titres of 2.7 and 1.7, respectively. Spleen cells from mice immunized to Listeria monocytogenes offered no protection. Serum from the mice donating the cells sensitized to Electromelia was ineffective, but serum from hyperimmunized animals did reduce virus log titres in liver (7.2 to 5.1) and spleen (6.5 to 4.4). The transfer of immunity by both hyperimmunized serum and immune cells was associated with the early appearance of mononuclear cell infiltrates in necrotic parenchymal foci of virus multiplication. Blanden reasoned that these mononuclear cells were responsible for virus resistance and contained macrophages derived from the bone marrow of the recipient. This was not elucidated directly, although it was observed that X irradiation of the recipients with 800 R prevented the ability of immune cells or serum to transfer resistance. This dose of X ray is known to impede production of blood monocytes and tissue macrophages from radiosensitive bone marrow precursors (van Furth and Cohn, 1968).

The conclusion of these studies is that sensitized thymus-derived lymphocytes mediate acquired resistance to Ectromelia by inducing an influx and/or activation of mononuclear phagocytic cells into infectious foci. At this point, many details in this attractive scheme need to be characterized more directly. In particular, it will be necessary to assess the relative importance of a variety of substances produced locally by sensitized lymphocytes, e.g., interferon, antibodies, and other effector molecules such as MIF.

C. Anticellular Defense

Macrophages are abundant in the inflammatory response that is mounted by the host against tumors (Gorer, 1956; Journey and Amos, 1962; Baker *et al.*, 1962) and grafts (Wiener *et al.*, 1969). These cells are also prominent in graft-*vs.*-host reactions where they appear to be of host (Elkins, 1971) and donor (graft) origin (Boak *et al.*, 1968). Although a good deal of attention has been given to the role of sensitized lymphocytes in tumor and graft immunity, a number of experiments are amplifying the role of mononuclear phagocytes in anticellular reactions.

1. IMMUNE SERA

Experiments performed within the peritoneal cavity (Baker *et al.*, 1962) and with *in vitro* systems (Bennett *et al.*, 1964; Evans, 1971) report the destruction of neoplastic cells by macrophage populations following phagocytosis. The mediator is a specific isoantibody which when added to normal or well-washed immune macrophages results in interiorization of target cells. "Immune macrophages," if not washed extensively, evidently contain enough associated antibody from the immunized peritoneal cavity to interiorize tumor cells effectively. The specific antibodies work at dilutions that do not directly lyse target cells in the presence of complement. Moreover, most of the phagocytosed cells appear to be viable at the time of interiorization This was determined on the basis of morphological criteria and the fact that the interiorized cells were not stained with trypan blue, when the experiment was performed in the presence of this dye. Normal mouse serum was found to have both heat-labile and heat-stable nonspecific opsonins that enhanced phagocytosis of tumor cells at limiting dilutions of specific antiserum.

2. IMMUNE MACROPHAGES

The experiments of Granger and Weiser (1964) have suggested the existence of a particularly interesting form of host resistance at the macrophage level. These authors obtained peritoneal cells from mice (of histocompatibility H_2d) injected intraperitoneally 10–14 days previously with normal (spleen) or malignant (sarcoma) cells of another histocompatibility type (H_2k). The resulting peritoneal exudate consisted mainly of macrophages (H_2d) and had only rare tumor cells and 3–5% lymphocytes, as assessed by Giemsa staining. If these exudate cells were plated on a target monolayer of the histocompatibility (H_2k) to which they were immunized, the macrophages promptly (4 minutes) adhered to the target cells. Phagocytosis apparently did not ensue. Instead, plaques began to appear within 12 hours as a result of damage to both the macrophages and target cells. Plaque formation was immunologically specific in that only immune macrophages were cytotoxic to target cells, and this cytotoxicity could be expressed only against cells manifesting the appropriate histocompatibility allele, e.g., if the target monolayer contained both HeLa and H_2k cells, only the latter were lysed. The ratio of macrophages to target cells is unclear from the published data.

Another type of immune macrophage phenomenon has been reported by Evans and Alexander (1970). Here purified peritoneal exudate cells from immunized animals specifically prevent the growth *in vito* of the murine lymphoma used during immunization. Since the lymphoma cells and macrophages are obtained from syngeneic animals, the macrophages somehow are recognizing tumor specific antigens. Neither lysis nor phagocytosis appears to be involved in inhibition of lymphoma growth. However, cell contact for many hours appears necessary. As few as 10 phagocytic cells per lymphoma cell are effective.

Several observations have been made which hopefully will elucidate the mechanism(s) whereby immune macrophages may kill malignant and histo-incompatible cells. The expression of cellular resistance is immunologically specific, unlike resistance to facultative intracellular parasites where the immune macrophage has enhanced microbicidal activity to antigenically unrelated organisms (see Section VI,A,3). Anticellular immunity is not expressed *in vitro* in the presence of puromycin or actinomycin D (Granger and Weiser, 1966) or 2×10^{-3} M sodium fluoride (McIvor and Weiser, 1971a), which itself does not block protein synthesis. Phagocytosis of whole cells does not occur (Granger and Weiser, 1964; Evans and Alexander, 1970). By electron microscopy (Chambers and Weiser, 1969), the cell membranes of macrophage and target cell are closely opposed, but specialized junctions and syncytia are not observed. Rather, portions of tumor-cell ctyoplasm are surrounded and/or engulfed by macrophage pseudopods. Granger and Weiser (1966) suggest that this cell-to-cell contact is mediated by a cytophilic antibody attached to the immune macrophage surface. They were able to isolate a hemagglutinin in an eluate of immune macrophages heated for 1 hour at 56°C, and this material conferred specific resistance on normal macrophages. This soluble factor was also cytotoxic *in vitro* to H_2k lymph node cells in the presence of complement. Using this same system, McIvor and Weiser (1971b) have also identified a heat-labile factor(s) which is released into the culture medium following cocultivation of immune macrophages and target cells for 2 hours. The factor(s) can inhibit target-cell growth and induce target-cell death. Its relation to complement is unclear. Thus several cytotoxic mechanisms are possible at this point, e.g., release of a specific cytotoxin, phagocytosis of small portions of target-cell cytoplasm which somehow leads to killing, and secretion of complement by macrophages resulting in cell lysis in the presence of antibody.

3. LYMPHOCYTE–MACROPHAGE INTERACTIONS

The specificity of the immune macrophage phenomenon implies that sensitized lymphocytes are somehow involved. This is a difficult problem to approach experimentally, because in most immune lymphoid populations there are sensitized lymphocytes which themselves are capable of specific cytotoxic activity (see Volume III, Chapter 1). An exception was recently reported by Grant *et al.* (1972). Thymocytes taken from animals immunized to a murine lymphoma do not themselves prevent the growth of the lymphoma *in vitro*. Nonimmune bone marrow or spleen cells are required in addition, and presumably the critical cooperating cell is a mononuclear phagocyte. It is radioresistant, glass adherent, and sensitive to antimacrophage serum. These nonimmune cooperating cells could be sensitized by a soluble factor obtained from mixed cultures of immune thymocytes and lymphoma cells. Thus a fruitful system may be available for studying the cooperation of lymphoid and phagocytic cells in the expression of anticellular immunity *in vitro*.

It is still not clear what role, if any, immune lymphocytes are playing in the other *in vitro* model where immune macrophages produce plaques in a target-cell monolayer. In Granger and Weiser's experiments (1964), only small numbers of lymphoid cells contaminated the immune macrophage populations, and enriched (73 %) immune peritoneal lymphocytes were not cytotoxic. In contrast, Bennett (1965), studying a similar system, reported that isolated immune peritoneal lymphocytes or heterogeneous peritoneal exudate populations were 16 times more effective than purified immune macrophages. Bennett reasoned that the numbers ·of lymphocytes in his purified macrophages were too small to account for the macrophage cytotoxicity. However, Koster *et al.* (1971) have shown that lymphocytes mediating antimicrobial immunity may selectively accumulate in exudates, so that it will be important to exclude a role for a small but specialized population of immune lymphocytes in the induction and/or expression of presumed macrophage-mediated anticellular immunity *in vitro*.

VII. Macrophage and the Immune Response

It is generally agreed that macrophages destroy at least some of the antigens with which they interact. Alveolar macrophages can destroy the antigenicity of *E. coli* agglutinogen *in vitro* (Cohn, 1964). Perkins and Makinodan (1965) carefully documented the exponential decay in the immunogenicity of ingested sheep red blood cells in tissue culture. More than 99 % of red cell antigenicity, as measured in an *in vitro* antibody-forming assay, was lost progressively over 1 day in culture, and there was no exocytosis of red cell antigens under the study conditions. Kölsch and Mitchison (1968) isolated lysosomal fractions from macrophages that had interiorized aggregated bovine serum albumin and again demonstrated a loss of immunogenicity.

A more controversial topic than the ability of macrophages to destroy antigens is the proposal that some of antigenic moieties, when bound to macrophages, are not in fact degraded but are somehow altered so as to enhance their immunogenicity. Several lines of evidence have been offered in support of the latter hypothesis.

A. Macrophages as a Source of Immunogenic RNA

The putative role of the macrophage in the induction of an immune response derived its initial impetus from the experiments of Fishman (1961) and Fishman and Adler (1963). Heterogeneous peritoneal exudate cells were homogenized shortly after exposure to antigen, and an RNA extract was prepared. This RNA, which has since been shown to contain small amounts of antigen (Askonas and Rhodes, 1965), was capable of inducing a specific antibody response in lymphoid tissue in vitro. In some experiments, animals of different allotypes provided the peritoneal exudate cells used to prepare the cell-free RNA extract and the lymphoid cells used for in vitro immunization. The initial antibody that was formed had the allotype of the RNA donor (Adler et al., 1966). As a result of these observations, it was proposed that macrophages process antigens yielding highly immunogenic antigen–RNA com-complexes.

Although antigens complexed to RNA behave as "superantigens," it has yet to be shown that this phenomenon occurs in intact macrophages or has any relevance to the development of most immune responses in vivo. The studies of Roelants and Goodman (1969) and Roelants et al. (1971) suggest that the formation of antigen–RNA complexes is a nonspecific event that follows the disruption of a variety of cell types in the presence of intact antigen. Many immunogenic and nonimmunogenic macromolecules will complex with RNA isolated from peritoneal exudate cells, HeLa cells, and even E. coli as long as divalent cations are present. It is improbable that even such nonspecific complexes are formed in intact macrophages. Most proteins interiorized by this cell are sequestered within the membranes of the lysosomal apparatus (Ehrenreich and Cohn, 1967; Steinman and Cohn, 1972a). Nonhydrophobic degradation products with molecular weights of more than 200–300 do not escape these lysosomes (Ehrenreich and Cohn, 1969). During homogenization and/or phenol extraction of living cells, it seems probable that some of the lysosomal contents could escape and thus artifactually be allowed to make contact with the "immunogenic" RNA of the cell sap.

B. Macrophage as an Antigen Reservoir

It is known that antigens can persist in lymphoid organs for weeks to months following their initial administration (Campbell and Garvey, 1963).

Many have assumed that this persistent antigen is localized within macrophages, and that it may constitute an antigen reservoir capable of inducing and sustaining an immune response (Unanue and Cerottini, 1970b). More recent studies on the fate of antigens in lymphoid organs *in situ* have demonstrated that the bulk of the persistent immunogen is not localized within typical macrophages; rather it is retained in an apparently extracellular location in association with the processes of dendritic reticular cells of lymphoid follicles (Hanna and Hunter, 1970). These dendritic cells, though sometimes termed "dendritic macrophages," clearly differ from macrophages morphologically (Szakal and Hanna, 1968) and are probably a distinct cell type. It remains to be shown directly that immunogenic, presumably non-degraded, moieties persist in macrophages, and if so, whether they ever function as immunogens. Indigestible macromolecules interiorized by the macrophage probably are sequestered for long periods of time within residual bodies (de Duve and Wattiaux, 1966).

The concept that macrophages serve as antigen reservoirs has been investigated *in vitro* as well. The data on so-called persistent antigens (Unanue and Askonas, 1968a,b) have been obtained in heterogeneous cell suspensions, so that the persistence of antigen in healthy macrophages was not directly demonstrated. Even if antigens can be detected for long periods following endocytosis, e.g., Pearson and Raffel (1971), the observations can be subject to overinterpretation. It seems that the degradation of macromolecules within lysosomes follows first-order kinetics (Steinman and Cohn, 1972a). Depending on the amount of antigen initially interiorized and on the antigen's half-life, one might expect to find intact antigen within viable cells for long periods of time, though the amount of such antigen would be decreasing steadily. Also, it remains to be proved that this long-lived antigen can be exocytosed in some form from live macrophages and serve as immunogens for lymphoid cells (see Section V, B, 4,).

C. Adoptive Transfer of Macrophage-Bound Antigens

Many investigators have administered soluble antigens to macrophage-rich cell suspensions and then adoptively transferred the cells into syngeneic recipients (Unanue and Askonas, 1968a,b; Mitchison, 1969). The presumed macrophage-bound antigen is up to 1000 times more potent than its freely soluble counterpart in priming the recipients for a secondary response. The cell populations that have been studied in this manner have been heterogeneous and were obtained from peritoneal cavities previously stimulated with an irritant to increase the yield of macrophages. The immune response that was observed may have originated from antigen bound to macrophages, to dying or dead cells, or just to the debris that is found in such preparations, or to other cell types such as so-called antigen-binding lymphocytes. Moreover, the fate of healthy, adoptively transferred macrophages is not clear at this time. Roser (reviewed 1970) has followed the distribution of macrophages that were labeled with endocytosed colloidal gold and injected intravenously or intraperitoneally into syngeneic mice. He found that 60% of the administered label localized to the liver, 20% to the spleen and less than 1% to bone marrow, lymph nodes, and lung. By autoradiography, the label was localized to tissue macrophages. However, these data still do not reveal the percentage of cells remaining intact following transfer. In the absence of double-label experiments, e.g., by labeling the nuclei of the gold-laden cells with thymidine, it is difficult to determine if the observed label in recipient tissues is present in the same live cells as it was at the time of injection.

It is conceivable, then, that the adoptive transfer of antigen in macrophages is followed by some cell disruption, releasing immunogenic aggregates of the once soluble protein. These concerns are particularly relevant, since it is well established that most soluble proteins are not good antigens unless aggregated, e.g., by heat denaturation or mixing with adjuvants. Adoptive transfer experiments of antigens bound to peritoneal exudate populations may simulate an adjuvant effect and may not be relevant to the development of most immune responses *in situ*.

D. *Antigens Bound to the Macrophage Surface*

Unanue *et al.* (1969) and Unanue and Cerottini (1970a,b) have proposed that macrophages can retain antigen attached to the external aspect of their cell surface for long periods of time (e.g., 3–4 days *in vitro*). This surface-bound material, rather than the interiorized protein, was considered to be highly immunogenic. Hemocyanins were administered to macrophage-rich cell suspensions for 1 hour, the noncell bound antigen was removed, and then the fate of the cell bound protein followed in tissue culture. The bulk of the hemocyanin was catabolized, but some 10–20% of the original cell-bound radiolabel "persisted" in the cells. About one-quarter of this persistent label could be released into the culture medium by gently trypsinization. The solubilized material was largely intact hemocyanin. Electron microscopic radioautograms prior to trypsin treatment revealed grains in the vicinity of the cell surface. Finally, trypsinization greatly impaired the ability of macrophage-bound material to adoptively transfer an immune response.

Although gentle trypsinization has been shown to release certain surface macromolecules from a variety of cell types (Winzler, 1970; Kornfeld and Kornfeld, 1970), the studies cited above failed to demonstrate directly that the trypsin-solubilized antigen was in fact originating from the surface of live macrophages. Since heterogeneous cell suspensions from stimulated animals were studied, it is difficult to assess the viability and relative contributions of the different cell types. We have been unable to confirm the existence of trypsin-releasable material in viable homogeneous macrophage monolayers that had been exposed to soluble horseradish peroxidase (HRP) (Steinman and Cohn, 1972a). Some intact enzyme was solubilized, however, from cells damaged by the incorporation of Tris buffer in the culture medium. Histochemical observations on the distribution of HRP in viable macrophages also did not reveal enzyme on the cell surface. Horseradish peroxidase was present in intracellular lysosomes. Antigen in lysosomes lying close to the cell surface could account in part for the porposed surface-bound radioautographic grains described by Unanue *et al.* (1969).

E. Macrophage–Lymphocyte Interactions

The nature of the cells required for the development of immune responses *in vitro* has been investigated in two types of system: the development of antibody-producing cells in unprimed mouse spleen cell suspensions (Mosier, 1967; Pierce, 1969) and the induction of cell division in primed lymphoid cells from a variety of species (Hersh and Harris, 1968; Cline and Sweet, 1968; Seeger and Oppenheim, 1970; Alter and Bach, 1970). In both instances, the cells which express the response to antigen, i.e., synthesize antibody or undergo blast transformation, are lymphoid in nature and do not stick to glass. However, a population of glass-adherent cells must be present in order to obtain this *in vitro* immunization. These glass-adherent cells are heterogeneous in nature, but in a few instances, highly purified macrophage monolayers have been utilized as the glass-adherent population and similar results were obtained (Hoffman and Dutton, 1971; Feldman and Palmer, 1971)

The physiological importance of these *in vitro* pehnomena are not clear. It seems probable that antigen handling by macrophages is not involved in their restorative role. Hoffman and Dutton (1971) have shown that non-adherent mouse spleen cells can be immunized to sheep red blood cells in the presence of a cell-free supernatant derived from cultures of macrophages that were not exposed to antigen. Bach *et al.* (1970) have also demonstrated that cell-free macrophage-conditioned media will suffice in the blastogenic response of highly purified human peripheral blood lymphocytes. The requirement for glass-adherent cells, or media conditioned by them, can be completely bypassed by adding small amounts of mercaptoethanol to the adherent cell populations (Chen and Hirsch, 1972). It is important to note that whether macrophages or mercaptoethanol (Chen and Hirsch, 1972) are used, the viability of the nonadherent cells is enhanced. The presence of macrophages in tissue cultures may thus provide some trophic influence required for the survival of lymphoid cells *in vitro*, an influence which does not involve processing of endocytosed antigen and which may not be related to events *in situ*.

F. Summary

We would urge that the proposed role of the macrophage in the induction of an immune response is still far from clear, in spite of the variety of experimental approaches that have been taken. In many *in vitro* studies, the cells examined have been heterogeneous cell suspensions. There is no direct evidence that healthy macrophages were responsible for the phenomena observed. In other instances, the applicability of *in vitro* observations to immunity *in situ* is either unclear and/or improbable.

In contrast, the evidence that macrophages destroy antigens is convincing and has been obtained in purified cell populations. *A priori* antigen uptake and degradation could serve just as important a role in the development of immunity and tolerance as the processing and release of "superantigens." The scavenger and destructive capacities of the macrophage in addition seem particularly well suited to function in the efferent limb of the immune response, i.e., in the events that follow rather than precede the differentiation of specific lymphoid cells. With respect to the humoral immune response, macrophages possess surface receptors that result in the rapid interiorization of antibody-coated materials. Interiorization is followed by thorough degradation as has been described for antibody-coated red cells (Perkins and Makinodan, 1965), microbial organisms (Cohn, 1963a,b; Silverstein, 1970; Jones and Hirsch, 1971), and protein antigens (Steinman and Cohn, 1972b). Macrophages seem to be specialized as well to participate in the efferent aspect of so-called "cellular," or nonantibody mediated, immunity. Here the critical sequel of lymphocyte sensitization by antigen is the enhanced resistance of the host's macrophages to that antigen (see Section VI).

References

Adler, F. L., Fishman, M., and Dray, S. (1966). *J. Immunol.* **97**, 554
Allen, W. P. (1962). *J. Exp. Med.* **115**, 411.
Alter, B. J., and Bach, F. H. (1970). *Cell. Immunol.* **1**, 207.
Armstrong, J. A., and D'Arcy Hart, P. (1971). *J. Exp. Med.* **134**, 713.
Aschoff, L. (1924). *Ergeb. Inn. Med. Kinderheilk.* **26**, 1.
Askonas, B. A., and Rhodes, J. M. (1965). *Nature (London)* **205**, 470.
Axline, S. G. (1968). *J. Exp. Med.* **128**, 1031.
Axline, S. G., and Cohn, Z. A. (1970). *J. Exp. Med.* **131**, 1239.
Bach, F. H., Alter, B. J., Solliday, S., Zoschke, D. C., and Janis, M. (1970). *Cell. Immunol.* **1**, 219.

Baker, P., Weiser, R. S., Jutila, J., Evans, C. A., and Blandau, R. J. (1962). *Ann. N.Y. Acad. Sci.* **101**, 46.

Balner, H. (1963). *Transplantation* **1**, 217.

Bang, F. B., and Warwick, A. (1957). *J. Pathol. Bacteriol.* **73**, 321.

Bang, F. B., and Warwick, A. (1960). *Proc. Nat. Acad. Sci. U.S.* **46**, 1065.

Baron, S. (1967). *In* "Modern Trends in Medicine and Virology" (R. B. Heath and A. P. Waterson, eds.), p. 77. Appleton, New York.

Beard, J. W., and Rous, P. J. (1938). *J. Exp. Med.* **67**, 883.

Bennett, B. (1965). *J. Immunol.* **95**, 656.

Bennett, B., Old, L. J., and Boyse, E. A. (1964). *Transplantation* **2**, 183.

Bennett, W. E., and Cohn, Z. A. (1966). *J. Exp. Med.* **123**, 145.

Berken, A., and Benacerraf, B. (1966). *J. Exp. Med.* **123**, 119.

Berry, D. M., and Almeida, J. D. (1968). *J. Gen. Virol.* **3**, 97.

Berthong, M., and Hamilton, M. A. (1959). *Amer. Rev. Tuberc. Pulm. Dis.* **79**, 221.

Bhisey, A. N., and Freed, J. J. (1971a). *Exp. Cell Res.* **64**, 419.

Bhisey, A. N., and Freed, J. J. (1971b). *Exp. Cell Res.* **64**, 430.

Blanden, R. V. (1970). *J. Exp. Med.* **132**, 1035.

Blanden, R. V. (1971a). *J. Exp. Med.* **133**, 1075.

Blanden, R. V. (1971b). *J. Exp. Med.* **133**, 1090.

Blanden, R. V., Mackaness, G. B., and Collins, F. M. (1966). *J. Exp. Med.* **124**, 585.

Bloom, B. R., and Bennett, B. (1970). *Semin. Hematol.* **7**, 215.

Boak, J. L., Christie, G. H., Ford, W. L., and Howard, J. G. (1968). *Proc. Roy. Soc. Ser. B* **169**, 307.

Bowden, D. H., Adamson, I. Y. R., Grantham, W. G., and Wyatt, J. P. (1969). *Arch. Pathol.* **88**, 540.

Brumfitt. W., and Glynn, A. A. (1961). *Brit. J. Exp. Pathol.* **42**, 408.

Bruns, R. R., and Palade, G. E. (1968). *J. Cell Biol.* **37**, 277.

Campbell, D. H., and Garvey, J. S. (1963). *Advan. Immunol.* **3**, 261.

Chambers, V. C., and Weiser, R. S. (1969). *Cancer Res.* **29**, 301.

Chen, C., and Hirsch, J. G. (1972). *J. Exp. Med.* **136**, 604.

Cline, M. J. (1970). *Infec. Immunity* **2**, 156.

Cline, M. J., and Sweet, V. C. (1968). *J. Exp. Med.* **128**, 1309.

Cohn, Z. A. (1962a). *Yale J. Biol. Med.* **35**, 12.

Cohn, Z. A. (1962b). *Yale J. Biol. Med.* **35**, 48.

Cohn, Z. A. (1963a). *J. Exp. Med.* **117**, 27.

Cohn. Z. A. (1963b). *J. Exp. Med.* **117**, 43.

Cohn, Z: A. (1964). *J. Exp. Med.* **120**, 869.

Cohn, Z. A. (1965). *In* "The Inflammatory Process" (B. W. Zweifach, L. Grant, and R. T. McCluskey, eds.), 1st ed., Chapter 8, p. 323. Academic Press, New York.

Cohn, Z. A. (1966). *J. Exp. Med.* **124**, 557.

Cohn, Z. A. (1968). *Advan. Immunol.* **9**, 163.

Cohn, Z. A. (1970). *In* "Mononuclear Phagocytes" (R. van Furth, ed.), p. 121. Blackwell, Oxford.

Cohn, Z. A., and Benson, B. (1965a). *J. Exp. Med.* **121**, 153.

Cohn, Z. A., and Benson, B. (1965b). *J. Exp. Med.* **121**, 279.

Cohn, Z. A., and Benson, B. (1965c). *J. Exp. Med.* **121**, 835.

Cohn, Z. A., and Ehrenreich, B. A. (1969). *J. Exp. Med.* **129**, 201.

Cohn, Z. A., and Fedorko, M. E. (1969). *In* "Lysosomes in Biology and Medicine" (J. T. Dingle and H. B. Fell, eds.), Vol. 1, p. 43. North-Holland Publ., Amsterdam.

Cohn, Z. A., and Parks, E. (1967a). *J. Exp. Med.* **125**, 213.

Cohn, Z. A., and Parks, E. (1967b). *J. Exp. Med.* **125**, 457.
Cohn, Z. A., and Parks, E. (1967c). *J. Exp. Med.* **125**, 1091.
Cohn, Z. A., and Wiener, E. (1963a). *J. Exp. Med.* **118**, 991.
Cohn, Z. A., and Wiener, E. (1963b). *J. Exp. Med.* **118**, 1009.
Cohn, Z. A., Fedorko, M. E., and Hirsch, J. G. (1966). *J. Exp. Med.* **123**, 747.
Cornforth, J. W., Hart, P. D., Rees, R. J. W., and Stock, J. A. (1951). *Nature (London)* **168**, 150.
Cotran, R. S., and Litt, M. (1970). *J. Immunol.* **105**, 1536.
Dales, S., and Kajioka, R. (1964). *Virology* **24**, 278.
Dannenberg, A. M. (1968). *Bacteriol. Rev.* **32**, 85.
Dannenberg, A. M., and Bennett, W. E. (1964). *J. Cell Biol.* **21**, 1.
Dannenberg, A. M., Walter, P. C., and Kapral, F. A. (1963). *J. Immunol.* **90**, 448.
de Duve, C., and Wattiaux, R. (1966). *Annu. Rev. Physiol.* **28**, 435.
Dumont, A., and Shelden, H. (1965). *Lab. Invest.* **14**, 2034.
Dvorak, H. F., Dvorak, A. M., Simpson, B. A., Richarson, M. B., Leskowitz, S., and Karnovsky, M. J. (1970). *J. Exp. Med.* **132**, 558.
Ebert, R. H., and Florey, H. W. (1939). *Brit. J. Exp. Pathol.* **20**, 342.
Ehrenreich, B. A., and Cohn, Z. A. (1967). *J. Exp. Med.* **126**, 941.
Ehrenreich, B. A., and Cohn, Z. A. (1968a). *J. Cell Biol.* **38**, 244.
Ehrenreich, B. A., and Cohn, Z. A. (1968b). *J. Reticuloendothel. Soc.* **5**, 230.
Ehrenreich, B. A., and Cohn, Z. A. (1969). *J. Exp. Med.* **129**, 227.
Elberg, S. S., Schneider, P., and Fong, J. (1957). *J. Exp. Med.* **106**, 545.
Elkins, W. L. (1971). *Prog. Allergy* **15**, 78.
Evans, R. (1971). *J. Immunol.* **20**, 67.
Evans, R., and Alexander, P. (1970). *Nature (London)* **228**, 620.
Fedorko, M. E., and Hirsch, J. G. (1970). *Semin. Hematol.* **7**, 109
Fedorko, M. E., Hirsch, J. G., and Cohn, Z. A. (1968a). *J. Cell Biol.* **38**, 377.
Fedorko, M. E., Hirsch, J. G., and Cohn, Z. A. (1968b). *J. Cell Biol.* **38**, 392.
Feldman, M., and Palmer, J. (1971). *Immunology* **21**, 685.
Fenner, F. (1948). *J. Pathol. Bacteriol.* **60**, 529.
Fenner, F. (1949). *J. Immunol.* **63**, 341.
Fishman, M. (1961). *J. Exp. Med.* **114**, 837.
Fishman, M., and Adler, F. L. (1963). *J. Exp. Med.* **117**, 595.
Fong, J., Schneider, P., and Elberg, S. S. (1957). *J. Exp. Med.* **105**, 25.
Frei, J., Borel, C., Horvath, G., Cullity, B., and Vanotti, A. (1961). *Blood* **18**, 317.
Gee, J. B. L., Vassallo, C. L., Bell, P., Kaskin, J., Basford, R. E., and Field, J. B. (1970). *J. Clin. Invest.* **49**, 1280.
Gelzer, J., and Suter, E. (1959). *J. Exp. Med.* **110**, 715.
Gentry, L. O., and Remington, J. S. (1971). *J. Infec. Dis.* **123**, 22.
Glasgow, L. A. (1966). *J. Bacteriol.* **91**, 2185.
Goldmann, E. (1909). *Beitr. Klin. Chir.* **64**, 192.
Goodman, J. W. (1964). *Blood* **23**, 18.
Gordon, S., and Cohn, Z. A. (1970). *J. Exp. Med.* **131**, 981.
Gordon, S., and Cohn, Z. A. (1971a). *J. Exp. Med.* **133**, 321.
Gordon, S., and Cohn, Z. A. (1971b). *J. Exp. Med.* **134**, 935.
Gordon, S., and Cohn, Z. A. (1971c). *J. Exp. Med.* **134**, 947.
Gorer, P. A. (1956). *Advan. Cancer Res.* **4**, 149.
Granger, G. A., and Weiser, R. S. (1964). *Science* **145**, 1427.
Granger, G. A., and Weiser, R. S. (1966). *Science* **151**, 97.
Grant, C. K., Currie, G. A., and Alexander, P. (1972). *J. Exp. Med.* **135**, 150.
Gravitz, E. (1890). *Verh. Int. Med. Congr. Berlin* **3**, 9.

Green, J. A., Cooperband, S. R., and Kibrick, S. (1969). *Science* **164**, 1415.

Gusek, W. (1964). *Med. Welt.* **15**, 850.

Hanna, M. G., Jr., and Hunter, R. L. (1970). *In* "Morphological and Functional Aspects of Immunity" (K. Lindahl-Kiessling, F. Alm, and M. G. Hanna, Jr., eds.), p. 257. Plenum, New York.

Harris, H. (1954). *Physiol. Rev.* **34**, 529.

Harris, H. (1966). *Proc. Roy. Soc. Ser. B* **166**, 358.

Hersh, E. M., and Harris, J. E. (1968). *J. Immunol.* **100**, 1184.

Hirsch, J. G. (1956). *J. Exp. Med.* **103**, 589.

Hirsch, J. G., Fedorko, M. E., and Dwyer, C. M. (1966). *In* "Proceedings of the 4th International Conference on Sarcoidosis" (J. Turiaf and J. Chabot, eds.), p. 59. Masson, Paris.

Hirsch, J. G., Fedorko, M. E., and Cohn, Z. A. (1968). *J. Cell Biol.* **38**, 629.

Hirsch, M. S., Zisman, B., and Allison, A. C. (1970). *J. Immunol.* **104**, 1160.

Hoffman, M., and Dutton, R. W. (1971). *Science* **172**, 1047.

Holland, J. J., and Pickett, M. J. (1958). *J. Exp. Med.* **108**, 343.

Holland, P., Holland, N. H., and Cohn, Z. A. (1972). *J. Exp. Med.* **135**, 458.

Howard, D. H., Otto, V., and Gupta, R. K. (1971). *Infec. Immunity* **4**, 605.

Howard, J. G. (1961). *Nature (London)* **191**, 87.

Huber, H., Polley, M. J., Linscott, W. D., Fudenberg, H. H., and Mueller-Eberhard, H. (1968) *Science* **162**, 1281.

Hurd, E. R., and Ziff, M. (1968). *J. Exp. Med.* **128**, 785.

Johnson, R. T. (1964). *J. Exp. Med.* **120**, 359.

Joklik, W. K., and Merigan, T. C. (1966). *Proc. Nat. Acad. Sci. U.S.* **56**, 558.

Jones, T. C., and Hirsch, J. G. (1971). *J. Exp. Med.* **133**, 231.

Journey, L. J., and Amos, D. B. (1962). *Cancer Res.* **22**, 998.

Kantock, M., Warwick, A., and Bang, F. B. (1963). *J. Exp. Med.* **117**, 781.

Karer, H. E. (1958). *J. Biophys. Biochem. Cytol.* **4**, 693.

Karthigasu, K., Reade, P. C., and Jenkins, C. R. (1965). *Immunology* **9**, 1.

Kiyono, K. (1914). "Die Vitale Carminspeicherung." Fischer, Jena.

Klebanoff, S. J. (1968). *J. Bacteriol.* **95**, 2131.

Kölsch, E., and Mitchison, N. A. (1968). *J. Exp. Med.* **128**, 1059.

Kornfeld, R., and Kornfeld, S. (1970). *J. Biol. Chem.* **245**, 2536.

Koster, F. T., and McGregor, D. D. (1971). *J. Exp. Med.* **133**, 864.

Koster, F. T., McGregor, D. D., and Mackaness, G. B. (1971). *J. Exp. Med.* **133**, 400.

Krahenbuhl, J. L., and Remington, J. S. (1971). *Infec. Immunity* **4**, 337.

Latta, J. S., and Gentry, R. P. (1958). *Anat. Rec.* **132**, 1.

Lay, W. H., and Nussenzweig, V. (1968). *J. Exp. Med.* **128**, 991.

Lewis, W. H. (1931). *Johns Hopkins Med. J.* **49**, 17.

Lo Buglio, A. F., Cotran, R. S., and Jandl, J. H. (1967). *Science* **158**, 1582.

Low, F. N., and Freeman, J. A. (1958). "Electron Microscopic Atlas of Normal and Leukemic Human Blood." McGraw-Hill, New York.

Lubaroff, D. M., and Waksman, B. H. (1968). *J. Exp. Med.* **128**, 1425.

Lurie, M. B. (1965). "Resistance to Tuberculosis." Harvard Univ. Press, Cambridge, Massachusetts.

McGregor, D. D., Koster, F. T., and Mackaness, G. B. (1971). *J. Exp. Med.* **133**, 389.

McIvor, K. L., and Weiser, R. S. (1971a). *J. Immunol.* **20**, 307.

McIvor, K. L., and Weiser, R. S. (1971b). *J. Immunol.* **20**, 315.

Mackaness, G. B. (1954). *Amer. Rev. Tuberc.* **69**, 690.

Mackaness, G. B. (1960). *J. Exp. Med.* **112**, 35.

Mackaness, G. B. (1962). *J. Exp. Med.* **116**, 381.

Mackaness, G. B. (1964a). *J. Exp. Med.* **120**, 105.
Mackaness, G. B. (1964b). *Symp. Soc. Gen. Microbiol.* **14**, 213.
Mackaness, G. B. (1969). *J. Exp. Med.* **129**, 973.
Mackaness, G. B. (1970). *Semin. Hematol.* **7**, 172.
Mackaness, G. B., and Blanden, R. V. (1967). *Progr. Allergy* **11**, 89.
Mackaness, G. B., and Hill, W. C. (1969). *J. Exp. Med.* **129**, 993.
Mandel, B. (1967a). *Virology* **31**, 238.
Mandel, B. (1967b). *Virology* **31**, 248.
Marchand, F. (1898). *Verh. Deut. Pathol. Ges.* **1**, 63.
Marchesi, V. T., and Florey, H. W. (1960). *Quart. J. Exp. Physiol.* **45**, 343.
Marcus, P. I., and Salb, J. M. (1967). *Virology* **30**, 248.
Metchnikoff, E. (1905). "Immunity in Infective Diseases." Cambridge Univ. Press, London and New York.
Miescher, P. A., and Jaffé, E. R. (1970). *Semin. Hematol.* **7**, 107.
Miki, K., and Mackaness, G. B. (1964). *J. Exp. Med.* **120** 93.
Mims, C. A. (1959a). *Brit. J. Exp. Pathol.* **40**, 533.
Mims, C. A. (1959b). *Brit. J. Exp. Pathol.* **40**, 543.
Mims, C. A. (1964). *Bacteriol. Rev.* **28**, 30.
Mitchison, N. A. (1969). *Immunology* **16**, 1.
Mosier, D. E. (1967). *Science* **158**, 1575.
Myrvik, Q. N., Leake, E. S., and Fariss, B. (1961). *J. Immunol.* **86**, 133.
Nachman, R. L., Ferris, B., and Hirsch, J. G. (1971a). *J. Exp. Med.* **133**, 785.
Nachman, R. L., Ferris, B., and Hirsch, J. G. (1971b). *J. Exp. Med.* **133**, 807.
Nakae, T., Nakano, M., and Saito, K. (1967). *Jap. J. Microbiol.* **11**, 189.
Nathan, C. F., Karnovsky, M. L., and David, J. R. (1971). *J. Exp. Med.* **133**, 1356.
Nelson, D. A. (1969). "Macrophages and Immunity." North-Holland Publ., Amsterdam.
Nichols, B. A., Bainton, D. F., and Farquhar, M. G. (1971). *J. Cell Biol.* **50**, 498.
Nishmi, M., and Niecikowski, H. (1963). *Nature (London)* **199**, 1117.
North, R. J. (1966). *J. Ultrastruct. Res.* **16**, 96.
North, R. J. (1969a). *J. Exp. Med.* **130**, 299.
North, R. J. (1969b). *J. Exp. Med.* **130**, 315.
North, R. J. (1970a). *J. Exp. Med.* **132**, 521.
North, R. J. (1970b). *J. Exp. Med.* **132**, 535.
North, R. J. (1970c). *Semin. Hematol.* **7**, 216.
North, R. J. (1971). *J. Exp. Med.* **134**, 1485.
Novikoff, A. B., and Essner, E. (1960). *Amer. J. Med.* **29**, 102.
Novikoff, A. B., Essner, E., and Quintana, N. (1964). *Fed. Proc.. Fed. Amer. Soc. Exp. Biol.* **23**, 1010.
Odartchenko, N., Lewerenz, M., Sordat, B., Roos, B., and Cottier, H. (1967). *In* "Germinal Centers in Immune Responses" (H. Cottier *et al.*, eds.), p. 212. Springer-Verlag, Berlin and New York.
Oren, R., Farnham, A. E., Saito, K., Milofsky, E., and Karnovsky. M. L. (1963). *J. Cell Biol.* **17**, 487.
Patterson, R. J., and Youmans, G. P. (1970). *Infec. Immunity* **1**, 600.
Pavillard, E. R., and Rowley, P. (1962). *Aust. J. Exp. Biol. Med. Sci.* **40**, 207.
Pearsall, N. N., and Weiser, R. S. (1970) "The Macrophage." Lea & Febiger, Philadelphia, Pennsylvania.
Pearson, M. N., and Raffel, S. (1971). *J. Exp. Med.* **133**, 494.
Perkins, E. H., and Makinodan, T. J. (1965). *Immunology* **94**, 765.
Pierce, C. W. (1969). J. *Exp. Med.* **130**, 345.

Pimstone, N. R., Tenhunen, R., Seitz, P. T., Marver, H. S., and Schmid, R. (1971). *J. Exp. Med.* **133**, 1264.

Pinkett, M. O., Cowdrey, C. R., and Nowell, P. C. (1966). *Amer. J. Pathol.* **48**, 859.

Pomales-Lebron, A., and Stinebring, W. R. (1957). *Proc. Soc. Exp. Biol. Med.* **94**, 78.

Rabinovitch, M. (1967a). *J. Immunol.* **99**, 232.

Rabinovitch, M. (1967b). *J. Immunol.* **99**, 1115.

Rabinovitch, M. (1967c). *Exp. Cell Res.* **46**, 19.

Rabinovitch, M. (1968). *Semin. Hematol.* **5**, 134.

Rabinovitch, M. (1969). *Exp. Cell Res.* **54**, 210.

Ramseier, H., and Suter, F. (1964). *J. Immunol.* **93**, 518.

Ranvier, L. (1900). *Arch. Anat. Microsc. Morphol. Exp.* **3**, 123.

Reaven, E. P., and Axline, S. G. (1973). *J. Cell Biol.* **59**, 12.

Remington, J. S., and Merigan, T. C. (1969). *Proc. Soc. Exp. Biol. Med.* **131**, 1184.

Robbins, D., Fahimi, H. D., and Cotran, R. S. (1971). *J. Histochem. Cytochem.* **19**, 571.

Roberts, J. A. (1964). *J. Immunol.* **92**, 837.

Robineaux, R., and Pinet, J. (1960). *Aspects Immunity, Ciba Found. Symp.*, 1959 p. 5.

Roelants, G. E., and Goodman, J. W. (1969). *J. Exp. Med.* **130**, 557.

Roelants, G. E., Goodman, J. W., and McDevitt, H. O. (1971). *J. Immunol.* **106**, 1222.

Roser, B. (1970). *In* "Mononuclear Phagocytes" (R. van Furth, ed.), pp. 166–174. Blackwell, Oxford.

Rossen, R. D., Kasel, J. A., and Couch, R. B. (1971). *Progr. Med. Virol.* **13**, 194.

Saito, K., Nakano, M., Akiyama, T., and Ushiba, D. (1962). *J. Bacteriol.* **84**, 800.

Sato, I., Tanaka, T., Saito, K., and Mitsuhashi, S. (1961). *Proc. Jap. Acad.* **37**, 261.

Seeger, R. C., and Oppenheim, J. J. (1970). *J. Exp. Med.* **132**, 44.

Seljelid, R., Silverstein, S. C., and Cohn, Z. A. (1973). *J. Cell Biol.* **57**, 484.

Sever, J. L. (1960). *Proc. Soc. Exp. Biol. Med.* **103**, 326.

Shorter, R. G., Titus, J. L., and Divertie, M. B. (1964). *Dis. Chest* **46**, 138.

Silverstein, S. C. (1970). *Semin. Hematol.* **7**, 185.

Silverstein, S. C., and Marcus, P. I. (1964). *Virology* **23**, 370.

Simon, H. B., and Sheagren, J. N. (1971). *J. Exp. Med.* **133**, 1377.

Smith, T. J., and Wagner, R. R. (1967). *J. Exp. Med.* **125**, 559.

Sorkin, E., Borel, J. F., and Stecher, V. J. (1970). *In* "Mononuclear Phagocytes" (R. van Furth, ed.), p. 347. Blackwell, Oxford.

Spector, W. G. (1967). *Brit. Med. Bull.* **23**, 35.

Spector, W. G., and Lyke, A. W. J. (1966). *J. Pathol. Bacteriol.* **90**, 589.

Spector, W. G., and Ryan, G. B. (1970). *In* "Mononuclear Phagocytes" (R. van Furth, ed.), p. 219. Blackwell, Oxford.

Spector, W. G., and Willoughby, D. A. (1963). *Bacteriol. Rev.* **27**, 117.

Spector, W. G., and Willoughby, D. A. (1968). *J. Pathol. Bacteriol.* **96**, 389.

Spector, W. G., Walters, M., and Willoughby, D. A. (1965). *J. Pathol. Bacteriol.* **90**, 181.

Stahelin, H., Karnovsky, M. L., and Suter, E. (1956). *J. Exp. Med.* **104**, 121.

Steinberger, A., and Rights, F. L. (1963). *Virology* **21**, 402.

Steinman, R. M., and Cohn, Z. A. (1972a). *J. Cell Biol.* **55**, 186.

Steinman, R. M., and Cohn, Z. A. (1972b). *J. Cell Biol.* **55**, 616.

Stevens, J. C., and Cook, M. L. (1971). *J. Exp. Med.* **133**, 19.

Stossel, T. P., Pollard, T. D., and Mason, R. J. (1971). *J. Clin. Invest.* **50**, 1745.

Suter, E. (1953). *J. Exp. Med.* **97**, 235.

Suter, E., and Hullinger, L. (1960). *Ann. N.Y. Acad. Sci.* **88**, 1237.

Suter, E., and Ramseier, H. (1964). *Advan. Immunol.* **4**, 117.

Sutton, J. S., and Weiss, L. (1966). *J. Cell Biol.* **28**, 303.

Svéhag, S. E. (1968). *Progr. Med. Virol.* **10**, 1.

Szakal, A. K., and Hanna, M. G., Jr. (1968). *Exp. Mol. Pathol.* **8**, 75.

Thalinger, K. K., Mandell, G. L. (1971). *Res, J. Reticuloendothel. Soc.* **9**, 393.

Thompson, J., and van Furth, R. (1970). *J. Exp. Med.* **131**, 429.

Tripathy, S. P., and Mackaness, G. B. (1969). *J. Exp. Med.* **130**, 17.

Tschaschin, S. (1913). *Folia Haematol. (Leipzig), Arch.* **17**, 317.

Uhr, J. W. (1965). *Proc. Nat. Acad. Sci. U.S.* **54**, 1599.

Unanue, E. R., and Askonas, B. A. (1968a). *Immunology* **15**, 287.

Unanue, E. R., and Askonas, B. A. (1968b). *J. Exp. Med.* **127**, 915.

Unanue, E. R., and Cerottini, J. C. (1970a). *J. Exp. Med.* **131**, 711.

Unanue, E. R., and Cerottini, J. C. (1970b). *Semin. Hematol.* **7**, 225.

Unanue, E. R., Cerottini, J. C., and Bedford, M. (1969). *Nature (London)* **222**, 1192.

van Furth, R. (1970a). *Semin. Hematol.* **7**, 125.

van Furth, R. (1970b). *In* "Mononuclear Phagocytes" (R. van Furth, ed.), p. 151. Blackwell, Oxford.

van Furth, R., and Cohn, Z. A. (1968). *J. Exp. Med.* **128**, 415.

van Furth, R., and Diesselhoff-Den Dulk, M. C. (1970). *J. Exp. Med.* **132**, 813.

van Furth, R., Hirsch, J. G., and Fedorko, M. E. (1970). *J. Exp. Med.* **132**, 794.

Vanotti, A. (1961). *Ciba Found. Study Group* **10**, 69.

Vickrey, H. M., and Elberg, S. S. (1971). *J. Immunol.* **106**, 191.

Virolainen, M. (1968). *J. Exp. Med.* **127**, 943.

Virolainen, M., and Defendi, V. (1967). *Wistar Inst. Symp. Monogr.* **7**, 67.

Vogt, M. T., Thomas, C., Vassallo, C. L., Basford, R. E., and Gee, J. B. L. (1971). *J. Clin. Invest.* **50**, 401.

Volkman, A. (1966). *J. Exp. Med.* **124**, 2411.

Volkman, A., and Gowans, J. L. (1965a). *Brit. J. Exp. Pathol.* **46**, 50.

Volkman, A., and Gowans, J. L. (1965b). *Brit. J. Exp. Pathol.* **46**, 62.

von Recklinghausen, F. (1863). *Arch. Pathol. Anat. Physiol. Klin. Med.* **28**, 157.

Wanstrup, J., and Christensen, H. E. (1966). *Acta Pathol. Microbiol. Scand.* **66**, 169.

Ward, P. A. (1968). *J. Exp. Med.* **128**, 1201.

Wattiaux, R., Wibo, M., and Bandhuin, P. (1963). *Lysosomes Ciba Found. Symp.*, 1963 p. 176.

Weiss, L., (1964). *Bull. Johns Hopkins Hosp.* **115**, 99.

Weiss, L. P., and Fawcett, D. W. (1953). *J. Histochem. Cytochem.* **1**, 47.

Werb, Z., and Cohn, Z. A. (1971a). *J. Exp. Med.* **134**, 1545.

Werb, Z., and Cohn, Z. A. (1971b). *J. Exp. Med.* **134**, 1570.

Werb, Z., and Cohn, Z. A. (1972). *J. Exp. Med.* **135**, 21.

West, J., Morton, D. J., Esman, V., and Stjernholm, R. (1968). *Arch. Biochem. Biophys.* **124**, 85.

Whitby, J. L., and Rowley, D. (1959). *Brit. J. Exp. Pathol.* **40**, 358.

Whitelaw, D. M. (1966). *Blood* **28**, 445.

Widmann, J. J., Cotran, R. S., and Fahimi, H. D. (1972). *J. Cell Biol.* **52**, 159.

Wiener, J., Lattes, R. G., and Pearl, J. S. (1969). *Amer. J. Pathol.* **55**, 295.

Winzler, R. J. (1970). *Int. Rev. Cytol.* **29**, 77.

Ziegler, E. (1890). *Verh. Int. Med. Congr. Berlin* **3**, 1.

Ziff, M., Hurd, E. R., Lemmel, E. M., and Jasin, H. E. (1970). *In* "Mononuclear Phagocytes" (R. van Furth, ed.), p. 282. Blackwell, Oxford.

Addendum

Further recent significant developments dealing with mononuclear phagocytes can be found in "Mononuclear Phagocytes" (R. van Furth, ed.), Vol. II. Blackwell Scientific Publ., Great Britain (1974).

Chapter 9

PLATELETS

MARJORIE B. ZUCKER

I. Introduction

Platelets play a pivotal role when blood or blood vessels are injured. If
inflammation, therefore, is viewed broadly as the response of tissue to injury,

the hemostatic function of platelets can be considered a component of an in-flammatory process. Hemostasis and thrombosis will be discussed in detail in Volume II, Chapters 10 and 11. With a much narrower definition of inflam-mation, platelets are rarely found to play a central role, but they influence the course of inflammatory responses, usually by releasing pharmacologically active substances. This effect can often be inhibited by nonsteroidal anti-inflammatory agents.

The relationship between platelets and inflammation has been discussed in several recent publications (Packham et al., 1968; Mustard et al., 1969; Ratnoff, 1969; Mustard and Packham, 1971). Des Prez and Marney (1971) reviewed immunological reactions involving platelets. Detailed reviews of platelet function may be found in a book by Marcus and Zucker (1965), reports of symposia (Jensen and Killman, 1970, 1971, 1973, 1974; Weiss, 1972; Spaet, 1972, 1974; Baldini and Ebbe, 1974), and articles by Marcus (1969), Mustard and Packham (1970), and Michal and Firkin (1969).

Studies in this area are beset by several difficulties. One is the poor cor-relation between results of research workers interested primarily in immuno-logy and of those interested primarily in platelet physiology. Only within the last year has coordination improved significantly; one purpose of this chapter is to acquaint workers in these two fields with each other's results and approaches.

Another difficulty relates to the platelets. Since they are profoundly affected by thrombin and adhere to strands of fibrin, the blood for experi-ments must be prevented from clotting. However, anticoagulants themselves can inhibit platelet function—citrate and ethylenediamine tetraacetate (EDTA) by chelating calcium and magnesium, and heparin by unknown means (Mustard and Packham, 1970, 1971; Zucker, 1972). When blood is added to one-ninth volume of 3.2 to 3.8% disodium citrate, the concentration of ionized calcium in plasma becomes too low to permit clotting but is adequate (though not optimal) to support platelet aggregation and release. Platelets are often studied in platelet-rich plasma, prepared by slow centri-fugation of anticoagulated blood. There is some evidence that this affects platelet function (Hampton and Mitchell, 1966; Friedberg and Zucker, 1972) but it can rarely be avoided during in vitro studies. To separate platelets from plasma, platelet-rich plasma must be centifuged rapidly to sediment the platelets. Platelets separated in this manner from citrated platelet-rich plasma are difficult to resuspend and undergo a partial release reaction unless centrifugation is carried out in the cold (Zucker, 1972). Use of EDTA, a more effective chelator of divalent cations than citrate, reduction of pH to about 6.5, or incubation of the sedimented platelets provides a platelet pellet which can be resuspended more readily. Methods which avoid centrifugation have been developed recently (Mannucci, 1972). Separation of platelets from plasma is necessary to study the role of plasma constituents in platelet function but undoubtedly affects platelet function in itself.

Unless otherwise noted, discussion in this chapter refers to the behavior of platelets in citrated human platelet-rich plasma. Platelet behavior varies considerably among species so that studies carried out in animals may not be relevant to human physiology and pathology. Unfortunately, human platelets were used in many studies of substances involved in hemostasis, and rabbit platelets in much of the work on immune agents.

II. Reactions in Hemostasis: Effects of Thrombin, Collagen, Subendothelial Microfibrils, ADP, and Epinephrine

Normally, platelets circulate through endothelium-lined blood vessels as discrete disk-shaped cells.* When blood vessels are injured and the endothelium is disrupted, the platelets contact other elements of the vascular wall, initiating a series of responses leading to the formation of either an effective hemostatic plug or a potentially dangerous intravascular thrombus (Brinkhous, 1970). Adhesion of the platelets is the first event, followed by aggregation and consolidation of the platelet mass with release of certain constituents from the platelets. These reactions will be discussed in some detail since they form the basis not only for the platelets' response to injury of blood and blood vessels, but also for their reaction to exogenous agents such as antigen–antibody complexes, latex particles, viruses, and bacteria.

A. Adhesion of Platelets to Physiological Surfaces

Platelets in flowing blood can adhere to strands of connective tissue (Hugues, 1962). Adhesion is also observed *in vitro*. It can occur in EDTA platelet-rich plasma, showing that divalent cations are not required (Spaet and Zucker, 1964).

Until recently, collagen was thought to be the only constituent of the blood vessel wall to which platelets adhered. Now it is clear that they adhere to the basement membrane of rabbit aorta after desquamation of the endothelial cells. Unlike collagen, the material to which platelets adhere is not destroyed by prolonged digestion with collagenase and is digested by trypsin (Stemerman *et al.*, 1971). It appears to consist of the subendothelial microfibrils described by Ross and Bornstein (1969) that differ chemically from both

---

*Strictly speaking, platelets are cell fragments without nucleus or DNA. Since they exhibit active metabolism and have varied organelles and a life span of about 10 days in man, they are usually called cells.

collagen and elastin. The mechanism of platelet adhesion to these micro-fibrils is just beginning to be explored. It differs from the platelet reaction to collagen because it is prevented by EDTA. An unusual feature is that adhesion can be demonstrated only in whole citrated or heparinized blood; few platelets adhere to exposed basement membrane when the aorta is perfused with platelet-rich plasma instead of whole blood (Baumgartner *et al.*, 1971).

B. Aggregation of Platelets

Aggregation in platelet suspensions can be followed by continuous recording of light transmission or optical density, usually at 37°C. Continuous stirring and a platelet count of more than about 100,000/mm³ are necessary.

ADP is a potent platelet aggregating agent (Gaarder *et al.*, 1961); when added to citrated or heparinized platelet-rich plasma in a final concentration of less than $1\mu M$, optical density begins to fall at once and reaches its lowest value in 2 to 3 minutes (Fig. 1). With low concentrations aggregation is reversible, with intermediate concentrations a double wave is often seen, and with high concentrations aggregation is irreversible. The second wave is associated with the release reaction and will be discussed in Section II,C.

Aggregation in hemostasis is stimulated by contact with collagen and microfibrils or exposure to thrombin. These substances cause aggregation partially or completely through the mediation of platelet ADP. Some ADP

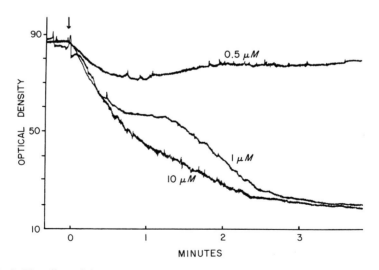

Fig. 1. The effect of three concentrations of ADP on the optical density of stirred human citrated platelet-rich plasma.

may be contributed by erythrocytes or cells of the vascular wall, but there is little evidence that these are important sources.

Aggregation can be induced by stirring fine particles of connective tissue with citrated or heparinized platelet-rich plasma, after a lag period which varies with the concentration of particles up to several minutes. Aggregation seems to be caused entirely by release of platelet ADP. The active material in the connective tissue is collagen because it is destroyed by incubation with collagenase (Zucker and Borrelli, 1962). Properly spaced polar groups, usually positively charged, are required for platelet adhesion and aggregation to collagen; different groups are necessary for activation of Hageman Factor (Factor XII) by collagen (Wilner *et al.*, 1968; Nossel *et al.*, 1969).

When low concentrations of thrombin (about 0.2 unit/ml) are stirred with citrated platelet-rich plasma, the resulting aggregation is often reversible. With higher concentrations, a double wave may be seen. Still higher concentrations induce coagulation. The second wave may be associated with release of catecholamines from platelets (Thomas, 1967). Exogenous epinephrine stimulates α-receptors on platelets and causes two waves of aggregation over a wide range of concentration. The second wave is associated with the release reaction (Section II,C). The cause of the first wave of aggregation with thrombin and epinephrine is unclear. There is some evidence that it is caused by ADP, presumably in or on the membrane (Haslam, 1967). Still another type of aggregation is observed when chilled platelet-rich plasma is shaken as it warms up. It is similar in many ways to aggregation induced by ADP, but there is no accompanying release of the nucleotide (Kattlove and Alexander, 1971).

Aggregation induced by any of these agents is prevented by EDTA and is absent in patients with the rare congenital hemorrhagic disorder known as thrombasthenia or Glanzmann's disease (Zucker *et al.*, 1966).

C. Release Reactions of Platelets

A number of stimuli besides collagen cause platelets to release ADP, and a number of constituents besides ADP are released. Some stimuli are particulate: collagen, antigen–antibody complexes, and latex particles; others are enzymatic: thrombin and trypsin; and still others are low molecular weight compounds such as ADP or, for primate platelets, epinephrine. In this section, we will discuss release induced by substances involved in hemostasis; in Section III, those more directly concerned with immune agents and inflammation will be considered. Three reviews of platelet-release reactions are highly recommended (Holmsen *et al.*, 1969; Day and Holmsen, 1971; Niewiarowski and Thomas, 1971) in addition to the specific references in this section.

1. Release Induced by Thrombin and Collagen

Release of a vasoconstrictor substance from platelets during clotting has been known for more than 70 years. The substance was shown to be 5-hydroxytryptamine or serotonin (Rapport, 1949), and thrombin was shown to be the clotting factor causing release (Zucker and Borrelli, 1955). Käser-Glanzmann and Lüscher (1962) demonstrated that thrombin also liberated ADP from washed platelets and in sufficient amount to account for thrombin's ability to aggregate platelets. Grette (1962) then showed that other substances were released as well and coined the term "release reaction." Soon after collagen particles were found to aggregate platelets, it was shown that here, too, that aggregation was induced by ADP liberated from the platelets (Hovig, 1963; Spaet and Zucker, 1964). To determine whether serotonin was also released, studies were carried out on platelets labeled with [14C]serotonin, an amine they take up rapidly (Born and Gillson, 1959). Release is studied simply by measuring the radioactivity of the supernatant plasma before and after exposing the labeled platelets to a releasing agent (Jerushalmy and Zucker, 1966). When platelets were exposed to connective tissue particles, [14C]serotonin was released in proportion to the concentration of adenine nucleotides released (Spaet and Zucker, 1964; Zucker, 1972). Parallel release of a third material, Platelet Factor 4, the antiheparin factor in platelets, was shown later (Harada and Zucker, 1971).

2. Release Induced by ADP, Epinephrine, and Propinquity

With guinea pig, cat, and human platelet-rich plasma, ADP produces two waves of aggregation (Thomas et al., 1970). In man, and presumably in the other species as well, the second wave is associated with release of ADP, ATP, [14C]serotonin (Zucker and Peterson, 1968; Mills et al., 1968), and Platelet Factor 4 (Youssef and Barkhan, 1968; Niewiarowski and Thomas, 1969). There is considerable evidence that all these are liberated together. The released material is not detected in plasma until the second wave is almost over. Either the second decrease in optical density results from contraction of already existing aggregates (Born and Hume, 1967) or the released ADP is at first trapped in the aggregates. With higher concentrations of ADP, only one wave of aggregation is seen, and measurement of the released material in the supernatant is the only indication of release.

When epinephrine is stirred with human platelet-rich plasma, two waves of aggregation also result (Mills et al., 1968). Animal platelets do not show this response (Thomas et al., 1970). The second wave is much easier to demonstrate with epinephrine than with ADP because it is caused by any concentration above 0.1–1.0 μM (Hardisty et al., 1970). As with ADP, adenine nucleotides, [14C]serotonin, and Platelet Factor 4 are also liberated. In the cat, platelets stirred with serotonin show the two-phased aggregation characteristic of release (Thomas *et al.*, 1970).

ADP and epinephrine do not induce release in unstirred platelet-rich plasma; the platelets must also come in contact with each other (Zucker and Peterson, 1968). Propinquity induced by centrifugation can also induce release, especially when carried out at 37°C at a somewhat elevated pH (O'Brien and Woodhouse, 1968; Massini and Luscher, 1971; Zucker, 1972). It has virtually no effect at 4°C.

3. CHARACTERISTICS OF RELEASE; SUBSTANCES RELEASED

The ADP and ATP freed during the release reaction come from a pool which is metabolically inert and not readily labeled with radioactive precursors (Holmsen *et al.*, 1969). These nucleotides, with serotonin, histamine in the rabbit, Platelet Factor 4, nonexchangeable potassium, and probably calcium, are normally held in special dense bodies in the platelets (Pletscher, 1968; Day *et al.*, 1969). These substances are thus released together. The number of dense bodies per platelet varies widely between species and presumably correlates with the serotonin content (Humphrey and Jaques, 1954).

Under some circumstances, certain platelet enzymes are also released. Thrombin, in particular, releases a considerable proportion of platelet β-glucuronidase, β-N-acetylglucosaminidase, and cathepsin, all hydrolytic enzymes shown to occur in so-called α-granules. These granules probably also contain acid phosphatase but little is released (Holmsen and Day, 1968, 1970; Day *et al.*, 1969). High concentrations of collagen also release hydrolytic enzymes, whereas epinephrine and ADP do not (Mills *et al.*, 1968; Holmsen *et al.*, 1969). It is notable that thrombin and other releasing agents do not free cytoplasmic enzymes such as lactic dehydrogenase or mitochondrial enzymes (Holmsen and Day, 1970).

It thus appears that nucleotides, serotonin, and other constituents of dense bodies can be released independently of enzymes in the α-granules. Day and Holmsen (1971) suggest calling the former Release I and the latter Release II. The latter may require a stronger stimulus than the former, but there may be a qualitative difference in the stimuli as well as in the response.

Release from platelets induced by stimuli concerned in hemostasis is very rapid—about 30 seconds for Release I and a few minutes for Release II. It is an active process, consuming ATP derived from glycolysis or oxidative phosphorylation. Grette (1962), Markwardt *et al.* (1968), and Day and Holmsen (1971) have proposed that the platelet contractile protein ejects the granules or their contents into the platelet surface-connected system or the surrounding medium.

Morphologically, release induced by ADP is not associated with striking degranulation. Since α-granules outnumber dense bodies, especially in human platelets, this is hardly surprising. Thrombin and collagen, on the other hand, can cause marked degranulation, but mitochondria remain. Rupture of the plasma membrane is not characteristic (Parmegianni, 1961), although it may occur after many minutes when fibrin is present (Rodman and Mason, 1967). Day and Holmsen (1971) provided biochemical evidence for lysis of 2–10% of the platelets after any type of release reaction.

D. Plasma Factors Necessary for Aggregation and Release

1. THROMBIN AND COLLAGEN

Washed human platelets aggregate when shaken with thrombin, provided the pH is above about 7.0 (Zucker and Borrelli, 1955). Phase microscopy reveals a tighter packing of the platelets within a few seconds after aggregation, resulting in homogeneous, glassy-looking clumps. This was called "fusion" or "viscous metamorphosis" until electron microscopy showed intact platelet membranes (Parmegianni, 1961). When concentrated suspensions of washed human platelets are exposed to thrombin (Bettex-Galland and Lüscher, 1964) or to collagen (Lackner et al., 1970), the entire mass is seen to contract, presumably through the action of the platelet contractile protein, thrombosthenin. Clot retraction appears to result from the contraction of platelets throughout a fibrin clot.

In contrast to earlier investigators, Taylor and Müller-Eberhard (1970) found that one or more plasma factors were necessary for the complete reaction of platelets with thrombin. Using platelets prepared with EDTA in the washing solutions, they observed that thrombin alone caused aggregation but no apparent "fusion." Serum or certain purified serum constituents restored so-called viscous metamorphosis. Unfortunately, no measurements of release were made. These varied results cannot be reconciled readily but suggest that with some techniques serum factors are necessary for thrombin-induced release.

Although Spaet and Zucker (1964) and Davey and Lüscher (1968) found that collagen induced release from washed platelets, Day and Holmsen (1971) have been unable to confirm this. The difference may result from differences in collagen concentration since high and low concentrations induce release by different mechanisms (Zucker and Peterson, 1970; Valdorf-Hansen and Zucker, 1971).

2. ADP

The pitfalls of technique again must be kept in mind. Under some conditions, washed platelets aggregate when shaken with calcium and ADP; under others, fibrinogen and perhaps another plasma factor are also needed (Mustard and Packham, 1970). Different conditions appear to be optimal for different species (Ardlie *et al.*, 1970). To undergo release with ADP or epinephrine, human platelets require a plasma factor other than fibrinogen (Cronberg *et al.*, 1971), perhaps citrate (Kinlough-Rathbone *et al.*, 1974).

E. Platelet Factor 3

Platelets contribute to blood clotting by behaving as a phospholipid, thus providing a surface necessary for several of the reactions in the coagulation cascade. This activity is known as Platelet Factor 3. Circulating platelets do not have Platelet Factor 3 activity, but it develops when platelets aggregate (Hardisty and Hutton, 1965, 1966). Little Platelet Factor 3 activity is released into the plasma; instead, it seems to represent a change in the membrane (Marcus and Zucker, 1965). The development of Platelet Factor 3 activity induced by ADP can be clearly differentiated from ADP-induced release of amines and adenine nucleotides. The former is not prevented by aspirin and occurs about as well at room temperature as at 37°C, whereas the latter is prevented by aspirin and fails to occur at room temperature (Atac *et al.*, 1970; Sixma and Nijessen, 1970; Valdorf-Hansen and Zucker, 1971).

Walsh (1972) and Walsh and Biggs (1972) recently reported that platelets play a role in several other reactions in coagulation which may be of great importance in hemostasis.

III. Reaction of Platelets with Foreign Materials

A. Glass

Platelets in human citrated or heparinized platelet-rich plasma adhere to and spread on glass slides. They do not adhere in the presence of EDTA, in this way resembling the reaction of platelets with microfibrils more than that with collagen. There is another resemblance between glass and microfibrils. When citrated or heparinized blood is passed through a column of glass beads at an appropriate rate, many platelets are retained, but when platelet-rich plasma is used rather than whole blood, virtually none are retained. Erythrocytes probably act by affecting the blood flow pattern (Zucker *et al.*, 1972).

These observations with glass bead columns may seem to be of purely academic interest. However, decreased retention is the only abnormal *in vitro* test of platelet function in the congenital hemorrhagic disorder known as von Willebrand's disease.* This disease is characterized by a prolonged bleeding time without obvious cause; aggregation and release with ADP, collagen, and thrombin are normal. It is tempting to think that the abnormal retention in glass bead columns reflects a similar abnormal reaction between platelets and subendothelial microfibrils and hence points to a role for these fibrils in hemostasis.

The role of plasma proteins in the reaction of platelets to glass has been explored. Washed human platelets suspended in isotonic saline or buffer adhere readily to glass, but this reaction is considered nonphysiological because platelets from thrombasthenic patients adhere when suspended in saline but not in blood or plasma (Braunsteiner and Pakesch, 1956). Washed human platelets resuspended in normal plasma or in fibrinogen solutions adhere to glass slides, but platelets resuspended in serum or defibrinated plasma do not (Zucker and Vroman, 1969). Platelets in platelet-rich plasma from patients with congenital afibrinogenemia show some impairment of release and aggregation (Weiss and Rogers, 1971), but their most striking abnormality is failure to adhere to glass slides (Zucker and Vroman, 1969). Retention in glass bead columns is also impaired (Weiss and Rogers, 1971).

There are striking similarities between the adhesion of platelets to glass slides and their reaction with ADP. In both cases, divalent cations and fibrinogen play a part, thrombasthenic platelets fail to react, and platelet energy must be produced. The adhesion of platelets to collagen differs in that divalent cations and fibrinogen are not important, and thrombasthenic platelets adhere normally (Spaet and Zucker, 1964).

Platelets also react with kaolin, a siliceous clay. It releases ADP (Weiss and Rogers, 1971) as well as serotonin (M. B. Zucker, unpublished) and induces Platelet Factor 3 activity (see Section II,E) in the presence of fibrinogen. Hageman Factor (Factor XII) is not required (Hardisty and Hutton, 1966).

B. Immune Agents; Phagocytosis

Unlike leukocytes, washed platelets from immunized animals do not react with antibody (Gocke and Osler, 1965). However, platelets from normal animals have a remarkable ability to react as "passive participants" (Gocke, 1965) when exposed to antigen and its antibody. Early experiments showed that histamine was released from platelets when antigen was added to the blood of immunized rabbits (Katz, 1940; McIntire et al., 1952) (see Section II,C), but it was soon shown that platelets from nonimmunized animals were similarly affected by antigen in the presence of antibody.

---

* Aggregation of platelets in vitro with the antibiotic Ristocetin is also abnormal and, like platelet retention in a glass bead column, is restored by a large-molecular-weight plasma factor (Weiss et al., 1973).

As pointed out by Barbaro (1961a), experiments can be carried out in three ways: (1) addition of antigen to blood or platelet-rich plasma from an immunized animal; (2) separate addition of soluble antigen and antibody; or (3) addition of insoluble antigen–antibody complexes to blood, platelet-rich plasma, or washed platelets from a nonimmunized animal. A fourth type of experiment utilizes an insoluble antigen (Henson and Cochrane, 1969a,b,c). Aggregated γ-globulin, which behaves in many ways as an antigen–antibody complex, also affects platelets, and so does endotoxin. As in platelet reactions with substances concerned with hemostasis, the platelet response with immune agents varies with the species, so they will be discussed separately.

Species differences are not the only obstacle to drawing comprehensive conclusions from a survey of the literature in this area. A variety of platelet responses has been measured: adherence, aggregation, contraction, release, and phagocytosis. Only rarely have more than one or two of these parameters been measured simultaneously; since they do not necessarily occur together, it is not meaningful to compare results of such studies.

The relationship of immunological mechanisms and platelets has been the subject of several valuable reviews (Ratnoff, 1969; Mustard *et al.*, 1969; DesPrez and Marney, 1971; Osler and Siraganian, 1972; Pfueller and Lüscher, 1972a).

1. HUMAN PLATELETS

Washed human platelets do not undergo mixed agglutination (i.e., "immune adherence") with antigen–antibody complexes in the presence of serum as a source of complement; under the same conditions, guinea pig or rabbit platelets adhere (Siqueira and Nelson, 1961; Henson, 1969b). In contrast, human and primate erythrocytes do undergo immune adherence, but red cells from other species do not.

Bettex-Galland and Lüscher (1964) showed that concentrated suspensions of washed human platelets incubated with preformed antigen–antibody complexes underwent contraction similar to the "viscous metamorphosis" produced by thrombin. Movat *et al.* (1965a) used an aggregometer to assess the response to such complexes and found that the reaction of native or citrated platelet-rich plasma did not differ from that of twice-washed platelets prepared from EDTA blood and suspended in Tyrode–gelatin solution. Aggregation developed during about 5 minutes, was not increased by fresh pig serum as a complement source, and was largely prevented by AMP, iodoacetate, or EDTA. It was associated with release of ADP, [^{14}C]serotonin, and [^{3}H]histamine in 10 minutes and degranulation in 1 hour. According to Mueller-Eckhardt and Lüscher (1968a), aggregation and release of adenine nucleotides was not altered by addition of complement (diluted fresh guinea pig or human serum). Ethylenediamine tetraacetate inhibited aggregation and contraction but only partially prevented nucleotide release. The reaction of platelets to immune agents and thrombin was abolished by N-ethylmaleimide, and inhibition was prevented by the simultaneous addition of L-cysteine. Iodoacetate inhibited release by immune agents but not by thrombin, and the inhibition was not prevented by cysteine (Mueller-Eckhardt and Lüscher, 1968c). Two-phased aggregation has not been demonstrated; release of platelet enzymes has not been measured; and the effects of aspirin, DFP, and agents which affect cyclic AMP have not been tested. In summary, it seems clear that human platelets react strongly with preformed antigen–antibody complexes without the addition of complement, but do not undergo immune adherence with such complexes even in the presence of complement.

There are very few experiments on the reaction of human platelets to soluble antigen–antibody complexes, yet, at least in rabbits, they differ considerably from the response to insoluble complexes (Des Prez and Marney, 1971). Humphrey and Jaques (1955), in their classic paper on release of amines, reported one experiment in which human platelets released serotonin when incubated with antigen and antibody, whereas platelets of a number of other species required the addition of plasma as well. Recent studies showed that plasma from patients hypersensitive to penicillin or equine antitetanus serum promoted release of [^{14}C]serotonin from labeled rabbit or human platelets in the presence of antigen. The test was positive when other tests for antibody were negative, but not all allergic subjects had a positive response, and the effective amount of antigen was very critical (Caspary and Comaish, 1967; Comaish, 1968).

Myllylä et al. (1969) observed that most preparations of washed human platelets aggregate when incubated in the cold with soluble (20–25 S) complexes of small-size viral antigen with human antibody. The test was more sensitive than the complement fixation test for detecting rubella antibodies, for example. Platelets also reacted with soluble haptene–bovine serum albumin–antibody complexes (Penttinen et al., 1969). It is noteworthy that, again, no plasma factors were required.

Two groups of investigators have pointed out that substances which react with human platelets are also able to bind complement. Thus, similar to antigen-antibody complexes, aggregated γ-globulin bound complement and caused platelets to aggregate, contract, and release adenine nucleotides. In contrast, nonaggregated γ-globulin or aggregated γ-globulin exposed to pH 4 failed to bind complement or react with platelets (Bettex-Galland and Lüscher, 1964; Mueller-Eckhardt and Lüscher, 1968a). Jobin and co-workers (Jobin and Tremblay, 1969; Jobin and Gagnon, 1970; Jobin et al., 1970) made similar observations but pointed out that collagen is a notable exception, since it does not bind complement. These investigators also observed that many complement inhibitors inhibited platelet aggregation although correlation was far from perfect.

The correlation, as well as the lack of requirement for added complement, could be explained if washed human platelets were coated with complement, but Mueller-Eckhardt and Lüscher (1968a) failed to demonstrate activity of C1,2,3, or 4 on human platelets either tested whole or after destruction mechanically or by freeze-thawing. Furthermore, platelets digested with chymotrypsin to dissolve possible bound-surface complement aggregated normally. Platelets treated with aggregated γ-globulin failed to split acetyl-L-tyrosine ethyl ester, which is hydrolyzed by C1 esterase (A. Siegel, unpublished, cited by Mueller-Eckhardt and Lüscher, 1968a). These workers therefore concluded that the correlation probably indicates the occurrence of similar chemical reactions or configurations rather than pointing to a role of complement itself in human platelet reactions. Nagaki et al. (1965) demonstrated the presence of C4 but not C1 or 2 on washed human and guinea pig platelets, although in an amount so small that only about 0.01 % of the C4 content of platelet-rich plasma could be attributed to platelets. Packham et al. (1968) reported that frozen and thawed washed human platelets of unspecified concentration can lyse sensitized erythrocytes.

A number of interesting observations have been made on the responses of human platelets recently. Pfueller and Luscher (1972b) showed that myeloma proteins from subclasses IgG1, IgG2, and IgG3 but not IgG4 bind complement when aggregated; in contrast, all IgG subclasses cause a release reaction with washed platelets (IgG3 only weakly). Structural requirements of the immunoglobulin were also studied; removal of 36% of the hexose from IgG abolished its effect on platelets with little reduction of its complement-fixing ability (Pfueller and Lüscher, 1972c). Immune complexes induced a biphasic release reaction in citrated platelet-rich plasma. The first phase, like that occurring with washed platelets, was not inhibited by EDTA. The second phase was inhibited by EDTA and adenosine and was associated with marked ADP-induced aggregation. (Pfueller and Lüscher, 1973). Zymosan particles incubated with plasma induced release of the second type (Zucker and Grant, 1974; Zucker et al., 1973; Pfueller and Luscher, 1974a,b). The complement by-pass (properdin) mechanism appeared to be involved but incubation of zymosan with serum rather than plasma did not induce activity unless fibrinogen was added (Pfueller and Luscher, 1974b; Zucker and Grant, 1974), and became bound to the zymosan (Zucker and Grant, 1974).

PHAGOCYTOSIS. When native or citrated human platelet-rich plasma was gently agitated at 37°C with polystyrene latex particles 0.3 μm in diameter, electron microscopy revealed phagocytosis of the particles by the platelets (Fig. 2) and, after 1 hour, marked degranulation (Movat et al.,

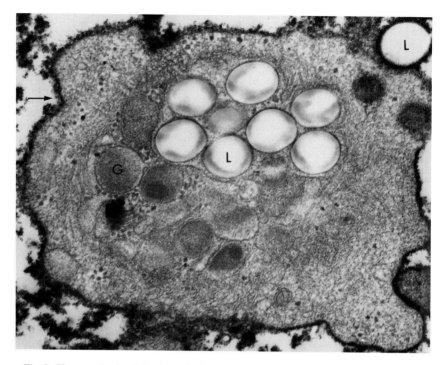

Fig. 2. Human platelet following 15-minute incubation with latex particles, fixed in the presence of ruthenium red to delineate the surface coat (arrow). Latex particles, L; granules, G. Magnification × 45,000. (Courtesy of Dr. Dorothea Zucker-Franklin.)

1965b). Platelet aggregation developed gradually and was associated with release of ADP and ATP (Glynn *et al.*, 1965). Adenosine or AMP prevented aggregation but not phagocytosis, whereas EDTA or a combination of iodoacetate and 2,4-dinitrophenol prevented both (Movat *et al.*, 1965b). Phagocytosis stimulated glycolysis and CO_2 production via the citric acid cycle (Kuramoto *et al.*, 1970). Particles from 0.088 μm to more than 1 μm in diameter were effective (Glynn *et al.*, 1965; Kuramoto *et al.*, 1970). Colloidal carbon also induced phagocytosis and aggregation of human platelets (Movat *et al.*, 1965b) and platelets can take up fat (Schulz and Wedell, 1962). A review of platelet phagocytosis has appeared (Mustard and Packham, 1968).

With washed human platelets, particles 0.796 μm in diameter were inactive but caused rapid aggregation, release, and contraction if they were coated with human γ-globulin. Coating with albumin, fibrinogen, or aggregated γ-globulin exposed to pH 4 was ineffective. Particles more than 22 μm in diameter coated with γ-globulin were inactive although they could activate complement (Mueller-Eckhardt and Lüscher, 1968b).

2. RABBIT PLATELETS

a. AGGREGATION; PHAGOCYTOSIS. Rabbit platelets aggregate with insoluble antigen–antibody complexes in the presence of plasma (immune adherence) (Siqueira and Nelson, 1961). Ishizaka and Ishizaka (1962) induced aggregation with such complexes or with aggregated γ-globulin without added plasma, but clumps were small and were probably observed only microscopically. Aggregated γ-globulin caused two waves of clumping when tested on heparinized platelet-rich plasma (1 unit/ml blood). The second wave was inhibited by 10 units/ml heparin and by adenosine; it may have been associated with release. Epinephrine, norepinephrine, and serotonin themselves caused only slight transient aggregation but potentiated the aggregation induced by low concentrations of aggregated γ-globulin. Histamine and bradykinin had no effect (Davis and Holtz, 1969).

Washed rabbit platelets stirred with γ-globulin-coated latex particles released ADP, ATP, and serotonin after a 2-minute latent period. Aggregation and release occurred without plasma addition and were inhibited by phenylbutazone and sulfinpyrazone (Packham et al., 1967). Release induced by other particulate material required a plasma factor. Platelets contain silicon dioxide or thorium oxide after these materials have been injected intravenously into rabbits (Ferreira, 1961; Schulz, 1961).

b. RELEASE AND OTHER EFFECTS INDUCED BY IMMUNE AGENTS. Rabbit platelets, dissimilar to those of other mammals tested, have a high concentration of histamine, and similar to some other species, of serotonin (Humphrey and Jaques, 1954). Washed platelets release histamine in the presence of antigen, antibody, and heparinized plasma (Humphrey and Jaques, 1955). According to Barbaro (1961a, b), antigen–antibody complexes preformed at equivalence or antibody excess also liberated histamine provided plasma was present.

Barbaro (1961a,b) concluded that the plasma did not act by supplying complement because the correlation between complement activity and histamine-releasing activity of plasma treated in various ways was imperfect. On the other hand, Gocke and Osler (1965) and Gocke (1965) favored the involvement of complement since pepsin-treated antibodies did not support release. They noted, however, as did Des Prez and Bryant later (1966), that guinea pig serum, rich in complement, could not restore the activity of rabbit plasma heated to 56°C for 30 minutes. They did not observe aggregation, presumably because the platelet count was only about 60,000/cm^3 and mixing was gentle. Serotonin release paralleled that of histamine. Releasing activity could be generated in plasma by antigen–antibody complex and had a half-life of 7 to 8 minutes at 37°C.

Recent studies by Henson and Cochrane have been summarized (Henson, 1969a). The mechanism of release with particulate antigen plus antibody (Henson and Cochrane, 1969a,b) or preformed antigen–antibody complexes (Des Prez and Bryant, 1969) is different from that observed when antigen and antibody are added separately and the complex is soluble. Both mechanisms may act simultaneously under certain circumstances, explaining some discrepancies in results (Des Prez and Bryant, 1969).

With particulate material, zymosan or sensitized erythrocytes, Henson and Cochrane concluded that the reaction was related to immune adherence. Aggregation and release required complement through C3 but was normal with plasma from rabbits congenitally deficient in C6. Further studies (Henson, 1970c) indicated that release was a rapid, selective, active mechanism: Vasoactive amines and adenine nucleotides were released but not rubidium-86; aggregation was induced; glucose was required; and the reaction was inhibited by DFP and ethyleneglycoldiaminoethyltetraacetic acid (EGTA), which binds calcium far more readily than magnesium. One millimolar adenosine or aspirin caused marked inhibition whereas sodium salicylate did not. Surprisingly, platelets became degranulated although only small amounts of β-glucuronidase were released without acid phosphatase or lactic dehydrogenase.

Sirganian's results (1972) differed since he found that C6 was necessary for release of histamine, serotonin, and potassium from washed platelets by inulin, zymosan, or antigen–antibody aggregates. Release induced by thrombin, collagen, or kaolin, however, did not require C6 or, in fact, any plasma. Different experimental conditions presumably explain the disparity between these results and those of the La Jolla group.

Des Prez and Bryant (1969), who also studied the reaction of rabbit platelets to particulate material, measured serotonin release caused by preformed antigen–antibody complexes in the presence of plasma. Since citrate and anticomplementary concentrations of heparin or sodium chloride were not inhibitory, and antibody digested with pepsin to remove the Fc fragment was active, they concluded that complement was not required. They postulated the need for an unidentified heat-labile factor which was removed from plasma by zymosan adsorption at 16°C in the presence of EDTA, conditions under which complement is not affected. This factor was previously shown to be necessary for endotoxin action (Des Prez, 1967).

Zimmerman and co-workers observed several interesting complement-induced reactions. A polypeptide was deleted from rabbit platelets treated with inulin in the presence of normal but not C6-deficient plasma (Zimmerman and Müller-Eberhard, 1973). Under these conditions, inulin and aggregated γ-globulin also shortened the clotting time and accelerated prothrombin consumption (Zimmerman and Müller-Eberhard, 1971). A possible role for complement in normal coagulation was suggested by the observation that prothrombin consumption was abnormal in C6-deficient rabbits (Zimmerman *et al.*, 1971).

These investigators and others have described another mechanism for release which occurs in the presence of a soluble antigen, antibody in about 20-fold excess, heparinized plasma, and washed platelets. According to Henson and Cochrane (1969a,b), aggregation but not release took place with plasma from C6-deficient rabbits. With normal plasma, histamine was released by means of platelet lysis; this was indicated by release of rubidium-86 in large amounts (Siraganian *et al.*, 1968) and of cytoplasmic (lactic dehydrogenase) as well as lysosomal enzymes (Henson, 1970c). Electron microscopy also revealed membrane lysis. Glucose was not necessary, and DFP and aspirin were not inhibitory. Magnesium appears to be the important cation in this reaction (Siraganian *et al.*, 1968).

In studies carried out under similar conditions, Des Prez and Bryant (1966) noted that citrate (10 mM) inhibited release when added to immune heparinized plasma plus platelets prior to antigen, but not when added after preincubation of the plasma and antigen but prior to the platelets. They assumed that citrate inhibited a complement-dependent step, but subsequent studies (Marney and Des Prez, 1971) showed that 10 mM citrate did not inhibit complement-dependent red cell lysis in plasma. Similarly, tosyl-L-arginine methyl ester (TAME) inhibited release from rabbit platelets (Shore and Alpers, 1963; Marney and Des Prez, 1971) but failed to affect complement-mediated red cell lysis. Thus the role of complement is again in question. Dissimilar to citrate, TAME or acetyl-L-tyrosine ethyl ester was inhibitory when added after preincubation of antigen, antibody, and plasma. Epsilon-aminocaproic acid and soybean trypsin inhibitor did not inhibit serotonin release under these circumstances.

Westerholm (1965) also characterized release induced by soluble antigen in the presence of antibody. The reaction was inhibited by heparin (100 units/ml), EDTA, salicylaldoxime, ninhydrin, allicin, and hypertonic sodium chloride. Platelets heated to 47°C were no longer active, and plasma lost its activity at 56°C.

The relationship of release and aggregation was poorly understood until recently. Henson (1970c) pointed out that insoluble antigen with antibody and complement through C3 produced both aggregation (presumably immune adherence) and release, whereas soluble antigen, antibody, and complement through C3 produced aggregation without release. C6 was necessary for release to occur. Marney (1971) used an aggregometer to assess aggregation induced by this system. Two waves of aggregation were evident when ovalbumin and rabbit antibody in a 1:20 ratio by weight were added to stirred heparinized plasma at 37°C. With 1.5 μg of antigen N, a maximal response was seen starting about 1 minute after challenge. The first wave was associated with development of platelet stickiness (measured with a glass bead column), but not with release of ADP or vasoactive amines; the second wave was accompanied by release of serotonin and ADP. The results therefore agree essentially with Henson's in separating aggregation from release. The experiments reveal a second wave similar to that occurring in release induced by nonimmunological stimuli (see Section II,C) and bridge the gap between the approaches of the immunologist and investigator primarily interested in hemostasis. AMP (10 mM) prevented the second wave of aggregation but not the associated release of ADP. As shown earlier (Des Prez and Bryant, 1966; Marney and Des Prez, 1971), citrate prevented release and also the second but not the first wave of aggregation. Perhaps an inhibitory action of the citrate is also responsible for failure of ADP to cause a second wave of aggregation in citrated rabbit platelet-rich plasma. When release was assessed with [^{14}C]serotonin, ADP sometimes induced release in heparinized but not citrated rabbit platelet-rich plasma (Zucker and Grant, cited in Peterson and Zucker, 1970).

In Marney's studies, heating plasma to 56°C for 30 minutes or adding a low concentration of cobra venom factor abolished the first wave of platelet aggregation, the associated stickiness, the second wave of aggregation, and the accompanying release. Preincubation of cobra venom factor with plasma was not required. The author concludes, as do Henson and Cochrane, that complement through C3 is necessary for aggregation, and complement through C6 for release when soluble antigen is added with a 20-fold antibody excess.

Anaphylatoxin from rat and rabbit plasma does not induce release from rabbit platelets (Henson and Cochrane, 1969b).

Complexes of soluble antigen and antibody also increase Platelet Factor 3 activity when added to citrated platelet-rich plasma (Horowitz *et al.*, 1962).

3. PLATELETS OF SPECIES OTHER THAN MAN AND RABBIT

Guinea pig platelets, just as rabbit platelets, can undergo immune adherence with antigen–antibody complexes in the presence of serum (Siqueira and Nelson, 1961). Henson (1969b) examined adherence to sheep red cells sensitized with IgM antibody and complement. Platelets from the rabbit, guinea pig, rat, mouse, horse, and cat exhibited immune adherence, but those from the ox, goat, sheep, and pig, also from the baboon and man, did not. The role of C3 was indicated by the observation that serum treated with cobra venom factor was inactive whereas serum from C6-deficient rabbits was active. Complement from man, rabbit, guinea pig, and horse effectively promoted adherence of guinea pig platelets and was ineffective with human platelets. Human complement was ineffective with rabbit platelets, and complement from the other three species was active. Ethylenediamine tetraacetate did not prevent adherence of platelets to coated particles.

Platelets from dogs and guinea pigs released serotonin in the presence of antigen, antibody, and plasma (Humphrey and Jaques, 1955).

The response of pig platelets has been investigated in Mustard's laboratory. It should be noted that ADP does not induce release from platelets in citrated platelet-rich plasma of this species (Thomas *et al.*, 1970). Pig platelets in platelet-rich plasma were only transiently aggregated by latex particles, perhaps because the released ADP was rapidly destroyed (Glynn *et al.*, 1965). Washed pig platelets reacted as rabbit platelets to γ-globulin-coated latex particles (Packham *et al.*, 1967).

C. Heterologous Antibody

When washed platelets of one species are injected into another species, antibodies are produced which can induce profound thrombocytopenia when injected into the first species. According to Mueller-Eckhardt and Lüscher (1968a), some samples of rabbit antibody to human platelets caused aggregation, contraction, and release without addition of complement and were able to fix complement. Other samples of antibody were much less effective in both respects. Treatment of human platelets with anti-platelet serum in the presence of complement revealed deletion of a polypeptide (Zimmerman and Müller-Eberhard, 1973).

Henson (1970b) found that antibody to rabbit platelets raised in sheep had two actions. It caused release of vasoactive amines by an energy-requiring DFP-inhibitable mechanism which did not require complement. Antibody with at least two combining sites was needed but the Fc piece could be removed without loss of activity. In the presence of complement, the antibody caused frank lysis of the platelets, with loss of internal contents including cytoplasmic enzymes.

D. Leukocytes

Henson and Cochrane (1969c; Henson, 1970d) showed that the presence of blood or peritoneal neutrophils enhanced the release of histamine, serotonin, and adenine nucleotides from rabbit platelets induced by zymosan or antigen–antibody complexes with particulate antigen. Mixed aggregates formed which contained leukocytes. As in the absence of neutrophils, plasma was necessary and plasma without C3 activity was inactive. Leukocytes were also active in the system with soluble antigen. Here, C6-deficient plasma could not support release in the absence of leukocytes but could do so in their presence although they did not supply C6. The reactions were inhibited by DFP, aspirin, and adenosine. In some experiments, fibrin formed despite the presence of 10 units heparin/ml. It was suggested that leukocytes may supply a proteolytic enzyme which enhances release or they may act via thrombin.

Basophilic leukocytes are involved in inducing release from platelets by an entirely different mechanism. Schoenbechler and Barbaro (1968) thought that lymphocytes from rabbits infected with *Schistosoma mansoni* caused histamine release from platelets in the presence of specific antigen but in the absence of complement or added antibody. Platelets could be obtained from either infected or normal animals. Initially, the platelets were believed to be sensitized (Barbaro and Zvaifler, 1966), but it was shown that antigen could release histamine from washed platelets of infected rabbits only if leukocytes were present (Schoenbechler and Sadun, 1968; Siraganian and Osler, 1969). According to Barbaro and Schoenbechler (1970), the reaction took place in two steps: a temperature-sensitive, calcium-dependent activation step and a reaction between platelets and activated leukocytes. The latter retained their activity when washed free of antigen or frozen and thawed. Henson (1970a) produced a similar reaction with bovine serum albumin or ferritin as antigen. He found that leukocytes from extravascular sources were much less active than those from blood. Platelets did not release cytoplasmic enzymes or ^{86}Rb and released only a very small amount of β-glucuronidase. Henson (1970a) and Henson and Cochrane (1970) found that a soluble factor, released when leukocytes and antigen were incubated together, caused release of amines from platelets, but Barbaro and Schoenbechler (1970) could not confirm this.

Recently, Siraganian and Osler (1971a) confirmed the earlier observations that when leukocytes from a sensitized rabbit were exposed to antigen, they released histamine and a soluble factor which acts on platelets. The reaction occurred in the absence of plasma, required calcium, and was inhibited by magnesium. The soluble factor(s) from the leukocytes, in turn, released histamine from washed rabbit platelets in a rapid, temperature- and calcium-dependent reaction which was described as cytotoxic since ^{86}Rb was also released. The leukocytes involved are basophils; when sensitized with IgE and exposed to antigen, they release histamine and platelet-aggregating factor (PAF) (Siraganian and Osler, 1971b; Benveniste *et al.*, 1972).

E. Bacteria; Endotoxin

Bacteria were thought to clump suspensions of rabbit but not human platelets (Roskam, 1923), suggesting a reaction similar to immune adherence.

However, recently Clawson and White (1971) found that staphylococci and other bacteria induced platelet aggregation when added to human citrated platelet-rich plasma in a 1:1 ratio (bacteria:platelets). Neither human nor rabbit platelets killed the bacteria in 2 hours under these conditions.

Endotoxin, the lipopolysaccharide(s) of the wall of gram-negative bacteria, also reacts with platelets and has been the subject of many experiments. Although the generalized Shwartzman reaction requires two injections of endotoxin and the intervention of polymorphonuclear leukocytes (Vol. II, Chap. 11), even a single intravenous injection of endotoxin into rabbits or dogs causes transient thrombocytopenia, and the plasma shows serotonin and Platelet Factor 3 activity which is normally confined to platelets (Davis *et al.*, 1960; Des Prez *et al.*, 1961; Horowitz *et al.*, 1962). *In vitro*, endotoxin accelerates coagulation by acting on the platelets (Robbins and Stetson, 1958), enhancing their phospholipid-like activity (Horowitz *et al.*, 1962). Aggregation and serotonin release also occurred *in vitro* after incubation of as little as 1.0 μg *E. coli* endotoxin/ml heparinized platelet-rich plasma. With citrate as anticoagulant, almost 100 times more endotoxin was required, and EDTA inhibited the reaction entirely (Des Prez *et al.*, 1961). Aggregation and release occurred gradually over a 60-minute period in citrated platelet-rich plasma (Des Prez, 1964), parallel with degranulation (Spielvogel, 1967). The suggestion that endotoxin reacts with a natural antibody (Robbins and Stetson, 1958; Spielvogel, 1967) is consistent with the observation of Des Prez *et al.* (1961) that aggregation and release are accelerated by prior incubation of plasma with endotoxin and diminished by prior adsorption of the plasma with endotoxin. Spielvogel (1967) provided evidence of immune adherence: Endotoxin in plasma adhered to primate red cells rather than to platelets, and to the platelets but not to red cells of rabbits, rats, dogs, and guinea pigs. Interestingly, degranulation was noted only with rabbit and rat platelets and was not abolished by incubation with combined inhibitors of glycolysis and respiration. Some phagocytosis of endotoxin particles by rabbit platelets was observed.

Rabbit platelets suspended in citrated plasma which had been heated to 56°C for 30 minutes did not respond to endotoxin, and plasma adsorbed with zymosan could not restore the response, suggesting the mediation of complement through C3 (Des Prez *et al.*, 1961; Spielvogel, 1967). However, Des Prez (1967) obtained clear evidence that the factor adsorbed by zymosan was not C3; adsorption in the cold in the presence of EDTA resulted in plasma with almost complete C3 activity but no ability to promote the action of endotoxin. (See discussion in Section III,B, 2.)

Endotoxin and staphyloccal protein A enhanced coagulation and prothrombin consumption of rabbit blood only when C6 was present (Zimmerman and Müller-Eberhard, 1971).

A study of aggregation, release of [^{14}C]serotonin, and development of Platelet Factor 3 activity in rabbit heparinized platelet-rich plasma revealed different relative activity of endotoxins from different bacterial species on each test (Nagayama et al., 1971).

Washed human platelets do not aggregate grossly with endotoxin (Mueller-Eckhardt and Lüscher, 1968d); however, they are not entirely inert. A small amount of [^{14}C]serotonin was slowly released but no macroscopic aggregation or Platelet Factor 3 activity was noted when human heparinized platelet-rich plasma was incubated with endotoxin from several species of bacteria (Nagayama et al., 1971). Ream et al. (1965) noted microscopic aggregation of washed platelets with several endotoxins, which occurred only with use of plasma containing coagulation Factor V.

F. Viruses

Washed human platelets adsorb myxoviruses, as do erythrocytes, but elute them much less readily. Adsorption is only partially inhibited by receptor-destroying enzyme under conditions which abolish the ability of red cells to take up virus (Jerushalmy et al., 1961). Retention may be the result of phagocytosis of the virus particles (Danon et al., 1959). Viruses also affect platelet function; viruses causing Newcastle disease and influenza inhibit clot retraction and enhance clot-promoting activity, and the Newcastle agent actually lyses platelets. These viruses are not known to cause viremia, however, and the concentrations used here were several orders of magnitude higher than the peak concentration of other viruses found in the blood (Jerushalmy et al., 1962).

IV. Inhibitors of Platelet Aggregation and Release: Similarities between the Reactions of Platelets and Other Cells

A number of investigators have referred to the "injury" to platelets caused by antigen–antibody complexes. However, some platelet reactions to such complexes appear to be identical with platelet-release reactions induced by agents involved in hemostasis. Release is a selective, specific process, dissimilar to frank lysis with loss of cytoplasmic contents such as lactic dehydrogenase.

Some insight into mechanisms can be obtained by use of inhibitors. Some inhibitors of reactions involved in hemostasis act only with certain stimulating agents rather than on a common mechanism of response, e.g., heparin with thrombin or α-receptor inhibitors with epinephrine. EDTA and

EGTA in concentrations sufficient to chelate ambient calcium ions prevent aggregation by all agents. TAME and related compounds are competitive inhibitors of ADP-induced aggregation (Salzman and Chambers, 1964). Release induced by ADP or epinephrine is coupled with primary ADP-induced aggregation since substances which inhibit the latter also inhibit the former. Examples are adenosine, agents which react with sulfhydryl groups (Valdorf-Hansen and Zucker, 1971), dibutyryl cyclic AMP, or cyclic AMP when elevated within the platelets by stimulation of adenyl cyclase or inhibition of phosphodiesterase (Salzman and Levine, 1971). On the other hand, release, but not primary aggregation, is prevented by aspirin and other nonsteroidal antiinflammatory compounds but not sodium salicylate (Zucker and Peterson, 1970; O'Brien *et al.*, 1970). DFP acted similarly (Zucker, 1972). Release induced by collagen and thrombin is less readily inhibited by antiinflammatory agents.

Many of these compounds have been shown to inhibit various aspects of the platelet response to immune agents. Unfortunately, studies on hemostasis have usually been carried out with human platelets and studies on immune agents with rabbit platelets. In contrast to human platelets, rabbit platelets fail to release readily with ADP, are not aggregated by epinephrine, and require plasma for reactions with immune agents. Comparison of their responses is therefore hazardous. Nevertheless, effects of some inhibitors on platelet reactions to immune and hemostatic stimuli are summarized in Table I. As pointed out by Henson and Cochrane, it is evident that the C3-dependent reaction to insoluble antigens is very similar to the release reaction induced by hemostatic agents.

The platelet release reaction resembles secretory activity or amine release in other types of cells, as noted by Stormorken (1969) and Day and Holmsen (1971). Notable among these are mast cells, which of course release histamine during immune reactions. Detailed discussion is beyond the scope of this chapter, but as in the case of platelets, release from mast cells or basophils is inhibited by DFP, cyclic AMP, EDTA, and diminished energy production and is much more active at 37°C than at room temperature. Aspirin, but not sodium salicylate, blocks release of a smooth muscle-contracting material from sensitized guinea pig lungs by antigen (Collier, 1969).

V. Platelets in Other Inflammatory Reactions

A. Bactericidal Activity

Hirsh (1960) confirmed Metchnikoff's early finding that rabbit serum prepared from whole blood had bactericidal activity on gram-positive organisms, whereas serum prepared from plasma did not. The active

TABLE I

CHARACTERISTICS OF AGGREGATION AND RELEASE INDUCED BY STIMULI INVOLVED IN IMMUNOLOGICAL AND HEMOSTATIC RESPONSES

			Substances released			Release or aggregation inhibited by					
Stimulus	Species	Response	Amines, adenine nucleotides	β-Glucu-ronidase	LDH, ^{50}Rb	EDTA	Cyclic AMP	TAME	Adenosine	Aspirin	DFP
C3 dep., insol. ag.	Rabbit	Agg. and Rel.	+	±	−	+			+	+	+
C3 dep., ag. + ab.	Rabbit	Agg.[a]	−	−	−	+		+			
C6 dep., ag. + ab.	Rabbit	Agg. and Rel.	+	+	+	+		+	−	−	−
Thrombin	Man or rabbit	Agg. and Rel.	+	+	−	±[b, c]	[d]	[e]	±[c]	±[c]	[e]
Collagen	Man or rabbit	Agg. and Rel.	+	±[c]	−	±[b, c]	+		±[c]	±[c]	
ADP	Man or rabbit	Agg.[a]	−	−		+	+	+	+	−	−
ADP	Man	Rel.	+	−	−	+	+		+		
Epinephrine	Man	Agg.[a]	−	−		+	+		+	+	+
Epinephrine	Man	Rel.	+	−	−	+	+		+	+	+

[a] First wave of two-phased aggregation.
[b] EDTA prevents aggregation but does not entirely prevent release.
[c] Dependent on concentration of stimulus.
[d] Disagreement.
[e] Inhibits by action against thrombin.

material was stable at 56°C and ineffective against gram-negative bacteria. Jago and Jacox (1961) found that two nondialyzable components in rat or rabbit platelets plus bicarbonate were required to kill *Bacillus subtilis*. At least one component was bound to particles in disrupted platelets. Both research groups observed that human serum and platelets were inactive against gram-positive organisms.

Endotoxin liberated bactericidal activity against *B. subtilis* when incubated with rabbit citrated platelet-rich plasma (Des Prez *et al.*, 1961). The material appeared to be a cationic protein liberated from platelet granules; its activity was inhibited by heparin (Weksler, 1971).

B. Increased Permeability and Vascular Damage

There is considerable evidence that local accumulation of platelets can cause vascular injury in rabbits and pigs. Hughes and Tonks (1959, 1962) prepared heparinized platelet-rich rabbit plasma which underwent spontaneous aggregation and reinjected the material into the animal's pulmonary or jugular vein. On sacrifice at intervals up to 3 weeks, intravascular thrombi were noted in the heart or lungs, with focal cellular infiltration of the vessel walls and, with large aggregates, frank necrosis of cardiac muscle. When aggregation was induced intravascularly by implanted metallic couples (Moore and Lough, 1970) or by infusion of ADP in pigs or rabbits (Jørgensen *et al.*, 1970), similar lesions were seen in renal arterioles. No endothelial cells were found beneath the emboli, leukocytes infiltrated the vascular wall, smooth muscle degenerated, and lipid accumulated. Whether the vascular damage results from ischemia or a more specific effect is not yet known.

Cochrane and his co-workers reported that in rabbits with serum sickness the antigen–antibody complexes are deposited only in the walls of blood vessels with increased permeability (Kniker and Cochrane, 1968; Cochrane and Dixon, 1968). In mice and guinea pigs, permeability was enhanced by release of tissue mast-cell constituents. In rabbits, which have few tissue mast cells, platelets were responsible, since localization was prevented by thrombocytopenia induced by injecting heterologous antiplatelet serum. Antihistamine plus antiserotonin agents also inhibited the deposition of complexes and the resultant vascular inflammation. Because serotonin has little effect on vascular permeability in rabbits, these investigators implicated local release of histamine from blood platelets. Experiments were then carried out to ascertain which immune mechanism was responsible (Henson and Cochrane, 1969c, 1970). Since complexes were deposited in blood vessels of rabbits depleted of C3 by injection of cobra venom factor, it was concluded that complement was unnecessary and that vascular damage was induced by the noncomplement-dependent reaction in which antigen plus sensitized basophilic leukocytes liberated the amines from rabbit platelets (Section III,D).

The mechanism by which permeability was increased in passive cutaneous anaphylaxis (PCA) in rabbits was entirely different (Henson and Cochrane, 1969a). Two types of antibody were found capable of inducing PCA when antigen was given intravenously 48 hours after introducing antibody intradermally. Homocytotropic antibody did not require complement and induced normal PCA in animals made thrombocytopenic with antiplatelet serum. The second type of antibody required complement (i.e., was ineffective in rabbits given cobra venom factor), platelets, and neutrophils and was inhibited by antihistamine but not by antiserotonin drugs. It was postulated that local antigen–antibody complexes reacted with complement, entrapped platelets by immune adherence, and caused them to release histamine. The Arthus reaction was not inhibited in thrombocytopenic rabbits.

Not all of the permeability-enhancing effect of platelets can be attributed to histamine. According to Mustard *et al.* (1965) and Packham *et al.* (1968), washed human and pig platelets gently agitated for 15 minutes with a variety of agents released material that increased permeability when injected intradermally into the guinea pig, pig, or rabbit. Amines in the platelets were not responsible since human and pig platelets contain very little histamine, and the material could be prepared from platelets depleted of serotonin by treatment with reserpine. Antigen–antibody complexes and thrombin (10 units/ml) were very active, while collagen, latex suspensions, and ADP (20 μM) were moderately active in inducing release. The active material had a molecular weight below 10,000. Since its action was blocked by antihistamine, it presumably liberated histamine in the recipient's skin. The active preparation of permeability factor also caused contraction of guinea pig ileum.

Nachman *et al.* (1970) identified a similar material in isolated granules of human platelets. It was a cationic protein which caused degranulation of mouse and rat mast cells and whose effect in mice was blocked by prior treatment with antihistamine, but not with an antiserotonin agent. The authors pointed out that platelets may be the only cellular source of permeability-enhancing agents in blood, since exudative, but not blood, leukocytes give rise to activity. The material has been further characterized (Nachman *et al.*, 1972).

Enzymes released from platelet granules may also cause vascular injury. Granules of human platelets contain cathepsin (Nachman and Ferris, 1968) and elastase (Robert *et al.*, 1969).

C. *Chemotaxis by Complement Activation*

Weksler and Coupal (1973) made the important observation that a granule protein released from human platelets during the release reaction or clotting is capable of producing chemotactic activity from C5.

D. *Anaphylaxis*

The role of platelets in anaphylactic reactions is best established in rabbits (Becker and Austen, 1968). Intravenous injection of antigen into sensitized rabbits caused thrombocytopenia and the immediate though transient appearance of histamine and serotonin in the plasma (Waalkes *et al.*, 1957a). Prior administration of reserpine depleted the platelets of these amines and prevented the rise in plasma serotonin but not histamine during anaphylaxis (Waalkes *et al.*, 1957b). It does not prevent shock (Fisher and Lecomte, 1956), nor do antihistamines do so (Reuse, 1956). Apparently the combination has not been tested. Movat *et al.* (1968) showed that antigen–antibody complex, neutrophils, and platelets were trapped in the pulmonary vessels. In nonfatal anaphylaxis, the trapping of platelets was reversible, much of their amine content being retained (Waalkes and Coburn, 1959). The relative roles of mechanical obstruction and release have not been established. Prior injection of a high concentration of heparin (plasma concentration estimated at 100 units/ml) prevented the thrombocytopenia and the decrease in serotonin level in whole blood (Johansson, 1960). Mustard *et al.* (1969) point out that certain antiinflammatory agents prevent shock and death when antigen–antibody complexes are injected into rabbits, but the mechanism is still unclear.

E. *Pulmonary Embolism*

Release of preformed clots into the lungs of rabbits caused rapid death in only 15% of the animals and little symptomatology in the others. In contrast, clots injected 30 minutes after 5 μg epinephrine proved fatal in 60% of the animals and caused serious respiratory distress in the others. The clots became coated with platelets. The increased mortality following epinephrine was prevented by heparin or methysergide. The platelets' markedly increased sensitivity to thrombin produced by the epinephrine could be directly demonstrated, and this was believed to be responsible for the enhancement. The epinephrine probably permits platelets to respond to thrombin on the surface of the clots (Thomas *et al.*, 1968).

F. Clearance by the Reticuloendothelial System

Cohen *et al.* (1965) observed that intravenous injection of carbon particles or endotoxin into dogs or rabbits caused thrombocytopenia. Platelets labeled before injection did not return to the circulation, and the authors concluded that platelet aggregation or phagocytosis may facilitate transport of injected particulate material to the reticuloendothelial system. Van Aken *et al.* (1968) showed that the rate of carbon clearance was reversibly decreased in rabbits during infusion of ADP, AMP, or adenosine and that transfusion of platelets increased the clearance rate. Fibrinolytic agents and products of fibrinolytic degradation decreased the rate of clearance; epsilon-amino-caproic acid first increased and then decreased the rate (Van Aken and Vreeken, 1969).

G. Renal Transplant Rejection

Intravascular platelet aggregates were seen in renal biopsies removed during clinical rejection episodes in man but not at other times (Porter *et al.*, 1967). The platelets also aggregated within minutes of transplanting kidneys into dogs sensitized with skin grafts. Degranulation was noted at 1 hour (Lowenhaupt and Nathan, 1968). The aggregates, which probably formed in response to local accumulations of antigen–antibody complex, could cause renal damage by release of vasoactive materials and by ischemia from mechanical vessel obstruction.

H. Thrombocytopenia in Man

The platelets' ability to respond to antigen-antibody interaction is a cause of thrombocytopenia in man. Shulman (1964), summarizing findings from his own and other laboratories, concluded that the thrombocytopenia produced by certain drugs (e.g., quinidine) is caused by the formation of an antibody to the drug which then reacts with quinidine. The complex is adsorbed onto the platelets and destroys them. He suggests that complexes with 7 S antibody may react with platelets, but complexes with 19 S antibody react with erythrocytes. Miescher and Pepper (1968) discuss drug purpura in detail.

In posttransfusion purpura, a patient lacking a common platelet antigen (PL[A1]) develops very severe thrombocytopenia about 5 days after a trans-fusion of PL[A1]-positive blood. Shulman suggests that a circulating complex of antibody with some finely divided or soluble form of antigen (donor platelets) is responsible. The reason that only a very small proportion of transfused PL[A1]-negative patients are affected is not clear. Finally, this investigator discussed the possibility that idiopathic thrombocytopenic purpura is not caused by the formation of antibodies to autologous platelets but by cellular injury caused by complexes of an unknown exogenous antigen with antibodies formed in response to it. Karpatkin *et al.* (1972), on the other hand, provided evidence of circulating antiplatelet antibody in idiopathic thrombocytopenic purpura as well as in systemic lupus erythematosis.

References

Ardlie, N. G., Packham, M. A., and Mustard, J. F. (1970). *Brit. J. Haematol.* **19**, 7.

Atac, A., Spagnuolo, M., and Zucker, M. B. (1970). *Proc. Soc. Exp. Biol. Med.* **133**, 1331.

Baldini, M. G., and Ebbe, S., eds. (1974). "Platelets: Production, Function, Transfusion and Storage." Grune and Stratton, New York and London.

Barbaro, J. F., (1961a). *J. Immunol.* **86**, 369.

Barbaro, J. F. (1961b). *J. Immunol.* **86**, 377

Barbaro, J. F., and Schoenbechler, M. J. (1970). *J. Immunol.* **104**, 1124.

Barbaro, J. F., and Zvaifler, N. J. (1966). *Proc. Soc. Exp. Biol. Med.* **122**, 1245.

Baumgartner, H. R., Stemerman, M., and Spaet, T. H. (1971). *Experientia* **27**, 283.

Becker, E. L., and Austen, K. F. (1968). *In* "Textbook of Immunopathology" (P. A. Miescher and H. J. Müller-Eberhard, eds.), Vol. 1, p. 76. Grune & Stratton, New York.

Benveniste, J., Henson, P. M., and Cochrane, C. G. (1972). *J. Exp. Med.* **136**, 1356.

Bettex-Galland, M., and Lüscher, E. F. (1964). *Pathol. Microbiol.* **25**, 553.

Born, G. V. R., and Gillson, R. E. (1959). *J. Physiol. (London)* **146**, 472.

Born, G. V. R., and Hume, M. (1967). *Nature (London)* **215**, 1027.

Braunsteiner, H., and Pakesch, F. (1956). *Blood* **11**, 965.

Brinkhous, K. M. (1970). *Thromb. Diath. Haemorrh., Suppl.* **40**.

Caspary, E. A., and Comaish, J. S. (1967). *Nature (London)* **214**, 286.

Clawson, C. C., and White, J. G. (1971). *Amer. J. Pathol.* **65**, 367 and 381.

Cochrane, C. G., and Dixon, F. J. (1968). *In* "Textbook of Immunopathology" (P. A. Miescher and H. J. Müller-Eberhardt, eds.). Vol. 1, p. 94. Grune & Stratton, New York.

Cohen, P., Braunwald, J., and Gardner, F. H. (1965). *J. Lab. Clin. Med.* **66**, 263.

Collier, H. O. J. (1969). *Nature (London)* **223**, 35.

Comaish, S. (1968). *Acta Dermato. Venereol.* **48**, 592

Cronberg, S., Kubitsz, P., and Caen, J. P. (1971). *Thromb. Diath. Haemorrh.* **24**, 409.

Danon, D., Jerushalmy, Z., and de Vries, A. (1959). *Virology* **9**, 719.

Davey, M. G., and Lüscher, E. F. (1968). *Biochim. Biophys. Acta* **165**, 490.

Davis, R. B., and Holtz, G. C. (1969). *Thromb. Diath. Haemorrh.* **21**, 65.

Davis, R. B., Meeker, N. R., and McQuarrie, D. G. (1960). *Circ. Res.* **8**, 234.

Day, H. J., and Holmsen, H. (1971). *Ser. Haematol.* **4**, 3.

Day, H. J., Holmsen, H., and Hovig, T. (1969). *Scand. J. Haematol., Suppl.* **7**.

Des Prez, R. M. (1964). *J. Exp. Med.* **120**, 305.

Des Prez, R. M. (1967). *J. Immunol.* **99**, 966.

Des Prez, R. M., and Bryant, R. E. (1966). *J. Exp. Med.* **124**, 971.

Des Prez, R. M., and Bryant, R. E. (1969). *J. Immunol.* **102**, 241.

Des Prez, R. M., and Marney, S. R., Jr. (1971). *In* "The Circulating Platelet" (S. A. Johnson, ed.), p. 415. Academic Press, New York.

Des Prez, R. M., Horowitz, H. I., and Hook, E. W. (1961). *J. Exp. Med.* **114**, 857.

Ferreira, J. F. D. (1961). Z. Zellforsch. Mikrosk. Anat. 55, 89.

Fisher, P., and Lecomte, J. (1956). C. R. Soc. Biol. 150, 1026.

Friedberg, N. M., and Zucker, M. B. (1972). J. Lab. Clin. Med. 80, 603.

Gaarder, A., Jonsen, J., Laland, S., Hellem, A., and Owren, P. A. (1961). Nature (London) 192, 531.

Glynn, M. F., Movat, H. Z., Murphy, E. A., and Mustard, J. F. (1965). J. Lab. Clin. Med. 65, 179.

Gocke, D. J. (1965). J. Immunol. 94, 247.

Gocke, D. J., and Osler, A. G. (1965). J. Immunol. 94, 236.

Grette, K. (1962). Acta Physiol. Scand., Suppl. 195.

Hampton, J. R., and Mitchell, J. R. A. (1966). Nature London 209, 470.

Harada, K., and Zucker, M. B. (1971). Thromb. Diath. Haemorrh. 25, 41.

Hardisty, R. M., and Hutton, R. A. (1965). Brit. J. Haematol. 11, 258.

Hardisty, R. M., and Hutton, R. A. (1966). Nature (London) 210, 644.

Hardisty, R. M., Hutton, R. A., Montgomery, D., Rickard, S., and Trebilcock, H. (1970). Brit. J. Haematol. 19, 307.

Haslam, R. J. (1967). In "Physiology of Hemostasis and Thrombosis" (S. A. Johnson and W. H. Seegers, eds.), p. 88. Thomas, Springfield, Illinois.

Henson, P. M. (1969a). Fed. Proc., Fed. Amer. Soc. Exp. Biol. 28, 1721.

Henson, P. M. (1969b). Immunology 16, 107.

Henson, P. M. (1970a). J. Exp. Med. 131, 287.

Henson, P. M. (1970b). J. Immunol. 104, 924.

Henson, P. M. (1970c). J. Immunol. 105, 476.

Henson, P. M. (1970d). J. Immunol. 105, 490.

Henson, P. M., and Cochrane, C. G. (1969a). J. Exp. Med. 129, 153.

Henson, P. M., and Cochrane, C. G. (1969b). J. Exp. Med. 129, 167.

Henson, P. M., and Cochrane, C. G. (1969c). In "Cellular and Humoral Mechanisms of Anaphylaxis and Allergy" (H. Z. Movat, ed.), p. 129. Karger, Basel.

Henson, P. M., and Cochrane, C. G. (1970). J. Reticulendothel. Soc. 8, 124.

Hirsh, J. G. (1960). J. Exp. Med. 112, 15.

Holmsen, H., and Day, H. J. (1968). Nature (London) 219, 760.

Holmsen, H., and Day, H. J. (1970). J. Lab. Clin. Med. 75, 840.

Holmsen, H., Day, H. J., and Stormorken, H. (1969). Scand. J. Haematol. Suppl. 8.

Horowitz, H. I., Des Prez, R. M., and Hook, E. W. (1962). J. Exp. Med. 116, 619.

Hovig, T. (1963). Thromb. Diath. Haemorrh. 9, 264.

Hughes, A., and Tonks, R. S. (1959). J. Pathol. Bacteriol. 77, 207.

Hughes, A., and Tonks, R. S. (1962). J. Pathol. Bacteriol. 84, 379.

Hugues, J. (1962). Thromb. Diath. Haemorrh. 8, 241.

Humphrey, J. H., and Jaques, R. (1954). J. Physiol. (London) 124, 305.

Humphrey, J. H., and Jaques, R. (1955). J. Physiol. (London) 128, 9.

Ishizaka, T., and Ishizaka, K. (1962). J. Immunol. 89, 709.

Jago. R., and Jacox, R. F. (1961). J. Exp. Med. 113, 701.

Jensen, K. G., and Killman, S. -A., eds. (1970). Ser. Haematol. 3, No. 4; (1971) 4, No. 1; (1973) 6, No. 3; (1974) 7, No. 1.

Jerushalmy, Z., and Zucker, M. B. (1966). Thromb. Diath. Haemorrh. 15, 413.

Jerushalmy, Z., Kohn, A., and de Vries, A. (1961). Proc. Soc. Exp. Biol. Med. 106, 462.

Jerushalmy, Z., Adler, A., Rechnic, J., Kohn, A., and de Vries, A. (1962). Pathol. Biol. 10, 41.

Jobin, F., and Gagnon, F. T. (1970). Can. J. Microbiol. 16, 63.

Jobin, F., and Tremblay, F. (1969). Thromb. Diath. Haemorrh. 22, 450 and 466.

Jobin, F., Tremblay, F., and Morisette, M. (1970). Thromb. Diath. Haemorrh. 23, 110.

Johansson, S. A. (1960). *Acta Physiol. Scand.* **50**, 95.

Jørgensen, L., Hovig, T., Rowsell, H. C., and Mustard, J. F. (1970). *Amer. J. Pathol.* **61**, 161.

Karpatkin, S., Strick, N., Karpatkin, M. B., and Siskind, G. W. (1972). *Amer. J. Med.* **52**, 776.

Käser-Glanzmann, R., and Lüscher, E. F. (1962). *Thromb. Diath. Haemorrh.* **7**, 480.

Kattlove, H. E., and Alexander, B. (1971). *Blood* **38**, 39.

Katz, G. (1940). *Science* **91**, 221.

Kinlough-Rathbone, R. L., Perry, D. W., and Mustard, J. F. (1974). *Fed Proc.* **33**, 611.

Kniker, W. T., and Cochrane, C. G. (1968). *J. Exp. Med.* **127**, 119.

Kuramoto, A., Steiner, M., and Baldini, M. G. (1970). *Biochim. Biophys. Acta* **201**, 471.

Lackner, H., Hunt, V., Zucker, M. B., and Pearson, J. (1970). *Brit. J. Haematol.* **18**, 625.

Lowenhaupt, R., and Nathan, P. (1968). *Nature (London)* **220**, 822.

McIntire, F. C., Roth, L. W., and Sproull, M. (1952). *Proc. Soc. Exp. Biol. Med.* **81**, 691.

Mannucci, P. M. (1972). *Advan. Exp. Med. Biol.* **34**, 281

Marcus, A. J. (1969). *N. Engl. J. Med.* **280**, 1213, 1278, and 1330.

Marcus, A. J., and Zucker, M. B. (1965). "The Physiology of Blood Platelets." Grune & Stratton, New York.

Markwardt, F., Barthel, W., and Glusa, E. (1968). *Med. Exp.* **18**, 176.

Marney, S. R., Jr. (1971). *J. Immunol.* **106**, 82.

Marney, S. R., Jr., and Des Prez, R. M. (1971). *J. Immunol.* **106**, 74.

Massini, P., and Lüscher, E. F. (1971). *Thromb. Diath. Haemorrh.* **25**, 13.

Michal, F., and Firkin, B. G. (1969). *Annu. Rev. Pharmacol.* **9**, 95.

Miescher, P. A., and Pepper, J. J. (1968). *In* "Textbook of Immunopathology" (P. A. Miescher and H. J. Müller-Eberhard, eds.). vol. 1, p. 278, Grune & Stratton, New York.

Mills, D. C. B., Robb, I. S., and Roberts, G. C. K. (1968). *J. Physiol. (London).* **195**, 715.

Moore, S., and Lough, J. (1970). *Amer. J. Pathol.* **58**, 283.

Movat, H. Z., Mustard, J. F., Taichman, N. S., and Uriuhara, T. (1965a). *Proc. Soc. Exp. Biol. Med.* **120**, 232.

Movat, H. Z., Weiser, W. J., Glynn, M. F., and Mustard, J. F. (1965b). *J. Cell Biol.* **27**, 531.

Movat, H. Z., Uriuhara, T., Taichman, N. S., Rowsell, H. C., and Mustard, J. F. (1968). *Immunology* **14**, 637.

Mueller-Eckhardt, C., and Lüscher, E. F. (1968a). *Thromb. Diath. Haemorrh.* **20**, 155.

Mueller-Eckhardt, C., and Lüscher, E. F. (1968b). *Thromb. Diath. Haemorrh.* **20**, 168.

Mueller-Eckhardt, C., and Lüscher, E. F. (1968c). *Thromb. Diath. Haemorrh.* **20**, 327.

Mueller-Eckhardt, C., and Lüscher, E. F. (1968d). *Thromb. Diath. Haemorrh.* **20**, 336.

Mustard, J. F., and Packham, M. A. (1968). *Ser. Haematol.* **1**, 168.

Mustard, J. F., and Packham, M. A. (1970). *Pharmacol. Rev.* **22**, 97.

Mustard, J. F., and Packham, M. A. (1971). *In* "Inflammation, Immunity and Hypersensitivity" (H. Z. Movat, ed.), p. 527. Harper, New York.

Mustard, J. F., Movat, H. Z., Macmorine, D. R. L., and Sényi, A. (1965). *Proc. Soc. Exp. Biol. Med.* **119**, 988.

Mustard, J. F., Evans, G., Packham, M. A., and Nishizawa, E. E. (1969). *In* "Cellular and Humoral Mechanisms in Anaphylaxis and Allergy" (H. Z. Movat, ed.), p. 151. Karger, Basel.

Myllylä, G., Vaheri, A., Vesikari, T., and Pentinnen, K. (1969). *Clin. Exp. Immunol.* **4**, 323.

Nachman, R. L., and Ferris, B. (1968). *J. Clin. Invest.* **47**, 2530.

Nachman, R. L., Weksler, B., and Ferris, B. (1970). *J. Clin. Invest.* **49**, 274.

Nachman, R. L., Weksler, B., and Ferris, B. (1972). *J. Clin. Invest.* **51**, 549.

Nagaki, K., Fujikawa, K., and Inai, S. (1965). *Biken J.* **8**, 129.

Nagayama, M., Zucker, M. B., and Beller, F. K. (1971). *Thromb. Diath. Haemorrh.* **26**, 467.

Niewiarowski, S., and Thomas, D. P. (1969). *Nature (London)* **222**, 1269.

Niewiarowski, S., and Thomas, D. P. (1971). *Thromb. Diath. Haemorrh.*, Suppl. **40**, 199.

Nossel, H. L., Wilner, G. D., and Leroy, E. C. (1969). *Nature (London)* **221**, 75.

O'Brien, J. R., and Woodhouse, M. A. (1968). *Exp. Biol. Med.* **3**, 90.

O'Brien, J. R., Finch, W., and Clark, E. (1970). *J. Clin. Pathol.* **23**, 522.

Osler, A. G., and Siraganian, R. P. (1972). *Progr. Allergy* **16**, 450.

Packham, M. A., Warrior, E. S., Glynn, M. F., Senyi, A. S., and Mustard, J. F. (1967). *J. Exp. Med.* **126**, 171.

Packham, M. A., Nishizawa, E. E., and Mustard, J. F. (1968). *Biochem. Pharmacol.*, Suppl. p. 171.

Parmeggiani, A. (1961). *Thromb. Diath. Haemorrh.* **6**, 517.

Pentinnen, K., Myllylä, G., Mäkelä, O., and Vaheri, A. (1969). *Acta Pathol. Microbiol. Scand.* **77**, 309.

Peterson, J., and Zucker, M. B. (1970). *Thromb. Diath. Haemorrh.* **23**, 148.

Pfueller, S. L., and Lüscher, E. F. (1972a). *Immunochemistry* **9**, 1151.

Pfueller, S. L., and Lüscher, E. F. (1972b). *J. Immunol.* **109**, 517.

Pfueller, S. L., and Lüscher, E. F. (1972c). *J. Immunol.* **109**, 526.

Pfueller, S. L., and Lüscher, E. F. (1974a). *J. Immunol.* **112**, 1201.

Pfueller, S. L., and Lüscher, E. F. (1974b). *J. Immunol.* **112**, 1211.

Pletscher, A. (1968). *Brit. J. Pharmacol. Chemother.* **32**, 1.

Porter, K. A., Dossetor, J. B., Marchiore, T. L., Peart, W. S., Rendall, J. M., Starzl, T. E., and Terasaki, P. I. (1967). *Lab. Invest.* **16**, 153.

Rapport, M. M. (1949). *J. Biol. Chem.* **180**, 961.

Ratnoff, O. D. (1969). *Advan. Immunol.* **10**, 145.

Ream, V. J., Deykin, D., Gurewich, V., and Wessler, S. (1965). *J. Lab. Clin. Med.* **66**, 244.

Reuse, J. J. (1956). Histamine, *Ciba Found. Symp., 1955* p. 150.

Robbins, J., and Stetson, C. A., Jr. (1958). *J. Exp. Med.* **109**, 1.

Robert, B., Legrand, Y., Pignaud, G., Caen, J., and Robert, L. (1969). *Pathol. Biol.* **17**, 615.

Rodman, N. F., and Mason, R. G. (1967). *Fed. Proc., Fed. Amer. Soc. Exp. Biol.* **26**, 95.

Roskam, J. (1923). *Arch. Int. Physiol.* **20**, 241.

Ross, R., and Bornstein, P. (1969). *J. Cell Biol.* **40**, 366.

Salzman, E. W., and Chambers, D. A. (1964). *Nature (London)* **204**, 698.

Salzman, E. W., and Levine, L. (1971). *J. Clin. Invest.* **50**, 131.

Schoenbechler, M. J., and Barbaro, J. F. (1968). *Proc. Nat. Acad. Sci. U.S.* **60**, 1247.

Schoenbechler, M. J., and Sadun, E. H. (1968). *Proc. Soc. Exp. Biol. Med.* **127**, 601.

Schulz, H. (1961). *Folia Haematol. (Frankfurt am Main).* [N.S.]. **5**, 195.

Schulz, H., and Wedell, J. (1962). *Klin. Wochenschr.* **40**, 1114.

Shore, P. A., and Alpers, H. S. (1963). *Amer. J. Physiol.* **205**, 348.

Shulman, N. R. (1964). *Ann. Intern. Med.* **60**, 506.

Siqueira, M., and Nelson, R. A. (1961). *J. Immunol.* **86**, 516.

Siraganian, R. P. (1972). *Nature New Biol. (London)* **239**, 208.

Siraganian, R. P., and Osler, A. G. (1969). *J. Allergy* **43**, 167.

Siraganian, R. P., and Osler, A. G. (1971a). *J. Immunol.* **106**, 1244.

Siraganian, R. P., and Osler, A. G. (1971b). *J. Immunol.* **106**, 1252.

Siraganian, R. P., Secchi, A. G., and Osler, A. G. (1968). *J. Immunol.* **101**, 1130, 1140, and 1148.

Sixma, J. J., and Nijessen, J. G. (1970). *Thromb. Diath. Haemorrh.* **24**, 206.

Spaet, T. H., ed. (1972), "Progress in Hemostasis and Thrombosis." Vol. 1. Grune and Stratton, New York.

Spaet, T. H., ed. (1974). "Progress in Hemostasis and Thrombosis." Vol. 2. Grune and Stratton, New York.

Spaet, T. H., and Zucker, M. B. (1964). *Amer. J. Physiol.* **206**, 1267.

Spielvogel, A. R. (1967). *J. Exp. Med.* **126**, 235.

Stemerman, M., Baumgartner, H. R., and Spaet, T. H. (1971). *Lab. Invest.* **24**, 179.

Stormorken, H. (1969). *Scand. J. Haematol., Suppl.* **9**.

Taylor, F. B., Jr., and Müller-Eberhard, H. J. (1970). *J. Clin. Invest.* **49**, 2068.

Thomas, D. P. (1967). *Nature (London)* **215**, 298.

Thomas, D. P., Gurewich, V., and Stuart, R. K. (1968). *J. Lab. Clin. Med.* **71**, 955.

Thomas, D. P., Niewiarowski, S., and Ream, V. J. (1970). *J. Lab. Clin. Med.* **75**, 607.

Valdorf-Hansen, J. F., and Zucker, M. B. (1971). *Amer. J. Physiol.* **220**, 105.

Van Aken, W. G., and Vreeken, J. (1969). *Thromb. Diath. Haemorrh.* **22**, 496.

Van Aken, W. G., Goote, T. M., and Vreeken, J. (1968). *Scand. J. Haematol.* **5**, 333.

Waalkes, T. P., and Coburn, H. (1959). *J. Allergy* **30**, 394.

Waalkes, T. P., Weissbach, H., Bozicevich, J., and Udenfriend, S. (1957a). *J. Clin. Invest.* **36**, 1115.

Waalkes, T. P., Weissbach, H., Bozicevich, J., and Udenfriend, S. (1957b). *Proc. Soc. Exp. Biol. Med.* **95**, 479.

Walsh, P. N. (1972). *Brit. J. Haematol.* **22**, 237 and 393.

Walsh, P. N., and Biggs, R. (1972). *Brit. J. Haematol.* **22**, 743.

Weiss, H. J., ed. (1972). Platelets and their role in hemostasis. *Ann. N.Y. Acad Sci.* **201**, 1.

Weiss, H. J., and Rogers, J. (1971). *N. Engl. J. Med.* **285**, 369.

Weis, H. F., Rogers, J., and Brand, H. (1973). *J. Clin. Invest.* **52**, 2697.

Weiss, H. F., Rogers, J., and Brand, H. (1973). *J. Clin. Invest.* In press.

Weksler, B. (1971). *J. Exp. Med.* **134**, 1114.

Weksler, B. B., and Coupal., C. E. (1973). *J. Exp. Med.* **137**, 1419.

Westerholm, B. (1965). *Acta Physiol. Scand.* **63**, 257.

Wilner, G. D., Nossel, H. L., and LeRoy, E. C. (1968). *J. Clin Invest.* **47**, 2616.

Youssef, A., and Barkhan, P. (1968). *Brit. Med. J.* **1**, 746.

Zimmerman, T. S., and Müller-Eberhard, H. J. (1971). *J. Exp. Med.* **134**, 1601.

Zimmerman, T. S., and Müller-Eberhard, J. (1973). *Science* **180**, 1183.

Zimmerman, T. S., Arroyave, C. M., and Müller-Eberhard, H. J. (1971). *J. Exp. Med.* **134**, 1591.

Zucker, M. B. (1972). *Thromb. Diath. Haemorrh.* **28**, 393.

Zucker, M. B., and Borrelli, J. (1955). *J. Appl. Physiol.* **7**, 432.

Zucker, M. B., and Borrelli, J. (1962). *Proc. Soc. Exp. Biol. Med.* **109**, 779.

Zucker, M. B., and Grant, R. A. (1974) *J. Immunol.* **112**, 1219.

Zucker, M. B., Grant, R. A., Alper, C. A., Lepow, I. H., and Goodkofsky, I. (1973). Proc. IV Internat, Congr. Thombosis and Haemostasis, Vienna.

Zucker, M. B., and Peterson, J. (1968). *Proc. Soc. Exp. Biol. Med.* **127**, 547.

Zucker, M. B., and Peterson, J. (1970). *J. Lab. Clin. Med.* **76**, 66.

Zucker, M. B., and Vroman, L. (1969). *Proc. Soc. Exp. Biol. Med.* **131**, 318.

Zucker, M. B., Pert, J. H., and Hilgartner, M. W. (1966). *Blood* **28**, 524.

Zucker, M. B., Rifkin, P. L., Friedberg, N. M., and Coller, B. S. (1972). *Ann. N.Y. Acad. Sci.* **201**, 138.

Chapter 10

STRUCTURAL AND BIOCHEMICAL CHARACTERISTICS OF MAST CELLS

GUNNAR D. BLOOM

I. Introduction

General interest in the tissue mast cell is well reflected in the literature. Between the years 1877 and 1935 only some 40 to 45 major reports pertaining to this subject were published. However, from this period and on, mast cell research assumed an epidemic nature. This has been pointed out by Goffman (1966), who within the area of mast cell research applied the mathematical theory of epidemics to the investigation of the spread of scientific ideas. As a basis for his investigation, Goffman (1966) used the Selye (1965) biblio-graphy covering roughly 2500 articles on mast cells from the time of Ehrlich's discovery of the mast cell in 1877 until 1963. That interest in this cell is still great is evident from a recent computerized literature search covering material from January 1966 through June 1970. This search retrieved close to 1000 articles.

The difficulty of reviewing even a portion of this vast literature is obvious; completeness is an impossibility. For more extensive discussions pertaining to the mast cell, the reader is referred to the monographs of Michels (1938), Jorpes (1946), Riley (1959), Kelsall and Crabb (1959), Selye (1965), and Sagher and Even-Paz (1967) as well as to the reviews of Asboe-Hansen (1954), Arvy (1955), Padawer (1957), Smith (1963a,b), Benditt and Lagunoff (1964), and the volume *Mast Cells and Basophils* (see Padawer, 1963).

During a period of time surrounding and following its discovery by Ehrlich (1877, 1879), the mast cell* was regarded as a relatively simple, immobile, large connective tissue element of unknown character which displayed a beautiful reddish or purple color when stained with certain triphenylmethane and thiazine dyes. Today, more than 90 years later, little is left of that early general and diffuse impression. On the contrary, the mast cell has proved to be so complex in nature and so elusive that in spite of generous contributions from numerous fields of science our knowledge of its qualities and functions is still far from complete.

II. Origin and Distribution of Mast Cells

The genesis of the mast cell constitutes a perplexing problem. There was a good deal of confusion among early investigators with regard to its classifica-tion. It is therefore not surprising to find suggestions in the literature that mast cells originate from almost every type of connective tissue element, including fixed cells, lymphocytes, large mononuclear cells, adventitial cells, leukocytes, wandering cells, and plasma cells (for example, see Michels, 1938). It should, however, be pointed out that several of these originally highly controversial hypotheses have in no way been refuted but rather they have received support in more recent investigations. Thus Downey's original report (1911) on the relationship between mast cells and lymphocytes, on the one hand, and plasma cells, on the other, has been substantiated by among others Ginsburg and Lagunoff (1967) and Hottendorf *et al.* (1966), respectively. Furthermore, considerable interest has been focused on the thymus and the spleen as locations for mast cell genesis. A direct transforma-

---

*In German, *mästen* means "to fatten."

tion of thymocytes into mast cells has been suggested by among others Csaba *et al.* (1961), Ginsburg (1963), and Burnet (1965), and in the spleen a differentiation of mast cells from the reticulum cells has been reported (Hill and Praslička, 1958; Viklicky, 1969). Parwaresch *et al.* (1971) maintain that mast cells may arise from emigrated blood monocytes. For a detailed discussion concerning mast cell formation and its regulation the reader is referred to the recent monograph on this subject by Csaba (1972).

In the literature, numerous cell types exhibiting metachromatic cytoplasmic granules have been termed mast cells. However, fibroblasts will readily ingest polysaccharides, especially heparin, as well as shed mast granules, and thereby develop into "quasimastcells" (Higginbotham and Dougherty, 1956). Among others, Landsberger (1964) considers fibroblasts and mast cells to be truly related. Macrophages and leukocytes will also phagocytize discharged mast cell granules and assume the appearance of mast cells (Smith and Lewis, 1958) (see Fig. 18, p. 565). Certain cells found in nevi, freckles, and melanosarcomas contain both metachromatic and pigment granules and have been designated "pigment mast cells" (Rheindorf, 1905, cited by Selye, 1965). It is interesting to note in this connection that whereas Smith and Lewis (1958) could not establish any relationship whatsoever between mast cells and pigment cells, Okun (1965, 1967) and Okun *et al.* (1970) are strongly of the opinion that mast cells are capable of melanin synthesis and that they are histogenetically related to melanocytes. An "atypical mast cell" (see Michels, 1938), the globule leukocyte, frequently observed within epithelia of mucous surfaces, has more recently been suggested to be derived from mast cells (Murray *et al.*, 1968; Veilleux and Cantin, 1972). However, Whur and Gracie (1967) consider these two cell types unrelated.

It is evident from the literature that a heteroplastic formation of mast cells from already differentiated cells may take place. However, by far the most common general view is that fixed, undifferentiated, mesenchymal cells are the chief source of mast cells.

Mast cells also proliferate by mitosis. Maximow, as early as 1904, suggested that mature mast cells increase primarily by mitosis, but Michels (1938) was the first to show a series of mitotic stages in mast cells. For a rather long period of time, however, isolated cases of mitosis in mast cells were mentioned in the literature merely as a curiosity.

Hunt and Hunt (1957) noticed mitotic figures in mast cells to be rather common in rats treated with a histamine-liberating compound and reported a mitotic index of 1.6 % among the mesenteric mast cells. Allen (1961, 1962) expressed the opinion that mast cells divide by mitosis much more frequently than was believed earlier. From his own work he concluded that mesenteric mast cells of rats normally undergo mitosis and that this activity is greatest in young rapidly growing rats. Although there is a divergence of opinion regarding the frequency of mitoses in normal granular mast cells, they certainly do occur (Fig. 4). According to Asboe-Hansen (1968), however, the majority of the mast cells divide mitotically at a nongranular, fibroblastlike, precursor cell stage.

Incorporation of tritiated thymidine into nuclei of mast cells has been demonstrated by Padawer (1961), Allen (1962), Asboe-Hansen and Levi (1962), and Asboe-Hansen *et al.* (1965). Allen (1962), utilizing autoradiography and the Feulgen-methyl-green technique, found that 5.7% of the mesenteric mast cells in 30-day-old rats contained labeled interphasic nuclei, and, of these, 75% were considered to have a doubled deoxyribonucleic acid content.

Although cells which are strikingly similar to the mast cells of higher vertebrates have been encountered in lower forms, such as sponges (Cotte, 1904) and simple coelenterates (Kollmann, 1908), it is at the level of fish and amphibians that tissue mast cells become conspicuous and appear in larger numbers.

Mast cells in the main are found in the loose connective tissue. With few exceptions, their presence in tissues and organs of higher vertebrates can be correlated to the connective tissue content. Cartilage and bone are devoid of mast cells, but the surrounding layers of dense connective tissue, the perichondrium and periosteum, may contain a fair number of cells. Parenchymatous organs such as liver, kidney, and adrenals contain relatively little connective tissue, and mast cells are rare in these organs. An exception, however, is the dog liver which is rather rich in mast cells. In the testes, ovaries, salivary glands, lymph glands, spleen, pancreas, and heart, mast cells occur more frequently. Organs rich in connective tissue such as mammary glands, tongue, prostate gland, lung, and omentum contain large numbers of mast cells. Mast cells also may be numerous in intermuscular connective tissue, in the various layers of the respiratory and digestive tract, in serous membranes, and in skin. Johnson (1957) states that the normal human skin has somewhere between 2000 and 7500 mast cells/cm^3, depending on the region from which specimens are taken.

As shown by numerous authors over the years, the localization and appearance of mast cells in various species and the evolution of the blood vascular system are closely correlated. This is not surprising, considering that the cells of the hemopoietic tissue and most of the formed elements of the connective tissue proper have a common origin, i.e., the primitive multipotent mesenchyme. In lower vertebrates, it has been possible to follow the development of the blood-forming organs and to observe that the originally active, diffusely scattered, hemopoietic tissue may turn into production sites for the granular cells of the connective tissue, i.e., the mast cells (Riley, 1959). A comprehensive comparative study of the mast cell in the vascular connective tissue of invertebrates and vertebrates has been presented by Grünberg and Kaiser (1964, 1965).

III. Normal Tissue Mast Cells; Neoplastic Mast Cells

By definition, an increase in the number of cells of an organ is termed hyperplasia, while a state in which cells proliferate with no restraint is referred to as a neoplasia. It is evident that the borderline between hyperplasia and the process of neoplasia is blurred.

Cell growth in tissues is undoubtedly regulated. However, our general knowledge of how it is regulated is scanty and with respect to the mast cell it is nil. Mast cell proliferation or hyperplasia is rather common in a wide variety of conditions, a few of which will be discussed later. Mast cell neoplasias also exist but are relatively rare. While our main dilemma is one shared with all workers in the field of neoplastic growth, i.e., our lack of understanding of the fine mechanisms underlying normal and abnormal growth at the cellular and subcellular level, we are also confronted with the need to determine where hyperplasia ends and neoplasia begins. The complex nature of this problem may be exemplified by the extensively studied proliferation of mast cells in the skin of mice after painting with 3-methylcholantrene. It is still not clear if this increase in mast cell numbers is simply a hyperplastic reaction associated with the development of skin cancer (Cramer and Simpson, 1944 a.o.) or a true neoplastic proliferation of mast cells in direct response to the carcinogen. On attempts at transplantation, mast cell tumors have generally not developed although this may be caused by, e.g., other cells in the area having a greater potential for growth (Dunn, 1969). On the other hand, the well-established transplantable murine mast cell tumor of Dunn and Potter (1957) arose subcutaneously in a mouse which had received repeated paintings of methylcholanthrene.

Morphologically, hyperplastic mast cells do not differ significantly from normal mast cells. Neoplastic mast cells, on the other hand, may show the general characteristics of neoplastic cells, such as polymorphism, a decrease in number and distribution of cytoplasmic granules, a shift in the nuclear–cytoplasmic ratio in favor of the nucleus, large nucleoli, an increase in number of cells in mitosis (although this increase may be slight), and sometimes giant multinucleated cell forms.

It is not known whether neoplastic mast cells arise from primitive nongranulated precursor cells. Such a development was suggested in some of the neoplasias of the mouse mast cell investigated by Deringer and Dunn (1947). However, these authors also observed mitoses and considered that such processes could explain the mast cell increase. Bloom (1942) favors a homoplastic regeneration, i.e., that neoplastic mast cells arise through proliferative stages from normal tissue mast cells. With respect to mast cell neoplasias, the observations of Lombard et al. (1963) and Rickard and Post (1968) are most interesting. These authors reported on the cell-free transmissibility of a canine mastocytoma and a canine mast cell leukemia, respectively. This important area awaits further study.

IV. Mast Cell Cytology

A. Morphology of the Mast Cell as Observed under the Light Microscope

In man and most other mammals, mast cells vary widely in shape and size. These cells are greatly influenced by surrounding tissue components; in loose or areolar connective tissue, they assume plump, rounded, shapes while in coarse fibrous tissue of skin or organ capsules, for example, they may appear as elongated, almost filiform elements.

Cell size varies in different species as well as within the same individual; and, according to the literature, cell diameters range from 3.5–24 μm (Michels, 1938). The mean diameter of rat peritoneal mast cells, as measured in the living state, is 13.5 $\pm$ 0.1 (Krüger et al., 1974). The mean area of fixed rat and mouse peritoneal mast cells is 128 and 78.4 μm^2, respectively, corresponding to mean diameters of 12.8 and 10 μm (Bloom, 1960). The volume of rat peritoneal mast cells as measured by packing a known number of cells averages $(1.32 \pm 0.2) \times 10^{-6}$ mm^3/cell (Benditt, 1958). It has been calculated in fixed and embedded rat peritoneal mast cells that the granule volume averages 0.3 μm^3 and that the total number of granules present in individual such cells is of the order of 1000 (Helander and Bloom, 1974).

Mast cells contain prominent nuclei which are round or oval in shape and are generally not lobated. Kidney- and horseshoe-shaped nuclei are seen in mast cells but most often in those of neoplastic type. The nuclear size is about 4–7 μm. The chromatin of the nucleus shows a wide variety of patterns. Some nuclei stain poorly and display little or no chromatin strands whereas others may be rather chromatin rich. One, two, or more well-defined nucleoli are generally present.

The cytoplasm of normal mast cells contains an abundance of spheroidal basophilic granules which often are so numerous that they partially or completely obscure other cytoplasmic structures (Figs. 1 and 2). The granules actually occupy 50–55% of the cytoplasmic volume in rat peritoneal mast cells (Helander and Bloom, 1974). The size of the granules varies somewhat in different species; there is also marked variation in mast cells from the same animal. In the literature, granule sizes have been reported to vary between 0.3 and 1 μm, an average being about 0.7 μm. A common finding,

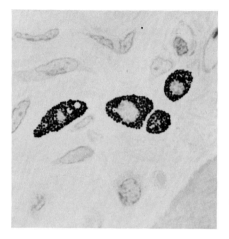

Fig. 1. Normal mast cells from rat tongue. The dense granule population fills the cytoplasm and obscures other cytoplasmic structures. Occasional vacuoles appear in the cytoplasm, some containing granule remnants. Glutaraldehyde fixation, Epon embedding. One-micron section stained with toluidine blue. Light micrograph. Magnification × 1000.

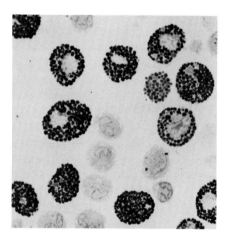

Fig. 2. Normal rat peritoneal mast cells obtained by centrifugation procedures. The richness of mast cells in these preparations facilitates their study by electron microscopy. Pellet fixed in glutaraldehyde and embedding performed in Epon. Staining as in Fig. 1. Light micrograph. Magnification × 1000.

especially in neoplastic mast cells, is a fusion of granules into larger aggregates or masses of basophilic metachromatic substance.

The question of whether mast cells contain such classic cytoplasmic organelles as mitochondria, Golgi apparatus, etc., is no longer pertinent, having been well established through electron microscopy. However, difficulty in demonstrating these structures under the light microscope led to much speculation and teleological dispute in the past which occasionally is still echoed in the literature. Suffice it to state here that Maximow (1906) reported on a centrosome, Nakajima (1928) described what he believed to be mitochondria, and Compton (1952) occasionally observed a Golgi apparatus in mast cells.

Mast cells easily discharge their granules. This degranulation may be evoked by such a wide variety of physicochemical factors that it has hitherto not been possible to specify any single basic mechanism by which this cell secretory process is brought about. The matter is further complicated by suggestions in the literature that release of active principles from mast cells may not require the expulsion of mast granules. The reader is referred to Selye's (1965) critical review on the subject of mast cell degranulation and to his extensive listing of the numerous physical factors and chemical agents reported to elicit a granule discharge and/or release of active substances from mast cells. Only a few characteristic features of the degranulation process will be dealt with in the following section.

B. Fine Structure of the Mast Cell as Revealed by the Electron Microscope

Mast cells of both normal and neoplastic types have by now been subjected to thorough investigation at the electron microscopic level. Although numerous under the light microscope, mast cells in the connective tissue are so widely separated from each other on a submicroscopic level that electron microscope studies of large numbers of these cells in this tissue meet with certain difficulties (Fig. 1). In the serous fluids of the peritoneal cavity of rodents, for example (rat, mouse, and hamster), mast cells are abundant (Fig. 2) and readily lend themselves to isolation in sufficient numbers to facilitate electron microscope studies. Much of our present knowledge of the fine structure of normal mast cells is therefore based on observations of such peritoneal mast cells (Fig. 3). Neoplastic mast cells may easily be studied in mast cell tumors, e.g., those of the mouse or the dog (Fig. 5). Human mast cells have most frequently been studied in urticaria pigmentosa lesions.

As a rule, the mast cell granules are delimited from the cytoplasmic ground substance by a perigranular membrane (Figs. 6, 7, and 8) (Benditt and Lagunoff, 1964; Bloom and Haegermark, 1965). Their internal fine structure, however, shows considerable variation not only species-wise but also within cells from the same animal (Fig. 6). Although some of the structural differences reported on earlier may be attributed to variations in the preparatory techniques applied in electron microscopy, others have proved to be so consistent that it appears evident that the complex biochemical nature of the granules may be reflected in different manners. Thus the matrix of mast cell

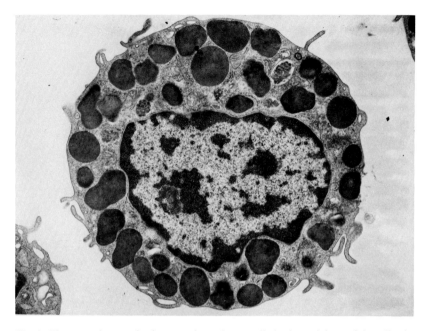

Fig. 3. Electron micrograph of a rat peritoneal mast cell. At the periphery of the cell, micro-villi and cytoplasmic folds are observed. The granules vary somewhat in size and shape and have a rather uniform, fairly homogeneous appearance. A few granules are in the stage of formation as visualized by small vacuolar structures containing minute progranules. Mito-chondria are few in numbers, and elements belonging to the rough endoplasmic reticulum are dispersed between the granules. Glutaraldehyde fixation followed by postfixation in osmium tetroxide. Thin sectioning performed with the LKB-Ultrotome. Section stained with uranyl acetate and lead citrate. Magnification × 8800.

granules from different species has been described as homogeneous and completely electron-dense, finely granular, reticular, beaded-reticular, filamentous, lamellated, or containing scroll-like lamellae and/or crystalline bodies.

In the rat, the majority of the mast cell granules generally appear fairly homogeneous (Figs. 3 and 4) but at higher magnification a substructure of a finely granular or filamentous nature may be revealed (Singleton and Clark, 1965; Bloom and Haegermark, 1965; Horsfield, 1965; Lagunoff, 1966; Yamasaki et al., 1970). This substructure may be very conspicuous in a few "altered" granules in normal rat peritoneal mast cells, and it becomes a characteristic feature of numerous granules in association with histamine release and the concomitant discharge of granules from cells subjected, e.g., to the effects of various histamine-releasing agents such as compound 48/80 and bee venom or treatment with antigen (Figs. 6l, 11, 13, and 14) (Bloom and

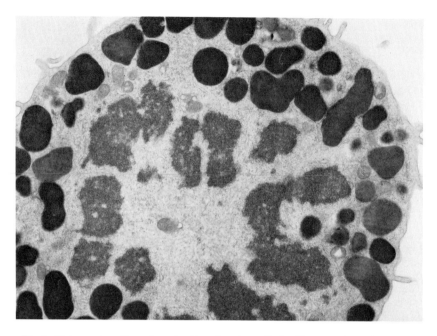

Fig. 4. Mature rat peritoneal mast cell undergoing mitosis. The metaphase chromosomes are centrally located and granules and organelles are displaced towards the periphery of the cells. Specimen processed as in Fig. 3. Electron micrograph. Magnification × 11,400.

Haegermark, 1965, 1967; Bloom *et al.*, 1967; Bloom and Chakravarty, 1970 a.o.).

Some intracellular granules in rat mast cells may show the presence of minute particles, dense clumps, or even cords of material arranged in a variety of fashions (Figs. 3 and 6). Such granules probably represent some of the stages in granule formation first reported on by Combs (1966) in the rat and Skalko *et al.* (1968) in the mouse. Granules very similar to those depicted in Figs. 6j and 6k have been observed further in the fowl, *Gallus domesticus* (Wight, 1970), and in developing guinea pig mast cells (Vollrath and Wahlin, 1970). However, in the guinea pig, mast cell granules may in addition to cordlike strands of material also exhibit a crystalloid-like substructure (Taichman, 1970). Myelinlike lamellae as well as crystalloidal subcomponents have been reported in mast cell granules of the hedgehog (Flood and Krüger, 1970). In mouse tumor mast cells, the granules greatly resemble those of normal rat and mouse mast cells (Bloom, 1963). Canine tumor mast cell granules vary considerably in size and shape (Fig. 5). They are often homogeneous in appearance but may also exhibit a granular–reticular substructure (Fig. 12).

The greatest complexity of, and variety in, mast granule fine structure is observed in human mast cells (Figs. 7, 8, and 9). In the latter the granules

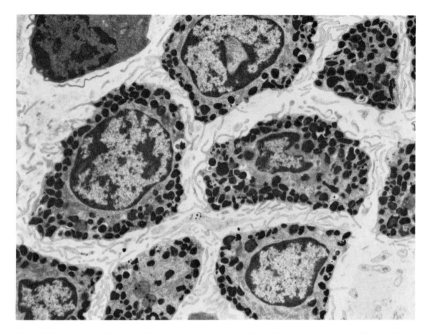

Fig. 5. Low magnification electron micrograph of a dog mastocytoma. Mast cells are abundant. The cells are rather irregular in shape and numerous long, slender microvilli project from the cell surfaces. Granule size and shape varies considerably. Specimen processed as in Fig. 3. Magnification × 4300.

may display a substructure of a highly ordered crystalline lattice (Fig. 9) or weirdly arranged scroll-like lamellae (Fig. 7) (Orfanos and Stüttgen, 1962; Iwamoto and Smelser, 1965; Weinstock and Albright, 1967; Fedorko and Hirsch, 1965; Brinkman, 1968; Bowyer, 1968; Kobayasi et al., 1968; Fujita et al., 1969; Dobbins et al., 1969; Dieterich, 1972). However, in some cases of urticaria pigmentosa, mast cells may be observed, the granules of which show more or less amorphous appearance or at the most only exhibit traces of internal lamellae (Fig. 8).

Mast cells contain mitochondria which show the classic appearance of these organelles as known from various other cell types. They are thus surrounded by a double-membrane structure and exhibit transverse membrane-delimited internal cristae or lamellae. Earlier, the presence of mitochondria in mast cells was questioned. The matter was, however, definitely settled when this organelle was consistently observed in electron microscope investigations of normal mast cells from mouse (Rogers, 1956) and man (Stoeckenius, 1956) and tumor mast cells from dog (Bloom et al., 1956). However, mitochondria are not numerous and in, e.g., rat peritoneal mast cells,

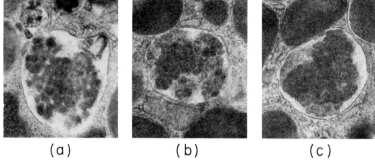

(a)   (b)   (c)

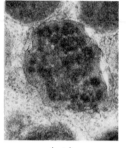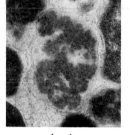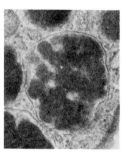

(d)   (e)   (f)

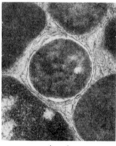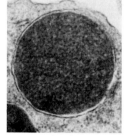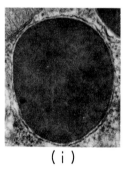

(g)   (h)   (i)

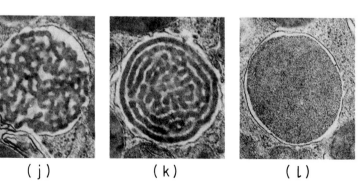

(j)   (k)   (l)

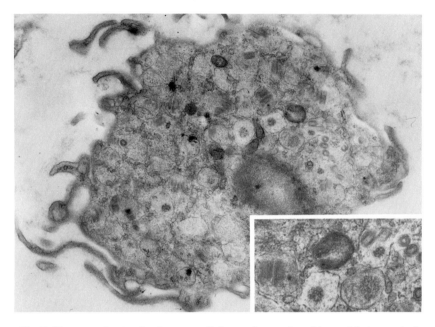

Fig. 7. Electron micrograph of a mast cell from a human lung biopsy. Mast granule fine structure is characterized by the presence of short cylindrical bodies which on sectioning at various angles give rise to lamellated figures with a whorled appearance. Other subcomponents of the granules are dense particles as well as minute vesicular structures. Long slender microvilli are seen at the periphery of the cells. Specimen fixed in osmium tetroxide and embedded in Maraglas. Stained with lead hydroxide. Magnification × 14,300. Inset shows details of granule structure at higher magnification (× 26,000).

they occupy only some 2% of the cytoplasmic volume of the cells (Helander and Bloom, 1974).

Electron microscope observations on the Golgi apparatus of mast cells were first reported in cells of a dog mastocytoma (Bloom *et al.*, 1956) and in normal mouse mast cells (Rogers, 1956). This organelle is characterized by a series of parallel membranes which correspond to cross sections of flattened

Fig. 6. Electron micrographs depicting various types of mast cell granules encountered in rat peritoneal mast cells. Micrographs (a–i) are arranged to simulate a possible sequence of events in the formation of granules. (i) Exhibits the features of the normal mast cell granule with its surrounding perigranular membrane. (j–k) Represents a type of granule only occasionally observed in normal rat mast cells but more frequently in cells subjected to the effects of stimulating agents, e.g., histamine dischargers. (l) Depicts the earliest stage of granule alteration which generally precedes histamine release and granule discharge. Subsequent stages of alteration are shown in Figs. 11–14. For further descriptions of mast granule formation and alteration see text. Specimens all processed as in Fig. 3. Magnifications (a–c) × 27,000; (d) × 33,000; (e) × 21,000; (f) × 33,000; (g) × 26,000; (h) × 33,000; (i) × 44,000; (j) × 30,000; (k) × 35,000; and (l) × 28,000.

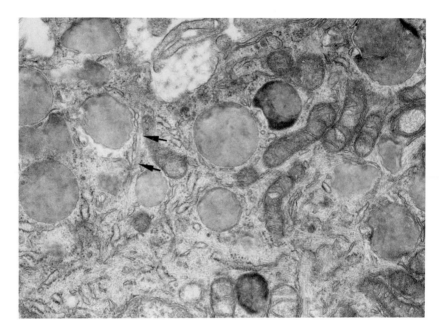

Fig. 8. Detail of a mast cell from human skin (urticaria pigmentosa lesion). The granules are fairly homogeneous and show only traces of intragranular lamellae. In the ground substance of the cytoplasm, filamentous structures are abundant and arrows indicate a cytoplasmic microtubule. Electron micrograph. Specimen processed as in Fig. 3. Magnification × 23,000. (From Bloom and Haegermark, unpublished observations.)

sacs or cisternae; associated with the membranes are clusters of vesicles, varying in size from 300–1000 Å or more and a few larger vacuoles. In a number of different cell types, the Golgi apparatus has been shown to be associated with the synthesis of cell secretory products. This is now documented on a structural basis also in mast cells (Fujita, 1965; Combs, 1966; Yamasaki *et al.*, 1970). A sequence of events for the development of mast cell granules has been postulated by Combs (1966) (see also Fig. 6): Granule synthesis is first visualized by the formation of progranules in the Golgi zone. Several progranules aggregate inside a common membrane. Finely granular material derived from the rough endoplasmic reticulum is added to the vacuoles containing aggregates of progranules. The latter then fuse, and material continues to accumulate inside the perigranular membrane until the granule reaches its maximum size. The dense and finely granular components reorganize to form electron-opaque strands 20–30 nm in diameter. The granule may then undergo compaction and perhaps further reorganization to form the dense, homogeneous and chemically complete mast

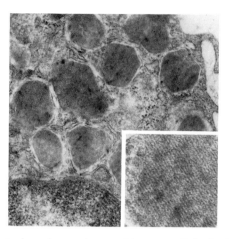

Fig. 9. Detail of cytoplasm from a human skin mast cell (urticaria pigmentosa lesion) the granules of which exhibit angular shapes. At higher magnification (inset) a regular crystalline pattern is revealed. Electron micrograph. Specimen fixed in osmium tetroxide and embedded in Epon. Staining as in Fig. 3. Magnification × 18,900 (inset × 62,000).

cell granule. However, it should be pointed out that there are authors who do not consider the Golgi apparatus to be involved in granule synthesis but rather that the granules develop *in situ* in the cytoplasm (Fernando and Movat, 1963; Vollrath and Wahlin, 1970).

The cytoplasm of normal as well as tumor mast cells shows the presence of a rough endoplasmic reticulum (Smith and Lewis, 1957; Bloom, 1960, 1963; Policard *et al.*, 1960; Klug, 1961; Smith, 1963a,b). In normal tissue mast cells, the endoplasmic reticulum is rather insignificant, compressed as it is into the narrow intergranular cytoplasmic spaces. In tumor mast cells of the mouse, which often contain a small number of mast granules, the endoplasmic reticulum is prominent, although it appears to be highly developed only in small areas of the cells (Bloom, 1963). Free ribosomes may be observed scattered throughout the cytoplasm. The actual relationship of the mast granules to elements of the endoplasmic reticulum is not clear. However, a direct continuity between membranes of the rough endoplasmic reticulum and perigranular membranes in mast cells of the rat has been observed (Combs, 1966).

Cytoplasmic microtubules have been reported in mast cells (Behnke, 1964; Padawer, 1967a,b,c) (Fig. 8). Colchicine treatment enhances cytoplasmic movements as observed in living mast cells but apparently removes the tubular elements; this indicates that the tubules are not involved in these cytoplasmic activities (Padawer, 1967c). A possible role of microtubules in mast cell-degranulation processes has been indicated (Gillespie *et al.*, 1968).

In the cytoplasmic ground substance of human mast cells, fine filamentous structures may be observed. They measure roughly 80–90 Å in diameter and traverse the cytoplasm apparently at random (Fig. 8). In rat mast cells, filamentous bundles exhibiting a striated pattern with a periodicity of roughly 300–400 Å have occasionally been observed in the close proximity of the mast cell granules (Fig. 10). Their significance has yet to be determined.

The process of granule discharge from mast cells has been studied with the electron microscope in a variety of experimental systems. Early investigations include hamster mast cells treated with protamine sulfate (Smith and Lewis, 1957), rat peritoneal mast cells treated with stilbamidine (Bloom *et al.*, 1957) or antirat serum (Keller and Mühlethaler, 1962), mouse mastocytoma cells treated with compound 48/80 (Sellyei and David, 1963), and human urticaria pigmentosa mast cells treated with 48/80 (Orfanos and Stüttgen, 1963). Only limited information was gained through these studies, since they were all impaired by lack of suitable fixation and embedding techniques for electron microscopy.

Subsequent investigations have indicated that release of active substances from mast cells may be reflected in structural changes within the cells which may vary somewhat in relation to the discharging stimuli. Most investigators have concerned themselves with the effects of the well-known histamine liberator 48/80. In rat peritoneal mast cells incubated with this agent (Fig. 11), the normally dense and rather homogeneous granules will alter their appearance; they will decrease in electron density, and as if unmasked in some way,

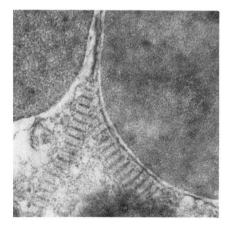

Fig. 10. Detail of cytoplasm from a rat peritoneal mast cell. Two typical granules are depicted. In close apposition to the perigranular membranes, two striated filamentous bundles are seen converging from different directions. Specimen processed as in Fig. 3. Electron micrograph. Magnification × 67,000.

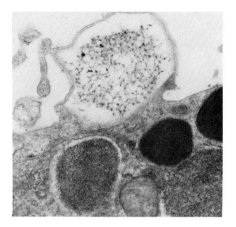

Fig. 11. Electron micrograph of a peripheral portion of a rat peritoneal mast cell incubated with 0.25 μg/ml of compound 48/80. Two normal, electron dense granules are seen as are other granules in different stages of alteration. Note the grossly altered granule in the membrane-delimited vacuole which is bulging out from the cell surface. The matrix of this granule appears as a fine, beaded, filamentous network. Specimen processed as in Fig. 3. Magnification × 16,800. (From the work of Bloom and Haegermark, 1965, 1967.)

the fine substructure of the granule matrix will appear. Such altered granules will also exhibit a more or less clear peripheral zone separating the granule matrix from the perigranular membrane. Furthermore, these vacuolar structures may merge, forming large membranous enclosures containing several altered granules. At the periphery of the cells the perigranular membranes will fuse with the plasma membrane, and the altered granules of these vacuoles may be expelled to the surrounding medium. Reports describing these features of rat mast cell degranulation by compound 48/80 were published independently by Singleton and Clark (1965), Bloom and Haegermark (1965), and Horsfield (1965).

More recent investigations applying similar experimental conditions have confirmed these observations (Bloom *et al.*, 1967; Yamasaki *et al.*, 1970). Furthermore, certain other histamine-releasing agents such as bee venom will produce similar changes in rat mast cells (Fig. 13) (Bloom and Haegermark, 1967). In addition, anaphylactic histamine release in rat mast cells is accompanied by structural changes in the cells closely resembling those observed with both 48/80 and bee venom (Fig. 14) (Bloom and Chakravarty, 1970; Anderson *et al.*, 1973). Alteration of mast-granule structure in connection with granule discharge has also been observed in dog mastocytoma mast cells (Fig. 12).

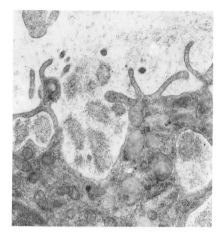

Fig. 12. Dog mastocytoma mast cell discharging granules to the intercellular space. One large membrane-delimited vacuole has opened onto the cell surface and several grossly altered mast granules are in the process of being expelled. Several other granule-containing vacuoles are also present. Note the homogeneous appearance of unaltered granules. Electron micrograph. Specimen processed as in Fig. 3. Magnification × 12,500.

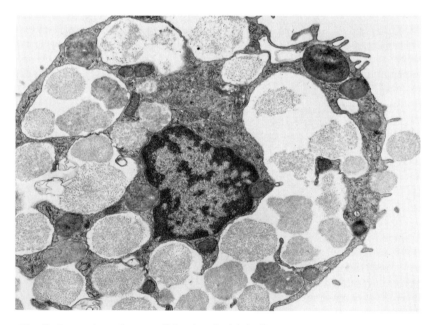

Fig. 13. Rat peritoneal mast cell incubated with buffer containing bee venom (5 μg/ml). Perigranular membranes of individual granules have fused and disintegrated; large vacuolar structures containing varying numbers of altered mast granules have developed. Discharged altered granules are seen extracellularly. Note the presence of single, intracytoplasmic, unaffected granules located at the periphery of the cell. Electron micrograph. Specimen processed as in Fig. 3. Magnification × 10,500. (From the work of Bloom and Haegermark, 1967.)

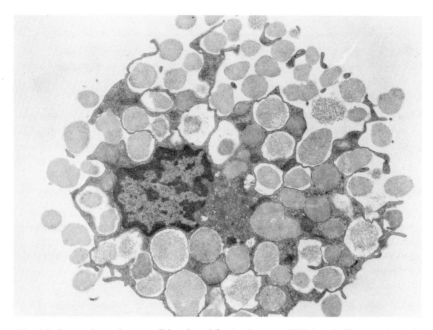

Fig. 14. Rat peritoneal mast cell incubated for 1 minute at 37°C in a buffer containing 0.1 mg/ml of antigen. Numerous vacuoles have formed as well as confluent, intracytoplasmic, membrane-delimited spaces which contain large numbers of altered granules and which communicate directly with the external environment. Numerous altered granules are being expelled from the cell. Electron micrograph. Specimen processed as in Fig. 3. Magnification × 8300. (From the work of Bloom and Chakravarty, 1970.)

The beaded reticular network which emerges in altered mast cell granules probably represents the heparin-protein skeleton of the granule matrix. From rats, injected with $Na_2{}^{35}SO_4$, mast cell granules have been isolated and subjected to treatment with aqueous KCl solutions. At low concentrations (0.05 to 0.7 M) the granules coalesced into a continuous mass and the beaded reticular network became prominent (Figs. 15, 16, and 17). Histamine is completely removed by such treatment, but only limited amounts of heparin were found in the supernatants after these serial extractions. However, approximately 25% of granule heparin was extracted with 1.0 M KCl and an additional 57% with 2.0 M KCl; the latter treatment caused a complete dissolution of the network (Lloyd et al., 1967a). Serafini-Fracassini et al. (1969) also suggest that the beaded filaments depicted in their electron micrographs of rat mast-cell granules may represent a network of heparin–protein macromolecules.

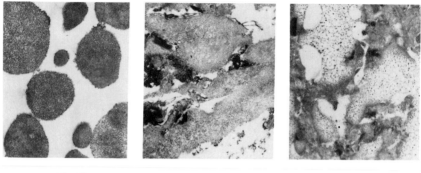

Fig. 15   Fig. 16   Fig. 17

Figs. 15–17. Rat peritoneal mast cell granules isolated according to the method of Lagunoff *et al.* (1964). Figure 15 shows the normal appearance of such granules; note the complete absence of any delimiting membrane and the faint granular-reticular pattern of the matrix. Figure 16 depicts the effects of suspending such granules in 0.05 *M* KCl solution. The granules have coalesced and their matrix has decreased markedly in electron density. The granule matrix substructure is more pronounced. Figure 17 shows the effect of suspension of the granules seen in Fig. 16 in 0.7 *M* KCl. In the fused granular masses, a beaded, reticular network is clearly seen. Sediments fixed, embedded, sectioned, and stained as in Fig. 3. Electron micrographs. Magnifications: Fig. 15, × 10,200; Figs. 16–17, × 7500. (From the work of Lloyd *et al.*, 1967a,b.)

The degranulation process in human mast cells has mainly been studied in urticaria pigmentosa lesions. The findings are not unequivocal. This is probably caused by the great variations in experimental conditions. However, after injecting 48/80 subcutaneously or treating excised urticaria pigmentosa specimens with the same compound, Orfanos (1966) observed granule alteration, vacuole formation, and the expulsion of altered granules into the surrounding environment. On the other hand, degranulation of human mast cells by stroking the skin of above-mentioned lesions leads to both intracellular dissolution of granules and extrusion of disintegrating as well as whole granules (Hashimoto *et al.*, 1966; Kobayasi and Asboe-Hansen, 1969).

Horsfield (1965) suggested that in 48/80-treated rat peritoneal mast cells, pores may exist between the plasma membrane and the perigranular membranes of the vacuoles, and that these pores may either normally be closed or be so small as to be regularly missed in sections of cells. Although no convincing evidence was presented at that time, it should be noted that in some very recent work it has been proposed that the vacuoles containing altered mast cell granules which appear after treatment of the cells with various histamine discharging agents, although seemingly intracellular, are in fact exocytoplasmic and in contact with the extracellular fluid via surface openings (Slorach, 1971; Röhlich *et al.*, 1971; Lagunoff, 1972a,b; Anderson *et al.*, 1973; Krüger and Bloom, 1973; Krüger *et al.*, 1974) (Fig. 19).

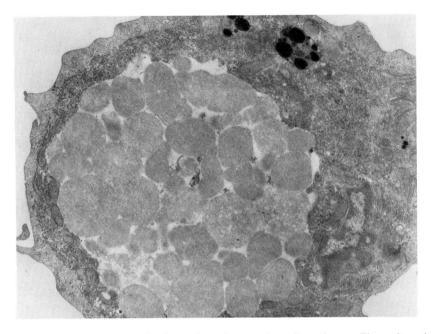

Fig. 18. Electron micrograph of a peritoneal macrophage from the rat. The peritoneal cells were incubated in a buffer containing 0.5 μg/ml of phospholipase; this caused extensive discharge of granules from mast cells. The cytoplasm of the depicted macrophage is occupied by numerous phagocytized mast cell granules which in the light microscope showed a metachromatic staining reaction. Specimen processed as in Fig. 3. Magnification × 10,500. (From Bloom and Haegermark, unpublished observations.)

C. Cytochemistry and Histochemistry of the Mast Cells

Mast cells and especially their cytoplasmic granules were found by early investigators to stain well with a variety of basic dyes such as thionine, methylene blue, azure, methylene violet, cresyl violet, acridine red, pyronine, saffranine, etc. Actually, it was their reaction toward certain basic dyes of the aniline family that brought about the discovery of the mast cells by Ehrlich (1877, 1879). When staining with Dahlia, a triphenylmethane dye, Ehrlich noticed that the mast cells were stained red with this blue-violet dye, a reaction which he was first to define as a metachromatic one. The physicochemical background of the metachromatic reaction is complex and was not understood by the early histologists. They nevertheless found it useful for identifying mast cells, cartilage, and amyloid. Particularly, dyes of the thiazine group such as the azure dyes, thionine, and toluidine blue have been widely used in histology.

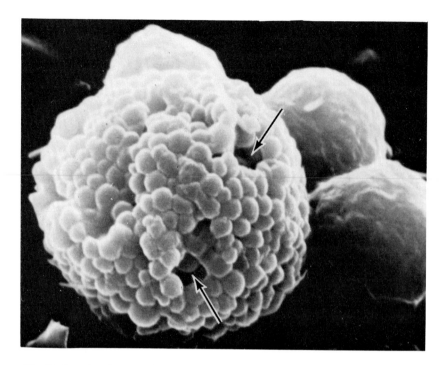

Fig. 19. Scanning electron micrograph of a rat peritoneal mast cell treated with 0.1 μg/ml of compound 48/80. Note the peripheral openings of intracytoplasmic caveolae (arrows). In lower opening an intravacuolar granule is seen. Magnification × 10,350.

An important contribution to the clarification of the metachromatic staining reaction was that of Lison (1935). From his studies he concluded that metachromasia was a specific chemical reaction provided only by sulfuric acid esters of high molecular weight. Although later this proved not to hold true, it in no way diminishes the importance of Lison's work. Subsequently, various investigators found that metachromasia was shown by a number of substances such as colloids bearing carboxyl and phosphoryl groups (Bank and Bungenberg de Jong, 1939), detergents with long hydrocarbon chains carrying anionic end groups (Michaelis, 1947), etc. For a thorough review of the metachromasia problem, the reader is referred to the monographs by Lison (1935) and Kelly (1956), as well as to the reports of Lennert and Schubert (1959) and Jaques (1961).

It is now well established that the mast cells contain sulfated mucopolysaccharides and that these substances are responsible for the metachromasia shown by the granules. The sulfated mucopolysaccharides are also demonstrable by their basophilia. When the pH of a basic staining fluid is lowered, fewer and fewer acidic groups in the tissue are dissociated and available for dye binding. The strongly acidic groups of sulfuric acid esters will bind certain basic dyes down to a pH of below 1.0. The basic copper phthalocyanine dye, Astrablau, used at a pH of 0.2 will specifically stain mast granules (Bloom and Kelly, 1960). It should be stressed, however, that Spicer (1963), employing several different staining techniques, found great variability in mast cell basophilia among different animal species.

The complex chemical nature of the mast granules is a major stumbling block in experiments where histochemical procedures are used to elucidate their components (see Fullmer, 1959; Stolk, 1961). These authors found in mast cells from mice and lower vertebrates that three stains, viz., the alde-hyde–fuchsin, the Hale (1946) stain, and azure-A, all normally stain mast cells. After peracetic acid oxidation, glucuronidase and lysozyme remove some component from the mast cells which, in turn, alters the aldehyde–fuchsin and the Hale stain but not the metachromasia.

Reports in the literature on the staining reaction of mast cells with the PAS-technique are divergent. Jorpes et al. (1948) found a strong PAS reaction in mast cells of young rats and suggested that it was caused by heparin monosulfuric acid, as heparin itself gave a negative Schiff color reaction. Similar findings were reported by Friberg et al. (1951). In adult rats, except in lymph nodes, no PAS-positive reaction was found in mast granules (Radden, 1962). Compton (1952) noted that in rats and hamsters, mast granules were generally PAS-negative and only occasionally positive, whereas Noback and Montagna (1946) as well as Lillie (1954) found all rat mast cells PAS-negative. A positive PAS reaction after pretreatment with amylase has been observed by, among others, Wislocki et al. (1949), Leblond (1950), and Friberg et al. (1951). Lennert and Schubert (1961) reported that 98 % of the human mast cells show a positive PAS reaction. Arvy (1955) observed a variability in staining with the PAS-technique among granules in one and the same mast cell.

Mast cells have been reported to contain glycogen (see Michels, 1938). This finding has not been verified, although several authors have applied varying techniques (Lehner, 1924; Nakajima, 1928; Wislocki et al., 1947; Kirkman, 1950). It has been stated further that nucleic acids are components of the mast granules (see Michels, 1938). Montagna (1957) found after ribonuclease (RNase) treatment that certain granules lost their stainability entirely, while in others metachromasia had changed to orthochromasia. Wislocki et al. (1947) and Zollinger (1950) found RNase to be without effect on toluidine blue staining of the granules.

Mast cells have also been reported to contain histochemically demon-strable lipids, as shown by Sudan black B staining (Wislocki and Dempsey,

1946; Montagna and Noback, 1948). Compton (1952) stated that only the granules in mast cells which were located in close proximity to tissue fat were positive. Lennert and Schubert (1961) observed no lipid staining of human mast cells with Sudan black B.

For a comprehensive comparative review of the staining histochemistry of mast cells in invertebrates as well as vertebrates, the reader is referred to the paper by Grünberg and Kaiser (1965).

Various histochemical techniques have been developed and proved suitable for demonstrating different amines in mast cells. Among the most sensitive and accurate methods are those employing the use of fluorescence microscopy and which are based on the formation of characteristic fluorophores on interaction between biogenic amines and certain aldehydes. In this way, histamine (Lagunoff et al., 1961; Juhlin and Shelley, 1966; Ehinger and Thunberg, 1967; Håkanson and Owman, 1967) 5-hydroxytryptamine (Riley, 1958; Coupland and Riley, 1960; Falck, 1962) and dopamine (Falck et al., 1964; Adams-Ray et al., 1964) have been histochemically demonstrated in mast cells although distinct species variations occur with respect to the amine(s) present in the cells. The value of these fluorescence techniques in mast cell-amine cytochemistry was vastly increased when it was shown that by careful standardization and utilization of microspectrophotometry they may yield quantitative data (Ritzén, 1967).

Numerous enzymes have been demonstrated in mast cells with both histochemical and biochemical techniques. These will be dealt with in Section V,E.

V. Biochemistry of the Mast Cells

For almost 60 years after Ehrlich's first report on the mast cells (1877), the work in the field was carried out primarily by histologists who were interested in the development of the cells, mapped out their locations, and studied their general habits. Unfortunately, during this era there was a complete lack of knowledge of the biochemical nature of the cells. It is now well established that the granules of the mast cells contain a broad spectrum of substances such as the mucopolysaccharide heparin and the biogenic amine histamine and occasionally 5-hydroxytryptamine and dopamine. The granules further contain structural protein and proteolytic enzymes. A strongly basic histonelike protein has been reported present (Spicer, 1963), and according to Uvnäs et al. (1970) the basic peptides of granule protein have a minimal molecular weight around 5600. The average dry weight of individual rat peritoneal mast cells has been estimated to roughly 500 pg (Diamant and Lowry, 1966; Diamant and Glick, 1967).

A. Mast Cells and Polysaccharides

The anticoagulant substance heparin was originally isolated from the liver of a dog in the laboratories of Howell (McLean, 1916). First characterized as a phosphatide, heparin was later shown by Jorpes (1936) to be an acid mucopolysaccharide,* a polymer of disaccharide units of glucuronic acid and glucosamine, highly esterified with sulfate. The fact that polysulfuric acid esters of high molecular weight gave metachromatic reactions with toluidine blue, for example (Lison, 1935), together with the finding of Jorpes (1936) that heparin in solution was precipitated by and stained metachromatically with toluidine blue, suggested to the Scandinavian group (Jorpes et al., 1937; Holmgren and Wilander, 1937; Wilander, 1938) that heparin might be responsible for the metachromatic reaction of mast cells with dyes of the thiazine type. These authors found a close correlation between the mast cell content of a tissue and the amount of heparin that could be extracted from it. The suggestion that mast cells contained heparin received strong support when it was shown by Oliver et al. (1947) that a mast cell tumor in a dog contained some 50 times the amount of heparin that could be extracted from the dog liver.

Asboe-Hansen (1950, 1954), however, found the mast cell population count to correspond better to the amount of hyaluronic acid in a tissue. Inasmuch as this nonsulfated mucopolysaccharide also proved to give a metachromatic reaction with toluidine blue, he concluded that the mast cells secreted the mesenchymal mucopolysaccharide hyaluronic acid, perhaps by way of a heparinlike precursor. The view that mast cells participate in the production of tissue hyaluronic acid is shared by among others Velican and Velican (1959) and Likar et al. (1964). Battezatti (1951) considers the possibility that the metachromatic substance of mast cells may not be heparin but some precursor, possibly hyaluronic acid, which is metabolized to heparin by the cells. A similar view is expressed by Hissard et al. (1951), who believe that the hyaluronic acid of the ground substance constitutes a large pool of material from which the mast cells can synthesize their heparin.

At the time Asboe-Hansen presented his hypothesis (1950), the mast cell was the only connective tissue cell which had been shown to contain muco-polysaccharide materials (Asboe-Hansen, 1957). It has since been established that the fibroblasts, which by far are the most numerous elements of the connective tissue, also secrete these substances (Grossfeld et al., 1957); and others.

---

* For practical purposes the term "mucopolysaccharide" will be applied throughout this chapter although in more recent work the authors cited may have used the term "glycosaminoglycan" for amino sugar-containing polysaccharides.

In the cornea, which normally contains an abundance of various muco-polysaccharides and is also capable of synthesizing these substances, wound healing may take place without vascularization and in the complete absence of mast cells. As Smith (1961) states in discussing the suggestions of Asboe-Hansen and co-workers that mast cells participate in the production of connective tissue ground-substance mucopolysaccharides, i.e., hyaluronate, in the cornea "other cells, such as fibroblasts, must do the job equally well."

No direct chemical evidence exists that mast cells contain hyaluronic acid. On the other hand, evidence is overwhelming with regard to the heparin content of mast cells.

Strong support for the mast cell–heparin relationship was obtained by radioisotope experiments. Jorpes and co-workers (1953) showed that mast cells of rat skin selectively incorporate and retain ^{35}S-labeled sulfate. Similar findings were made on isolated rat peritoneal mast cells (Lagunoff et al., 1960). Higginbotham and co-workers (1956) demonstrated radioactivity in isolated mast granules from the skin of mice previously injected with $Na_2^{35}SO_4$.

Direct proof of the presence of large amounts of heparin in mast cells has been obtained by chemical analyses of tissues rich in mast cells and of isolated mast cells. The nature and content of polysaccharides in dog and mouse mastocytomas has been studied by Furth et al. (1957), Barrnett et al. (1958), Korn (1959b), Spolter and Marx (1959), Green and Day (1960), Ringertz and Bloom (1960), Ringertz (1960a,b, 1963), and others. These investigations have all shown that heparin is the major mucopolysaccharide present in these tumors. Varying amounts of heparin monosulfate and chondroitin sulfate as well as small amounts of hyaluronic acid have also been reported.

Analyses of mucopolysaccharides in tissues and organs rich in mast cells are all complicated by the heterogeneity of the material analyzed; numerous tissue components other than mast cells contribute their mucopolysaccharides to the extracts. However, pure mast cell samples may be obtained from peritoneal cavities of rodents, for example, by differential centrifugation procedures (Padawer and Gordon, 1955; Glick et al., 1956; Uvnäs and Thon, 1959). Mast cell granules may be subsequently isolated from purified mast cell samples by, e.g., sonication of the cells followed by further centrifugation procedures (Lagunoff et al., 1964).

Analyses of mucopolysaccharides in isolated rat and mouse peritoneal mast cells have shown heparin to constitute 80–100% of the total polysaccharide content; no hyaluronic acid has been found (Schiller and Dorfman, 1959; Bloom and Ringertz, 1960; Parekh and Glick, 1962). The amount of heparin present in rat peritoneal mast cells has recently been calculated to about 95 $\mu g/10^6$ cells (Slorach, 1971). If this value is applied to results from a quantitative analysis of mast cell structure a rough figure of 95×10^{-3} pg of heparin per mast cell granule is obtained (Helander and Bloom, 1974).

Owing to lack of suitable isolation procedures, certain controversies arose early regarding the state of native heparin in the mast cell granules (see Engelberg, 1963). However, Green and Day (1961) detected the presence of residual amino acids in heparin hydrolysates. Furthermore, it was found that extensively purified samples of commercial heparin were still firmly associated with residual peptide materials in which serine predominated (Lindahl et al., 1965). After mild acid hydrolysis of these preparations, xyloserine could be isolated, and it was suggested that heparin in the native state was covalently bound to a protein (Lindahl and Rodén, 1965). That mast granule heparin exists as a macromolecular complex with protein through covalent linkage is also suggested by the work of Lloyd et al. (1967b) and Serafini-Fracassini and Durward (1968).

B. Mast Cells and Histamine

Histamine is formed from the amino acid histidine by decarboxylation processes. The fact that this biologically active amine is present in tissues and organs under normal circumstances was shown by Best and co-workers (1927), but the actual sites of histamine localization, at least at the cellular level, were long to remain a secret.

In 1938, Wilander observed that the release of heparin in peptone shock in the dog was accompanied by marked damage of liver mast cells. Similar changes were described after anaphylactic shock (Jacques and Waters, 1941). Rocha e Silva et al. (1947) showed that injections with peptone caused a simultaneous release of heparin and histamine in the dog.

Different investigators have reported that a number of simple bases such as adrenaline, atropine, strychnine, and curare cause varying degrees of histamine release from its sites in tissues and organs. In 1949, the interesting report of MacIntosh and Paton appeared in which these authors showed that a number of substituted amines, diamines, diamidines, and diguanidines caused extensive and seemingly specific histamine release in the cat or the dog. The fact that, in the dog, histamine releasers brought about a simultaneous discharge of histamine and heparin from the liver of this animal led MacIntosh and Paton (1949) to state that it "could perhaps be supposed that histamine and heparin are associated in some tissue complex and that the displacement of the former mobilizes the latter as well, but we know of no evidence for such an association."

The availability of specific histamine releasers offered a direct approach to the problem of localizing cellular sites of histamine in tissues. Tracing the fluorescent liberator stilbamidine, Riley (1953b) found that it entered mast cells which subsequently disintegrated. Furthermore, Riley and West (1953), in their classic investigation, showed that there was a striking parallel between histamine content and the numbers of mast cells in various tissues. Fawcett (1955), in a simple experiment with injections of distilled water into the peritoneal cavity of the rat, showed a positive correlation between mast cell disruption and histamine release. After the serous tissues had been depleted of their normal mast cell population, little or no histamine could be released by the potent histamine-releaser compound 48/80.

The presence of histamine in mast cells is now well established (Riley, 1953a, 1959; West, 1956; Benditt et al., 1956; Keller, 1957; Sjoerdsma et al., 1957). Furthermore, this amine is located in the mast granule (Mota et al., 1954; Hagen et al., 1959; Green and Day, 1960). Although it has been generally considered probable that the positively charged histamine is ionically linked in a loose fashion to the negatively charged heparin of the heparin–protein complex in the mast cell granule (e.g., Benditt and Lagunoff, 1964), the Uvnäs group (Åborg et al., 1967; Uvnäs et al., 1970) have recently clearly demonstrated that histamine is actually ionically bound to the protein COO-groups of the heparin–protein complex, the strongly acid sulfate groups of heparin being masked by electrostatic binding to basic groups of the granule protein.

Histamine in mammalian tissues seems to be produced from histidine through the action of histidine decarboxylase; there is no known evidence that it is synthesized from smaller molecules or is formed from histidine in vitro by nonenzymatic processes (Schayer, 1963a). According to the literature, the amount of histamine present in mast cells may vary considerably. Among the values reported for rat peritoneal mast cells are 10 $\mu g/mm^3$ of concentrated cells (Benditt et al., 1955) and roughly 30 pg per cell (Moran et al., 1962; Slorach, 1971). West (1956) found a dog mastocytoma to contain 1.29 mg of histamine per gram of tissue, and Furth and collaborators (1957), in their transplantable mouse mastocytoma, obtained values of about 3–4 mg/gm tissue.

Normal as well as neoplastic mast cells not only synthesize histamine but also take up this amine (Day and Green, 1962b; Furano and Green, 1964). This uptake is a passive process (Day and Stockbridge, 1964) and the exogenous histamine is bound to the mast granules (Thon and Uvnäs, 1966; Cabut and Haegermark, 1966). However, it has also been stated that when the mast granules are rich in endogenous amines, i.e., saturated, the exogenous histamine may be found in the soluble portion of the cell (cf. Green, 1966, 1967). Such "free" histamine in mast cells may be artifactual (Uvnäs et al., 1970).

There seem to be different pathways along which histamine may be released from mast cells. The degranulation phenomenon and histamine release induced by some liberating agents, e.g., compound 48/80 or bee venom, are evidently dependent on energy-requiring enzymatic processes in the cells, since they are blocked by metabolic inhibitors (Junqueira and Beiguelman, 1955; Högberg and Uvnäs, 1957; Mota and Ishii, 1960; Fredholm and Haegermark, 1967) and by anoxia in the absence of glucose (Diamant and Uvnäs, 1961). However, some other substances, e.g., decylamine, are able to degranulate mast cells and release histamine by a different mechanism. Their action is not blocked by enzyme inhibitors (Högberg and Uvnäs, 1960; Moran et al., 1962). Histamine release may also be brought about in a simple way by osmotic disruption of the cells in hypotonic salt solutions (Fawcett, 1955). With the aid of the electron microscope it has been demonstrated that n-decylamine and hyposmotic solutions bring about histamine release simply by affecting the integrity of mast cell fine structure, resulting in a breakdown of plasma membrane and cellular compartments (Bloom and Haegermark, 1967).

Numerous theories have been advanced as to how histamine release is brought about under normal and pathological conditions. These theories include simple physical permeability mechanisms as well as more complicated intra- and extracellular enzymatic processes. Thon and Uvnäs (1967) propose a two-stage process: a primary energy-requiring transport of granules to the outside of the cell and a secondary nonenergy-requiring physicochemical process involving an exchange between histamine and cations of the extracellular fluid. This ionic exchange-histamine release concept has received additional support from continued work by the Uvnäs group (Röhlich et al., 1971; Bergendorff and Uvnäs, 1972; Anderson et al., 1973).

An interesting approach to the problems concerning histamine-release mechanisms has recently been made. Baxter and co-workers (1970) observed that epinephrine, theophylline, and dibutyryl-cyclic-AMP (DB-c-AMP) seemed to protect mast cells *in vivo* from the anaphylactoid reaction caused by administration of dextran. Loeffler et al. (1971), studying 48/80-induced histamine release from rat mast cells, found that the release was inhibited by DB-c-AMP, phosphodiesterase inhibitors, and prostaglandin E_1. Their data were viewed as circumstantial evidence in support of a role for c-AMP in the histamine release process of the mast cell.

C. Mast Cells and Serotonin

The presence of 5-hydroxytryptamine (5-HT) or serotonin in mast cells was first shown in the rat by Benditt and co-workers (1955). Parratt and West (1957) studied mast cells from different species and noticed that although 5-HT appeared to be a common component of rat and mouse mast cells, it was not present in significant amounts in mast cells of guinea pig, dog, man, rabbit, cow, hamster, or cat.

Through the use of fractionation–separation procedures, 5-HT has been shown to reside in the mast granules along with heparin and histamine (Hagen et al., 1959). It has been suggested that both 5-HT and histamine may be synthesized in the intergranular cytoplasm and then stored in the granules in an inactive form (Hagen, 1961).

A histochemical approach toward localization and identification of 5-HT in mast cells was made by Coupland and Riley (1960). These authors correlated various staining reactions and the formaldehyde-induced fluorescence of mast cells in precancerous mouse skin with direct assays of 5-HT amounts in the same tissue and concluded that this amine was concentrated in the mast cell granules.

Rat peritoneal mast cells are capable of producing 5-HT by decarboxylation of available 5-hydroxytryptophan (5-HTP) (Lagunoff and Benditt, 1959; Hagen, 1961). A similar mechanism exists in the neoplastic mast cells of mouse mastocytomas, which have been extensively studied by numerous investigators (Furth et al., 1957; Hagen and Lee, 1958; Schindler, 1958; Green and Day, 1960; Hagen, 1961). Furthermore, mouse tumor mast cells can produce 5-HT from tryptophan, indicating that they can hydroxylate this amino acid (Schindler, 1958; Day and Green, 1962a). Isolated rat peritoneal mast cells, however, although capable of decarboxylating 5-HTP and also dihydroxyphenylalanine (DOPA), were unable to hydroxylate either tryptophan, phenylalanine, or tyrosine (Slorach and Uvnäs, 1968).

Other mast cell tumors, such as those in dogs and cows, do not contain significant amounts of 5-HT (Sjoerdsma et al., 1957; Meier, 1959; West, 1959). In urticaria pigmentosa in man, the skin lesions, which contain numerous mast cells, have not been found to contain 5-HT. These patients do not show any significant urinary output of the excretory metabolic product of serotonin, 5-hydroxyindole acetic acid (Sjoerdsma et al., 1957). Although 5-HT is not concentrated in the mast cells of man (Parratt and West, 1957), Enerbäck (1963) observed strongly fluorescent mast cells in the connective tissue of an appendiceal carcinoid and suggested that under conditions of enhanced serotonin secretion human mast cells may store this amine.

The 5-HT content of mast cells is variable, even within the same animal (Bhattacharya and Lewis, 1956). The amount of 5-HT in mast cells has been reported as 0.6–0.7 μg 5-HT base/mm^3 of rat peritoneal mast cells (Benditt et al., 1955) or roughly 1 μg per million of the same cells (Moran et al., 1962). In mouse mastocytomas, Furth et al. (1957) obtained 5-HT values varying from 8 to 140 μg/g of tissue.

Both neoplastic and normal mast cells take up exogenous 5-HT. This uptake, dissimilar to that of histamine, appears to be both an active and a passive process (Day and Stockbridge, 1964; Green, 1966; Jansson, 1968). The observations of Furano and Green (1964) that when the granules of neoplastic mast cells are rich in amines, exogenous 5-HT is stored in the intergranular cytoplasm as a soluble pool could not be confirmed in normal rat peritoneal mast cells (Jansson, 1970).

D. Mast Cells and Other Amines

The natural occurrence of dopamine in mast cells of certain animal species has only recently been established. Bertler and co-workers (1959) reported on the presence of large amounts of dopamine in granular cells of the gut and liver capsule of ox and sheep. These cells were later identified as mast cells (Coupland and Heath, 1961; Coupland, 1963). The introduction of fluorescence techniques for localization and identification of intracellular amines has proved of utmost value in establishing the relationship between mast cells and various amines. Thus mast cells in the hamster, cat, and rabbit appear to normally contain only small amounts of the monoamines 5-HT and dopamine but are able to store large amounts of these amines after administration of dihydroxyphenylalanine (DOPA) or 5-hydroxytryptophan (5-HTP) (Adams-Ray et al., 1964, 1965, 1966). Peritoneal mast cells of the mouse are capable of concentrating not only 5-HT and DOPA but also dopamine and noradrenaline (Eränkö and Kauko, 1965; Eränkö and Jansson, 1967). Mast cells within one and the same species may vary with respect to monoamine-storing capacity. The rat gastrointestinal mucosa has been reported to contain a specific type of mast cell which normally does not contain significant quantities of 5-HT but will take up DOPA as well as 5-HTP and accumulate both dopamine and 5-HT (Enerbäck, 1966; Enerbäck and Häggendal, 1970).

E. Enzymes of Mast Cells

Mast cells contain a battery of enzymes which function in processes that take place intra- and possibly also extracellularly.

Some of these enzymes are common to all cell types, whereas others are peculiar to the mast cell. Only a few can be demonstrated by common histochemical staining techniques. For a review on mast cell enzymes, see Arvy (1968).

The presence of "stable" cytochrome oxidase in the granules of mast cells from the rat, mouse, dog, hamster, and man was reported by Noback and Montagna (1946) and Montagna and Noback (1948). They used frozen sections and the *M. nadi* reagent according to Lison (1936). Compton (1952) was unable to confirm this observation in hamster mast cells, and Kirkman (1950) did not observe any reaction in rat mast cells with either the *M. nadi* or the *G. nadi* reagent. Using the Gomori (1945) method for lipase, Montagna and Noback (1948) found that mast granules in several species showed a positive reaction.

Acid as well as alkaline phosphatase in the granules of mammalian mast cells have been reported by numerous investigators (Montagna and Noback, 1948; Wislocki and Dempsey, 1946; Compton, 1952; Eder and Schauer, 1961; Vetter, 1970).

There is little doubt that mast cells not only store mucopolysaccharides but are also capable of synthesizing them. It has been demonstrated that glucose can serve as a precursor in this biosynthesis (Eiber and Danishefsky, 1958; Korn, 1959a). A prerequisite for synthesis is the necessary complement of enzymes. Some of these have been identified with certainty; the presence of others is as yet only conjectural.

Much of the work on the polysaccharide-synthesizing processes has been performed on mast cell tumors, especially the transplantable mouse mastocytomas. Nucleoside diphosphate glucose pyrophosphorylase, which catalyzes an early step in heparin biosynthesis, viz., formation of a nucleoside diphosphate glucose from D-glucose 1-phosphate and nucleoside triphosphate, has been demonstrated in the Furth mastocytoma (Danishefsky and Heritier-Watkins, 1967). These tumors have also been found to contain the enzymes (adenosine triphosphate sulfurylase and adenosine phosphosulfate kinase) necessary for the formation of nucleotide "active sulfate" (adenosine 3'-phosphate 5'-phosphosulfate) (Ringertz, 1960b) as well as polysaccharide sulfotransferases, enzymes which participate actively in the transfer of sulfate from "active sulfate" to carbohydrate acceptor molecules (Korn, 1959b; Spolter and Marx, 1959; Ringertz, 1960a, 1963; Rice *et al.*, 1967). Furthermore, certain possible intermediates in polysaccharide synthesis such as uridine diphosphate-linked hexosamines (Silbert and Brown, 1961) as well as a series of glucosamine- and galactosamine-containing polysaccharides with a varying degree of sulfation have been found in these tumors (Ringertz, 1963). It has recently been shown that mast cells contain an aminotransferase which catalyzes the formation of glucosamine-6-P from fructose-6-P and glutamine (Danishefsky and Deutsch, 1968).

Gomori (1953), applying chloroacylesters as histochemical substrates, found that mast cells show a strong hydrolytic activity. Similar findings were reported by Benditt and Arase (1958, 1959), who thoroughly studied this esterase and found it to show a close resemblance to chymotrypsin. Lagunoff and Benditt (1963) proposed the name mast cell chymase for this proteolytic enzyme. It has further been reported that this enzyme may constitute at least 10% of the total dry mass of the rat mast cell; its active centers are fully available in the intact cell, and serotonin (but not histamine) has a high affinity for these active centers, indicating a role for serotonin in inhibiting protease activity (Darzynkiewicz and Barnard, 1967). A chymotrypsin-like enzyme with a pH optimum of 7.8 and a molecular weight of 23,000 has been isolated from the rat thyroid and has been traced to the mast cells of this organ (Pastan and Almqvist, 1966).

Another esterase, resembling trypsin in substrate specificity, has been reported in mast cells of dogs and man and has been demonstrated by histochemical methods (Glenner and Cohen, 1960; Glenner et al., 1962). The latter authors also observed the above-mentioned chymotrypsin-like enzyme in their material.

A proteolytic enzyme which splits leucyl naphthylamide has been demonstrated in mast cells of the rat, mouse, guinea pig, hamster, and man (Braun-Falco and Salfeld, 1959; Eder and Schauer, 1961). These authors' claim that this enzyme is leucine aminopeptidase has been seriously questioned by Patterson et al. (1961). Enerbäck and Hansson (1968), applying histochemical techniques to rat mast cells, consider it doubtful that mast cells have any aminopeptidase activity at all.

In splenic mastocytosis in man and in the dog mastocytoma, Ende and Auditore (1961b) found a plasminlike substance, the fibrinolytic activity of which was observed and measured on standard bovine fibrin plates. It has been suggested that this fibrinolytic activity may correspond to the tryptase activity demonstrated histochemically (Lagunoff and Benditt, 1963).

Amino acid decarboxylases occur in mast cells. It was shown by Schayer (1956) that rat peritoneal mast cells, incubated with $[^{14}C]$L-histidine, formed and bound $[^{14}C]$histamine, indicating the presence of histidine decarboxylase. Pyridoxal phosphate has been shown to be the coenzyme (Rothschild and Schayer, 1958; Ono and Hagen, 1959; Hagen, 1961). These findings have been confirmed in many laboratories, and investigations on mast cell tumors in particular have contributed much to our knowledge of the histamine metabolism of mast cells.

Lagunoff and Benditt (1959), in isolated rat peritoneal cells, were able to demonstrate 5-hydroxytryptophan decarboxylase activity. It was found that this activity, too, was enhanced by pyridoxal-5-phosphate. In mouse tumor mast cells, Hagen and Lee (1958) found not only histidine and 5-hydroxytryptophan decarboxylases but also dopa decarboxylase, although no dopamine was detected in the tumor. Also in neoplastic murine mast cells, tryptophan hydroxylase (Day and Green, 1962a) and phenylalanine hydroxylase (Levine et al., 1964a,b) activity have been reported. Furthermore, a tryptophan hydroxylase, free of 5-HTP decarboxylase and phenylalanine hydroxylase activity, has been prepared from a Dunn-Potter original line of neoplastic mast cells (Hosoda and Glick, 1966). Sato *et al.* (1967) consider phenylalanine and tryptophan hydroxylase activities to be associated with a single enzyme.

The presence in mast cells of phosphatidase A, a hydrolytic enzyme which splits off unsaturated fatty acids from phospholipids, has been demonstrated by Uvnäs and co-workers (Högberg and Uvnäs, 1957; Uvnäs and Thon, 1961; Uvnäs, 1963). The specificity of this enzyme for lecithin was demonstrated by Giacobini *et al.* (1965), who further interpreted their results as compatible with a location of the enzyme at the mast cell membrane.

The enzyme β-glucuronidase has been demonstrated in mast cells of rat, mouse, hamster, guinea pig, and man (Montagna, 1957; Eder and Schauer, 1961; Lutzner, 1964 a.o.). β-Xylosidase and β-galactosidase activity has been reported for tissue cultures of murine mast cells (Fisher *et al.*, 1967).

In spite of the fact that discharge of mast cell granules, presumably the very basis of the biological activity of these cells (Selye, 1965), is an energy requiring process, only a few investigators have concerned themselves with the enzymes of energy-supplying reactions in mast cells. Glick and Potha-pragada (1961) have shown that isolated rat peritoneal mast cells are rich in succinic dehydrogenase. Fumarase was demonstrated in the nongranule fraction of malignant mouse mast cells by Hagen and co-workers (1959). Whereas glucose 6-phosphate, 6-phosphogluconate, and isocitric dehydro-genase activities are high in neoplastic mouse mast cells, they are not de-monstrable in normal rat peritoneal mast cells; lactic dehydrogenase activity per unit weight of protein is 19 times higher in neoplastic as compared to normal mast cells (Diamant and Glick, 1967). Based on the histochemical demonstration of various phosphate-hydrolyzing enzymes, Schauer and Eder (1961) postulated a high content and turnover of adenosine 5′-tri-phosphate (ATP) in rat mast cells. Diamant (1967a) measured the ATP con-tent and obtained a value of about 8.7×10^{-16} moles of ATP per rat mast cell. The same author also found that when rat mast cells were incubated with ATP, hydrolysis occurred indicating an ATPase activity of the cells (Di-amant, 1967b). It should be noted that ATP is an effective histamine releasing agent (Diamant and Krüger, 1967; Krüger *et al.*, 1974).

VI. Functional View of the Tissue Mast Cell

The mast cell has been proposed as participating in such a variety of roles in normal as well as in pathological conditions that it would be presumptuous even to try to summarize all these suggestions and postulates. Up to the time of Michels' classic monograph (1938), some 25 hypothetical functions of the mast cell had been advanced.

The characteristic perivascular distribution of mast cells led numerous early investigators to suggest a hemic function for the cells. Evidence that heparin is localized in the mast cells has supplied strong support for such an hypothesis. When a correlation between mast cells and heparin was established, it was taken for granted that the mast cells, through the secretion of heparin, participated in regulating hemostatic mechanisms. It is therefore somewhat surprising that thus far there has been so little evidence to indicate that heparin is secreted from mast cells into the bloodstream. Furthermore, in numerous cases when mast cells are disrupted and at a time when liberated histamine is easily demonstrated, heparin is rarely found in increased amounts in the bloodstream, even in animals with large mast cell tumors. In such cases, heparin appears to leave the cells but apparently remains trapped in the surrounding connective tissue.

Observations of any kind of direct transfer of mast granules from the connective tissue into the blood vessels are almost completely lacking. This fact is often used as an argument against the possibility that heparin from the mast cells reaches the bloodstream. Furthermore, the macromolecular dimensions of the heparin molecule alone would, from a physicochemical point of view, complicate any kind of diffusion phenomenon. These simple facts strongly suggest that mast cell mucopolysaccharides exert their functions mainly in and around the cell itself. It *has*, however, been reported that numerous mast granules from ruptured peritoneal mast cells of the rat find their way into lymphatics and eventually into the bloodstream of these animals, where they appear as one of the components of hemoconia (Adams and Paff, 1962). Furthermore, despite the failure to demonstrate the presence of heparin in blood, considerable caution should be exercised before concluding that this biological material does not normally occur within the circulatory system. Assay of small amounts of heparin is difficult, and many methods applied in the past are inaccurate. Applying a radioisotope technique, Eiber and Danishefsky (1957) contend that heparin is a normal constituent of blood and is, for example, present in dog blood in concentrations of 0.5 mg/100 ml. Engelberg (1963), in his monograph, has extensively reviewed the subject and considers it indisputable that heparin is normally present in human blood in the general range 1–2 mg/liter of plasma.

The capacity of heparin to form loose complexes with proteins at physiological pH and ionic strength (Godal, 1960) suggests the possibility that in both plasma and tissue heparin functions homeostatically to regulate many protein interactions, shifting its bonds to combine with and inactivate proteins which have accumulated in excess (Engelberg, 1963). The ability of heparin to act as an ion exchange agent led Higginbotham and Dougherty

(1957) to suggest that, in the environment of mast cells, noxious substances carrying cationic groups may be inactivated by complex formation with acid polysaccharide.

It is also believed that the mast cell contributes to lipid metabolism (see, e.g., Selye, 1965). There is evidence in the literature of a relationship between heparin and the so-called "clearing factor," an enzyme of a lipase nature. It is, however, still not clear whether, or to what extent, mast cell heparin takes part in clearing hyperlipemia. Although Fodor and Lojda (1956) reported that alimentary lipemia could cause activity of the mast cells as judged by histologically observed changes in the cells, their results could not be verified by Jennings et al. (1960). In addition, isotope techniques in the hands of these authors showed no increase in the rate of mobilization of sulfated substance from mast cells either on repeated maximal alimentary lipemia or repeated starvation. Furthermore, it has been shown that mast cell granules inhibited a heparin-activated lipase extracted from rat adipose tissue, whereas purified rat heparin extracted from the granules activated the lipase (Lagunoff et al., 1966). Evidently mast cell chymase was responsible for the inhibition, and considering the stability of the chymase–heparin complex in extracellular and intravascular compartments, the authors found it unlikely that mast cell heparin modulates lipase activity in tissue or plasma.

The physiological role of mast cell histamine is not clear. Rocha e Silva (1955) stated that "here we have a powerful endogenous, active agent, present in almost every organ or tissue of the body in amounts that can produce not only physiological but also drastic pathological effects, and yet it appears to be devoid of physiological significance." However, histamine activates the reticuloendothelial system, and through its vascular effects causes a flooding of the tissues with protein-rich edema fluid. This would promote removal of foreign protein and enhance processes of repair (West, 1958).

The suggestion that histamine has a greater physiological role in circulatory regulation than believed earlier was advanced by Schayer (1963b). The histamine concerned has been designated "induced histamine" to distinguish it from the histamine bound in the tissues. Newly synthesized in free pharmacologically active form, it is thought to be formed in or near the vascular endothelial cells by the action of an inducible form of histidine decarboxylase. According to the same author, mast cell histamine serves more of an emergency function (Schayer, 1963a).

With regard to serotonin, almost nothing is known of its function in relation to tissue mast cells. It should be kept in mind that this amine, from all available evidence, is not a common component of mast cells in general. Histamine exerts a different biological effect in the rat and mouse than in the guinea pig. In these species, serotonin evokes responses which are ordinarily obtained with histamine. This led Benditt and co-workers (1963) to suggest that 5-HT in the rat and mouse is analogous to histamine in other species and that it constitutes the major activator of increased capillary permeability and smooth muscle contraction in the two mentioned species. When liberated, 5-HT has been reported to exert an even greater phagocytosis-stimulating action than histamine (Northover, cited by West, 1962).

Riley (1962) raised the question of whether the dramatic pharmacological effects of heparin and the biogenic amines, histamine and serotonin, had diverted attention from other less obvious physiological functions of the mast cell. He advocated a reexamination of the original suggestion by Ehrlich (1877, 1879) that the mast cells are concerned with events in the connective tissue and advanced a hypothesis of a "local mast cell cycle" in the tissues. According to his theory, histamine, released from mast cells, could activate nearby mesenchymal cells to phagocytize subsequently released heparin granules. Digestion of such material could stimulate the connective tissue cells to produce fresh mucopolysaccharide of their own. Having served its purpose, this extracellular material could again be broken down and utilized synthetically by mast cells (Riley, 1962).

Unfortunately, our knowledge of the mast cell proteases is still at a primitive level. It has been speculated that liberated mast cell chymase may act on extracellular mucoproteins of the ground substance and may also destroy antigens locally (Lagunoff and Benditt, 1963). The proteolytic enzyme(s) of human and dog mastocytoma mast cells show strong fibrinolytic activities (Ende and Auditore, 1961a,b, 1964) and may act on fibrin, e.g., in the wound-healing process. Another interesting aspect of the proteases is that on the basis of substrate specificity at least the rat mast cell enzyme also qualifies as a possible kininase (Lagunoff, 1968). Finally, it has been suggested that these enzymes may extend and perpetuate vascular responses in, e.g., inflammatory processes (Smith, 1963b). Whether or not the mast cell proteases have any specific intracellular function is still an open question.

As is evident from the above discussion, main interest has been focused on the role of the mast cell as a secretory cell. However, the possibility that mast cells may have important absorptive functions must not be overlooked. Evidence of such a role may be found in the numerous uptake studies reported in the literature. The great capacity of the cells to take up, e.g., biogenic amines, indicates that this may possibly be one of their normal functions. It has also clearly been suggested that with respect to, e.g., histamine, the mast cells may primarily be involved with detoxicating this substance rather than ejecting it (Chayen et al., 1966 a.o.). Padawer (1969) is also of the opinion that absorptive processes may be of prime importance.

His viewpoint is based on the fact that mast cells, although generally considered to be nonphagocytic (Selye, 1965), readily ingest various particulates such as zymosan, colloidal thorium dioxide, and gold (Padawer and Fruhman, 1968; Padawer, 1968, 1969). Furthermore, these particles were observed to become gradually intimately associated with, and even incorporated into, the mast cell granules. A more conventional type of phagocytosis by mast cells has been reported by Sato et al. (1969). When studying mast cells of skin lesions of dermal melanocytosis and blue nevus, those authors observed melanosomes in the cytoplasm of mast cells. The melanosomes were, however, all confined within phagocytic vacuoles outside the mast cell granules. It would be presumptuous to speculate on these findings at the present stage. However, as stated by Padawer (1968), any observations on phagocytic properties of mast cells would seem to have broad significance with respect to mast cell function.

VII.   Mast Cells in Pathological Disorders

A. The Mast Cell in Inflammatory Processes

Although less evident in acute inflammation, mast cells are invariably increased in chronic inflammatory processes. This observation was made by Maximow (1904), among others, and was subsequently confirmed by numerous investigators. Although many suggestions have been advanced to explain this phenomenon, they were essentially speculative since at that time nothing was known of the nature of the substances synthesized and stored within the cells.

The disappearance of mast cells during acute inflammation is preceded by degranulation. This process results in a displacement of heparin, histamine, and other substances (enzymes, occasionally 5-HT) from intact mast cells into the surrounding ground substance of the connective tissue. However, the biological effects of the liberated substances will vary widely, depending on the degree of liberation, detoxification processes, rate of removal, etc. The mediators of this degranulation process are at present unknown, although it has been suggested that an enzyme-free basic protein from the lysosomes of exudate polymorphonuclear leukocytes may act as an endogenous liberator of histamine (Janoff and Zweifach, 1964; Janoff and Schaeffer, 1967; Keller, 1968).

Cardinal features of an acute inflammatory reaction in a tissue are hyperemia, increased vascular permeability, formation of edema, and repairative processes. It is highly probable that products of mast cells provoke some of the above-mentioned features.

The work of Eder and Schauer (1961) and Sheldon and Bauer (1960) strongly supports this theory. Following the histological changes that take place in response to experimental cutaneous mucormycosis, the latter authors observed within minutes a discharge of mast granules at the site of infection. This event appeared to initiate the rapid onset of edema and congestion. Two hours after intial degranulation, regranulation began to appear in mast cells at the periphery of the lesion. After 12 hours, their incidence and appearance were normal. In animals whose mast cells were already degranulated by compound 48/80, the onset and intensity of the inflammatory process was decreased and fungus growth increased. Lastly, in rats with severe alloxan diabetes with acidosis, normal mast cell function appeared to be inhibited, resulting in complete failure of the cells to discharge their granules. In these animals, the onset and intensity of the inflammatory reaction was significantly delayed, and infection progressed rapidly and severely.

It is relatively simple to establish a parallel between certain features of the local inflammatory process and the effects of biologically active substances known to reside in mast cells and to be released on degranulation and/or disintegration of the cells. It is much more difficult, however, to assign specific roles to these substances. Whether or not an actual degranulation of mast cells is necessary to discharge these active substances is not entirely clear. In studies on the acute inflammatory response to corneal wounds, Garden and Sherk (1968) were unable to observe any change whatsoever in mast cell morphology or numbers even when the inflammatory reaction was severe.

Histamine and serotonin, liberated from mast cells, are believed to play an important part in the mechanisms by which capillary permeability is increased in inflammatory processes, thereby promoting the local leakage of protein-rich plasma into the tissues at the site of the inflammatory reaction. Furthermore, these amines, through their phagocytosis-stimulating effect, may enhance the elimination of noxious matter which arises in the tissue or which is introduced. The proteolytic enzymes of the mast cells may perpetuate the vascular responses (Smith, 1963b) possibly by reacting with tissue fluid proteins to form kinins (Keller, 1967). Mast cell heparin with its strong electric charge can react in numerous ways with proteins, enzyme systems, etc., and by complexing with noxious substances and toxins, it may participate in the local physiological defense reaction.

B. Mast Cells and Anaphylaxis

Anaphylaxis has been defined by Dragstedt (1941) as an autointoxication produced by the release of endogenous toxic principles, following union of antigen with antibody. Among those principles, histamine is the most important (Rocha e Silva, 1955).

It was shown in 1938 by Waters *et al.*, that heparin was responsible for the incoagulability of blood in dog anaphylaxis and, shortly afterwards, Ojers *et al.* (1941) demonstrated that histamine was discharged from the dog liver in anaphylactic shock. Morphological evidence for mast cell participation in anaphylaxis was found by Jaques and Waters (1941) in the same animal. The granules of mast cells in the liver diminished in numbers and showed altered staining properties. In spite of the above findings, the possible role of the mast cell as carrier of both heparin and histamine was overlooked for some time.

The findings of Riley and West (1953), implicating the mast cells as storage sites for both heparin and histamine, led to a renewed interest in the possible role of these cells in anaphylaxis.

In experimental anaphylaxis, utilizing egg albumen as an antigen, mast cells were found to be severely damaged in the rabbit, guinea pig, dog, and mouse (Stuart, 1952). Mota and co-workers (1953; Mota and Vugman, 1956) studied the mast cell reaction in rats and guinea pigs extensively. They found that the histamine content of the guinea pig lung is closely correlated to its mast cell population. Anaphylactic shock brings about a simultaneous drop in histamine content and a reduction of mast cells. Degranulation and a decrease of the metachromasia of the remaining cells also takes place (Mota and Vugman, 1956).

The occurrence of both histamine and lipid-soluble smooth muscle-stimulating principle (probably the same as the "slow reacting substance" of Kellaway and Trethewie, 1940) in guinea pig anaphylaxis was reported by Chakravarty and Uvnäs (1960). They showed a quantitative correlation between the two substances under various experimental conditions. Boréus and Chakravarty (1959), studying the anaphylactic reaction produced *in vitro* in isolated guinea pig tissue, could correlate both histamine and "slow reacting substance" (SRS) to the mast cell population. However, Eilbeck and Smith (1967) who also studied the guinea pig lung concluded that "whilst mast cells might also be the source of SRS, evidence for its occurrence in them is lacking." It has seriously been questioned whether the mast cell in general is the source of SRS (Austen, 1965). In isolated rat peritoneal mast cells, Austen and Humphrey (1962) using rabbit antirat γ globulin obtained an 80 % release of histamine without any concomitant release of SRS. In a more recent investigation, Orange *et al.* (1967) further studied the antigen-induced release of SRS in rats. Their findings indicated that the crucial cell type for optimum release of this substance was the polymorphonuclear leukocyte, whereas mast cells were not required.

The actual mechanism of mast cell damage in anaphylactic reactions has mainly been studied by *in vitro* experiments with isolated rat mast cells. When such cells from a sensitized animal are exposed to the antigen, they become degranulated and release their histamine (Uvnäs and Thon, 1959; Mota and Dias da Silva, 1960; Bloom and Chakravarty, 1970). Hence, the conclusion may be drawn that the antigen–antibody reaction is localized in the mast cell itself and in all probability takes place on the surface of the cell. The reaction between antigen and antibody is temperature dependent, influenced by pH and ionic milieu, and is inhibited by numerous enzyme inhibitors (Uvnäs and Thon, 1961; Keller and Schwarz, 1961). This would indicate that enzyme mechanisms are concerned with the release of histamine and serotonin in anaphylactic reactions (Uvnäs, 1961; Mongar and Schild, 1962). Oxidative energy metabolism has been shown to be directly involved in the process of anaphylactic histamine release (Chakravarty, 1968).

When the time course of anaphylactic histamine release is compared with that obtained by certain histamine releasers such as compound 48/80 or bee venom, there is a much longer initial lag period for the anaphylactic release. This may be caused by specific antibody sites in the mast cells with which antigen must combine to initiate the chain of reactions that finally leads to histamine release (Bloom and Chakravarty, 1970).

It has been shown that the guinea pig intestine differs from other tissues in having a high mast cell count which is unaffected during anaphylactic reactions. Intestinal mast cells are thus more resistant to disintegration when incubated with antigen (Boréus and Chakravarty, 1959). Furthermore, it seems evident that there are considerable variations in the anaphylactic pattern between different animal species. Some of these variations may be due to differences in the chemical composition and enzymatic contents of the tissue mast cells (Keller, 1962).

Current concepts of the "mast cell anaphylaxis complex" are far from clear. Whereas contact with antigen in passively sensitized guinea pigs duplicates the mast cell damage seen in active anaphylaxis, this is not the case in rats. These and other findings suggest the possibility, at least in the rat, that anaphylaxis may be brought about by different antigen–antibody reactions: (a) the reaction of antigen with precipitating antibodies that do not cause mast cell damage, and (b) the reaction of antigen with "mast cell lytic" antibodies (Mota, 1961, 1962, 1963). To further complicate the situation, Keller (1966) presents data indicating that histamine does not play an important role in rat anaphylaxis and further states that "if histamine release and mast cell alterations do occur this is not always due directly to a cellular antigen–antibody reaction."

There is also increasing evidence that induced histamine from other sources than mast cells is involved in allergic reactions. During anaphylaxis in guinea pigs and rats, nascent histamine is rapidly formed in most tissues, even those poor in mast cells, and Kahlson and Rosengren (1968) conclude that the newly formed histamine in anaphylaxis is largely of nonmast cell origin.

C. The Mast Cell in Mastocytosis

Mastocytoses are fairly rare pathological conditions which are characterized by proliferation of non-neoplastic and/or neoplastic mast cells in the skin (cutaneous mastocytosis) and/or in other tissues and organs such as bone marrow, lymph nodes, liver, and spleen (systemic mastocytosis). A wealth of pertinent information on the subject of mastocytosis is gathered in the monograph by Sagher and Even-Paz (1967). Comparative aspects of the mastocytoses have recently been discussed by Lingeman (1969).

Urticaria pigmentosa, the most common form of mastocytosis in man, had been known since almost 30 years before Unna's (1896) classic description of its histopathological features appeared. In tissue sections stained with dyes of the aniline family, he observed the metachromatic reaction of numerous tissue elements, the mast cells of Ehrlich. For more than 50 years, the disease was looked on as an isolated, purely cutaneous, benign condition characterized by skin lesions, either typically urticarial in type or appearing as heavily pigmented macules. Although the degree of pigmentation was found to vary in the affected skin areas, mast cell hyperplasia in the corium of the lesions was a pathognomonic feature.

The fact that the triple response of Lewis (1927) is easily elicited on mechanical irritation of the urticarial lesions indicates that these lesions are rich in histamine which is easily released. Actual analyses of skin lesions from urticaria pigmentosa patients have shown that they contain many times the histamine in normal skin (Riley and West, 1953; Sjoerdsma et al., 1957). Not only is histamine present in the lesions in increased amounts, but elevated levels of this amine are found in the blood and urine of patients with urticaria pigmentosa (Brogren et al., 1959). Bloom et al. (1958) reported the case of a 10-month-old child in which mechanical irritation of the skin lesions evoked such a massive release of histamine as to lead to spells of unconsciousness.

Hemorrhagic lesions of the skin are not common in cutaneous mastocytosis (Sagher and Even-Paz, 1967). Still rarer are the reports on general systemic affects of heparin supposedly released from the lesions. Increased coagulation time, prolonged bleeding time, and abnormal heparin tolerance tests have, however, been observed and attributed to heparin action (Poppel et al., 1959).

Serotonin (5-HT) has been reported to be lacking in the human mast cell (Parratt and West, 1957). Serotonin has not been detected either in skin lesions (Sjoerdsma et al., 1957) or in affected organs (Gardner et al., 1958) of patients with urticaria pigmentosa. Furthermore, while urinary histamine may be greatly increased, the output of the serotonin metabolite 5-hydroxyindoleacetic acid is normal (Bloom et al., 1958; Brogren et al., 1959).

However, conclusive evidence that a mast cell disease may affect internal tissues and organs and may prove fatal was first presented by Ellis (1949). He performed an autopsy on a case of urticaria pigmentosa in a 1-year-old child and found splenomegaly, hepatomegaly, and extensive mast cell proliferation throughout the reticuloendothelial system. It is apparent from the increasing evidence in the literature that mastocytoses are not as benign as earlier believed (Berlin, 1955; Sagher and Schorr, 1956; Poppel *et al.*, 1959). In their review of 71 cases of "proved" systemic mastocytosis, Sagher and Even-Paz (1967) reported that almost one-third proved fatal. Furthermore there is no effective treatment for mastocytosis.

Bigelow (1961), on the basis of his own observations and data from the literature, has pointed out many similarities between systemic mast cell disease (mastocytosis) and other reticuloses, particularly the reactive histiocytoses. He also stresses the fact that the functional capacities of the mast cell may well make it possible to distinguish between the two diseases from a clinical point of view. Nevertheless, he believes that a nosological relationship exists. His viewpoints are shared by numerous clinicians and pathologists. Solitary lesions of urticaria pigmentosa, classified as "mastocytomas" by Sézary (1936), are not to be considered as reticuloses (Lennert, 1962).

The term "mastocytoma" was originally suggested by Fabris (1927) for the nodular aggregations of mast cells which appeared in the subepithelial connective tissue in experimental tar cancers. In retrospect it may be stated that Fabris' suggestion was unfortunate since it has led to great confusion in the literature. The term has often been indiscriminantly used for mast cell aggregations whether of neoplastic nature or not.

Spontaneous "true" mast cell tumors (mastocytomas) are most common in dogs (F. Bloom, 1942; Mulligan, 1948; Head, 1953; G. D. Bloom *et al.*, 1956). They comprise 7–15 % of all canine skin tumors (Cook, 1969). These tumors are subcutaneous and may be either benign or malignant (F. Bloom, 1942). In malignant cases, there is systemic involvement, and neoplastic mast cells may occur in the liver, spleen, lung, bone marrow, and regional lymph nodes. It has been reported that canine mastocytoma may be caused by a viral agent (Lombard *et al.*, 1963). Occasional reports have appeared of mast cell tumors in the horse (Sabrazés and Lafon, 1908), cat (Sabrazés *et al.*, 1908), cattle (Head, 1958; Migaki, 1969), and pig (Migaki, 1969).

In mice, two classic mast cell tumor lines have been established. One arose in the subcutaneous tissue of a DAB/2 mouse after local skin treatment with methylcholanthrene (Dunn and Potter, 1957) and the other in a mouse of the LAF$_1$ strain after total body irradiation with 475 R (Furth *et al.*, 1957). Both the Dunn-Potter mastocytoma and that of Furth and collaborators proved to be transplantable and have survived in solid as well as ascitic form.

An interesting finding made in the Furth mastocytoma was the presence of large numbers of viruslike particles in the cytoplasm of the tumor mast cells (Bloom, 1963). Another transplantable mastocytoma which arose in a $(CBA \times DBA/2)F_1$ mouse inoculated subcutaneously with leukemic tissue from a transplantable plasma cell leukemia has been reported (Rask-Nielsen and Christensen, 1963). The mouse mastocytomas have proved extremely valuably for experimental purposes. Actually, much of our present knowledge of mast cell biochemistry is based on work with such tumors. It should, however, be pointed out that Green (1968) has reported that when clones are isolated and grown from descendants of the original Furth tumor line, for example, certain intrinsic genetic differences appear. He also considers that genetic variants must account for various discrepancies in biochemical data obtained with neoplastic murine mast cells in different laboratories. The latter supposition is strongly supported by the work of Lewis *et al.* (1973). Studying mastocytoma cells of a newly derived line, termed P815S, it was found not only that the amounts of sulfated mucopolysaccharides synthesized exceeded those of mastocytoma cells of long-established lines, but that the major mucopolysaccharide produced was chondroitin 4-sulfate.

Mast cell tumors in man are considered to be rare. One reason for this is undoubtedly the difficulty in distinguishing between mast cell hyperplasia and mast cell neoplasia. Another factor stems from the previous lack of agreement regarding classification of human mast cell disorders. As mentioned earlier, numerous pathological conditions involving mast cells, and with a definitely malignant trend, have been classified as atypical cases of urticaria pigmentosa. A reevaluation of the whole concept of mast cell disease is necessary to determine which cases are to be considered as true mast cell neoplasias and which are not.

If the solitary lesions of urticaria pigmentosa are classified as mastocytomas, some 80–90 cases have thus far been recorded in man (Holmberg, 1970). Mastocytomas apparently unrelated to cutaneous mastocytosis are extremely rare in man. Bloom *et al.* (1960) described a case believed to be a malignant mastocytoma in a 47-year-old female in which there were no cutaneous manifestations (urticaria pigmentosa) or disorders of the blood (tissue mast cell leukemia). The case proved fatal. Aggregations of presumably metastatic mast cells were found in the spleen, lung, liver, kidney, ovary, and lymph nodes, and enormous tumor masses were encountered in the bone marrow. Values of histamine excretion in the patient were among the highest ever to be reported ($600 \mu g/24$ hours), and histamine and heparin were found in increased amounts in all organs involved. The first solitary mast cell tumor of the lung (judged as a histiocytoma) was reported by Sherwin *et al.* (1965). In a second such case, 18 months after lobectomy, the patient showed no local or systemic evidence of mast cell disease (Charrette *et al.*, 1966).

D. The Mast Cell in Carcinogenesis

The close association of mast cells to developing tumors was noted by Ehrlich (1879) and Westphal (1880). These cells are particularly numerous in the connective tissue bordering the neoplasias (Bierich, 1922; Fabris, 1927; Sylvén, 1941; Cramer and Simpson, 1944). Since nothing is known of the factor(s) causing mast cell hyperplasia or the mechanism by which mast cells act on developing neoplastic growths, it is not surprising to find widely divergent opinions in the literature regarding the role of the cell in such conditions. Some investigators (Cramer and Simpson, 1944; Holmgren and Wohlfart, 1947; Csaba et al., 1961) are of the opinion that the mast cell reaction is an expression of a defense mechanism in an organism directed against the growing neoplasm. There are others, however (Borrel et al., 1923; Scott et al., 1958), who conclude that mast cells and/or their cellular products enhance the development of neoplasias. Peyron (1923, cited by Kelsall and Crabb, 1959) considers the increase of mast cells to be of no significance with respect to either the genesis of cancer or the defense against it.

Landsberger (1966) ascribes a tumor-inhibiting effect to the heparin of discharged mast cell granules. Mere increase of tissue mast cells without signs of degranulation was not accompanied by any inhibition of tumor growth.

It has long been known that heparin is an inhibitor of mitosis (Heilbrunn and Wilson, 1949; Lippman, 1957), possibly exerting its effect through interference with the metabolism of nucleoproteins (Anderson and Wilbur, 1951; Paff et al., 1952). In a human cancer of the cervix material, a close association was found between cancer cells in mitosis and mast cells, and it was suggested that mast cells may participate in a defense reaction against the tumor cells by interfering with the cell division process (Graham and Graham, 1966).

It has been suggested that the function of the mast cell in the process of skin carcinogenesis may be an inhibition of growth or a restoration to normal of the increased permeability of the connective tissue, both functioning by virtue of the mucopolysaccharide substance carried by the cells (Cramer and Simpson, 1944). Kelsall and Crabb (1959) do not consider the stimulating effects of chemical carcinogens on mastocytogenesis to be directly related to the carcinogen, but to its ability to produce conditions in the tissues similar to those characteristic of subchronic inflammation. Riley (1966), studying the two-stage process of methylcholanthrene-induced carcinogenesis, viz., initiation followed by promotion (co-carcinogenesis), has established that the mast cell is involved in the promotion phase. In addition, an index of the trend toward cancer is the gradual and progressive development of a mast cell reaction in the "basement membrane zone" (Riley, 1968). Wózniak and

Wranicz (1968) found no correlation between degree of malignancy in epithelial tumors and numbers of mast cells in surrounding connective tissue.

Scott and co-workers (1958), in studies with subcutaneous tumor implants in the rat, found that a tumor polypeptide readily diffused from the tumor and caused the release of histamine and 5-HT. They also found that administration of tumor polypeptide to normal rats resulted in a significant reduction in mast cells in mesentery spreads. From their experiments it was concluded that histamine and 5-HT release are beneficial to tumor growth and that the tumor cell may obtain some of its nourishment by influencing surrounding normal cells. On the other hand, Fisher and Fisher (1965) found that subcutaneous Walker carcinoma tumors in an inital phase grew more rapidly in rats depleted of mast cells than in controls. Local injections of serotonin inhibited subsequent growth whereas heparin and histamine were without effects. The results were considered consonant with a defensive role for mast cells in tumor growth, and serotonin was suggested as a possible inhibitory factor.

Csaba et al. (1961) have proposed that mast cells antagonize tumor growth by taking up, and thus depriving tumor cells of, heparin. They go so far as to state that "mast cells do not produce heparin but absorb and neutralize this substance." Unfortunately, these authors give no clue as to where the heparin "absorbed by mast cells" is supposed to originate. This would seem to be critical since, according to Jorpes (1946), no source of heparin other than mast cells is known.

VIII. Concluding Remarks

It is somewhat frustrating that the concluding remarks to this chapter in the first edition still appear to be valid. It was stated therein that we have yet to convincingly furnish the tissue mast cell with some specific physiological function(s). It is doubtful if any other single cell type has attracted the amount of attention that has been given to the mast cell. Yet, a unifying concept of the various functions, which have been suggested for this cell in different animal species and in man under normal as well as numerous pathological conditions, is still withholding. However, there appears to be no immediate call for pessimism, since according to Goffman (1966), mast cell research as a whole has not yet attained its maximum and will not do so until the latter part of this decade.

References

Åborg, C., Novotny, J., and Uvnäs, B. (1967). Acta Physiol. Scand. **69**, 276.
Adams, J. P., and Paff, G. H. (1962). Anat. Rec. **144**, 19.

Adams-Ray, J., Dahlström, A., Fuxe, K., and Hillarp, N.-Å. (1964). *Experientia* **20**, 80.
Adams-Ray, J., Dahlström, A., Fuxe, K., and Häggendal, J. (1965). *J. Pharm. Pharmacol.* **17**, 252.
Adams-Ray, J., Dahlström, A., and Sachs, C. (1966). *Acta Physiol. Scand.* **67**, 295.
Allen, A. M. (1961). *Anat. Rec.* **139**, 13.
Allen, A. M. (1962). *Lab. Invest.* **11**, 188.
Anderson, N. G., and Wilbur, K. M. (1951). *J. Gen. Physiol.* **34**, 647.
Anderson, P., Slorach, S. A., and Uvnäs, B. (1973). *Acta Physiol. Scand.* **88**, 359.
Arvy, L. (1955). *Rev. Hematol.* **10**, 55.
Arvy, L. (1968). *Annee biol.* **7**, 287.
Asboe-Hansen, G. (1950). *Acta Dermato-Venereol.* **30**, 221.
Asboe-Hansen, G. (1954). *Int. Rev. Cytol.* **3**, 399.
Asboe-Hansen, G. (1957). *In* "Connective Tissue: A Symposium" (R. E. Tunbridge, ed.), pp. 12–26. Blackwell, Oxford.
Asboe-Hansen, G. (1968). *Bull. N. Y. Acad. Med.* **44**, 1048.
Asboe-Hansen, G., and Levi, H. (1962). *Acta Pathol. Microbiol. Scand.* **56**, 241.
Asboe-Hansen, G., Levi, H., Nielsen, A., and Weis Bentzon, M. (1965). *Acta Pathol. Microbiol. Scand.* **63**, 533.
Austen, K. F. (1965). *In* "The Inflammatory Process" (B. W. Zweifach, L. Grant, and R. T. McCluskey, eds.), 1st ed., pp. 587–612. Academic Press, New York.
Austen, K. F., and Humphrey, J. H. (1962). *In* "Mechanism of Cell and Tissue Damage Produced by Immune Reactions" (P. Grabar and P. Miescher, eds.), pp. 93–106. Schwabe, Basel.
Bank, O., and Bungenberg de Jong, H. G. (1939). *Protoplasma* **32**, 489.
Barrnett, R. J., Hagen, P., and Lee, F. L. (1958). *Biochem. J.* **68**, 36P.
Battezatti, M. (1951). *Presse Med.* **59**, 1628.
Baxter, J. H., Horokova, Z., and Beaven, M. A. (1970). *Fed. Proc., Fed. Amer. Soc. Exp. Biol.* **29**, 618 (abstr.).
Behnke, O. (1964). *J. Ultrastruct. Res.* **11**, 139.
Benditt, E. P. (1958). *Ann. N. Y. Acad. Sci.* **73**, 204.
Benditt, E. P., and Arase, M. (1958). *J. Histochem. Cytochem.* **6**, 413.
Benditt, E. P., and Arase, M. (1959). *J. Exp. Med.* **110**, 451.
Benditt, E. P., and Lagunoff, D. (1964). *Progr. Allergy* **8**, 195.
Benditt, E. P., Wong, R. L., Arase, M., and Roeper, E. (1955). *Proc. Soc. Exp. Biol. Med.* **90**,303.
Benditt, E. P., Arase, M., and Roeper, E. (1956). *J. Histochem. Cytochem.* **4**, 419.
Benditt, E. P., Holcenberg, J., and Lagunoff, D. (1963). *Ann. N. Y. Acad. Sci.* **103**, 179.
Bergendorff, A., and Uvnäs, B. (1972). *Acta Physiol. Scand.* **84**, 320.
Berlin, C. (1955). *AMA Arch. Dermatol.* **71**, 703.
Bertler, E. P., Falck, B., Hillarp, N.-Å., Rosengren, E., and Torp, A. (1959). *Acta Phyiol. Scand.* **48**, 261.
Best, C. H., Bale, H. H., Duddley, H. W., and Thorpe, W. V. (1927). *J. Physiol. (London)* **62**, 397.
Bhattacharya, B., and Lewis, G. P. (1956). *Brit. J. Pharmacol. Chemother.* **11**, 411.
Bierich, R. (1922). *Virchows Arch. Pathol. Anat. Physiol.* **239**, 1.
Bigelow, E. L. (1961). *J. Pediat.* **58**, 499.
Bloom, F. (1942). *Arch. Pathol.* **33**, 661.
Bloom, G. D. (1960). Dissertation Med., Karolinska Institutet, Stockholm.
Bloom, G. D. (1963). *Ann. N. Y. Acad. Sci.* **103**, 53.
Bloom, G. D., and Chakravarty, N. (1970). *Acta Physiol. Scand.* **78**, 410.
Bloom, G. D., and Haegermark, Ö. (1965). *Exp. Cell Res.* **40**, 637.
Bloom, G. D., and Haegermark, Ö. (1967). *Acta Physiol. Scand.* **71**, 257.
Bloom, G. D., and Kelly, J. W. (1960). *Histochemie* **2**, 48.
Bloom, G. D., and Ringertz, N. (1960). *Ark. Kemi* **16**, 51.

Bloom, G. D., Friberg, U., and Larsson, B. (1956). *Nord. Veterinärmed.* **8**, 43.
Bloom, G. D., Larsson, B., and Smith, D. E. (1957). *Acta Pathol. Microbiol. Scand.* **40**, 309.
Bloom, G. D., Dunér, H., Pernow, B., Winberg, J., and Zetterström, R. (1958). *Acta Paediat. (Stockholm)* **47**, 152.
Bloom, G. D., Franzén, S., and Sirén, M. (1960). *Acta Med. Scand.* **168**, 95.
Bloom, G. D., Fredholm, B., and Haegermark, Ö. (1967). *Acta Physiol. Scand.* **71**, 270.
Boréus, L. O., and Chakravarty, N. (1959). *Acta Physiol. Scand.* **48**, 1.
Borrel, A., Boez, L., and de Coulon, A. (1923). *C. R. Soc. Biol.* **88**, 402.
Bowyer, A. (1968). *Acta Dermato-Venereol.* **48**, 574.
Braun-Falco, O., and Salfeld, K. (1959). *Nature (London)* **183**, 51.
Brinkman, G. L. (1968). *J. Ultrastruct. Res.* **23**, 115.
Brogren, N., Dunér, H., Hamrin, B., Pernow, B., Theander, G., and Waldenström, J. (1959). *Acta Med. Scand.* **163**, 223.
Burnet, F. M. (1965). *J. Pathol. Bacteriol.* **89**, 271.
Cabut, M., and Haegermark, Ö. (1966). *Acta Physiol. Scand.* **68**, 206.
Chakravarty, N. (1968). *Exp. Cell. Res.* **49**, 160.
Chakravarty, N., and Uvnäs, B. (1960). *Acta Physiol. Scand.* **48**, 302.
Charrette, E. E., Mariano, A. V., and Laforet, E. G. (1966). *Arch. Intern. Med.* **118**, 358.
Chayen, J., Darracott, S., and Kirby, W. W. (1966). *Nature (London)* **209**, 887.
Combs, J. W. (1966). *J. Cell Biol.* **31**, 563.
Compton, A. S. (1952). *Amer. J. Anat.* **91**, 301.
Cook, J. E. (1969). *Nat. Cancer Inst., Monogr.* **32**, 267.
Cotte, J. (1904). *Bull. Scient. France et Belg.* **38**, 420.
Coupland, R. E. (1963). *Ann, N. Y. Acad. Sci.* **103**, 139.
Coupland, R. E., and Heath, I. D. (1961). *J. Endocrinol.* **22**, 71.
Coupland, R. E., and Riley, J. F. (1960). *Nature (London)* **187**, 1128.
Cramer, W., and Simpson, W. L. (1944). *Cancer Res.* **4**, 601.
Csaba, G. (1972). "Regulation of Mast-Cell Formation," Studia Biologica Hungarica, Budapest.
Csaba, G., Acs, T., Horváth, C., and Mold, K. (1961). *Brit. J. Cancer* **15**, 327
Danishefsky, I., and Deutsch, L. (1968). *Biochim. Biophys. Acta* **151**, 529.
Danishefsky, I., and Heritier-Watkins, O. (1967). *Biochim. Biophys. Acta* **139**, 349.
Darzynkiewicz, Z., and Barnard, E. A. (1967). *Nature (London)* **213**, 1119.
Day, M., and Green, J. P. (1962a). *J. Physiol. (London)* **164**, 210.
Day, M., and Green, J. P. (1962b). *J. Physiol. (London)* **164**, 227.
Day, M., and Stockbridge, A. (1964). *Brit. J. Pharmacol. Chemother.* **23**, 405.
Deringer, M. K., and Dunn, T. B. (1947). *J. Nat. Cancer Inst.* **7**, 289.
Diamant, B. (1967a). *Acta Physiol. Scand.* **71**, 283.
Diamant, B. (1967b). *Acta Pharmacol. Toxicol.* **25**, suppl. 4, 33.
Diamant, B., and Glick, D. (1967). *J. Histochem. Cytochem.* **15**, 695.
Diamant, B., and Krüger, P.-G. (1967). *Acta Physiol. Scand.* **71**, 291.
Diamant, B., and Lowry, O. H. (1966). *J. Histochem. Cytochem.* **14**, 519.
Diamant, B., and Uvnäs, B. (1961). *Acta Physiol. Scand.* **53**, 315.
Dieterich, C. E. (1972). *Virch. Arch. Abt. B, Zellpath.* **11**, 358.
Dobbins, W. O., Tomasini, J. T., and Rollins, E. L. (1969). *Gastroenterology* **56**, 268.
Downey, H. (1911). *Anat. Anz.* **38**, 74.
Dragstedt, C. A. (1941). *Physiol. Rev.* **21**, 563.
Dunn, T. B. (1969). *Nat. Cancer Inst., Monogr.* **32**, 285.
Dunn, T. B., and Potter, M. (1957). *J. Nat. Cancer Inst.* **18**, 587.
Eder, M., and Schauer, A. (1961). *Beitr. Pathol. Anat. Allg. Pathol.* **124**, 251.
Ehinger, B., and Thunberg, R. (1967). *Exp. Cell Res.* **47**, 116.

Ehrlich, P. (1877). *Arch. Mikrosk. Anat. Entwicklungsmech.* **13**, 263.
Ehrlich, P. (1879). *Arch. Anat. Physiol. (Leipzig)* **3**, 166.
Eiber, H. B., and Danishefsky, I. (1957). *Proc. Soc. Exp. Biol. Med.* **94**, 801.
Eiber, H. B., and Danishefsky, I. (1958). *AMA Arch. Intern. Med.* **102**, 189.
Eilbeck, J. F., and Smith, W. G. (1967). *J. Pharmacol.* **19**, 374.
Ellis, J. M. (1949). *Arch. Pathol.* **48**, 426.
Ende, N., and Auditore, J. V. (1961a). *Nature (London)* **189**, 593.
Ende, N., and Auditore, J. V. (1961b). *Amer. J. Clin. Pathol.* **36**, 16.
Ende, N., and Auditore, J. V. (1964). *Amer. J. Physiol.* **206**, 567.
Enerbäck, L. (1963). *Nature (London)* **197**, 610.
Enerbäck, L. (1966). Dissertation Med., University of Gothenburg, Gothenburg.
Enerbäck, L., and Häggendal, J. (1970). *J. Histochem. Cytochem.* **18**, 803.
Enerbäck, L., and Hansson, C. G. (1968). *J. Histochem. Cytochem.* **16**, 441.
Engelberg, H. (1963). "Heparin" pp. 1–218. Thomas, Springfield, Illinois.
Eränkö, O., and Jansson, S.-E. (1967). *Acta Physiol. Scand.* **70**, 449.
Eränkö, O., and Kauko, L. (1965). *Acta Physiol. Scand.* **64**, 283.
Fabris, A. (1927). *Pathologica* **19**, 157.
Falck, B. (1962). *Acta Physiol. Scand.* **56**, Suppl., 197.
Falck, B., Nystedt, T., Rosengren, E., and Stenflo, J. (1964). *Acta Pharmacol. Toxicol.* **21**, 51.
Fawcett, D. W. (1955). *Anat. Rec.* **121**, 29.
Fedorko, M. E., and Hirsch, J. G. (1965). *J. Cell Biol.* **26**, 973.
Fernando, N. V. P., and Movat, H. Z. (1963). *Exp. Mol. Pathol.* **2**, 450.
Fisher, D., Whitehouse, M. W., and Kent, P. W. (1967). *Nature (London)* **213**, 204.
Fisher, E. R., and Fisher, B. (1965). *Arch. Pathol.* **79**, 185.
Flood, P. R., and Krüger, P. G. (1970). *Acta Anat.* **75**, 443.
Fodor, J., and Lojda, Z. (1956). *Physiol. Bohemoslov.* **5**, 275.
Fredholm, B., and Haegermark, Ö. (1967). *Acta Physiol. Scand.* **71**, 357.
Friberg, U., Graf. W., and Åberg, B. (1951). *Acta Pathol. Microbiol. Scand.* **29**, 197.
Fujita, H., Asagami, C., Murozumi, S., Yamamoto, K., and Kinoshita, K. (1969). *J. Ultrastruct. Res.* **28**, 353.
Fujita, T. (1965). *Z. Zellforsch. Mikrosk. Anat.* **66**, 66.
Fullmer, H. M. (1959). *Nature (London)* **183**, 1274.
Furano, A. V., and Green, J. P. (1964). *J. Physiol. (London)* **170**, 263.
Furth, J., Hagen, P., and Hirsch, E. I. (1957). *Proc. Soc. Exp. Biol. Med.* **95**, 824.
Garden, J. W., and Sherk, T. (1968). *Exp. Eye Res.* **7**, 619.
Gardner, L. I., Artelissa, A., and Tice, B. A. (1958). *Pediatrics* **21**, 805.
Giacobini, E., Sedvall, G., and Uvnäs, B. (1965). *Exp. Cell Res.* **37**, 368.
Gillespie, E., Levine, R. J., and Malawista, S. E. (1968). *J. Pharmacol. Exp. Ther.* **164**, 158.
Ginsburg, H. (1963). *Ann. N. Y. Acad. Sci.* **103**, 20.
Ginsburg, H., and Lagunoff, D. (1967). *J. Cell Biol.* **35**, 685.
Glenner, G. G., and Cohen, L. A. (1960). *Nature (London)* **185**, 846.
Glenner, G. G., Hopsu, V. K., and Cohen, L. A. (1962). *J. Histochem. Cytochem.* **10**, 109.
Glick, D., and Pothapragada, S. (1961). *Proc. Soc. Exp. Biol. Med.* **106**, 359.
Glick, D., Bonting, S. L., and DenBoer, D. (1956). *Proc. Soc. Exp. Biol. Med.* **92**, 357.
Godal, H. C. (1960). *Scand. J. Clin. Lab. Invest.* **12**, 56.
Goffman, W. (1966). *Nature (London)* **212**, 449.
Gomori, G. (1945). *Proc. Soc. Exp. Biol. Med.* **58**, 362.
Gomori, G. (1953). *J. Histochem. Cytochem.* **1**, 469.
Graham, R. M., and Graham, J. B. (1966). *Surg., Gynecol. Obstet.* **123**, 3,
Green, J. P. (1966). *Yale J. Biol. Med.* **39**, 21.

Green, J. P. (1967). *Fed. Proc., Fed. Amer. Soc. Exp. Biol.* **26**, 211.

Green, J. P. (1968). *Eur. J. Pharmacol.* **3**, 68.

Green, J. P., and Day, M. (1960). *Biochem. Pharmacol.* **3**, 190.

Green, J. P., and Day, M. (1961). *Fed. Proc., Fed. Amer. Soc. Exp. Biol.* **20**, 136.

Grossfeld, H., Meyer, K., Godman, G. and Linker, A. (1957). *J. Biophys. Biochem. Cytol.* **3**, 391.

Grünberg, W., and Kaiser, E. (1964). *Zentralbl. Veterinärmed., Reihe A* **11**, 729.

Grünberg, W., and Kaiser, E. (1965). *Zentralbl. Veterinärmed., Reihe A* **12**, 18.

Hagen, P. (1961). *Can. J. Biochem. Physiol.* **39**, 639.

Hagen, P., and Lee, F. L. (1958). *J. Physiol. (London)* **143**, 7.

Hagen, P., Barrnett, R. J., and Lee, F. L. (1959). *J. Pharmacol. Exp. Ther.* **126**, 91.

Håkanson, R., and Owman, C. (1967). *Life Sci.* **6**, 759.

Hale, C. W. (1946). *Nature (London)* **157**, 802.

Hashimoto, K., Gross, B. G., and Lever, W. F. (1966). *J. Invest. Dermatol.* **46**, 139.

Head, K. W. (1953). *Vet. Rec.* **65**, 926.

Head, K. W. (1958). *Brit. J. Dermatol.* **70**, 389.

Heilbrunn, L. V., and Wilson, W. L. (1949). *Proc. Soc. Exp. Biol. Med.* **70**, 179.

Helander, H. F., and Bloom, G. D. (1974). *J. Micros.* (London). In press.

Higginbotham, R. D., and Dougherty, T. F. (1956). *Res. Bull.* **2**, 27.

Higginbotham, R. D., and Dougherty, T. F. (1957). *Res. Bull.* **3**, 19.

Higginbotham, R. D., Dougherty, T. F., and Jee, W. S. S. (1956). *Proc. Soc. Exp. Biol. Med.* **92**, 256.

Hill, M., and Praslička, M. (1958). *Acta Haematal.* **19**, 278.

Hissard, R. Moncourier, L., and Jacquet, J. (1951). *Ann. Med. (Paris)* **52**, 583.

Högberg, B., and Uvnäs, B. (1957). *Acta Physiol. Scand.* **41**, 345.

Högberg, B., and Uvnäs, B. (1960). *Acta Physiol. Scand.* **48**, 133.

Holmberg, L. (1970). *Acta Paediat. Scand.* **59**, 558.

Holmgren, H., and Wilander, O. (1937). *Z. Mikrosk. Anat. Forsch.* **42**, 242.

Holmgren, H., and Wohlfart, G. (1947). *Cancer Res.* **7**, 686.

Horsfield, G. I. (1965). *J. Pathol. Bacteriol.* **90**, 599.

Hosoda, S., and Glick, D. (1966). *J. Biol. Chem.* **241**, 192.

Hottendorf, G. H., Nielsen, S. W., and Kenyon, A. J. (1966). *Nature (London)* **212**, 829.

Hunt, T. E., and Hunt, E. A. (1957). *Proc. Soc. Exp. Biol. Med.* **94**, 166.

Iwamoto, T., and Smelser, G. K. (1965). *Invest. Ophthalmol.* **4**, 815.

Janoff, A., and Schaeffer, S. (1967). *Nature (London)* **213**, 144.

Janoff, A., and Zweifach, B. W. (1964). *J. Exp. Med.* **120**, 747.

Jansson, S.-E. (1968). *Acta Physiol. Scand.* **73**, 196.

Jansson, S.-E. (1970). *Acta Physiol. Scand.* **80**, 345.

Jaques, L. B. (1961). *Can. J. Biochem.* **39**, 643.

Jaques, L. B., and Waters, E. T. (1941). *J. Physiol. (London)* **99**, 454.

Jennings, M. A., Florey, H. W., and Robinson, D. S. (1960). *Quart. J. Exp. Physiol.* **45**, 298.

Johnson, H. H. (1957). *AMA Arch. Dermatol.* **76**, 726.

Jorpes, E. (1936). *Acta Med. Scand.* **88**, 427.

Jorpes, E. (1946). "Heparin in the Treatment of Thrombosis," 2nd ed. Oxford Univ. Press, London and New York.

Jorpes, E., Holmgren, H., and Wilander, O. (1937). *Z. Mikrosk.-Anat. Forsch.* **42**, 279.

Jorpes, E., Werner, B., and Åberg, B. (1948). *J. Biol. Chem.* **176**, 277.

Jorpes, E., Odeblad, E., and Boström, H. (1953). *Acta Haematol.* **9**, 273.

Juhlin, L., and Shelley, W. B. (1966). *J. Histochem. Cytochem.* **14**, 525.

Junqueira, L. C. U., and Beiguelman, B. (1955). *Tex. Rep. Biol. Med.* **13**, 69.

Kahlson, G., and Rosengren, E. (1968). *Physiol. Rev.* **48**, 155.

Kellaway, C. H., and Trethewie, E. R. (1940). *Quart. J. Exp. Physiol. Cog. Med. Sci.* **30**, 121.
Keller, R. (1957). *Helv. Physiol. Pharmacol. Acta* **15**, 371.
Keller, R. (1962). *Experientia* **18**, 286.
Keller, R. (1966). *Int. Arch. Allergy Appl. Immunal.* **29**, 298.
Keller, R. (1967). *Med. Klin.* **62**, 1453.
Keller, R. (1968). *Int. Arch. Allergy Appl. Immunal.* **34**, 139.
Keller, R., and Mühlethaler, K. (1962). *Pathol. Microbiol.* **25**, 115.
Keller, R., and Schwarz, M. (1961). *Schweiz. Med. Wochenschr.* **91**, 1196.
Kelly, J. W. (1956). *Protoplasmatologia* **2**, p. 1.
Kelsall, M. A., and Crabb, E. D. (1959). "Lymphocytes and Mast Cells." Williams & Wilkins, Baltimore, Maryland.
Kirkman, H. (1950). *Amer. J. Anat.* **86**, 91.
Klug, H. (1961). *Acta Biol. Med. Ger.* **6**, 545.
Kobayasi, T., and Asboe-Hansen, G. (1969). *Acta Dermato-Venereol.* **49**, 369.
Kobayasi, T., Midtgård, K., and Asboe-Hansen, G. (1968). *J. Ultrastruct. Res.* **23**, 153.
Kollmann, M. (1908). *Ann. Sci. Natur., [Zool.]* **8**, 1.
Korn, E. D. (1959a). *J. Biol. Chem.* **234**, 1321.
Korn, E. D. (1959b). *J. Biol. Chem.* **234**, 1325.
Krüger, P.-G., and Bloom, G. D. (1973). *Experientia* **29**, 329.
Krüger, P.-G., Bloom, G. D., and Diamant, B. (1974). *Intern. Arch. Allergy.* In press.
Lagunoff, D. (1966). *In* "Mechanisms of Release of Biogenic Amines" (U.S. von Euler, S. Rosell, and B. Uvnäs, eds.), Vol. 5, pp. 79–94. Pergamon, Oxford.
Lagunoff, D. (1968). *Biochem. Pharmacol., Spec. Suppl.* pp. 221–227.
Lagunoff, D. (1972a). *Biochem. Pharmacol.* **21**, 1889.
Lagunoff, D. (1972b). *J. Invest. Dermatol.* **58**, 296.
Lagunoff, D., and Benditt, E. P. (1959). *Amer. J. Physiol.* **196**, 993.
Lagunoff, D., and Benditt, E. P. (1963). *Ann. N. Y. Acad. Sci.* **103**, 195.
Lagunoff, D., Calhoun, R., and Benditt, E. P. (1960). *Proc. Soc. Exp. Biol. Med.* **104**, 575.
Lagunoff, D., Phillips, M. T., and Benditt, E. P. (1961). *J. Histochem. Cytochem.* **9**, 534.
Lagunoff, D., Phillips, M. T., Iseri, O. A., and Benditt, E. P. (1964). *Lab. Invest.* **13**, 1331.
Lagunoff, D., Benditt, E. P., and Arase, M. (1966). *Proc. Soc. Exp. Biol. Med.* **121**, 864.
Landsberger, A. (1964). *Anat. Anz.* **115**, 243.
Landsberger, A. (1966). *Acta Anat.* **64**, 245.
Leblond, C. P. (1950). *Amer. J. Anat.* **86**, 1.
Lehner, J. (1924). *Ergeb. Anat. Entwicklungsgesch.* **25**, 67.
Lennert, K. (1962). *Klin. Wochenschr.* **40**, 61.
Lennert, K., and Schubert, J. C. F. (1959). *Frankfurt. Pathol.* **69**, 579.
Lennert, K., and Schubert, J. C. F. (1961). *Verh. Dtsch. Ges. Inn. Med.* **66**, 1061.
Levine, R. J., Lovenberg, W., and Sjoerdsma, A. (1964a). *Biochem. Pharmacol.* **13**, 1283.
Levine, R. J., Lovenberg, W., and Sjoerdsma, A. (1964b). *Fed. Proc., Fed. Amer. Soc. Exp. Biol.* **23**, 563.
Lewis, R. G., Spencer, A. F., and Silbert, J. E. (1973). *Biochem. J.* **134**, 455.
Lewis, T. (1927). "The Blood Vessels of the Human Skin and their Responses." Shaw, London.
Likar, I. N., Likar, L. J., and Robinson, R. W. (1964). *Nature (London)* **203**, 730.
Lillie, R. D. (1954). "Histopathologic Technic and Practical Histochemistry." McGraw-Hill (Blakiston). New York.
Lindahl, U., and Rodén, L. (1965). *J. Biol. Chem.* **240**, 2821.
Lindahl, U., Cifonelli, J. A., Lindahl, B., and Rodén, L. (1965). *J. Biol. Chem.* **240**, 2817.
Lingeman, C. H. (1969). *Nat. Cancer Inst., Monogr.* **32**, 289.
Lippman, M. (1957). *Cancer Res.* **17**, 11.
Lison, L. (1935). *Arch. Biol.* **46**, 599.

Lison, L. (1936). "Histochemie animale." Gauthier-Villars, Paris.
Lloyd, A., Bloom, G. D., Balazs, E. A., and Haegermark, Ö. (1967a). *Biochem. J.* **103**, 75P.
Lloyd, A., Bloom, G. D., and Balazs, E. A. (1967b). *Biochem. J.* **103**, 76P.
Loeffler, L. J., Lovenberg, W., and Sjoerdsma, A. (1971). *Biochem. Pharmacol.* **20**, 2287.
Lombard, L. S., Moloney, J. B., and Rickard, C. G. (1963). *Ann. N. Y. Acad. Sci.* **108**, 1086.
Lutzner, M. A. (1964). *Fed. Proc., Fed. Amer. Soc. Exp. Biol.* **23**, 441.
MacIntosh, F. C., and Paton, W. D. M. (1949). *J. Physiol. (London)* **109**, 190.
McLean, J. (1916). *Amer. J. Physiol.* **41**, 250.
Maximow, A. (1904). *Beitr. Pathol. Anat. Allg. Pathol.* **35**, 93.
Maximow, A. (1906). *Arch. Mikrosk. Anat. Entwicklungsmech.* **67**, 680.
Meier, H. (1959). *Proc. Soc. Exp. Biol. Med.* **100**, 815.
Michaelis, L. (1947). *Cold Spring Harbor Symp. Quant. Biol.* **12**, 131.
Michels, N. (1938). *In* "Handbook of Hematology" (H. Downey, ed.), Vol. 1, p. 231. Harper (Hoeber), New York.
Migaki, G. (1969). *Nat. Cancer Inst., Monogr.* **32**, 121.
Mongar, J. L., and Schild, O. H. (1962). *Physiol. Rev.* **42**, 226.
Montagna, W. (1957). *J. Biophys. Biochem. Cytol.* **3**, 343.
Montagna, W., and Noback, C. R. (1948). *Anat. Rec.* **100**, 535.
Moran, N. C., Uvnäs, B., and Westerholm, B. (1962). *Acta Physiol. Scand.* **56**, 26.
Mota, I. (1961). *Nature (London)* **192**, 1201.
Mota, I. (1962). *Immunology* **5**, 11.
Mota, I. (1963). *Ann. N. Y. Acad. Sci.* **103**, 264.
Mota, I., and Dias da Silva, W. (1960). *Nature (London)* **186**, 245.
Mota, I., and Ishii, T. (1960). *Brit. J. Pharmacol. Chemother.* **15**, 82.
Mota, I., and Vugman, I. (1956). *Nature (London)* **177**, 427.
Mota, I., Beraldo, W. T., and Junqueira, L. C. U. (1953). *Proc. Soc. Exp. Biol. Med.* **83**, 455.
Mota, I., Beraldo, W. T., Ferri, A. G., and Junqueira, L. C. U. (1954). *Nature (London)* **174**, 698.
Mulligan, R. M. (1948). *AMA Arch. Pathol.* **45**, 216.
Murray, M., Miller, H. R., and Jarrett, W. F. (1968). *Lab. Invest.* **19**, 222.
Nakajima, Y. (1928). *Trans. Jap. Pathol. Soc.* **18**, 150.
Noback, C. R., and Montagna, W. (1946). *Anat. Rec.* **96**, 279.
Ojers, G., Homes, C. A., and Dragstedt, C. A. (1941). *J. Pharmacol. Exp. Ther.* **73**, 33.
Okun, M. R. (1965). *J. Invest. Dermatol.* **44**, 285.
Okun, M. R. (1967). *J. Invest. Dermatol.* **48**, 424.
Okun, M. R., Edelstein, L. M., Or, N., Hamada, G., and Donnellan, B. (1970). *J. Invest. Dermatol.* **55**, 1.
Oliver, J., Bloom, F., and Mangieri, C. (1947). *J. Exp. Med.* **86**, 107.
Ono, S., and Hagen, P. (1959). *Arch. Klin. Exp. Dermatol.* **214**, 521.
Orange, R. P., Valentine, M. D., and Austen, K. F. (1967). *Science* **157**, 318.
Orfanos, C. (1966). *Klin. Wochenschr.* **44**, 1177.
Orfanos, C., and Stüttgen, G. (1962). *Arch. Klin. Exp. Dermatol.* **214**, 521.
Orfanos, C., and Stüttgen, G. (1963). *Z. Zellforsch. Mikrosk. Anat.* **61**, 622.
Padawer, J. (1957). *Trans. N. Y. Acad. Sci.* [2] **19**, 630.
Padawer, J. (1961). *Angiology* **12**, 538.
Padawer, J., (1963). *Ann. N. Y. Acad. Sci.* **103**, 1-492.
Padawer, J. (1967a). *Anat. Rec.* **157**, 380.
Padawer, J. (1967b). *J. Cell Biol.* **35**, 180A.
Padawer, J. (1967c). *J. Cell Biol.* **35**, 181A.
Padawer, J. (1968). *Proc. Soc. Exp. Biol. Med.* **129**, 905.
Padawer, J. (1969). *J. Cell Biol.* **40**, 747.

Padawer, J., and Fruhman, G. J. (1968). *Experientia* **24**, 471.
Padawer, J., and Gordon, A. S. (1955). *Proc. Soc. Exp. Biol. Med.* **88**, 29.
Paff, G. H., Suguira, H. T., Bocher, C. A., and Roth, J. S. (1952). *Anat. Rec.* **114**, 499.
Parekh, A. C., and Glick, D. (1962). *J. Biol. Chem.* **237**, 280.
Parratt, J. R., and West, G. B. (1957). *J. Physiol.* (*London*) **137**, 169.
Parwaresch, M. R., Müller-Hermelink, H. K., Desaga, J. F., Zakari, V., and Lennert, K. (1971). *Virchows Arch.*, *B* **8**, 20.
Pastan, I., and Almqvist, S. (1966). *J. Biol. Chem.* **241**, 5090.
Patterson, E. K., Keppel, A., and Hsiao, S. (1961). *J. Histochem. Cytochem.* **9**, 609.
Peyron, A. (1923). *C. R. Soc. Biol.* **88**, 151.
Policard, A., Collet, A., and Prégermain, S. (1960). *Rev. Hematol.* **15**, 374.
Poppel, M. H., Gruber, W. E., Silber, R., Holder, A. K., and Christman, R. O. (1959). *Amer. J. Roentgenol., Radium Ther. Nucl. Med.* **82**, 239.
Radden, B. G. (1962). *Aust. J. Exp. Biol. Med. Sci.* **40**, 9.
Rask-Nielsen, R., and Christensen, H. E. (1963). *J. Nat. Cancer Inst.* **30**, 743.
Rheindorf, A. (1905). Thesis, University of Berlin.
Rice, L. I., Spolter, L., Tokes, Z., Eisenman, R., and Marx, W. (1967). *Arch. Biochem. Biophys.* **118**, 374.
Rickard, C. G., and Post, J. E. (1968). In "Leukemia in Animals and Man" (H. J. Bendixen, ed.), pp. 279–281. Karger, Basel.
Riley, J. F. (1953a). *Science* **118**, 332.
Riley, J. F. (1953b). *J. Pathol. Bacteriol.* **65**, 471.
Riley, J. F. (1958). *Experientia* **14**, 141.
Riley, J. F. (1959). "The Mast Cells." Livingstone, Edinburgh.
Riley, J. F. (1962). *Lancet* **2**, 40.
Riley, J. F. (1966). *Lancet* **2**, 1457.
Riley, J. F. (1968). *Experientia* **24**, 1237.
Riley, J. F., and West, G. B. (1953). *J. Physiol.* (*London*) **120**, 528.
Ringertz, N. R. (1960a). Dissertation Med., Karolinska Instituet, Stockholm.
Ringertz, N. R. (1960b). *Ark. Kemi* **16**, 67.
Ringertz, N. R. (1963). *Ann. N. Y. Acad. Sci.* **103**, 209.
Ringertz, N. R., and Bloom, G. D. (1960). *Ark. Kemi.* **16**, 57.
Ritzén, M. (1967). Dissertation Med., Karolinska Institutet, Stockholm.
Rocha e Silva, M. (1955). "Histamine." Thomas, Springfield, Illinois.
Rocha e Silva, M., Scroggie, A. E., Fidlar, E., and Jaques, L. B. (1947). *Proc. Soc. Exp. Biol. Med.* **64**, 141.
Rogers, G. E. (1956). *Exp. Cell Res.* **11**, 393.
Röhlich, P., Anderson, P., and Uvnäs, B. (1971). *J. Cell Biol.* **51**, 465.
Rothschild, A. M., and Schayer, R. W. (1958). *Fed. Proc., Fed. Amer. Soc. Exp. Biol.* **17**, 136.
Sabrazés, J., and Lafon, C. (1908). *Folia Haematol.* (*Leipzig*) **6**, 3.
Sabrazés, J., Muratet, L., and Antoine, H. (1908). *C. R. Soc. Biol.* **64**, 292.
Sagher, F., and Even-Paz, Z. (1967). "Mastocytosis and the Mast Cell." Karger, Basel.
Sagher, F., and Schorr, S. (1956). *J. Invest. Dermatol.* **26**, 431.
Sato, S., Kukita, A., and Sato, S.-I. (1969). *J. Invest. Dermatol.* **53**, 183.
Sato, T. L., Jequier, E., Lovenberg, W., and Sjoerdsma, A. (1967). *Eur. J. Pharmacol.* **1**, 18.
Schauer, A., and Eder, M. (1961). *Klin. Wschr.* **39**, 76.
Schayer, R. W. (1956). *Amer. J. Physiol.* **186**, 199.
Schayer, R. W. (1963a). *Ann. N. Y. Acad. Sci.* **103**, 164.
Schayer, R. W. (1963b). *Progr. Allergy* **7**, 187.
Schiller, S., and Dorfman, A. (1959). *Biochim. Biophys. Acta* **31**, 287.

Schindler, R. (1958). *Biochem. Pharmacol.* **1**, 323.
Scott, K. G., Scheline, R. R., and Stone, R. S. (1958). *Cancer Res.* **18**, 927.
Sellyei, M., and David, H. (1963). *Z. Mikroskop.-Anat. Forsch. (Leipzig)* **70**, 103.
Selye, H. (1965). "The Mast Cell." Butterworth, London.
Serafini-Fracassini, A., and Durward, J. J. (1968). *Biochem. J.* **109**, 693.
Serafini-Fracassini, A., Durward, J. J., and Crawford, J. (1969). *J. Ultrastruct. Res.* **28**, 131.
Sézary, M. (1936). *Bull. Soc. Fr. Dermatol. Syphiligr.* **43**, 1069.
Sheldon, W. H., and Bauer, H. (1960). *J. Exp. Med.* **112**, 1069.
Sherwin, R. P., Kern, W. H., and Jones, J. C. (1965). *Cancer* **18**, 634.
Silbert, J. E., and Brown, D. H. (1961). *Biochim. Biophys. Acta* **54**, 590.
Singleton, E. M., and Clark, S. L., Jr. (1965). *Lab. Invest.* **14**, 1744.
Sjoerdsma, A., Waalkes, T. P., and Weissbach, H. (1957). *Science* **125**, 1202.
Skalko, R. G., Ruby, J. R., and Dyer, R. F. (1968). *Anat. Rec.* **161**, 459.
Slorach, S. A. (1971). *Acta Physiol. Scand.* **82**, 91.
Slorach, S. A., and Uvnäs, B. (1968). *Acta Physiol. Scand.* **73**, 457.
Smith, D. E. (1963a). *Ann. N. Y. Acad. Sci.* **103**, 40.
Smith, D. E. (1963b). *Int. Rev. Cytol.* **14**, 327.
Smith, D. E., and Lewis, Y. (1957). *J. Biophys. Biochem. Cytol.* **3**, 9.
Smith, D. E., and Lewis, Y. (1958). *Anat. Rec.* **132**, 93.
Smith, R. S. (1961). *Arch. Ophthalmol.* **66**, 383.
Spicer, S. S. (1963). *Ann. N. Y. Acad. Sci.* **103**, 322.
Spolter, L., and Marx, W. (1959). *Biochim. Biophys. Acta* **32**, 291.
Stoeckenius, W. (1956). *Exp. Cell Res.* **11**, 656.
Stolk, A. (1961). *Nature (London)* **190**, 360.
Stuart, E. G. (1952). *Anat. Rec.* **112**, 394.
Sylvén, B. (1941). *Acta Chir. Scand.* **86**, 1.
Taichman, N. S. (1970). *J. Ultrastruct. Res.* **32**, 284.
Thon, I., and Uvnäs, B. (1966). *Acta Physiol. Scand.* **67**, 455.
Thon, I., and Uvnäs, B. (1967). *Acta Physiol. Scand.* **71**, 303.
Unna, P. G. (1896). "The Histopathology of the Diseases of the Skin." Macmillan, New York.
Uvnäs, B. (1961). *Chemotherapia* **3**, 137.
Uvnäs, B. (1963). *Ann. N. Y. Acad. Sci.* **103**, 278.
Uvnäs, B., and Thon, I. (1959). *Exp. Cell Res.* **18**, 512.
Uvnäs, B., and Thon, I. (1961). *Exp. Cell Res.* **23**, 45.
Uvnäs, B., Åborg, C.-H., and Bergendorff, A. (1970). *Acta Physiol. Scand.* **78**, Suppl. 336,3–26.
Veilleux, R., and Cantin, M. (1972). *Rev. Can. Biol.* **31**, 287.
Velican, C., and Velican, D. (1959). *Acta Haematol.* **21**, 109.
Vetter, W. (1970). *Z. Anat. Entwicklungsgesch.* **130**, 153.
Viklicky, V. (1969). *Folia Biol. (Prague)* **15**, 361.
Vollrath, L., and Wahlin, T. (1970). *Z. Zellforsch. Mikrosk. Anat.* **111**, 286.
Waters, E. T., Markowitz, J., and Jaques, L. B. (1938). *Science* **87**, 582.
Weinstock, A., and Albright, J. T. (1967). *J. Ultrastruct. Res.* **17**, 245.
West, G. B. (1956). *Histamine, Ciba Found. Symp.*, 1955 pp. 14–19.
West, G. B. (1958). *Brit. J. Dermatol.* **70**, 409.
West, G. B. (1959). *J. Pharm. Pharmacol.* **11**, 513.
West, G. B. (1962). *J. Pharm. Pharmacol.* **14**, 618.
Westphal, E. (1880). *In* "Farbenanalytische Untersuchungen" (P. Ehrlich, ed.), pp. 17–41. Hirschwald, Berlin.
Whur, P., and Gracie, M. (1967). *Experientia* **23**, 655.
Wight, P. A. L. (1970). *Acta Anat.* **75**, 100.

Wilander, O. (1938). *Skand. Arch. Physiol.* **81**, Suppl. 15, 1–89.

Wislocki, G. B., and Dempsey, E. W. (1946). *Anat. Rec.* **96**, 249.

Wislocki, G. B., Bunting, H., and Dempsey, E. W. (1947). *Amer. J. Anat.* **81**, 1.

Wislocki, G. B., Reingold, J. J., and Dempsey, E. W. (1949). *Blood* **4**, 562.

Wózniak, L., and Wranicz, A. (1968). *Hautarzt* **19**, 158.

Yamasaki, H., Fujita, T., Ohara, Y., and Komoto, S. (1970). *Arch. Histol.* **31**, 393.

Zollinger, H. U. (1950). *Experientia* **6**, 384.

AUTHOR INDEX

Numbers in italics refer to the pages on which the complete references are listed.

SUBJECT INDEX

A

Acetylcholinesterase, in nerve-end plasma
    membrane, 76
Acid hydrolases, 469
Acrasin, in chemotaxis of cellular slime
    molds, 305 *et seq.*
Acridine orange, lysosome accumulation 133
Adami, on role of blood vessels in inflam-
    mation, 24
Adenosine, induction of pinocytosis, 480
Adenylcyclase, membrane-bound, 85
ADP, aggregation of platelets, 514
    in cell injury, 122 *et seq.*
    in platelet release, 516 *et seq.*
Agranulocytosis, 443
Alcoholic hyaline, 175
Alcoholism, chronic, mitochondrial changes,
    147
Aleutian mink trait, 170
Algae, chemotaxis, 304
Alkaline phosphatase deficiency, 443
Allomyces, chemotaxis, 309
Amines, having inflammatory action, 38
    in mast cell, 575
Amino acid decarboxylases, of mast cells,
    577
Amino acids, effect on chemotaxis, 302
Amoeba, chemotaxis, 310
AMP, cyclic, in autophagocytosis, 168
    in chemotaxis of cellular slime mold, 306
    in membrane movement, 154
Anaphylactic hypersensitivity, 20
Anaphylaxis, 537, 583
Ancient peoples, knowledge of inflammation,
    9
Angioblastic theory, of embryonic endo-
    thelium, 35
Anthracosis, 166
Antibody, and macrophage, 494

heterologous, 529
Anticoagulants, inhibition of platelet
    function, 512
Antigen(s), destruction by macrophage, 34,
    499
    macrophage–bound, 502
        adoptive transfer, 501
    processing, lysosomal digestion, 167
Antigenic property, of lysosomal membrane,
    267
Arthritis, role of lysosomes, 279
Arthus reaction, 20
Arylamidases, lysosomal, 271
Atherosclerosis, as acquired storage disease,
    168
ATP, in cell injury 122 *et seq.*, 204, 205
    release from platelets, 517
ATPase, of liver-cell plasma membrane, 63
Atrophy, disuse, mitochondrial changes, 149
Autolysis, definition, 116
Autophagic vacuoles, 172, 264
Autophagocytosis, 168
Autophagy, 154
    physiological and pathological function,
    169

B

Bacteria, avoiding reaction, 297
    chemotaxis, 296
    degradation by phagocytosis, 371
    inactivation by macrophage, 487
    platelet reaction to, 530
    tumbling action, in chemotaxis, 297
    virulence, and phagocytosis, 402
Bacterial hypersensitivity, tuberculin type.
        See Hypersensitivity, delayed
Bactericidal agents, of polymorphonuclear
    leukocyte, 32

637